Type 1 Diabetes

CONTEMPORARY ENDOCRINOLOGY

P. Michael Conn, *Series Editor*

Androgens in Health and Disease, edited by CARRIE BAGATELL AND WILLIAM J. BREMNER, 2003
Endocrine Replacement Therapy in Clinical Practice, edited by A. WAYNE MEIKLE, 2003
Early Diagnosis of Endocrine Diseases, edited by ROBERT S. BAR, 2003
Type 1 Diabetes: *Etiology and Treatment,* edited by MARK A. SPERLING, 2003
Handbook of Diagnostic Endocrinology, edited by JANET E. HALL AND LYNNETTE K. NIEMAN, 2003
Pediatric Endocrinology: *A Practical Clinical Guide,* edited by SALLY RADOVICK AND MARGARET H. MACGILLIVRAY, 2003
Diseases of the Thyroid, 2nd ed., edited by LEWIS E. BRAVERMAN, 2003
Developmental Endocrinology: *From Research to Clinical Practice,* edited by ERICA A. EUGSTER AND ORA HIRSCH PESCOVITZ, 2002
Osteoporosis: *Pathophysiology and Clinical Management,* edited by ERIC S. ORWOLL AND MICHAEL BLIZIOTES, 2002
Challenging Cases in Endocrinology, edited by MARK E. MOLITCH, 2002
Selective Estrogen Receptor Modulators: *Research and Clinical Applications,* edited by ANDREA MANNI AND MICHAEL F. VERDERAME, 2002
Transgenics in Endocrinology, edited by MARTIN MATZUK, CHESTER W. BROWN, AND T. RAJENDRA KUMAR, 2001
Assisted Fertilization and Nuclear Transfer in Mammals, edited by DON P. WOLF AND MARY ZELINSKI-WOOTEN, 2001
Adrenal Disorders, edited by ANDREW N. MARGIORIS AND GEORGE P. CHROUSOS, 2001
Endocrine Oncology, edited by STEPHEN P. ETHIER, 2000
Endocrinology of the Lung: *Development and Surfactant Synthesis,* edited by CAROLE R. MENDELSON, 2000
Sports Endocrinology, edited by MICHELLE P. WARREN AND NAAMA W. CONSTANTINI, 2000
Gene Engineering in Endocrinology, edited by MARGARET A. SHUPNIK, 2000
Endocrinology of Aging, edited by JOHN E. MORLEY AND LUCRETIA VAN DEN BERG, 2000
Human Growth Hormone: *Research and Clinical Practice,* edited by ROY G. SMITH AND MICHAEL O. THORNER, 2000
Hormones and the Heart in Health and Disease, edited by LEONARD SHARE, 1999
Menopause: *Endocrinology and Management,* edited by DAVID B. SEIFER AND ELIZABETH A. KENNARD, 1999
The IGF System: *Molecular Biology, Physiology, and Clinical Applications,* edited by RON G. ROSENFELD AND CHARLES T. ROBERTS, JR., 1999
Neurosteroids: *A New Regulatory Function in the Nervous System,* edited by ETIENNE-EMILE BAULIEU, MICHAEL SCHUMACHER, AND PAUL ROBEL, 1999
Autoimmune Endocrinopathies, edited by ROBERT VOLPÉ, 1999
Hormone Resistance Syndromes, edited by J. LARRY JAMESON, 1999
Hormone Replacement Therapy, edited by A. WAYNE MEIKLE, 1999
Insulin Resistance: *The Metabolic Syndrome X,* edited by GERALD M. REAVEN AND AMI LAWS, 1999
Endocrinology of Breast Cancer, edited by ANDREA MANNI, 1999
Molecular and Cellular Pediatric Endocrinology, edited by STUART HANDWERGER, 1999
Gastrointestinal Endocrinology, edited by GEORGE H. GREELEY, JR., 1999
The Endocrinology of Pregnancy, edited by FULLER W. BAZER, 1998
Clinical Management of Diabetic Neuropathy, edited by ARISTIDIS VEVES, 1998
G Proteins, Receptors, and Disease, edited by ALLEN M. SPIEGEL, 1998
Natriuretic Peptides in Health and Disease, edited by WILLIS K. SAMSON AND ELLIS R. LEVIN, 1997
Endocrinology of Critical Disease, edited by K. PATRICK OBER, 1997
Diseases of the Pituitary: *Diagnosis and Treatment,* edited by MARGARET E. WIERMAN, 1997
Endocrinology of the Vasculature, edited by JAMES R. SOWERS, 1996

TYPE 1 DIABETES

ETIOLOGY AND TREATMENT

Edited by

MARK A. SPERLING, MD

Professor of Pediatrics and Chair Emeritus, Department of Pediatrics,
University of Pittsburgh School of Medicine; and
Division of Endocrinology,
Children's Hospital of Pittsburgh, Pittsburgh, PA

HUMANA PRESS
TOTOWA, NEW JERSEY

999 Riverview Drive, Suite 208
Totowa, New Jersey 07512

www.humanapress.com

This publication is printed on acid-free paper. ∞

ANSI Z39.48-1984 (American National Standards Institute) Permanence of Paper for Printed Library Materials.

Editorial Coordinator: Sandra K. Arjona

Production Editor: Jessica Jannicelli

Cover design by Patricia F. Cleary.

For additional copies, pricing for bulk purchases, and/or information about other Humana titles, contact Humana at the above address or at any of the following numbers: Tel: 973-256-1699; Fax: 973-256-8341; E-mail: humana@humanapr.com or visit our website at http://humanapress.com

Printed in the United States of America. 10 9 8 7 6 5 4 3 2 1

Library of Congress Cataloging-in-Publication Data

Type 1 diabetes : etiology and treatment / edited by Mark A. Sperling.
p. ; cm. -- (Contemporary endocrinology)
Includes bibliographical references and index.
ISBN 0-89603-931-5 (alk. paper) eISBN: 1-59259-310-0
1. Diabetes--Etiology. 2. Diabetes--Treatment. I. Title: Type one diabetes. II. Sperling, M. III. Contemporary endocrinology (Totowa, N.J.)
[DNLM: 1. Diabetes Mellitus, Insulin-Dependent--therapy. 2. Diabetes Mellitus, Insulin-Dependent--complications. 3. Diabetes Mellitus, Insulin-Dependent--etiology. 4. Insulin--therapeutic use. WK 815 T991 2003]
RC660.T966 2003
616.4'62071--dc21

2002191326

Preface

This volume of the *Contemporary Endocrinology* series focuses on type 1 diabetes mellitus, an entity whose incidence is increasing worldwide, particularly in children aged less than five. Affected individuals carry a life-long burden of dependence on daily insulin administration that provides imperfect metabolic control with significant acute consequences of hypoglycemia and more insidious micro- and macrovascular complications linked to chronic hyperglycemia. Despite intensive research, the disease remains enigmatic. Although evidence for an autoimmune basis is compelling, not all cases of type 1 diabetes have autoimmune markers, and not all autoimmune forms have the same genetic basis. Nevertheless, as recently demonstrated in the parenteral arm of the Diabetes Prevention Trial-1 (DPT-1), a combination of immune markers and consistently diminished first-phase insulin response to glucose can reliably predict the likelihood of developing clinical diabetes. However, current intervention with parenteral insulin is not effective in preventing progression at this stage. A reliably effective intervention would spur population-wide surveys for at-risk individuals, now a practical possibility. Cure by transplantation of the pancreas or islets is showing great promise as better means become available to modulate immunity and prevent rejection.

In parallel with these wide-ranging and fundamental basic and clinical investigations, there is an ongoing transfer of technological innovations in designer insulins, insulin delivery systems, and the monitoring of glucose. These innovations permit refinement in managing diabetes mellitus under various circumstances, all aimed at improving the quality of life and preventing or delaying vascular complications.

The aim of *Type 1 Diabetes: Etiology and Treatment* is to fuse these contemporary investigational and practical issues and make them available to those involved in the research and practice of type 1 diabetes. This volume is not intended to be a comprehensive or exhaustive treatise on the subject of diabetes. As in many such endeavors, the pace of discovery often exceeds the ability to incorporate the latest knowledge into printed text. Nevertheless, we believe that this volume presents contemporary information on contemporary issues by recognized authorities in the field. We hope it stimulates thought and action in the research and care of patients with type 1 diabetes mellitus.

Mark A. Sperling, MD

Contents

Contributors

RODOLFO ALEJANDRO, MD, *Diabetes Research Institute, University of Miami School of Medicine, Miami, FL*
STEPHANIE A. AMIEL, BSc, MD, FRCP, *Guy's, King's, and St. Thomas' School of Medicine, King's College, London, UK*
TIMOTHY G. BARRETT, PhD, MB, *Diabetes Unit, Birmingham Children's Hospital, Birmingham, UK*
CHRISTINE A. BEEBE, MS, RD, LD, CDE, *Department of Human Nutrition, University of Illinois at Chicago, Chicago, IL*
THIERRY BERNEY, MD, MSc, *Visceral and Transplantation Surgery, Geneva University Hospital, Geneva, Switzerland*
ELIZABETH A. BOLAND, MSN, APRN, PNP, CDE, *Department of Pediatrics, Yale School of Medicine, New Haven, CT*
JEAN L. BOLOGNIA, MD, *Department of Dermatology, Yale Medical School, New Haven, CT*
IRWIN M. BRAVERMAN, MD, *Department of Dermatology, Yale Medical School, New Haven, CT*
MICHAEL BROWNLEE, MD, *Diabetes Research Center, Albert Einstein College of Medicine, Bronx, NY*
FERGUS J. CAMERON, MD, *Department of Endocrinology and Diabetes, Royal Children's Hospital, Parkville, Australia*
PETER A. CAMPOCHIARO, MD, *Departments of Ophthalmology and Neuroscience, Johns Hopkins University School of Medicine, Baltimore, MD*
ANA CEBRIAN, PhD, *Division of Endocrinology, University of Pittsburgh School of Medicine, Pittsburgh, PA*
CHOON HEE CHUNG, MD, PhD, *Division of Endocrinology, Wonju College of Medicine, Yonsei University, Seoul, Korea*
JOHN M. COURT, MBBS, *Centre for Adolescent Health, Royal Children's Hospital, Parkville, Australia*
PHILIP E. CRYER, MD, *Division of Endocrinology, Diabetes and Metabolism, and the General Clinical Research Center and Diabetes Research and Training Center, Washington University School of Medicine, St. Louis, MO*
PAUL CZERNICHOW, MD, *Department of Pediatric Endocrinology and Diabetology, Robert Debré Hospital, Paris, France*
FREDERICK DERUBERTIS, MD, *VA Pittsburgh Healthcare System, Pittsburgh, PA*
NICOLAI M. DOLIBA, PhD, DSci, *Department of Biochemistry/Biophysics, University of Pennsylvania, Philadelphia, PA*
JANICE S. DORMAN, PhD, *Department of Endocriniology, University of Pittsburgh, Pittsburgh, PA*
SHIMON EFRAT, PhD, *Human Genetics and Molecular Medicine, Sackler School of Medicine, Tel Aviv University, Tel Aviv, Israel*

WAEL EMAD EID, MD, *Department of Endocrinology, Baylor College of Medicine, Houston, TX*
GEORGE S. EISENBARTH, MD, PhD, *Barbara Davis Center for Childhood Diabetes, University of Colorado Health Sciences Center, Denver, CO*
EVA L. FELDMAN, MD, PhD, *Department of Neurology, University of Michigan, Ann Arbor, MI*
ALAN J. GARBER, MD, PhD, *Department of Medicine, Baylor College of Medicine, Houston, TX*
ADOLFO GARCIA-OCAÑA, PhD, *Division of Endocrinology, University of Pittsburgh School of Medicine, Pittsburgh, PA*
SAUL GENUTH, MD, *Division of Clinical and Molecular Endocrinology, Case Western Reserve University, Cleveland, OH*
MARGARET GREY, DRPH, FAAN, CDE, *Yale School of Nursing, New Haven, CT*
LUCA INVERARDI, MD, *Diabetes Research Institute, University of Miami School of Medicine, Miami, FL*
NIRMAL JOSHI, MD, FACP, *Department of Medicine, Pinnacle Health Hospitals, Harrisburg, PA*
LOIS JOVANOVIC, MD, *Sansum Medical Research Institute, Santa Barbara, CA*
FINNBOGI KARLSSON, MD, *Department of Medicine, Baylor College of Medicine, Houston, TX*
DAVID KENT, MD, *Unit of Ophthalmology, University of Liverpool, Liverpool, UK*
NORMA SUE KENYON, PhD, *Diabetes Research Institute, University of Miami School of Medicine, Miami, FL*
RONALD E. LAPORTE, PhD, *Disease Monitoring and Telecommunications, WHO Collaborating Center, University of Pittsburgh, Pittsburgh, PA*
ÅKE LERNMARK, MD, *Department of Medicine, University of Washington, Seattle, WA*
JUAN CARLOS LOPEZ-TALAVERA, MD, PhD, *Division of Endocrinology, University of Pittsburgh School of Medicine, Pittsburgh, PA*
ARISTIDES K. MANIATIS, MD, *Barbara Davis Center for Childhood Diabetes, University of Colorado Health Sciences Center, Denver, CO*
FRANZ M. MATSCHINSKY, MD, *Department of Biochemistry/Biophysics, University of Pennsylvania, Philadelphia, PA*
KRYSTYNA MATYKA, MRCP, MD, *Division of Medical Sciences, University of Birmingham, Birmingham, UK*
SIRIPOOM MCKAY, MD, *Children's Nutrition Research Center, Houston, TX*
RAM K. MENON, MD, *Division of Endocrinology, University of Michigan Medical School, Ann Arbor, MI*
DANIEL H. MINTZ, MD, *Diabetes Research Institute, University of Miami School of Medicine, Miami, FL*
JAAKKO PERHEENTUPA, MD, PhD, *The Hospital for Children and Adolescents, University of Helsinki, Helsinki, Finland*
JOHN C. PICKUP, MA, BM, BCh, DPhil, FRCPath, *Metabolic Unit, Guy's, King's, and St. Thomas' School of Medicine, Guy's Hospital, London, UK*
MASSIMO PIETROPAOLO, MD, *Division of Immunogenetics, Diabetes Institute, Rangos Research Center, Pittsburgh, PA*
CAMILLO RICORDI, MD, *Diabetes Research Institute, University of Miami School of Medicine, Miami, FL*

ROBERT A. RIZZA, MD, *Endocrinology and Metabolism, Mayo Clinic and Foundation, Rochester, MN*

R. PAUL ROBERTSON, MD, *Pacific Northwest Research Institute, Seattle, WA*

JEAN BETSCHART ROEMER, MN, MSN, CPNP, CDE, *Department of Endocrinology, Diabetes and Metabolism, Children's Hospital of Pittsburgh, Pittsburgh, PA*

JAMES W. RUSSELL, MD, MS, *Department of Neurology, University of Michigan, Ann Arbor, MI*

KENYA SAKAMOTO, MD, PhD, *Diabetes Research Center, Albert Einstein College of Medicine, Bronx, NY*

BAIJU R. SHAH, MD, FRCPC, *Department of Medicine, University of Toronto, Toronto, Ontario, Canada*

LINDA SIMINERIO, RN, PhD, CDE, *Children's Hospital of Pittsburgh, Pittsburgh, PA*

ERICA M. SOMMERMANN, BS, *Sansum Medical Research Institute, Santa Barbara, CA*

THOMAS J. SONGER, PhD, *Center for Injury Research and Control, University of Pittsburgh, Pittsburgh, PA*

MARK A. SPERLING, MD, *Division of Endocrinology, Children's Hospital of Pittsburgh, Pittsburgh, PA*

DAVID L. STEED, MD, *Wound Healing/Limb Preservation Clinic, University of Pittsburgh Medical Center, Pittsburgh, PA*

MARTIN J. STEVENS, MD, *Department of Internal Medicine, University of Michigan, Ann Arbor, MI*

ANDREW F. STEWART, MD, *Division of Endocrinology, University of Pittsburgh School of Medicine, Pittsburgh, PA*

KAREN K. TAKANE, PhD, *Division of Endocrinology, University of Pittsburgh School of Medicine, Pittsburgh, PA*

WILLIAM V. TAMBORLANE, MD, *Department of Pediatrics, Yale School of Medicine, New Haven, CT*

MASSIMO TRUCCO, MD, *Rangos Research Center, Children's Hospital of Pittsburgh, Pittsburgh, PA*

NADIA TUBIANA-RUFI, MD, *Department of Pediatric Endocrinology and Diabetology, Robert Debré Hospital, Paris, France*

TIINAMAIJA TUOMI, MD, PhD, *Department of Diabetology, Helsinki University Central Hospital, Helsinki, Finland*

ERIN K. VAN METER, BA, *Sansum Medical Research Institute, Santa Barbara, CA*

RUPANGI C. VASAVADA, PhD, *Division of Endocrinology, University of Pittsburgh School of Medicine, Pittsburgh, PA*

ABHAY VATS, MD, *Pediatric Nephrology, Children's Hospital of Pittsburgh, Pittsburgh, PA*

ADRIAN VELLA, MD, MRCP (UK), *Endocrinology and Metabolism, Mayo Clinic and Foundation, Rochester, MN*

GEORGE A. WERTHER, MD, MSc, *Department of Endocrinology and Diabetes, Royal Children's Hospital, Parkville, Australia*

BERNARD ZINMAN, MDCM, FRCPC, FACP, *Leadership Sinai Centre for Diabetes, Mount Sinai Hospital, Toronto, Ontario, Canada*

I

ETIOLOGY

1 Epidemiology of Type 1 Diabetes

Janice S. Dorman, PhD, *Ronald E. LaPorte,* PhD,
and Thomas J. Songer, PhD

CONTENTS

INTRODUCTION

Epidemiology is defined as "the study of the distribution and determinants of health-related states and events in populations, and the applications of this study to the control of health problems" *(1)*. Epidemiology is the scientific basis of public health. One might wonder why we should even consider epidemiology for disorders such as type 1 diabetes, as remarkable advances have occurred in basic research during the past few decades. However, epidemiology has proven to be the mainstay of prevention for infectious and chronic diseases in the United States and across the world during the past century. To cite an example, life expectancy has increased by approx 25 yr since 1950 *(2)*. The vast majority of this increase (24 of the 25 yr) has been the result of public health applications of epidemiologic research *(3)*. We believe that the same will hold true for type 1 diabetes.

Epidemiology will continue as the core science for public health during the new millennium, in combination with advances in genetics, immunology, and the environmental sciences. Should it become possible to modify potential etiologic determinants of type 1 diabetes or implement new interventions (e.g., dietary modifications, islet cell transplants, gene therapy, etc.), epidemiologic data based on these and other characteristics will be essential for assessing the efficacy and economic impact of implementing such strategies. A discussion of these issues, which serve as a model for other multifactorial diseases, forms the basis of this chapter.

From: *Contemporary Endocrinology: Type 1 Diabetes: Etiology and Treatment*
Edited by: M. A. Sperling © Humana Press Inc., Totowa, NJ

INCIDENCE OF TYPE 1 DIABETES BY PERSON, PLACE, AND TIME

A typical first step for studying the epidemiology of any disorder is the evaluation of geographic and temporal variations in disease incidence. These investigations require the development of a standardized epidemiologic approach, for reasons similar to those that justify the utilization of laboratory standards. To compare results among laboratories, one needs to employ comparable and standardized methodologies. Thus, a standardized epidemiologic protocol was developed to permit accurate comparisons of the incidence of type 1 diabetes worldwide. This began in 1983 at an important meeting held in Philadelphia, PA by the Juvenile Diabetes Foundation *(4)*. At that time, the first standardized protocol for the development of incidence registries for type 1 diabetes was outlined. Since then, this protocol has been used by essentially all of the registries for type 1 diabetes in the world and has permitted direct comparisons of standardized data regarding the epidemiology of the disease.

Once a standardized protocol was available, the next step was to establish a philosophy of data sharing. Data sharing is rare among most scientists in diabetes, but it has become the norm among diabetes epidemiologists. These collaborations began with early studies conducted by the Diabetes Epidemiology Research International (DERI) Group. In the mid-1980s, all researchers who had existing data participated in DERI by comparing the epidemiology of type 1 diabetes from their registries. Over 20 registries worldwide participated. This effort resulted in one of the largest global collaborations ever seen in medical research. Although the initial findings were extremely interesting, it became evident by the late 1980s that there were broad gaps in our knowledge about the distribution of type 1 diabetes in children worldwide *(5)*.

By 1990, two international groups working on the epidemiology of type 1 diabetes had been developed. The first was the EURODIAB Project *(6)*, which represented standardized type 1 diabetes incidence registries in Europe. The second was the World Health Organization (WHO) Multinational Project for Childhood Diabetes, also known as Diabetes Mondiale, or the DiaMond Project *(7)*. The DiaMond Project included type 1 diabetes incidence registries from all continents. Because of these two important projects, the descriptive epidemiology of type 1 diabetes has been mapped for most of the world, and we now know more about the international variation in the incidence of type 1 diabetes than practically any other chronic disease. Within a short 15-yr time period, the epidemiology of type 1 diabetes rose from a "black hole" of ignorance to one of the best characterized chronic diseases worldwide because of this remarkable global cooperation. Here, we describe some of these results and their implications for disease prevention.

Geographic Variation in Incidence

The variation in the incidence of type 1 diabetes worldwide is greater than that observed for any other chronic disease in children. Currently, there are incidence data from more than 60 countries around the world. As illustrated by Fig. 1, the global variation in risk is enormous. A child in Helsinki, Finland is almost 400 times more likely to develop diabetes than a child in Sichuan, China *(8)*. To put this in perspective, consider the following example. If children in the United States had the same risk of developing type 1 diabetes as children in China, then instead of 13,000 newly diagnosed children each year, there would be only 56. In other words, over 99% of the annual new cases of type 1 diabetes in the United States would be avoided.

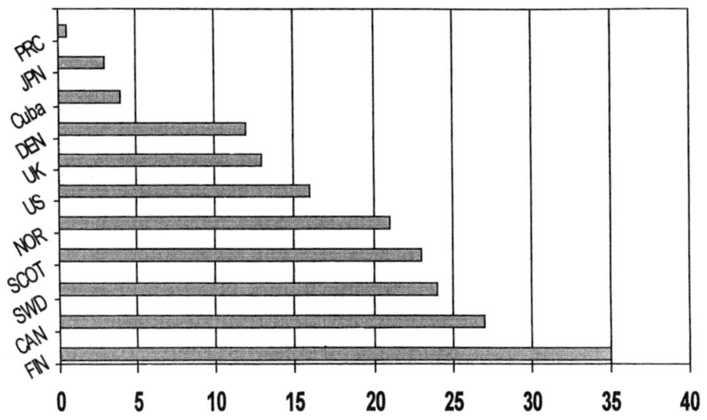

Fig. 1. Type 1 diabetes incidence rates per 100,000/yr worldwide. *Note:* PRC, People's Republic of China; JPN, Japan; DEN, Denmark; UK, United Kingdom; US, United States; NOR, Norway; SCOT, Scotland; SWD, Sweden; CAN, Canada; FIN, Finland.

Interestingly, the other epidemiologic features of type 1 diabetes are remarkably similar across populations, despite the enormous variation in disease risk *(9)*. Incidence rates among males and females do not differ significantly, and the peak age at onset for both sexes occurs near the time of puberty. Thus, compared to all other risk factors, including human leukocyte antigen (HLA) haplotypes, viral infections, or the presence of autoantibodies, the place where a child lives is the most potent determinant of type 1 diabetes risk, excluding genetic/racial differences. If we knew what was causing the geographic patterns of type 1 diabetes, we would be well on our way to preventing the disease.

Not unexpectedly, the epidemiology of type 1 diabetes is the result of both genetic and environmental processes. Most of the low-incidence populations are Asian (i.e., Japanese, Chinese). The genetic characteristics of these groups are somewhat different than those for Caucasians, African-Americans, and Hispanics. Moreover, much is known about the genetic determinants of type 1 diabetes, and these are discussed in the next section. Here, we focus on the evidence for an environmental etiology. Epidemiologic data, including studies of temporal trends and migrants, provide very strong support for an environmental role in the development of the disease.

Temporal Trends in Incidence

Temporal trends in chronic disease incidence rates are almost certainly environmentally induced. If one observes a 50% increase in the incidence of a disorder over 20 yr, it is most likely the result of changes in the environment because the gene pool cannot change that rapidly. Type 1 diabetes is a very dynamic disease. Throughout Europe, there has been an approx 3% rise in disease incidence since the mid-1960s, making type 1 diabetes an important and very costly disorder *(10)*. In the United States, the temporal trends are less clear, primarily because of the lack of monitoring. The longest ongoing type 1 diabetes registry is from Allegheny County, Pennsylvania, the region surrounding the city of Pittsburgh *(11)*; a rapid increase in disease incidence has been observed since 1965. This trend was most apparent during the 1990s. These results

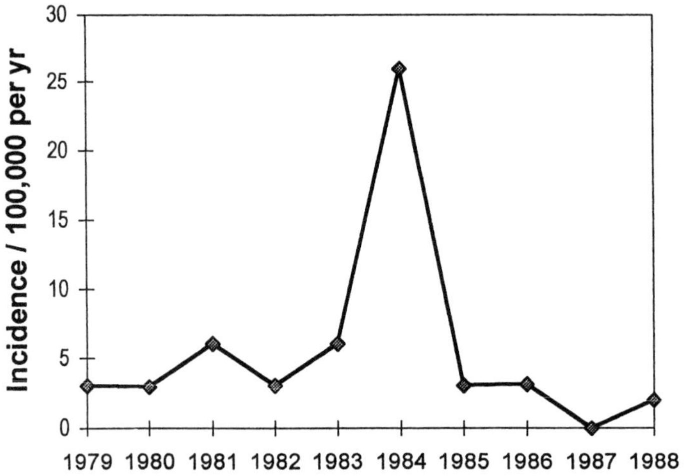

Fig. 2. Type 1 diabetes incidence rates per 100,000/yr in the US Virgin Islands.

clearly demonstrate that the incidence of type 1 diabetes is rising, bringing with it a large public health problem. Moreover, these findings indicate that something in our environment is changing to trigger a disease response.

Perhaps an even more interesting pattern is the epidemic nature of type 1 diabetes. Epidemics, which are rarely observed for chronic diseases, have been reported for type 1 diabetes. The first epidemic that appeared was in midwest Poland in 1984 *(12)*. Then, the epidemic moved east. During 1985–1986, similar trends were observed in Latvia, Lithuania, and Estonia *(13)*. If one examined the descriptive epidemiology of type 1 diabetes without knowing that it was a chronic disease, it would appear to be an infectious disorder.

In the 1980s, we reviewed all of the available temporal trend data for type 1 diabetes *(14)*. The results were striking. More than 30% of the population-based registries worldwide exhibited epidemic trends. Most remarkable was a global pandemic of childhood diabetes that occurred between 1983 and 1984 in geographically distant populations, including Hokkaido, Japan, Auckland, New Zealand, and Poznan, Poland. Thus, epidemics of type 1 diabetes were not only focal, but they also were global.

Figure 2 presents a classic epidemic pattern from the US Virgin Islands, where the incidence of type 1 diabetes rose almost fourfold during a 1-yr period of time *(15)*. Before the epidemic, the incidence of type 1 diabetes among these African-American children was similar to the rates observed in low-incidence populations. Then suddenly, the incidence rose to that of one of the highest rates in the world, for reasons which are not known. The following year, the incidence returned to the baseline rate. Epidemics have received little attention because they appear in retrospect. However, the locations of epidemics are likely the best places to evaluate the environmental etiology of type 1 diabetes.

Migrant Studies of Type 1 Diabetes

Migrant studies are one of the purest designs for examining the contribution of the environment to chronic diseases. Migrant studies are based on groups of individuals that move from a source population to a host population. The magnitude and speed at

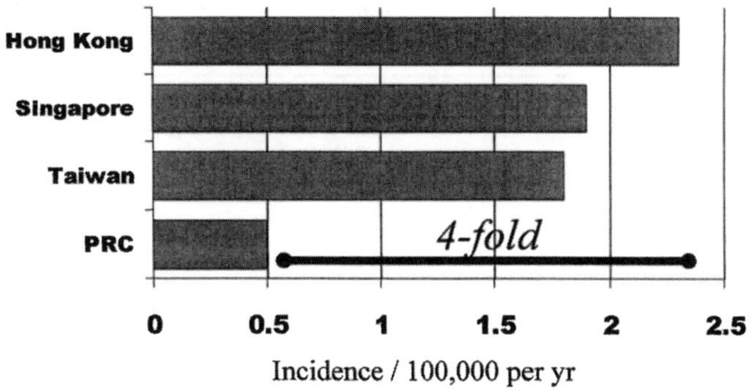

Fig. 3. Type 1 diabetes incidence rates per 100,000/yr among Chinese migrants.

which the disease incidence patterns among migrants become similar to those observed for the host population provide insight regarding potential environmental risk factors for the disease. Migrant studies have been very beneficial for studying the etiology of chronic disorders, such as cardiovascular disease and breast cancer.

The most dramatic effect of migration on type 1 diabetes incidence rates has been observed among the Chinese. There is an approximate fourfold difference in the incidence of type 1 diabetes among Chinese children living in the People's Republic of China, Taiwan, Singapore, and Hong Kong (*see* Fig. 3) *(6)*. This variation may even be greater if data for Chinese migrants to the United States, the United Kingdom, or Australia were available. Similar, but less dramatic, patterns were reported for Jewish and French children living in Israel and France, respectively, compared to those who migrated to Canada *(16)*. Interestingly, Japanese children do not appear to have been affected by migration; rates in host and source populations are similar. Thus, barring this example, temporal trend and migration data suggest that, at a minimum, 75% of all newly diagnosed type 1 diabetes cases might be prevented by modifying the environmental risk factors for the disease. If the factors contributing to the migratory effects for type 1 diabetes could be identified, the development of disease prevention strategies would be greatly facilitated.

There is now a critical need to integrate the findings of basic research into epidemiologic research. A primary reason for this is that the missions of both basic science and epidemiology are the prevention of disease. Prevention is defined by Last as "a reduction in the incidence of a disease" *(1)*. We also need to have epidemiologists develop systems for monitoring disorders such as type 1 diabetes. Without these approaches, we will never know whether any attempts at prevention are successful. What is even more important is that we will never know whether purported prevention strategies are doing harm.

RISK FACTORS FOR TYPE 1 DIABETES

The data just described clearly indicate that environmental factors are involved in the etiology of type 1 diabetes. With the exception of a possible role for viruses and infant nutrition, the specific environmental determinants that initiate or precipitate the onset of type 1 diabetes remain unclear. Type 1 diabetes is also, in large part, genetically determined *(17)*. Evidence of a genetic component for type 1 diabetes has been

Table 1
Susceptibility Loci for Type 1 Diabetes

Name	*Location*	*Candidate genes or markers*
IDDM1	6p21.3	HLA
IDDM2	11p15.5	INS-VNTR
IDDM3	15q26	D15S107
IDDM4	11q13.3	ICE, CD3, MDU1, ZFM1, RT6, LRP5, FADD, FGF3, D11S1917
IDDM5	6q15	ESR, MnSOD
IDDM6	18q21–q21	D18S487, D18S64
IDDM7	2q31–33	D2S152
IDDM8	6q25–27	D6S281, D6S264, D6S446
IDDM9	3q21–25	D3S1303
IDDM10	10p11–q11	D10S193, D10S208
IDDM11	14q24–q31	D14S67
IDDM12	2q33	CTLA-4, CD28
IDDM13	2q34	D2S137–D2S164, IGFBP2, IGFBP5
IDDM14	Unknown	Unknown
IDDM15	6q21	D6S283, D6S434, D6S1580

Source: Data from refs. *21–24.*

provided by studies showing a significantly increased risk for first-degree relatives of affected individuals *(18,19).* In addition, twin studies have revealed stronger disease concordance rates among monozygotic than dizygotic twins, although rates among monozygotic twins are less than 50% *(20).* In terms of specific genetic markers, type 1 diabetes is determined primarily by genes in the HLA region of chromosome 6. However, recent genome screens have identified at least 15 additional loci that may also contribute to disease risk (*see* Table 1) *(21–24).* Here, we describe our current knowledge about the major genetic and environmental risk factors for type 1 diabetes.

Genetic Susceptibility (see also Chapter 2)

HLA Region

The HLA region of chromosome 6 (6p21.3) encompasses approx 3500 kb of DNA, and contains at least 150 genes *(25).* It is the primary region of susceptibility for type 1 diabetes, as well as other autoimmune disorders. Recent genomewide screens have defined the class II subregion, particularly the HLA-DR and DQ loci, as insulin-dependent diabetes mellitus 1 *(IDDM1).* However, these results do not exclude a potential contribution for other genes in the HLA region (e.g., class I genes).

When evaluated as haplotypes, DQA1*0501–DQB1*0201 and DQA1*0301–DQB1*0302 confer the highest risk for type 1 diabetes in most Caucasian populations. DQA1*0501–DQB1*0201 is in linkage disequilibrium with DRB1*03, and DQA1*0301–DQB1*0302 is in linkage disequilibrium with DRB1*04. Specific DRB1*04 alleles also appear to modify the risk associated with the DQA1*0301–DQB1*0302 haplotype. Other reported high risk haplotypes for type 1 diabetes include DRB1*07–DQA1*0301–DQB1*0201 among African-Americans *(26),* DRB1*09–DQA1*0301–DQB1*0303 among Japanese *(27),* and DRB1*04–DQA1*0301–DQB1*0401

Table 2
Estimated Relative Risks, Absolute Risks, and Population Attributable Fractions for Individuals with Two, One, or Zero Susceptible Haplotypes from the WHO DiaMond Molecular Epidemiology Project

	Relative risk by no. of susceptible haplotypes			*Absolute risk[a] by no. of susceptible haplotypes*			*Attributable fraction by no. of susceptible haplotypes*	
Population	*2*	*1*	*0*	*2*	*1*	*0*	*2*	*1 or 0*
Caucasian	15.9*	4.0	1.0	2.6%	0.2%	0.7%	36.2%	66.6%
African-American	44.8*	7.3	1.0	3.1%	0.1%	0.5%	43.5%	74.9%
Asian	10.7*	3.6	1.0	0.2%	0.02%	0.1%	18.8%	53.3%

Note: Caucasian population from Jefferson County, AL and Allegheny County, PA. African-American population from Jefferson County, AL and Allegheny County, PA. Asian population from Hokkaido, Japan and Seoul, Korea.

* $p < 0.001$, test for trend.

[a] Absolute risks are expressed as % through age 30 yr.

Source: ref. *23*.

among Chinese *(28)*. The DRB1*15–DQA1*0102–DQB1*0602 is protective and associated with a reduced risk for type 1 diabetes in most populations.

Because of the geographic differences in the incidence of type 1 diabetes, as well as population variation in the frequency of DR-DQ haplotypes, the WHO DiaMond Project began a standardized international case-control molecular epidemiology study of type 1 diabetes in 1990 *(29)*. More than 20 participating centers were involved in this collaboration. Cases were selected from DiaMond incidence registries, and nondiabetic controls were identified from corresponding populations at risk. This approach permitted the estimation of relative risks, absolute risks, and population attributable fractions for individuals with two, one, and zero high-risk HLA-DQ haplotypes for each area. As illustrated in Table 2, relative-risk estimates revealed statistically significant dose-response relationships in all populations studied *(25)*. These data indicate that worldwide, susceptibility for type 1 diabetes is determined, in part, by high-risk HLA-DQ haplotypes *(30)*.

Although these data present useful information in terms of the strength of genetic associations, cumulative incidence rates for specific haplotype combinations can be more meaningful from a clinical and public health perspective *(25)*. These rates reflect the absolute risk of developing type 1 diabetes given two, one, or zero high-risk haplotypes. As illustrated in Table 2, Caucasians from moderate–high-incidence countries, such as Finland, the United States, and New Zealand, with two "susceptible" haplotypes had cumulative type 1 diabetes incidence rates that approached those typically observed for first-degree relatives (i.e., approx 5% through age 30 yr). However, corresponding estimates for the low-incidence populations, such as Korea, Japan, and China, were much less striking (0.1%). Thus, HLA-DQ haplotypes appear to be better predictive markers for type 1 diabetes in Caucasian than Asian populations.

Using these data, population attributable fractions (PAFs) can also be estimated. PAFs provide important information regarding the potential public health implications for disease-prevention strategies. They reflect the proportion of disease incidence that can be attributed to specific risk factors. In this context, they estimate the proportion of cases that could be prevented by modifying the environment for "susceptible" individuals. As shown in Table 2, PAFs were lower for Asian compared to Caucasian or African-American groups *(25)*. This indicates that disease interventions in "susceptible" individuals would likely have greater impact among Caucasians or African-Americans than Asians. However, even among the latter groups, no more than half of the disease would be prevented, assuming a successful intervention in all "susceptible" individuals.

Insulin Gene Polymorphisms

In Caucasians, it has been demonstrated that the insulin gene region (INS), located on chromosome 11p15.5, contains the second major susceptibility locus for type 1 diabetes (i.e., *IDDM2*) *(31,32)*. Positive associations have been observed with a nontranscribed minisatellite (variable number of tandem repeats [VNTR]) region in the 5′ flanking region. There are two common alleles. The shorter class I allele predisposes to type 1 diabetes, whereas the longer class III allele appears to be protective. The biological plausibility of these associations may relate to the expression of insulin mRNA in the thymus *(32)*. Class III alleles appear to generate higher levels of insulin mRNA than class I alleles. Such differences could contribute to a better immune tolerance for class III positive individuals by increasing the likelihood of negative selection for autoreactive T-cell clones.

The effect of the insulin gene also appears to vary by ethnicity. Undlien et al. found that class I alleles were significantly associated with type 1 diabetes in Caucasians. However, they only reached borderline significance in Tanzanian blacks and were not associated with the disease in Japanese *(33)*. However, other studies found a significant positive association between INS class I alleles and type 1 diabetes in the Japanese *(34)*. Methodological differences, such as heterogeneous case and control groups and variations in allele frequencies in the general populations, may be responsible for the inconsistencies in the literature. There also may be an interaction between the insulin gene and the HLA-DR, DQ loci, which varies by ethnicity *(35,36)*. This may also contribute to the geographic patterns of type 1 diabetes.

Beta Cell Autoantibodies

Evidence that type 1 diabetes is an autoimmune disorder is based on the presence of lymphocytic infiltrates of the pancreas at the onset of the diseases *(37)*, as well as the occurrence of autoantibodies to islet cell antigens (ICAs), tyrosine phosphatase IA-2 (IA-2), glutamic acid decarboxylase (GAD), and insulin autoantibodies (IAA) *(38,39)*. The presence of these autoantibodies indicates that tissue damage has likely been initiated by other etiologic agents. Thus, they represent important preclinical markers rather than risk factors for the disease.

Numerous studies have reported high prevalence rates for ICAs (65–100%) and GAD autoantibodies (60–68%) among Caucasian children at disease onset *(38,39)*. Data from Allegheny County, PA have also revealed that Caucasian children with type 1 diabetes are significantly more likely to have β-cell autoantibodies at disease onset than affected African-American children (45% vs 30%, $p < 0.05$) *(40)*. This may reflect etiologic differences because some African-American children are able to discontinue daily insulin injections after stabilization of their metabolic control.

Although most type 1 diabetes cases have β-cell autoantibodies at disease onset, they decrease in prevalence over time. In addition, they are rarely observed among first-degree relatives (2–5%) or in the general population (approx 1%) *(41–43)*. Moreover, not all autoantibody positive individuals develop the disease. However, first-degree relatives who are positive for multiple autoantibodies appear to be at very high risk for developing type 1 diabetes. Some clinical studies have estimated the positive predictive values associated with two and three autoantibodies at 65% and >90%, respectively *(43,44)*. It has been suggested that β-cell autoantibodies are as predictive in the general population as they are in high-risk families *(45)*. However, most studies have found them to be better markers among first-degree relatives *(41,42)*. This has important implications regarding potential disease interventions, which will be discussed in greater detail later in this chapter.

Data from our research group have also shown that HLA-DQ haplotypes modify type 1 diabetes risk in the absence of β-cell autoantibodies *(46)*. Among our first-degree relatives who were negative for autoantibodies to GAD, IA-2, and ICA, 32% of those who carried two high-risk HLA-DQ haplotypes developed the disease after 12.5 yr of follow-up. These results emphasize the importance of both genetic and autoantibody markers in estimating type 1 diabetes risk.

Viruses

Many epidemiologic investigations have supported the involvement of viruses in the etiology of type 1 diabetes *(47,48)*. They are thought to act as initiators, accelerators, or precipitators of the disease. They may function by direct or indirect mechanisms. However, it is not clear whether they are necessary (or sufficient) to cause type 1 diabetes.

The viruses that have received the most attention include the enteroviruses, especially Coxsackie virus B (CVB). Sequence homology between a highly conserved nonstructural CVB4 protein (P2C) and GAD has been reported *(49)*. In addition, several investigations indicated that antibodies to P2C and GAD crossreacted *(50,51)*. However, other studies failed to confirm these results *(52)* or observed P2C antibodies among healthy GAD-negative controls *(53)*. T-Cell proliferation studies have also been conflicting *(54–56)*. Moreover, two reports *(55,57)* noted that reactivity was strongest in subjects with DR4, which contrasts with other investigations showing that the CVB associations with type 1 diabetes occurred among individuals with DR3 *(58,59)*. Because CVB infections are frequent during childhood and are known to have systemic effects on the pancreas, they are likely to remain considered as important risk factors for type 1 diabetes.

Other viruses have also been associated with type 1 diabetes. Finnish investigators observed an increase in the incidence of diabetes 2–4 yr after a mumps epidemic *(60)*. Studies of cytomegaloviruses (CMVs) have shown an increased prevalence of integrated viral genome in DNA extracted from lymphocytes when comparing cases with type 1 diabetes to controls without the disease *(61)*. CMV antibody studies, however, have been inconsistent *(62,63)*, suggesting that persistent, rather than acute, CMV infections during childhood may increase type 1 diabetes risk. In addition, rotaviruses, which are common causes of childhood gastroenteritis, contain peptide sequences similar to T-cell epitopes in IA-2 and GAD *(64)*. A recent prospective study showed that high-risk children who developed β-cell autoantibodies or type 1 diabetes were significantly more likely to show serological evidence of rotavirus infections than those who did not develop diabetes autoimmunity *(65)*. These data suggest that infections with rotavirus may also trigger β-cell autoimmunity in genetically susceptible children.

Epidemiologic studies have revealed that the time of exposure to viruses may be important. Approximately 10–20% of children with congenital rubella syndrome (CRS), particularly those who carry high-risk HLA alleles, develop autoimmune type 1 diabetes *(66)*. Recently, T-cell-stimulation studies revealed that rubella virus peptides with binding motifs for HLA-DR3/DR4 were recognized by clones specific to GAD in type 1 diabetics, particularly those with CRS *(67)*. These data provide additional evidence for the importance of early exposures in the etiology of the disease.

Other investigations have shown that enteroviral infections *in utero* increase the risk of developing the disease *(68,69)*. Most recently, a prospective study of infants at high genetic risk revealed that enterovirus infections were more common among those who developed β-cell autoimmunity than those who remained antibody negative *(70)*. In more than half of the infants, the infections occurred 6 mo prior to the appearance of autoantibodies. These data indicate that enteroviral infections during pregnancy or in early infancy may be related to the development of diabetes autoimmunity in susceptible infants.

Human endogenous retroviruses (HERVs) received considerable attention after a study provided evidence for the involvement of a superantigen in the etiology of type 1 diabetes *(71)*. Superantigens can be products of bacteria, viruses, or endogenous retroviral genes and function by stimulating T-cell families rather than specific clones. One investigator reported that human endogenous retrovirus K ($IDDMK_{1,2}22$) RNA was present in 10 other type 1 diabetic cases, but not in controls *(72)*. Other investigators failed to replicate these findings and observed $IDDMK_{1,2}22$ sequences and expression among both type 1 diabetic and non diabetic individuals *(73,74)*. However, one group reported HLA-DQA1*0301-DQB1*0302 haplotypes carrying HERV-K long-terminal repeat (LTR3) sequences were preferentially transmitted to type 1 diabetics than those without the LTR3 *(75)*. In contrast, the absence of LTR3 in HLA-DQA1*0201-DQB1*0501 haplotypes conferred increased risk of the disease. The authors hypothesized that these sequences may affect transcription or tissue-specific regulation of DQB1 and, therefore, influence disease risk.

Infant Nutrition

Another hypothesis that has received considerable attention in recent years relates to early exposure to cow's milk protein and the subsequent development of type 1 diabetes *(76–79)*. Experimental studies in rodents revealed that the frequency of type 1 diabetes could be modified by altering the cow's milk protein composition of dietary chows *(80)*. This led investigators to speculate about the role of diet in the etiology of type 1 diabetes in humans.

The first epidemiologic observation of such a relationship was by Borch-Johnsen et al., who found that diabetic children were breast-fed for shorter periods of time than healthy siblings or children from the general population *(81)*. The authors postulated that lack of immunologic protection from insufficient breast-feeding may lead to type 1 diabetes later during childhood. It was also hypothesized that the protective effect of breast feeding may indirectly reflect early exposure to dietary proteins.

Numerous case-control studies subsequently investigated this issue. Results of a meta-analysis revealed a weak positive association between exposure to cow's milk at an early age (< 3 mo) and type 1 diabetes (odds ratio = 1.4; 95% confidence interval =

1.2–1.6) *(82)*. These data were supported by investigations that showed associations with elevated levels of antibodies to cow's milk peptides among cases compared to controls *(83,84)*. However, T-cell proliferation studies in response to cow's milk antigens have been negative or lacked specificity for type 1 diabetes *(85,86)*. Concern has also been raised by short-term natural history studies that showed no association between infant feeding patterns and the development of β-cell autoimmunity *(87,88)*. Moreover, consumption of milk or other dietary proteins later in childhood appears to increase risk of developing the disease *(89)*. Thus, the contribution of the infant diet to the development of type 1 diabetes is far from clear.

Because of recent data showing that GAD-reactive lymphocytes express the gut-specific $\alpha_4\beta_7$ homing receptor *(90)*, investigators have proposed a unifying hypothesis that focuses on the gut immune system *(91–93)*. It has been hypothesized that the protective effect of breast-feeding against the development of type 1 diabetes may be, in part, the result of its role in gut maturation. Breast milk contains growth factors, cytokines, and other substances necessary for the maturation of the intestinal mucosa. Breast-feeding also protects against enteric infections during infancy, and promotes proper colonization of the gut. In contrast, early exposure to dietary antigens, such as cow's milk peptides, may contribute to the loss of tolerance to self-antigens through molecular mimicry. In addition, cow's milk contains bovine insulin, which differs from human insulin by three amino acids *(94)*. Oral exposure to cow's milk formulas appears to induce the formation of antibodies that crossreacts with human insulin. It also increases cellular responses to bovine insulin in high-risk infants, which is evident at age 3 mo *(95)*. Thus, immune response to dietary bovine insulin may be another early environmental trigger of diabetes autoimmunity. Interesting, enteroviral infections can also interfere with gut immunoregulation, which may explain the epidemiologic associations between viral infections and type 1 diabetes.

The lack of specificity for a particular antigen suggests that type 1 diabetes may involve a general defect in the gut immune system *(91–93)*. Enhanced immune response to early dietary and/or viral exposures may reflect a failure to induce immune tolerance in the gut. Such effects are likely to be mediated by genetic predisposition. Higher levels of antibodies to cow's milk proteins *(96)* and GAD *(97)* have been associated with DQB1*0201, which also increases susceptibility to celiac disease *(98)*. Moreover, the relative risk associated with early introduction of cow's milk *(99)* and milk consumption in childhood *(91)* appears to be stronger among individuals with high-risk DQB1 susceptibility alleles than those with low-risk genotypes. These results emphasize the need to match cases and controls by HLA haplotypes in epidemiologic studies of type 1 diabetes.

FINANCIAL AND SOCIAL IMPACT OF TYPE 1 DIABETES

The burdens of type 1 diabetes provide the rationale for current discussions regarding disease prevention. These burdens include medical, social, psychological, and financial elements. Several studies on costs have noted a large financial burden related to diabetes *(100)*, and the most current estimate in the United States places the annual medical and social costs of diabetes at $97 billion *(101)*. Estimates focused solely on type 1 diabetes appear less frequently in the literature. Reports from England and

Wales *(102),* Israel *(103),* and Spain *(104)* note meaningful expenses in type 1 diabetes both in the short-term and on a lifetime basis.

Studies that describe the economic costs of diabetes often consider the direct or medical costs of the disease and, less frequently, the indirect costs of diabetes. Examples of indirect costs include the value assigned to morbidity, disability, and premature mortality associated with type 1 diabetes. From an economic perspective, the most important medical costs in type 1 diabetes include those related to the daily management of the disease and those related to the treatment of late-stage complications. The annual costs of treatment for type 1 diabetes have been shown to range between $1500 per person for standard (twice a day) insulin regimens, to $3000 for intensive regimens (multiple daily injections), and nearly $6000 for insulin pump protocols *(105).* Out-of-pocket health care costs for families with type 1 diabetic children in the United States exceed $1000 per year *(106).* The onset of complications generally leads to a marked increase in the use of hospital and outpatient services *(107).* The treatment of complications in England and Wales in 1992 accounted for one-half of the total medical costs of type 1 diabetes *(102).*

Estimating the economic value of the social costs of type 1 diabetes is often difficult. Several arguments exist over the most appropriate method to value human life. Several studies, though, note higher rates of disability and work-related absenteeism in persons with type 1 diabetes, particularly in those with late-stage complications *(108–111).* Together with higher rates of mortality, preliminary indications are that these indirect costs are larger than the direct costs of type 1 diabetes.

The impact of diabetes may also be felt in ways that are less easily quantifiable. The presence of type 1 diabetes, for example, is known to influence the insurance and employment experiences of affected individuals. Health, life, and sometimes automobile insurance are generally more difficult to obtain for a person with type 1 diabetes *(106,112,113).* Individuals may also face discrimination in the job application process *(106,114)* and often face limitations in the types of jobs available to them. Employment in commercial driving, for example, is limited out of concern for hypoglycemia *(115).*

Recent evidence suggests that the economic impact of type 1 diabetes does not affect all individuals equally. Financial barriers exist to appropriate implementation of diabetes management protocols. Individuals with inadequate health insurance coverage, for example, have been shown to test blood sugar levels less frequently *(106,116)* and have poorer levels of glycemic control *(117).* Out-of-pocket health care costs are also proportionately greater in the poor *(112).*

EPIDEMIOLOGY AND THE PREVENTION OF TYPE 1 DIABETES

Intervention Trials

Because of the tremendous burden of type 1 diabetes, the rationale for seeking prevention programs is fairly straightforward. Currently, several large clinical trials have begun to evaluate a variety of primary (i.e., the Trial to Reduce Type 1 Diabetes in the Genetically At-Risk [TRIGR] *(118)*) and secondary interventions (i.e., the European Nicotinamide Diabetes Intervention Trial [ENDIT] *(119),* the Diabetes Prevention Trial-1 [DPT-1] *(120)*) in family members of affected individuals (*see* Table 3). Eligible relatives are identified by either genetic screening for high-risk HLA-DQ alleles (i.e., TRIGR) or autoantibody screening for β-cell antibodies (i.e., DPT-1, ENDIT). Those who carry disease susceptibility genes or are autoantibody positive are eligible for randomization.

Table 3
Type 1 Diabetes Prevention Trials in Progress

Study[a]	*Intervention*	*Target group*	*Screening*
TRIGR *(118)*	Nutramigen (Mead Johnson)	First degree relatives, newborns	HLA-DQ
ENDIT *(120)*	Nicotinamide	First degree relatives, 5–40 yr	ICA
DPT-1 *(119)*	Parenteral and oral insulin	First degree relatives, 5–40 yr	ICA
DIPP *(121)*	Nasal insulin	General population, newborns	HLA-DQ

[a]TRIGR, Trial to Reduce Type 1 Diabetes in the Genetically At-Risk; ENDIT, European Nicotinamide Diabetes Intervention Trial; DPT-1, Diabetes Prevention Trial-1; DIPP, Diabetes Prediction and Prevention Project.

Note: HLA-DQ Screening

TRIGR, Positive for DQB1*0302 and/or *0201; negative for DQB1*0602/3 or *0301.
ENDIT, no genetic screening.
DPT-1, done for ICA+ individuals only; negative DQA1*0102-DQB1*0602.
DIPP, DQB1*02/*0302 or DQB1*0302/X (X = allele other than *02, *0301, or *0602).

ICA Screening

TRIGR, no ICA screening, β-cell autoantibodies are endpoints.
ENDIT, ICA titrs > 20 JDF units on two occasions.
DPT-1, ICA titrs > 20 JDF units; if positive, continue with additional screening tests.
DIPP, no ICA screening, β-cell autoantibodies are endpoints.

Several of these studies are now closed to recruitment *(119,120)*. Although these trials are based on first-degree relatives, about 90% of individuals who develop type 1 diabetes have a negative family history of the disease. For interventions to have a public health impact, they must be based on the general population. Unfortunately, the genetic and autoantibody screening strategies used in families of affected individuals are not as effective in the general population *(41,42)*. However, one primary prevention trial based on genetic screening in the general population has recently been initiated [i.e., Diabetes Prediction and Prevention Project (DIPP) *(121)*].

Although the potential therapies being offered to eligible high-risk individuals are controversial and others may be associated with acute or long-term complications, positive preliminary results are now appearing in the literature *(122–124)*. Thus, there is a critical need to reconsider, from an epidemiologic perspective, the risks and benefits of genetic/autoantibody screening and possible participation in prevention trials for type 1 diabetes. It is also necessary to develop thoughtful approaches for translating the findings from epidemiology into public health practice. This begins with public education, continues with an assessment of the efficacy of the intervention, and includes an evaluation of the effectiveness of the program.

Education and Screening

The final report of the Task Force on Genetic Testing recently noted that "a knowledge base on genetics and genetic testing should be developed for the general public. Without a sound knowledge base, informed decisions are impossible and claims of autonomy and informed consent are suspect" *(125)*. Because genetic screening for type 1 diabetes is currently being performed, it is essential that we begin to address this issue in epidemiology.

Translation involves the utilization of epidemiologic data for public health practice and the development of appropriate policy recommendations. For type 1 diabetes, data collected from population-based epidemiologic studies, such as the WHO DiaMond Molecular Epidemiology Project, provide an excellent foundation for translation. We currently know that for individuals with two HLA-DQ susceptibility haplotypes, the cumulative risk of type 1 diabetes in the general Caucasian population is approximately 5% *(25)*. However, it may range from 0.1% to >90%, depending on one's risk factor profile, which includes age, ethnic, familial, genetic, environmental, and autoimmune determinants. Population-based epidemiologic studies that have investigated these potential determinants are able to generate risk-factor-specific rates. These data can be used to "individualize" risk estimates for those who carry (or do not carry) particular susceptibility genes and have had (or have not had) specific exposures or life experiences. The availability of this information to investigators and potential participants in current type 1 diabetes intervention trials would facilitate education and counseling, before and after genetic/autoantibody screening. In this manner, individuals would be able to make more informed decisions about the risks and benefits of genetic and autoantibody screening and participation in intervention trials.

Economic and Social Issues

The real value of the effect of any prevention program is not just its ability to prevent type 1 diabetes but also its impact on a range of economic, public health, and ethical issues. Concerns that merit strenuous debate include not just the efficacy of a particular prevention program but also its efficiency, equity, and protection of human subjects. At the moment, with yet incomplete data regarding the efficacy of prevention, several alternatives are being discussed: Screening in high-risk populations or screening in the community? Screening with genetic or immunologic or metabolic markers? Treatment with immunologic vaccines or dietary supplements? Each alternative poses different questions regarding the implementation and effect of the prevention program. Several investigators recognize the need to assess the relative costs and benefits (or efficiency) of the programs. It is not clear, though, that equity, accessibility, or privacy issues are included in the requested evaluations. These are the hidden risks that underlie any subsequent program. The privacy of screening data is of noted importance in type 1 diabetes. We have highlighted that persons and families living with type 1 diabetes face meaningful insurance and employment issues. Disregarding this impact is short-sighted.

Equity issues remain one of the most important considerations for determining the success of any intervention program. The data showing the economic influences on the use of diabetes care raise questions about the availability of health care to all. Will diabetes prevention even be available to those who could benefit from it, or will we have another situation of "boutique medicine" (of benefit to a selected few)? There are serious concerns regarding the viability of prevention programs in type 1 diabetes in the whole population and a noted need for more information to more completely evaluate their impact.

Several potential risks of prevention programs are not yet fully understood. Reports in other diseases note a psychological stress or anxiety impact related to screening itself and to false positives in screening tests in particular. At this point, we do not adequately know what impact this may have in screening for type 1 diabetes. What are the ramifications of being falsely told that your son or daughter is very likely to develop diabetes? How will it affect the lifestyle decisions in these families?

Other considerations relate to the desire for information and perceptions of risk. For example, some family members or individuals from the general population actively solicit information regarding their type 1 diabetes risk. However, others prefer not to know their likelihood of developing the disease. This is an extremely important ethical issue because there is currently no cure for diabetes. In addition, the interventions being tested are not appropriated for all individuals at risk. A wide variety of factors may influence one's perception of risk *(126,127)*.

Thus, education programs must be developed with considerable input from those for whom they are targeted. Participation from lay organizations and health departments would be invaluable. Possible strategies for the development of education programs include focus groups and personal interviews conducted in accordance with existing behavioral models, such as the Expanded Health Belief Model *(128)*. Once created, these programs must be made widely available. Self-education packets could be distributed to potential participants in the intervention trials. In addition, an interactive website could be developed. This could not only increase knowledge of type 1 diabetes risk but also improve perception and awareness of the risk and benefits of potential therapies that may become available in the near future.

SUMMARY

Epidemiology will continue to play a central role in preventing chronic diseases in the new millennium. It is the only field that can be used to evaluate the risks and benefits of prevention programs on a population basis. At present, we are extremely close to being able to apply the results of current clinical trials for the prevention of type 1 diabetes. However, the scientific and medical communities have not, as yet, begun to prepare for this important step. There are many unanswered questions regarding actual risk of disease, perceptions of risk, ethics, confidentiality, potential complications, costs, and insurance or employment discrimination based on genetic and autoantibody testing and the various approaches to intervention. We are in the position to be able to begin to address these issues based on current epidemiologic research. The translation of epidemiologic research, from the laboratory to the community, will help prepare individuals in our community to meet these challenges for type 1 diabetes and other chronic diseases in the years to come.

ACKNOWLEDGMENTS

The authors would like to acknowledge the assistance of Ms. Cathy Sobocinski in the preparation of this manuscript. This work was supported by NIH grant R01-DK44590.

REFERENCES

1. Last JM. A Dictionary of Epidemiology. Oxford University Press, New York; 1983.
2. World Bank. The World Bank overview. In: World Development Report 1993. Oxford University Press, Oxford, 1993, pp. 1–16.
3. World Health Report 1999. http://www.who.int/whr/1999/en/report.htm.
4. LaPorte RE, Tajima N, Akerblom HR, et al. Geographic differences in the risk of insulin-dependent diabetes mellitus: the importance of registries. Diabetes Care 1985;8(Suppl 1):17–23.

5. Diabetes Epidemiology Research International Group (DERI). Geographic patterns of childhood diabetes mellitus. Diabetes 1988;37:1113–1119.
6. Eurodiab ACE Study Group. Variation and trends in incidence of childhood diabetes in Europe. Lancet 2000;355:873–876.
7. WHO DiaMond Project Group. WHO multinational project for childhood diabetes. Diabetes Care 1990;13:1062–1068.
8. Yang Z, Wang K, Li T, et al. Childhood diabetes in China. Diabetes Care 1998;21:525–529.
9. Karvonen M, Viik-Kajander M, Moltchanova E, et al. Incidence of childhood type 1 diabetes worldwide. Diabetes Care 2000;23:1516–1526.
10. Onkamo P, Väänänen S, Karvonen MJ, Tuomilehto I. Worldwide increase in incidence of type 1 diabetes—the analysis of the data on published incidence trends. Diabetologia 1999;42:1395–1403.
11. Dokheel TM. Pittsburgh Diabetes Epidemiology Research Group. An epidemic of childhood diabetes in the United States? Diabetes Care 1993;16:1606–1611.
12. Rewers M, LaPorte RE, Walczak M, Dmochowski K, Bogacznska E. Apparent epidemic of insulin-dependent diabetes mellitus in midwestern Poland. Diabetes 1987;36:106–113.
13. Padaiga Z, Tuomilehto J, Karvonen M, et al. Incidence trends in childhood onset IDDM in four countries around the Baltic sea during 1983–1992. Diabetologia 1997;40:187–192.
14. WHO DiaMond Project Group. Childhood diabetes, epidemics and epidemiology: an approach for controlling diabetes. Am J Epidemiol 1992,135:803–816.
15. Tull ES, Roseman JM, Christian CLE. Epidemiology of childhood IDDM in the U.S. Virgin Islands from 1979 to 1988. Diabetes Care 1991;14:558–564.
16. Siemiatycki J, Colle E, Campbell S, Dewar R, Aubert D, Belmonte MM. Incidence of IDDM in Montreal by ethnic group and by social class and comparisons with ethnic groups living elsewhere. Diabetes 1988;37:1096–1102.
17. Dorman JS. Molecular epidemiology of insulin-dependent diabetes mellitus. Epidemiol Rev 1997;19:91–98.
18. WHO Multinational Project for Childhood Diabetes Group. Familial insulin-dependent diabetes mellitus (IDDM) epidemiology: standardization of data for the DIAMOND project. WHO Bull 1991;69:767–777.
19. Eurodiab ACE Study Group and Eurodiab Ace Substudy 2 Study Group. Familial risk of type 1 diabetes in European children. Diabetologia 1998;41:1151–1156.
20. Redondo MJ, Rewers M, Yu L, et al. Genetic determination of islet cell autoimmunity in monozygotic twin, dizygotic twin, and non-twin siblings of patients with type 1 diabetes: prospective twin study. Br Med J 1999;318:698–702.
21. Concannon P, Gogolin-Ewens KJ, Hinds DA, et al. A second-generation screen of the human genome for susceptibility to insulin-dependent diabetes mellitus. Nat Genet 1998;19:292–296.
22. Mein CA, Esposito L, Dunn MG, et al. A search for type 1 diabetes susceptibility genes in families from the United Kingdom. Nat Genet 1998;19:297–300.
23. Buzzetti R, Quattrocchi CC, Nistico L. Dissecting the genetics of type 1 diabetes: relevance for familial clustering and differences in incidence. Diabetes Metab Rev 1998;14:111–128.
24. Pugliese A. Unraveling the genetics of insulin-dependent type 1A diabetes: the search must go on. Diabetes Rev 1999;7:39–54.
25. Dorman JS, Bunker CH. HLA-DQ locus of the human leukocyte antigen complex and type 1 diabetes mellitus: a HuGE review. Epidemiol Rev 2000;22:218–227.
26. Todd JA, Mijovic C, Fletcher J, Jenkins D, Bradwell AR, Barnett AH. Identification of susceptibility loci for insulin-dependent diabetes mellitus by trans-racial gene mapping. Nature 1989;388;587–589.
27. Awata T, Kuzuya T, Matsuda A, Iwamoto Y, Kanazawa Y. Genetic analysis of HLA class II alleles and susceptibility to type 1 (insulin-dependent) diabetes mellitus in Japanese subjects. Diabetologia 1992;35:419–424.
28. Huang HS, Peng JT, She JY, et al. HLA-encoded susceptibility to insulin-dependent diabetes mellitus is determined by DR and DQ genes as well as their linkage disequilibria in a Chinese population. Hum Immunol 1995;44:210–219.
29. Dorman JS, McCanlies E. WHO DiaMond Molecular Epidemiology Sub-Project Group. Molecular type 1 diabetes epidemiology: international studies. Diabetes Res Clin Pract 1996;34:107–116.
30. Dorman JS, LaPorte RE, Stone RA, et al. Worldwide differences in the incidence of type 1 diabetes are associated with amino acid variation at position 57 of the HLA-DQ β chain. PNAS 1990;87:7370–7374.

31. Bennett ST, Wilson AJ, Esposito L, et al. Insulin VNTR allele-specific effect in type 1 diabetes depends on identity of untransmitted paternal allele. Nat Genet 1997;17:350–352.
32. Pugliese A, Zeller M, Fernandez A Jr, et al. The insulin gene is transcribed in human thymus and transcription levels correlated with allelic variation at the INS VNTR-IDDM 2 susceptibility locus for type 1 diabetes. Nat Genet 1997;15:293–297.
33. Undlien DE, Hamaguchi K, Kimura A, et al. Type 1 diabetes susceptibility associated with polymorphism in the insulin gene region: a study of blacks, Caucasians, and orientials. Diabetologia 1994;37:745–749.
34. Kawaguchi Y, Ikegami H, Shen GO. Insulin gene region contributes to genetic susceptibility to, but may not to, low incidence of insulin-dependent diabetes mellitus in Japanese. Biochem Biophys Res Commun 1997;233:283–287.
35. Van der Auwera B, Schuit F, Lyaruu I, et al. Genetic susceptibility for insulin-dependent diabetes mellitus in Caucasians revisited: the importance of diabetes registries in disclosing interactions between HLA-DQ and insulin gene-linked risk. J Clin Endocrinol Metab 1995;80:2567–2573.
36. Metcalf KA, Hitman GA, Fennessy MJ, et al. In Finland insulin gene region encoded susceptibility to IDDM exerts maximum effect when there is low HLA-DR associated risk. Diabetologia 1995;38:1223–1229.
37. Trucco M. To be or not to be ASP57: that is the question. Diabetes Care 1992;15:705–715.
38. Bach JF. Insulin-dependent diabetes mellitus as an autoimmune disease. Endocrinol Rev 1994;15:516–542.
39. Schranz DB, Lernmark A. Immunology in diabetes: an update. Diabetes Metab Rev 1998;14:3–29.
40. Libman M, Pietropaolo M, Trucco M, Dorman JS, LaPorte RE, Becker D. Islet cell autoimmunity in white and black children and adolescents with IDDM. Diabetes Care 1998;21:1824–1827.
41. Bingley PJ, Bonifacio E, Williams AJK, Genovese S, Bottazzo GF, Gale EAM. Prediction of IDDM in the general population. Diabetes 1997;46:1701–1710.
42. Knip M, Karjalainen J, Akerblom HK, et al. Islet cell antibodies are less predictive of IDDM among unaffected children in the general population than in sibs of children with diabetes. Diabetes Care 1998;21:1670–1673.
43. Verge CF, Gianani R, Kawasaki E, et al. Prediction of type 1 diabetes in first-degree relatives using a combination of insulin, GAD, and ICA512/IA-2 autoantibodies. Diabetes 1996;45:926–933.
44. Dittler J, Seidel D, Schenker M, Ziegler AG. GADIA2-combi determination as first-line screening for improved prediction of type 1 diabetes in relatives. Diabetes 1998;47:592–597.
45. Schatz D, Krischer J, Horne G, et al. Islet cell antibodies predict insulin-dependent diabetes in United States school age children as powerfully as in unaffected relatives. J Clin Invest 1994;93:2403–2407.
46. Pietropaolo M, Becker D, Dorman JS, et al. Are GAD 65 & IA-2 autoantibodies sufficient to predict type 1 diabetes? Diabetes 1999;48(Suppl 1):A45.
47. Foulis K. The pathology of the endocrine pancreas in type 1 (insulin dependent) diabetes mellitus. APMIS 1996;104:161–167.
48. von Herrath MG, Holz A, Homann D. Role of viruses in type 1 diabetes. Semin Immunol 1998;10:87–100.
49. Kaufman DL, Erlander MG, Clare-Salzler M, et al. Autoimmunity to two forms of glutamic decarboxylase in insulin-dependent diabetes mellitus. J Clin Invest 1992;89:283.
50. Hou J, Sid C, Franchi D. Antibodies to glutamic acid decarboxylase and P2-C peptides in sera from coxsackie virus B4-infected mice and IDDM patients. Diabetes 1994;43:1260–1266.
51. Lönnrot M, Hyöty H, Knip M, et al. Antibody cross-reactivity induced by the homologous regions in glutamic acid decarboxylase (GAD65) and 2C protein of coxsackievirus B4. Clin Exp Immunol 1996;104:398–405.
52. Richter W, Mertens T, Schoel B, et al. Sequence homology of the diabetes-associated autoantigen glutamate decarboxylase with coxsackie B4–2C protein and heat shock protein 60 mediates no molecular mimicry of autoantibodies. J Exp Med 1994;180:721–726.
53. Vreugdenhil GR, Batstra MR, Aanstoot HJ, Melchers WJG, Galama JMD. Analysis of antibody responses against coxsackie virus B4 protein 2C and the diabetes autoantigen GAD_{65}. J Med Virol 1999;59:256–261.
54. Atkinson MA, Bowman MA, Campbell L, Darrow BL, Kaufman DL, Maclaren NK. Cellular immunity to a determinant common to glutamate decarboxylase and coxsackie virus in insulin-dependent diabetes. J Clin Invest 1994;94:2125–2129.

55. Schloot NC, Roep BO, Wegmann DR, Yu L, Wang TB, Eisenbarth GS. T-cell reactivity to GAD65 peptide sequences shared with coxsackie virus protein in recent-onset IDDM, post-onset IDDM patients and control subjects. Diabetologia 1997;40:332–338.
56. Juhela S, Hyöty H, Roivainen M, et al. T-cell responses to enterovirus antigens in children with type 1 diabetes. Diabetes 2000;49:1308–1313.
57. Jones DB, Crosby I. Proliferative lymphocyte responses to virus antigens homologous to GAD65 in IDDM. Diabetologia 1996;39:1318–1324.
58. D'Alessio DJ. A case-control study of group B coxsackievirus immunoglobulin M antibody prevalence and HLA-DR antigens in newly diagnosed cases of insulin-dependent diabetes mellitus. Am J Epidemiol 1992;135:1331–1338.
59. Vreugdenhil GR, Geluk A, Ottenhoff THM, Melchers WJG, Roep BO, Galama JMD. Molecular mimicry in diabetes mellitus: the homologous domain in coxsackie B virus protein 2C and islet autoantigen GAD65 is highly conserved in the coxsackie B-like enteroviruses and binds to the diabetes associated HLA-DR3 molecule. Diabetologia 1998;41:40–46.
60. Hyöty H, Hiltunen M, Reuranen A. Decline of mumps antibodies in type 1 (insulin-dependent) diabetic children with a plateau in the rising incidence of type 1 diabetes after introduction of the mumps-measles-rubella vaccine in Finland. Diabetologia 1993;36:1303–1308.
61. Pak CY, McArthur RG, Eun HM, Yoon JW. Association of cytomegalovirus infection with autoimmune type 1 diabetes. Lancet 1988;2:1–4.
62. Nicoletti F, Scalia G, Lunetta M, et al. Correlation between islet cell antibodies and anti-cytomegalovirus IgM and IgG antibodies in healthy first-degree relatives of type 1 (insulin-dependent) diabetic patients. Clin Immunol Immunopathol 1990;55:139–147.
63. Hiltunen M, Hyöty H, Karjalainen J, et al. Serological evaluation of the role of cytomegalovirus in the pathogenesis of IDDM: A prospective study. Diabetologia 1995;38:705–710.
64. Honeyman MC, Coulson BS, Stone NL, et al. Association between rotavirus infection and pancreatic islet autoimmunity in children at risk of developing type 1 diabetes. Diabetes 2000;49:1319–1324.
65. Serreze DV, Ottendorfer EW, Ellis M, Gauntt CJ, Atkinson MA. Acceleration of type 1 diabetes by a coxsackievirus infection requires a preexisting critical mass of autoreactive t-cells in pancreatic islets. Diabetes 2000;49:708–711.
66. McIntosh EDG, Menser M. A fifty-year follow-up of congenital rubella. Lancet 1992;340:414–415.
67. Ou D, Mitchell LA, Metzger DL, Gillam S, Tingle AJ. Cross-reactive rubella virus and glutamic acid decarboxylase (65 and 67) protein determinants recognised by T cells of patients with type 1 diabetes mellitus. Diabetologia 2000;43:750–762.
68. Hyöty H, Hiltunen M, Knip M, et al. A prospective study of the role of coxsackie B and other enterovirus infections in the pathogenesis of IDDM. Diabetes 1995;44:652–657.
69. Dahlquist G, Frisk G, Ivarsson SA, Svanberg L, Forsgren M, Diderholm H. Indications that maternal coxsackie B virus infection during pregnancy is a risk factor for childhood-onset IDDM. Diabetologia 1995;38:1371–1373.
70. Lönnrot M, Korpela K, Knip M, et al. Enterovirus infection as a risk factor for β-cell autoimmunity in a prospectively observed birth cohort. Diabetes 2000;49:1314–1318.
71. Conrad B, Weldmann E, Trucco G, et al. Evidence for superantigen involvement in insulin-dependent diabetes mellitus aetiology. Nature 1994;371:351–355.
72. Conrad B, Weissmahr RN, Böni J, Arcari R, Schüpbach, J, Mach B. A human endogenous retroviral superantigen as candidate autoimmune gene in type 1 diabetes. Cell 1997;90:303–313.
73. Jaeckel E, Heringlake S, Berger D, Brabant G, Hunsmann G, Manns MP. No evidence for association between IDDMK1,2 22, a novel isolated retrovirus, and IDDM. Diabetes 1999;48:209–214.
74. Muir A, Ruan QG, Marron MP, She JX. The IDDMK1,2 22 retrovirus is not detectable in either mRNA or genomic DNA from patients with type 1 diabetes. Diabetes 1999;48:219–222.
75. Donner H, Tönjes RR, VanderAuwera B, et al. The presence or absence of a retroviral long terminal repeat influences the genetic risk for type 1 diabetes conferred by human leukocyte antigen DQ haplotypes. J Clin Endo Metab 1999;84:1404–1408.
76. Scott FW. Cow milk and insulin-dependent diabetes mellitus: is there a relationship? Am J Clin Nutr 1990;51:589–591.
77. Akerblom HK, Savilahti E, Savkkonen TT. The case for elimination of cow's milk in early infancy in the prevention of type 1 diabetes: the Finnish experience. Diabetes Metab Rev 1993;9:269–278.
78. Kostraba JN. What can epidemiology tell us about the role of infant diet in the etiology of IDDM? Diabetes Care 1994;17:87–91.

79. Gerstein HC. Cow's milk exposure and type 1 diabetes mellitus. Diabetes Care 1994;17:13–19.
80. Elliott RB, Martin JM. Dietary protein: a trigger of insulin-dependent diabetes in the BB rat? Diabetologia 1984;26:297–299.
81. Borch-Johnsen K, Joner G, Mandrup-Poulsen T, et al. Relation between breast-feeding and incidence rates of insulin-dependent diabetes mellitus. Lancet 1984;2:1083–1086.
82. Norris JM, Scott FW. A meta-analysis of infant diet and insulin-dependent diabetes mellitus: do biases play a role? Epidemiology 1996;7:87–92.
83. Karjalainen J, Martin JM, Knip M. A bovine albumin peptide as a possible trigger of insulin-dependent diabetes mellitus. N Engl J Med 1992;327:302–307.
84. Füchtenbusch M, Karges W, Standl E, Dosch HM, Ziegler AG. Antibodies to bovine serum albumin (BSA) in type 1 diabetes and other autoimmune disorders. Exp Clin Endocrinol Diabetes 1997;105:86–91.
85. Cavallo MG, Fava D, Monetini L, Barone F, Pozzilli P. Cell-mediated immune response to β casein in recent-onset insulin-dependent diabetes: implications for disease pathogenesis. Lancet 1996;348: 926–928.
86. Atkinson MA, Bowman MA, Kao KJ, et al. Lack of immune responsiveness to bovine serum albumin in insulin-dependent diabetes. N Engl J Med 1993;329:1853–1858.
87. Norris JM, Beaty B, Klingensmith G, et al. Lack of association between early exposure to cow's milk protein and β-cell autoimmunity. JAMA 1996;276:609–614.
88. Couper JJ, Steele C, Beresford S, et al. Lack of association between duration of breast-feeding or introduction of cow's milk and development of islet autoimmunity. Diabetes 1999;48:2145–2149.
89. Virtanen SM, Läärä E, Hyppönen E, et al. Cow's milk consumption, HLA-DQB1 genotype, and type 1 diabetes. Diabetes 2000;49:912–917.
90. Paronen J, Klemetti P, Kantele JM, et al. Glutamate decarboxylase-reactive peripheral blood lymphocytes from patients with IDDM express gut-specific homing receptor α4 β7-intergrin. Diabetes 1997;46:583–588.
91. Kolb H, Pozzilli P. Cow's milk and type 1 diabetes: the gut immune system deserves attention. Immunol Today 1999;20:108–110.
92. Harrison LC, Honeyman MC. Cow's milk and type 1 diabetes. Diabetes 1999;48:1501–1507.
93. Vaarala O. Gut and the induction of immune tolerance in type 1 diabetes. Diabetes Metab Res Rev 1999;15:353–361.
94. Paronen J, Knip M, Savilahti E, et al. Effect of cow's milk exposure and maternal type 1 diabetes on cellular and humoral immunization to dietary insulin in infants at genetic risk for type 1 diabetes. Diabetes 2000;49:1657–1665.
95. Vaarala O, Knip M, Paronen J, et al. Cow's milk formula feeding induces primary immunization to insulin in infants at genetic risk for type1 diabetes. Diabetes 1999;48:1389–1394.
96. Saukkonen T, Virtanen SM, Karppinen M, et al. Significance of cow's milk protein antibodies as risk factor for childhood IDDM: interactions with dietary cow's milk intake and HLA-DQB1 genotype. Diabetologia 1998;41:72–78.
97. Hagopian WA, Sanjeevi CB, Kockum, I, et al. Glutamate decarboxylase-, insulin-, and islet cell-antibodies and HLA typing to detect diabetes in a general population-based study of swedish children. J Clin Invest 1995;95:1505–1511.
98. DeBlock CEM, DeLeeuw IH, Van Gaal LF, Belgian Diabetes Registry. High prevalence of manifestations of gastric autoimmunity in parietal cell antibody-positive type 1 (insulin-dependent) diabetic patients. J Clin Endocrinol Metab 1999;84:4062–4067.
99. Kostraba JN, Cruickshanks KJ, Lawler-Heavner J, et al. Early exposure to cow's milk and solid foods in infancy, genetic predisposition, and risk of type 1 diabetes. Diabetes 1993;42:288–295.
100. Songer TJ, Ettaro L. Studies on the Cost of Diabetes. Centers for Disease Control, Atlanta, GA, 1998.
101. American Diabetes Association. Economic consequences of diabetes mellitus in the U.S. in 1997. Diabetes Care 1998;21:296–309.
102. Gray A, Fenn P, McGuire A. The cost of insulin-dependent diabetes mellitus (IDDM) in England and Wales. [see comments]. Diabet Med 1995;12:1068–1076.
103. Stern Z, Levy R. The direct cost of type 1 diabetes mellitus in Israel. Diabet Med 1994;11:528–533.
104. Hart WM, Espinosa C, Rovira J. A simulation model of the cost of the incidence of IDDM in Spain. Diabetologia 1997;40:311–318.
105. The DCCT Study Research Group. Resource utilization and costs of care in the diabetes control and complications trial. Diabetes Care 1995;18:1468–1478.

106. Songer TJ, LaPorte RE, Lave JR, Dorman JS, Becker DJ. Health insurance and the financial impact of IDDM in families with a child with IDDM. Diabetes Care 1997;20:577–584.
107. Guo JJ, Gibson JT, Gropper DM, Oswald SL, Barker KN. Empiric investigation on direct costs-of-illness and healthcare utilization of Medicaid patients with diabetes mellitus. Am J Manag Care 1998;4:1433–1446.
108. Songer TJ, LaPorte RE, Dorman JS, Orchard TJ, Becker DJ, Drash AL. Employment spectrum of IDDM. Diabetes Care 1989;12:615–622.
109. Songer TJ. Disability in diabetes. In: Diabetes in America. National Diabetes Data Group, ed. US Government Printing Office, Washington, DC, 1995, pp. 259–282.
110. Ingberg CM, Palmer M, Aman J, Larsson S. Social consequences of insulin-dependent diabetes mellitus are limited: a population-based comparison of young adult patients vs healthy controls. Diabet Med 1996;3:729–733.
111. Mayfield JA, Deb P, Whitecotton L. Work disability and diabetes. Diabetes Care 1999;22:1105–1109.
112. Songer TJ, LaPorte RE, Dorman JS, et al. Health, life, and automobile insurance characteristics in adults with IDDM. Diabetes Care 1991;14(4):318–324.
113. Borch-Johnsen K. Improving prognosis of type 1 diabetes. Mortality, accidents, and impact on insurance. Diabetes Care 1999;22(Suppl 2):B1–B3.
114. Matsushima M, Tajima N, Agata T, Yokoyama J, Ikeda Y, Isogai Y. Social and economic impact on youth-onset diabetes in Japan. Diabetes Care 1993;16:824–827.
115. DIAMOND Project Group on Social Issues. Global regulations concerning insulin-treated diabetes and commercial motor vehicle operation. Br Med J 1993;307:250–253.
116. Karter J, Ferrara A, Darbinian JA, Ackerson LM, Shelby JV. Self-monitoring of blood glucose: language and financial barriers in a managed care population with diabetes. Diabetes Care 2000;23:477–483.
117. The DCCT/EDIC Research Group. Health insurance affects care in type 1 diabetes. JAMA 2003, in press.
118. Gerstein HC, Simpson JR, Atkinson S, Taylor D, Van der Meulen J. Feasibility and acceptability of a proposed infant feeding intervention trial for the prevention of type 1 diabetes. Diabetes Care 1995;18:940–942.
119. Gale EAM. Nicotinamide: potential for the prevention of type 1 diabetes? Horm Metab Res 1996;28:361–364.
120. DPT-1 Study Group. The Diabetes Prevention Trial—Type 1 Diabetes (DPT-1): implementation of screening and staging of relatives. Transplant Proc 1995;27:3377.
121. Ilonen J, Simell O, Knip M, Akerblom HK. Screening for genetic IDDM risk and prevention trials in infancy. Diabetes Metab Rev 1998;14:188.
122. Pozzilli P, Dolb H, Browne PD. The Nicotinamide Trialists. Meta-analysis of nicotinamide treatment in patients with recent-onset IDDM. Diabetes Care 1996;19:1357–1363.
123. Keller RJ, Eisenbarth GS, Jackson RA. Insulin prophylaxis in individuals at high risk of type 1 diabetes. Lancet 1993;341:927–928.
124. Füchtenbusch M, Rabl W, Grassl B, Bachmann W, Standl E, Ziegler AG. Delay of type 1 diabetes in high risk, first degree relatives by parenteral antigen administration: the Schwabing Insulin Prophylaxis Pilot Trial. Diabetologia 1998;41:536–541.
125. Holtzman NA, Watson S. Promoting Safe and Effective Genetic Testing in the United States. Johns Hopkins University Press, Baltimore, MD, 1998.
126. Johnson SB, Tercyak KP Jr. Psychological impact of islet cell antibody screening for IDDM on children, adults, and their family members. Diabetes Care 1995;18:1370–1372.
127. Tercyak KP, Johnson SB, Schatz DA. Patient and family reflections on the use of subcutaneous insulin to prevent diabetes: a retrospective evaluation from a pilot prevention trail. J Diabetes Complic 1998;12:279–286.
128. Strecher V, Rosenstock I. The health belief model. In: Health Behavior and Health Education (Glanz K, Lewis FM, Rimer, BK, eds.). Jossey-Bass, San Francisco, 1997, pp. 41–59.

2 Genetics of Type 1 Diabetes

Massimo Pietropaolo, MD
and Massimo Trucco, MD

CONTENTS

INTRODUCTION

Type 1 diabetes mellitus (T1DM) is an autoimmune disease arising through a complex interaction of both genetic and environmental factors. Similar to the majority of autoimmune diseases, T1DM is characterized by both humoral and cellular immunological abnormalities, which precede the clinical onset of the disease process *(1,2)*. In T1DM, the presence of multiple antibodies to islet autoantigens can serve as a surrogate marker of disease in primary intervention strategies among first-degree relatives *(3–5)*. As a general rule, in the bulk of chronic autoimmune disorders, antibody laboratory testing in addition to genetic typing can facilitate decision-making for disease management based on the identification of disease activity *(6)*.

Familial clustering is indicated by the observation that the overall risk for developing T1DM in North American Caucasian siblings, parents, and offspring of individuals with T1DM ranges from 1% to 15% *(7–13)*, as compared to less than 1% for individuals without T1DM relatives and 1.2/1000 of the general population *(14)* (*see* Table 1). It is noteworthy that an increased risk of T1DM seems to be present also in first-degree relatives of individuals with non-insulin-dependent diabetes mellitus *(15–20)*. How-

From: *Contemporary Endocrinology: Type 1 Diabetes: Etiology and Treatment*
Edited by: M. A. Sperling © Humana Press Inc., Totowa, NJ

Table 1
Empiric Risk of Type 1 Diabetes

	Empiric risk
First-degree relatives of T1DM probands*	5–7%[a]
Individuals without relatives with T1DM*	<1%
Children of affected father**	~6%
Children of affected mother**	~2%

Note: Estimates are for North American Caucasian (*) and Scandinavian (**) populations. T1DM, type 1 diabetes mellitus.
[a] 1–15% range depending on the populations.
Source: ref. *12.*

ever, over 80% of cases of T1DM occur in individuals with no apparent family history of the disease. In the remaining 20%, this disease aggregates in families.

Specific human leukocyte antigen (HLA) haplotypes account for susceptibility to both T1DM and to a subtype of type 2 diabetes *(21–24).* The latter finding is supported by the occurrence of β-cell humoral autoimmunity in 10–33% of Caucasian adult-onset diabetic patients not treated with insulin *(15–18,25).* Therefore, a subset of patients with type 2 diabetes manifests similar genetic susceptibility and immunologic abnormalities to those characteristic of classical T1DM. Because of the peculiar characteristics of this subgroup of type 2 diabetes, the term "latent autoimmune diabetes in adults" (LADA) has been coined.

Studies conducted in the United States and Scandinavia have shown that offspring of parents with T1DM have a higher risk to progress to T1DM if thc father, rather than the mother, is affected by the disease *(13,26–30).* In fact, the risk is increased to about 1/40 in offspring of fathers with T1DM and to 1/66 in offspring of type 1 diabetic mothers *(31).* A number of explanations have been proposed for this finding, including genomic imprinting of genes involved in the susceptibility to T1DM, leading to an increase in spontaneous abortion by T1DM mothers of fetuses that might develop T1DM *(7,12),* maternal environmental factors that allow the fetus to remain tolerant to islet autoantigens *(7),* or a preferential paternal transmission of HLA diabetogenic alleles *(32).*

Not only genetic but also environmental factors may contribute to determine the risk of progression to the clinical stage of the disease. A discordance rate of greater than 50% between monozygotic twins indicates a potential involvement of environmental factors on disease development *(33,34).* This aspect of the disease is supported by the observed tendency to develop T1DM after exposure to viral agents. Viral antigens may, in fact, play a role in the generation of β-cell autoimmunity *(35–40).* These observations are supported by the increasing seasonal incidence of T1DM in many Western countries *(41,42)* and that enteroviruses may be involved in the autoimmune pathogenesis of T1DM *(36,43,44).*

WHAT ARE THE GENES?

Although it has been suggested that multiple genes play a role in disease susceptibility, there is strong evidence that at least two chromosomal regions are closely associated with and linked to T1DM: the HLA region on chromosome 6p21 *(IDDM1),* and the

Table 2
Summary of Human *IDDM* Susceptibility Loci

Chromosome	*Locus*	*Linkage status (according to ref. 45)*
6p21	*IDDM1;* HLA-DQB	Confirmed
11p15.5	*IDDM2;* INS 5′ VNTR	Confirmed
15q26	*IDDM3;* IGF1R	Suggestive ($p < 0.001$, MLS > 2.2)[d]
11q13	*IDDM4;* FGF3	Confirmed ($p < 2.2 \times 10^{-5}$, MLS > 3.6)
6q25	*IDDM5;* ESR1	Confirmed ($p < 2.2 \times 10^{-5}$, MLS > 3.6)
18q21	*IDDM6*	
2q31	*IDDM7;* IL-1, HOXD8	Suggestive ($p < 0.001$, MLS > 2.2)
6q27	*IDDM8;* IGF2R	Confirmed ($p < 2.2 \times 10^{-5}$, MLS > 3.6)
3q21-q25 *IDDM9*		
10p11.21-q11.2	*IDDM10*	
14q24.3	*IDDM11*	Significant ($p < 2.2 \times 10^{-5}$, MLS > 3.6)
2q33	*IDDM12;* CTLA-4	
2q34	*IDDM13;* IGFBP2, IGFBP5	
6p21	*IDDM15* (distinct from HLA)	
10q25[a]	*IDDM17*	Significant (NPL: $p < 0.002$)
7p	Not assigned; GCK, IGFBP1, IGFBP3	
Xq	Not assigned	
Xp[b]	Not assigned	Significant ($p = 2.7 \times 10^{-4}$; MLS > 3.6)
1q[c]	Not assigned	Suggestive (MLS = 3.31)

Note: The IDDM nomenclature is assigned to a locus after linkage has been formally demonstrated, replicated, and confirmed in at least three different datasets. Where functional candidate genes are flanked by or very close to susceptibility markers, they are indicated.

[a] The evidence for linkage increased substantially ($p = 0.00004$) with the higher density of markers and the inclusion of data for additional affected relatives and all unaffected siblings *(46);* NPL, nonparametric linkage.

[b] In major histocompatibility complex (MHC) human leukocyte antigen (HLA)-DR3 positive patients *(47).*

[c] This locus *(48)* colocalizes with loci for systemic lupus erythematosus (SLE) *(49)* and ankylosing spondylitis *(50).*

[d] MLS, maximum logarithm of odds score.

insulin gene region on chromosome 11p15 *(IDDM2).* The contribution of these two loci to familial inheritance is approx 42% for *IDDM1* and 10% for *IDDM2.* As a result of genomewide searches, many other putative loci have been proposed to be related with T1DM. These loci, along with some potential candidate genes, are listed in Table 2. The fact that, in humans, the highest risk-conferring locus linked to the disease is the HLA cluster, and, in particular, HLA genes encoding specific class II alleles, strongly indicates an important role of the immune cells in both the development and the activation of the autoimmune response leading to disease onset *(51,52).* Interestingly, the same HLA locus seems to have the same susceptibility influence in a mouse model of T1DM, the nonobese diabetic (NOD) mouse *(53)* (*see* Table 3). The immune-mediated processes of β-cell destruction are mainly T-cell dependent and chronic in the NOD mouse *(54),* the Bio-Breeding (BB) rat *(55),* and, more than likely, in humans *(51)* (*see* Table 3). Comparative mapping of human and NOD mouse insulin-dependent diabetes *(Idd)* genes and phenotype/functions controlled by *Idd* loci are shown in Tables 3 and 4.

Table 3
Comparative Mapping of Human *(IDDM)* and Murine *(Idd)* Genes

Human locus (Chr)	*Marker/ candidate*	*Potential NOD "Idd" homolog (Chr)*	*Marker*
IDDM1 (6p21)	HLA	*"Idd1"* (17)	H2g7
IDDM2 (11p15.5)	INS/VNTR	? NOD.DR-2 (Chr.7 region from C57L)	?Ins2
IDDM3 (15q26)	D15S107	*"Idd2"* (9)	Cyp19
IDDM4 (11q13)	FGF3	None yet identified (distal 7)	
IDDM5 (6q25)	ESR	None yet identified (proximal 10)	
IDDM6 (18q)	D18S64	?*"Idd5"* (1)	Bcl2
IDDM7 (2q31–33)	D2S326	?*"Idd5"* (1)	Il1r/Stat1
IDDM8 (6q25–27)	D6S264	None yet identified (proximal 10 or 17)	
IDDM9 (3q21–q25)	D3S1303	None yet identified (middle 6)	
IDDM10 (10p11.2–q11.2)	GAD2	None yet identified (proximal 2)	
IDDM11 (14q24.3–q31)	D14S67	None yet identified (middle 12)	
IDDM12 (2q31-33)		?*"Idd5.1"* (1)	Ctla4
IDDM13 (2q34)	IGFBP-2,5	? *"Idd5.2"* (1)	Slc11a1 (Nramp)
GCK (7p)	GCK	None yet identified (proximal 11)	
IDDM15 (6q21)	D6S283	? *"Idd14"* (13)	D13Mit61
IDDM16? (1p36.1–p35)	NHE1	? *"Idd11"* (4)	Slc9a1 (Nhe1)

Note: "Idd5" nomenclature placed in quotation marks because there are multiple *"Idd"* loci on mouse Chr 1.

Source: Modified from ref. *194*. Genes and cellular requirements for autoimmune diabetes susceptibility in NOD mice. In: von Herrath H, ed. Molecular Pathology of Insulin Dependent Diabetes Mellitus. Karger, New York, 2001, pp. 31–67.

THE HLA COMPLEX

The short arm of human chromosome 6 (6p21) accommodates an approximate 3.5-megabase genetic segment containing a group of immune response genes termed the major histocompatibility complex (MHC) (*see* Fig. 1). The principal genes located within the MHC code for human leukocyte antigens, or HLA, two molecular classes of cell surface glycoproteins differing in structure, function, and tissue distribution (*see* Table 5 and Fig. 1).

The class I HLA molecule exists as a heterodimer, consisting of a polymorphic 44-kDa MHC-encoded α-chain or heavy chain in noncovalent association with β_2-microglobulin, a 12-kDa protein encoded by a nonpolymorphic gene on chromosome 15. The class I molecule is anchored to the cell membrane only by the heavy chain.

Table 4
Phenotypes/Functions Controlled by *Idd* Loci

Locus or provisional designation	*Chr (region)*	*Phenotype/function*
MHC/Idd1	17 (entire H2 haplotype)	Insulitis, T1DM, diabetogenic T-cell repertoire selection, strong TH1 responses to islet antigens
Idd2	9 (Thy1)	Time of T1DM onset (T-cell activation?)
Idd3	3 (Il2)	Insulitis, T1DM
Idd5a	1 (Il1r1-Vil)	Insulitis, T1DM
Idd5b	1 (Bcl2)	Peri-insulitis, sialitis, T-cell resistance to apoptosis, hypergammaglobulinemia
Idd10	3 (Tshb)	Bone marrow-derived macrophage developmental and functional defects, T1DM
Idd11	11 (Acrb-Scya-Mpo)	T-cell proliferative unresponsiveness

This chain contains 338 amino acids and, beginning from the amino terminus, is functionally divided into three regions: an extracellular hydrophilic region (amino acid residues 1–281), a transmembrane hydrophobic region (amino acid residues 282–306), and an intracytoplasmic hydrophilic region (amino acid residues 307–338). The extracellular region is further subdivided into three domains, designated α_1, α_2, and α_3, each of approx 90 amino acid residues (*see* Fig. 2). The α_1 and α_2 domains comprise the peptide- or antigen-binding region of the molecule.

Class II HLA molecules consist of two glycoprotein chains, α-chain of approx 34 kDa and a β-chain of approx 29 kDa, both encoded within the MHC. As with the class I heavy chain, each class II chain can be divided into three regions (extracellular, transmembrane, and intracytoplasmic), but, in contrast, both class II chains span the cell membrane. Each extracellular region of the class II α- and β-chains has been further divided into two domains of approx 90 amino acid residues each, termed α_1, α_2 and β_1, β_2 respectively. The α_1 and β_1 domains form the peptide-binding region of class II HLA molecules (*see* Fig. 3). Also of note, the class II α_2 and β_2 domains, class I α_3 domain, and β_2-microglobulin all show homology to the constant region of immunoglobulins and are therefore classified as members of the immunoglobulin superfamily.

The genes that encode class I MHC are located at the HLA-A, B, and C loci, whereas class II molecules are encoded by the DR, DQ, and DP genes (*see* Fig. 1). Other genes in this cluster include TAP *(56,57)* and LMP (low-molecular-weight proteins), both involved in antigen processing *(58)*. A third region of the MHC, denoted as class III, codes instead for several molecules having a variety of functions, namely complement components (C4A, C4B, factor B, and C2), tumor necrosis factor (TNF-α and TNF-β) and the 21-hydroxylase genes (CYP21P and CYP21) (*see* Fig. 1).

Whereas class I MHC molecules are expressed in virtually all nucleated cells, class II molecule expression is restricted to B-lymphocytes, dendritic cells, macrophages, and activated T-lymphocytes. Both class I and class II antigens are involved in the presentation of antigen to T-cells. Cytotoxic T-cells ($CD8^+$) mainly recognize antigen in

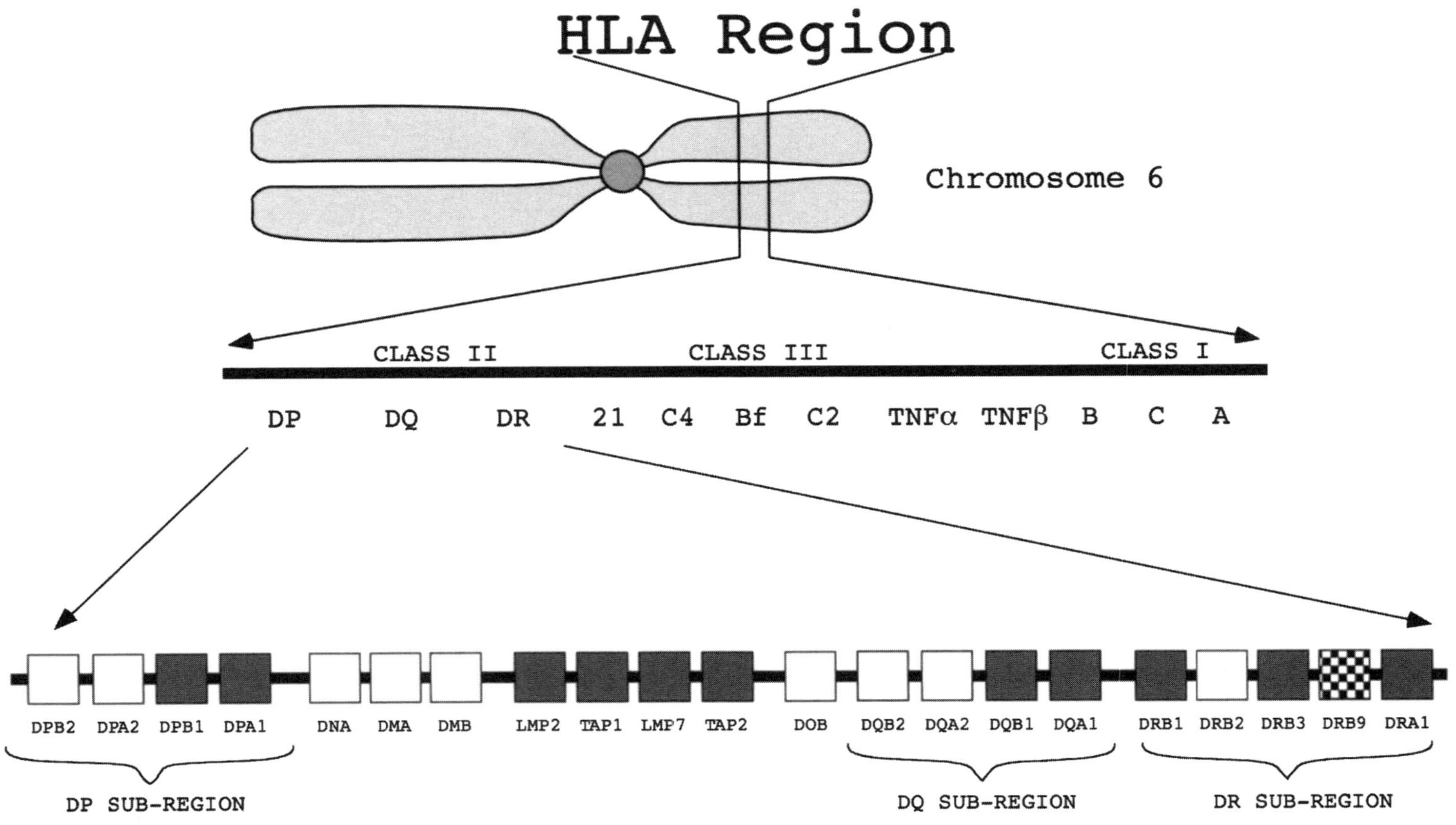
HLA Region
Chromosome 6
CLASS II
CLASS III
CLASS I
DP
DQ
DR
21
C4
Bf
C2
TNFα
TNFβ
B
C
A
DPB2
DPA2
DPB1
DPA1
DNA
DMA
DMB
LMP2
TAP1
LMP7
TAP2
DOB
DQB2
DQA2
DQB1
DQA1
DRB1
DRB2
DRB3
DRB9
DRA1
DP SUB-REGION
DQ SUB-REGION
DR SUB-REGION

Fig. 1. The HLA complex present on human chromosome 6, can be subdivided into three regions. The genes present in each region encode class I, class III, and class II molecules, respectively. The class II region, which is closest to the centromere of the chromosome, is conventionally subdivided into three additional subregions. Among the genes contained in each subregion are some that encode functional molecules (in black), genes that are not functioning (i.e., pseudogenes) (in white), or genes that encode proteins not yet characterized (also in white). Although DQA1 and DQB1 genes encode for the α- and β-chains of a functional HLA-DQ molecule (like DPA1 and DPB1 genes for the chains of a functional HLA-DP molecule), the DRA1 gene encodes for a nonpolymorphic α-chain able to pair with the products of each of the functional DRB genes. In the example, a DR3-positive haplotype of an individual is shown. The DRB1 gene encodes for the DR3 allele, DRB2 is a pseudogene, and DRB3 encodes for the so-called DR52 molecule, which is always found associated with DR3. The DRB9 gene has not been well studied yet but seems to be able to encode for a nonfunctionally stable protein chain. Transporter associated with antigen processing (TAP) 1 and 2 genes are cytoplasmic transporters of antigenic peptides, whereas LMP 2 and 7 are genes encoding proteasome subunits. Both of these molecules are involved in the antigenic peptide transport from the cytoplasm to the cell surface. Tumor necrosis factor (TNF)-α and TNF-β genes, located between class I and class III regions, are also indicated. The 21-hydroxylase locus encompassing CYP21P and CYP21 genes is simply indicated as "21". (Modified from ref. *192.*)

Table 5
Comparison Between Class I and Class II Molecules

	Class I	*Class II*
Molecules	HLA-A, B, C	HLA-DR, DQ, DP
Structure	44,000-MW	~34,000-MW α-chain
heavy chain	12,000-MW β_2-microglobulin	~29,000-MW β-chain
Tissue distribution	Virtually on every nucleated cell	Restricted to B-cells, macrophages, activated T-cells
Function	Bind and present antigenic peptides to CD8+ T-cells	Bind and present antigenic peptides to CD4+ cells

the context of class I, whereas helper/inducer cells ($CD4^+$) usually recognize antigen in the context of the class II molecules.

Many immunologically mediated diseases, including certain endocrine syndromes, are genetically associated with specific HLA molecules and several hypotheses have been suggested to explain HLA-disease associations *(59,60)*. Four of these general hypotheses apply to diseases associated with both class I and class II molecules. First, the antigen-binding cleft of a specific HLA molecule can accept antigenic peptides that other molecules cannot accept. These peptides can be either exogenous (e.g., a viral particle) or endogenous (e.g., an autoantigen). Those peptides that can be processed by the antigen-presenting cell (APC) are ultimately responsible for the generation of an immune response directed against the antigenic peptide. If this is a self peptide, an anti-self (e.g., autoimmune) reaction will be activated. The second hypothesis suggests that α- and β-chains of the T-cell receptor (TCR) are the target of foreign molecules capable of potently stimulating T-cells by binding the TCR outside the HLA–peptide–TCR complex. Because the TCR carrying a certain β-chain is recognized by specific proteins

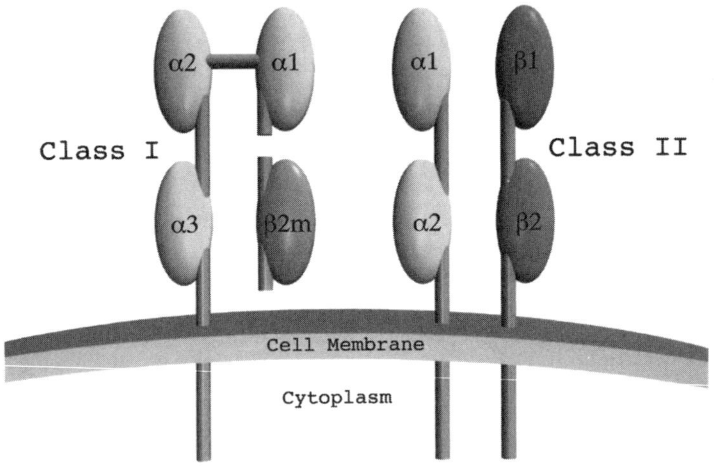

Fig. 2. Secondary structure of HLA class I and class II molecules in comparison. As is the case for immunoglobulins, peptidic sequences that show similarities and are present more than once in the same polypeptidic chain are called "domains." α_1, α_2, and α_3 constitute the domains of the class I α-chain, whereas β_1 and β_2 are the domains of the class II β-chain as α_1 and α_2 are the domains characteristic of the class II α-chain. Both class I and class II molecules are composed of noncovalently bound and somewhat different α- and β-chains. These heterodimers form, at their most external end, a peptide-combining site composed of the α_1 and α_2 domains for class I and α_1 and β_1 domains for class II molecules. The nonpolymorphic β_2-microglobulin completes the structure of class I molecules. (Modified from ref. *193.*)

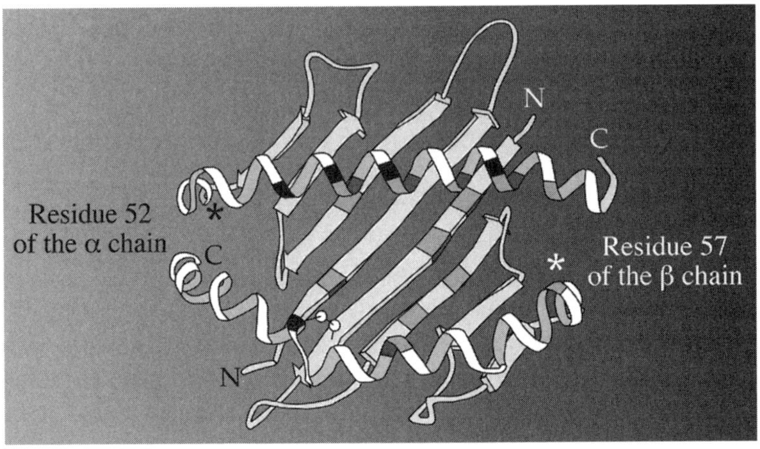

Fig. 3. The two outermost domains of HLA class I and class II molecules fold together to form their antigen-combining sites in which the processed antigenic peptide can find appropriate lodging. The polymorphic regions of the HLA molecule seen from the top, present on the floor, and on the α-helices of its groove, are indicated in different nuances of color from gray to black. The antigenic peptides found in HLA class I molecule grooves are normally nine amino acids long, whereas the antigenic peptides most frequently found associated with HLA class II molecules are longer than nine amino acids and can vary considerably in size. The position of the amino acid 52 of the α-chain and that of the β-chain in position 57 are indicated. (Modified from ref. *22.*)

that are products of bacterial or viral invaders (e.g., superantigens) in the context of a particular HLA molecule, these superantigens may trigger the generation of an immune response directed against self antigens, by nonspecifically activating autoreactive T-cell clones. The third hypothesis postulates that a TAP gene product, which normally transports antigenic peptides from the cytoplasm to the endoplasmic reticulum, is defective and, therefore, this predisposes to disease susceptibility. As a result of a defective TAP gene product, few peptides become available for binding to class I molecules, leading to a low surface density of class I–peptide complexes and to a high surface density of empty class I molecules. A high density of empty surface class I molecules may bind peptides to which they would otherwise not be exposed intracellularly—for instance, viral or bacterial peptides. These newly formed class I–exogenous peptide complexes may account for an induction of an immune response that can be responsible for disease. The fourth hypothesis, termed "molecular mimicry," implies that a foreign antigen such as a viral or bacterial antigen shares similarities with a self molecule, and because of this similarity, the immune response is turned against self target tissues, causing an autoimmune response.

Alleles at multiple loci on a single chromosome are usually inherited in combination as a unit. This combination of multiple genes inherited together is termed "haplotype." Because each individual inherits one set of chromosomes from each parent, each individual has two haplotypes for a given physical genetic interval. HLA genes are codominant and follow a simple Mendelian form of transmission in families (*see* Fig. 4). Therefore, as a consequence of HLA codominance, both alleles (one on each chromosome) are expressed from a given HLA locus. There is a 25% chance that two siblings share both haplotypes and are immunologically compatible, a 50% chance that they will share only one haplotype, and a 25% chance that they share no haplotype and, thus, are HLA different.

Certain combinations of HLA alleles are found with a frequency greater than expected and, consequently, they are not randomly distributed within the general population. This phenomenon is known as linkage disequilibrium and it is quantified by the difference (Δ) between the observed and the expected frequencies of a certain allele. One example is given by the HLA-A*0101 and the HLA-B*0801 alleles, which are found in Caucasian populations with frequencies of 0.161 and 0.104, respectively. Thus, the expected frequency of the HLA-A*0101, HLA-B*0801 haplotype should be $0.161 \times 0.104 = 0.0167$, but the frequency of this haplotype is instead 0.0592, which is almost four times the expected frequency ($\Delta = 0.0592 - 0.0167 = 0.0425$).

The observation of linkage disequilibrium and extended haplotype inheritance is still a subject of discussion regarding the reason for its existence. One hypothesis that could explain linkage disequilibrium is that some haplotypes are preferentially protected from genetic recombination and, therefore, are preserved (ancestral haplotypes) *(61,62)*. The mechanism underlying preservation of HLA haplotypes is not clear, but inhibition of crossing over during gametic meiosis may, in part, explain the cause of gene haplotype associations. Another hypothesis to explain the phenomenon of linkage disequilibrium is that certain haplotypes are preferentially reconstituted by recombination, even though this hypothesis may not completely explain the phenomenon *(63)*. A third, evolution-based "Darwinian" hypothesis holds that certain HLA haplotypes confer a certain advantage and are favored by natural selection *(64)*.

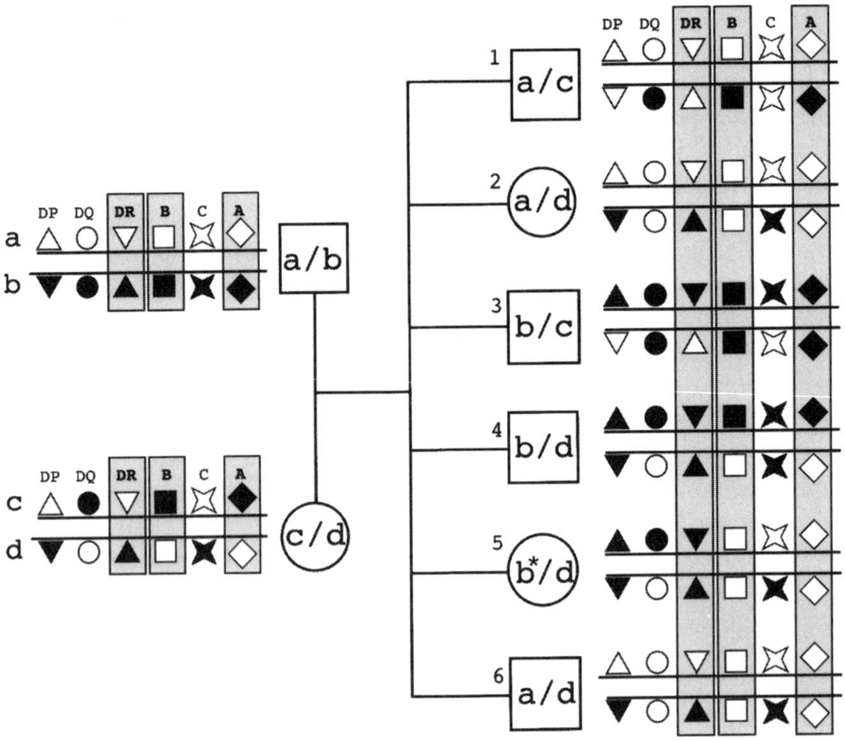

Fig. 4. The study of the segregation of HLA alleles through a family is based on the determination of the HLA phenotypes on at least the two parents and a child or on three HLA-different members of the same family. Segregation analysis allows the definition of the four haplotypes (normally called a, b, c, and d) present in the family and, consequently, the definition of individuals heterozygous or homozygous at certain loci (e.g., sibling 1 is homozygous at C, DR, and DP loci, both alleles are white; but heterozygous at A, B, and DQ loci, 1 white and 1 black allele), together with the recognition of individuals who share one haplotype only (e.g., siblings 1 and 2 are haploidentical because they share the "a" haplotype), or two haplotypes (e.g., siblings 2 and 6 are HLA identical because they share the "a" and the "d" haplotypes), or none (e.g., siblings 2 and 3, or 1 and 4 are HLA different). Although it is considered a very rare event, it is possible to find individuals, represented here by sibling 5, in which a crossing over between class I and class II gene regions, involving the paternal and maternal haplotypes of the father of this family, cause the "a–b" recombination flagged here with an asterisk (b*). (Modified from ref. *193*.)

HLA GENES AND T1DM

Many factors play a role in determining the risk of progression to T1DM. These include family history of diabetes, genotype (e.g., HLA haplotype), age, environmental factors, the residual insulin secretory capacity, the presence of cytoplasmic islet cell antibodies (ICAs), and antibodies to characterized islet autoantigens *(65,66)*. The presence or absence of the others may modify the prognostic significance of any of these risk factors *(67)*.

T1DM and corresponding animal models of the disease such as the NOD mouse *(54)* have a strong association with specific alleles of the MHC *(53)*. Alleles encoding the class II antigens DQ and DR account for the principal HLA-linked susceptibility to disease *(22,33,34,68)*. This notion is supported by transracial studies that have consistently shown the influence of HLA genotypes in the risk of developing T1DM *(69)*, by conservation of a MHC class II effect between human and murine autoimmune diabetes *(70)* and by studies in MHC transgenic mice *(71)*.

As indicated by case-control studies, significant differences in polymorphic HLA marker frequencies between affected and nonaffected individuals suggest that a chromosomal region defined by markers on chromosome 6 is involved in the disease. In genetically and clinically heterogeneous diseases such as T1DM, between 70–95% of affected individuals in different populations carry a specific HLA susceptibility allele (*IDDM1* locus) *(72–74)*. *IDDM1* represents the major T1DM-related susceptibility locus and susceptibility to T1DM is mostly conferred by alleles of the DQ region located within the HLA complex. Diabetogenic alleles are not fully penetrant, so that not every individual who inherits the gene has the disease.

The association between the HLA region and T1DM susceptibility was first documented in case-control studies in the mid-1970s *(75,76)*, when it was observed that the HLA B8, B15, and B18 were increased in frequency in patients as compared to a nondiabetic control population. Subsequently, serological typing for class II HLA loci revealed a more significant association between HLA-DR and T1DM *(72,77,78)*. Approximately 95% of patients with T1DM in most populations had DR3 and/or DR4, and individuals with heterozygosity for DR3/4 appeared to be the most susceptible to progression to T1DM. In contrast, expression of the HLA-DR2 allele was initially considered to be associated with protection from T1DM.

The advent of the polymerase chain reaction (PCR) techniques *(79–81)* has provided researchers with more rapid means of arriving at T1DM susceptibility estimates than those provided by serological techniques. PCR amplification of individuals' HLA alleles in a variety of racial and ethnic groups have revealed that the presence of a specific human DQβ-chain variant encoding a neutral amino acid (alanine, valine, or serine) other than aspartic acid at position 57 (non-Asp-57) is strongly associated with T1DM *(21,82)*. In contrast, a negatively charged aspartic acid at position 57 of the DQβ chain (Asp-57) appears to confer "resistance" to T1DM progression *(21,22,82)*. This association is much stronger than the association between HLA-DR3 and DR4 and the presence of the disease (*see* Tables 6 and 7). Studies aimed at investigating the contribution of the DQα-chain to T1DM susceptibility or resistance were initially performed by a group from France. They conducted molecular typing in 50 unrelated T1DM patients and 75 randomly selected volunteers using PCR and specific oligonucleotide probes. Their results not only confirmed the importance of DQβ non-Asp-57 in disease susceptibility but also implicated a role for the Arg-52 amino acid residue of the DQα-chain in the pathogenesis of type 1 diabetes *(83)*. It should be mentioned that the discovery of these two disease-associated HLA polymorphisms represents a refinement of the IDDM relative risk assessments for the HLA-DR3 and HLA-DR4 disease associations. Because of linkage disequilibrium, the class II HLA-extended haplotypes inherited with the HLA-DR3 and the HLA-DR4 alleles include DQα alleles with the Arg-52 associated with non-Asp-57 DQβ alleles. The refinement of the DR locus data lies in the fact that the genetically linked DQ associations with T1DM are much stronger than the associations with HLA-DR3 and DR4. A DQ molecule composed of an Arg-52 α-chain and a non-Asp57 β-chain, can then be defined as a "diabetogenic" heterodimer.

Because T1DM is an autoimmune disease with a long preclinical course *(1)*, the identification of individuals prior to the onset of the disease process provides a real opportunity for predictive testing and for therapeutic intervention. The relative risk for T1DM using both genetic and antibody markers has been calculated in a study of 151 first-degree rela-

Table 6
Genetic Risk Estimates for HLA Class II in T1DM

High-risk genotypes	*Risk in an individual with this genotype*
DQB1*0302 (DQ3.2)	1 in 60
DQ3.2/DQ2 (DR3)	1 in 25
DQB1*0302 + family history of IDDM	1 in 10
DQ3.2/DQ2 (DR3) + family history of IDDM	1 in 4

Source: Adapted from ref. *195*.

Table 7
Effect of HLA Alleles on T1DM Susceptibility

DQ alleles	*Effect*	*Associated DR*
B1*0302, A1*0301	Susceptible	DR4
B1*0201, A1*0501	Susceptible	DR3
B1*0501, A1*0101	Susceptible	DR1
B1*0201, A1*0301	Susceptible (African-Americans)	DR7
B1*0502, A1*0102	Susceptible (Sardinians)	DR2 (DR16)
B1*0303, A1*0301	Susceptible (Japanese)	DR4
B1*0303, A1*0301	Susceptible (Japanese)	DR9
B1*0602, A1*0102	Protective	DR2 (DR15)
B1*0301, A1*0501	Protective	DR5
B1*0600, ?	Neutral	DR6
B1*0201, A1*0201	Neutral	DR7
B1*0303, A1*0301	Neutral	DR4
B1*0301, A1*0301	Neutral	DR4

tives of probands from the Children's Hospital/Allegheny County registry *(84)*. In this prospective study, using a multivariate model, an enhanced relative risk for T1DM was estimated for having 4 HLA-DQ diabetogenic heterodimers as compared to one or two heterodimers, independently of the islet cell antibody status. Therefore, the greater the potential to generate HLA diabetogenic heterodimers, the higher the likelihood of developing diabetes is during a prospective follow-up in first-degree relatives of diabetic patients. This observation was proposed in several case-control studies *(83,85)*. The frequencies of diabetogenic heterodimers were analyzed in a population of the Madrid area in 102 individuals with T1DM and compared with those of 87 randomly selected nondiabetic control subjects from the general population. These findings provide evidence that a quantitative effect promoted by DQα Arg 52 and DQβ non-Asp 57 alleles may account for an enhanced susceptibility to T1DM. In other words, the genetic predisposition to T1DM increases as the number of susceptibility alleles in a given individual increases. These data support the molecular hypothesis proposed by Khalil et al. in which the expression of the heterodimers DQα Arg 52 along with DQβ non-Asp 57 at the cell surface increases the diabetogenic effect *(83,86,87)*. Susceptibility dose effect increases with the number of heterodimers that can be formed. Highest risk was determined for subjects with four diabetogenic heterodimers (odds ratio [OR] 41; 95% confidence interval [CI]: 17–96) *(87)*. Simultaneous expression of four different diabetogenic heterodimers explains the very high risk of Caucasian DR3/4 *(84)*, although HLA-DQA1*0301/DQB*0302 and -DQA1

0501/DQB*0201 heterodimers appear to have the strongest association with diabetes in the context of the high-risk HLA-DR4 and DR3 haplotypes *(21,82,88–92,95)* (*see* Table 4).

At our institution, a prospective study in first-degree relatives of type 1 diabetic probands has been in progress since 1979 and has served as the foundation for investigating the etiology and prediction of T1DM *(93)*. To date, we have longitudinally followed 6177 first-degree relatives of T1DM patients, 82 of whom developed the disease. ICA testing was performed in all relatives as first screening for islet cell autoimmunity. A hospital-based registry, which identifies all children (≥ 17 yr of age) who were diagnosed at our children's hospital or seen within 1 yr of diagnosis since January 1, 1950, was utilized to identify study subjects *(93)*. A subgroup of 500 of 6711 nondiabetic first-degree relatives of diabetic probands from this registry was evaluated to measure ICA, autoantibodies to GAD65, IA-2, and insulin and to evaluate HLA-DQ genotyping. The demographics of these 500 relatives evaluated in the present analyses were not statistically different from those of all relatives included in the registry with regard to age (median 30.5 vs 30 yr, respectively), percentage of affected parents (53% vs 50%, respectively), percentage of affected siblings (47% vs 50%, respectively), and race (percentage of blacks: 4% vs 5%, respectively). Therefore, the subgroup evaluated is likely representative of the whole population of first-degree relatives of the registry. Males and females were nearly equally represented in this subgroup of relatives, with 56% being female. In addition, these demographic criteria in seronegative individuals were not statistically different from those of seropositive relatives. Diabetes was diagnosed according to standard National Diabetes Data Group criteria *(94)*. A survival analysis of the above-mentioned subset of relatives indicated a markedly increased cumulative risk for T1DM in those first-degree relatives who carry two HLA-DQ high-risk haplotypes as compared to relatives who have no or one HLA-DQ high-risk haplotypes (*see* Fig. 5). Moreover, in seronegative relatives who developed what is termed "idiopathic" type 1 diabetes according to the current classification *(96)*, which is based on autoantibody testing alone, the presence of 2 HLA-DQ high-risk haplotypes conferred an increased cumulative risk of developing insulin requirement of 27% at 12.5 yr of follow-up, compared to a risk of 6% for nondiabetic relatives who were antibody negative and had no or one HLA-DQ high-risk haplotype (log rank $p = 0.01$) *(97)*. These conclusions are particularly important in light of the criteria for classification of diabetes and design of future diabetes-prevention trials that include autoantibody assessment alone to enroll high-risk subjects. Our data strongly indicate that the classification of diabetes should be revised.

There is still controversy as to whether DR molecules are also important in T1DM susceptibility *(68)*. Whereas some investigators have argued that DR alleles are not the primary factors in conferring T1DM susceptibility *(98)* because they are in linkage disequilibrium with DQ alleles *(99,100)*, others believe that the DR locus play a role in T1DM susceptibility independently from DQ alleles *(86,92,101–104)*. At least three studies have shown an independent effect of the DRB1 alleles in T1DM *(23,66,92,101,105–111)*. In Oriental populations (Chinese and Japanese), susceptibility appears to be conferred by the DRB1*0405 haplotype, whereas DRB1*0403 and DRB1*0406 confer protection in Japanese *(106,112)*, Sardinians *(101)* and Spaniards *(113)*. However, the DRB1*0405 haplotype seems to confer strong susceptibility and DRB1*0403 or DRB1*0406 protection in all ethnic groups *(66)*. The protection conferred by DRB1*0403 and DRB1*0406 might overcome the strong susceptibility effect of DQ*0301/*0302. A study by a Belgian group described that DRB1*0403 protects against T1DM in the high-risk DR3/4 heterozygotes *(114)*.

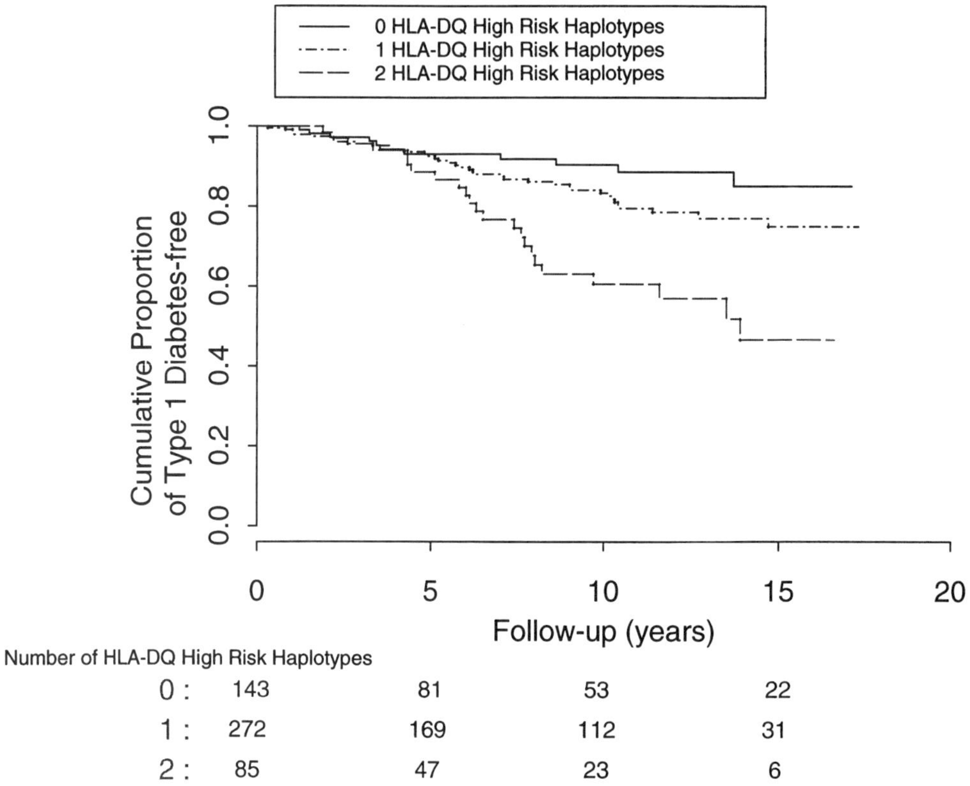

Fig. 5. Cumulative risk of developing insulin-requiring diabetes for different years of follow-up among 500 relatives by number of high HLA-DQ high-risk haplotypes (2 vs 0 or 1) 95% [confidence intervals] (DQA1*0501-DQB1*0201 and DQA1*0301-DQB1*0302). The number of HLA-DQ high-risk haplotypes was assigned as 0, 1, or 2. First-degree relatives of type 1 diabetic probands were initially evaluated by autoantibody screening at the Children's Hospital of Pittsburgh, as previously reported *(84,95)*. For the present study, 74 prediabetics (who developed overt diabetes in a prospective follow-up) before the onset of T1DM were analyzed and compared with 426 relatives who did not develop diabetes over time. The genetic susceptibility to TIDM increases as the number of HLA-DQ high-risk haploytpes increases.

Number of HLA-DQ high-risk haplotypes		*IDDM cases*	*Cumulative risk of diabetes within 5 yr*	*Cumulative risk of diabetes within 8 yr*	*Cumulative risk of diabetes within 10 yr*	*Cumlative risk of diabetes within 12.5 yr*
0	143	11	7 [4–10]	8 [5–11]	0 [7–13]	11 [7–15]
1	272	39	8 [6–10]	14 [11–17]	17 [14–20]	22 [19–25]
2	85	23	11 [7–15]	35 [28–42]	40 [33–47]	43 [35–51]

The HLA class II DPB1 locus (*see* Fig. 1) may also influence susceptibility to T1DM. Analysis of 269 multiplex families from the Human Biological Data Interchange suggest that HLA-DPB1*0301 and HLA-DPB1*0202 alleles are predisposing for T1DM, whereas HLA-DPB1*0402 appears protective *(115)*. Interestingly, the effect of the class II locus DPB1 appears to be more apparent in patients with this genotype than in patients carrying the highest-risk DR3/DR4-DQB1*0302 genotype *(115)*.

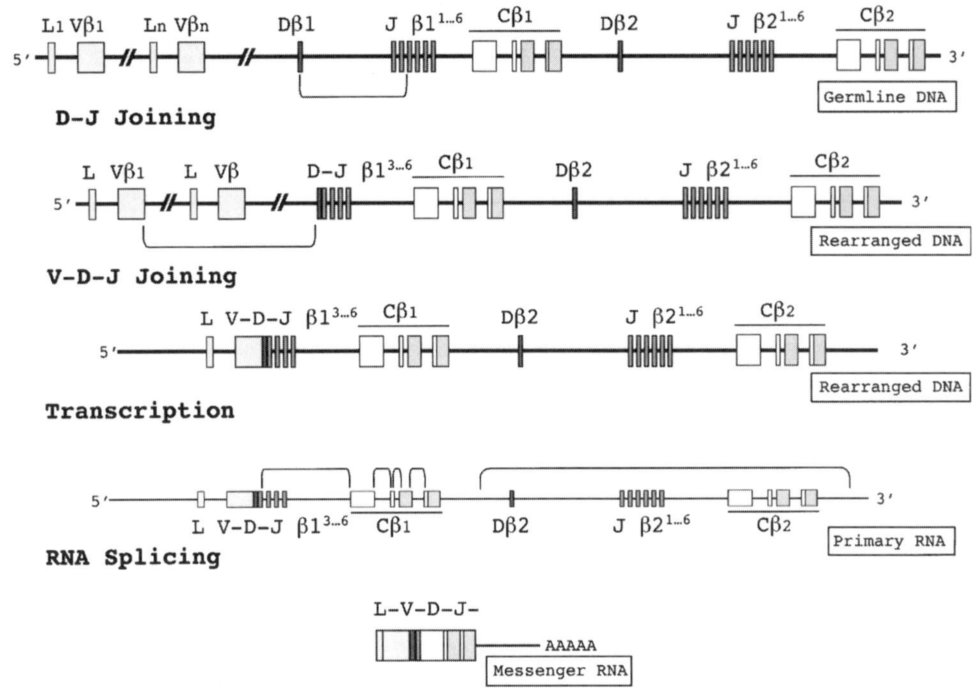

Fig. 6. The human TCR β-chain locus on chromosome 7 encompasses 75 different variable segments, each with its own leader sequence (Vβ1–Vβ*n* and L1–L*n*). These are associated with two gene clusters, one composed of one diversity segment (Dβ1), six joining segments ($J\beta1^{1 \cdots 6}$), and one constant segment (Cβ1) encoding the β_1-chain, and the other with the $D\beta2/D\beta2^{1 \cdots 6}/C\beta2$ segment encoding the β_2 chain. Two somatic recombination events take place to generate the version of the rearranged DNA that is eventually transcribed. The D-J joining event occurs first, followed by the V-D-J event. The rearranged DNA is then transcribed into the primary RNA transcript. This transcript is converted into messenger RNA (mRNA) through an RNA splicing event. The TCR β-chain protein will be made after translation, processing, and glycosylation. The leader sequence is removed once the TCR β-chain is in place on the cell membrane. (Modified from ref. *51.*)

The prevalence of HLA-DR2 is decreased *(116,117)* in patients with T1DM, and the DQA1*0102/DQB1*0502/DRB1*1601 haplotype accounts for the most part of disease susceptibility in DR2-associated cases of T1DM *(118–123)*. Therefore, the originally described effect of the DR2 allele in conferring resistance to diabetes is considered to be neutral rather than protective, whereas the real protective effect is provided by the DQ alleles, generally found in linkage disequilibrium with DR2. The effects of HLA alleles on T1DM susceptibility are summarized in Table 6.

HLA COMPLEX AND MECHANISMS OF SUSCEPTIBILITY TO OR PROTECTION FROM T1DM

Amino acid polymorphism at position 57 the HLA-DQβ-chain could influence the interaction between the class II molecule on the antigen-presenting cell, the peptide antigen, and the TCR of the helper T-cell. Consequently, this influences the control of the specificity of the immune response to foreign and/or self antigens (*see* Fig. 6) *(22)*.

However, other residues in the DQβ-chain as well as the DQα-chain *(124–126)* also appear to be involved in the susceptibility to T1DM. As discussed earlier, genetic susceptibility to autoimmune diabetes is strongly conferred by DQ DQA1*0501-DQB1*0201 and DQA1*0301-DQB1*0302 haplotypes. This concept is strengthened by recently published results obtained in vivo providing experimental evidence for the contribution of HLA-DQ molecules to autoimmune-related diabetes development. Using a unique "humanized" animal model of diabetes, the replacement of human HLA-DQ6 for human HLA-DQ8 molecules completely prevented the disease *(127)*.

The importance of class II molecules in playing a role in the pathogenesis of T1DM is also indicated by studies in a transgenic NOD mouse model, in which the expression of an I-A (the equivalent to the human class II DQB1 locus) β-chain transgene carrying Asp 57 instead of Ser 57 protects these mice from developing diabetes *(128,129)*. Moreover, expression of Pro56 instead of the normal His56 in the I-A α-chain has the same effect *(130)*. Finally, expression of certain I-E (the equivalent of the human HLA-DR locus) transgenes appears to confer resistance to the disease *(130,131)*. Of note, the treatment of NOD mice with a monoclonal antibody reacting with the murine class II molecule, also prevents the progression to overt diabetes *(132)*. These findings obtained in an animal model of T1DM certainly support the role of both HLA-DQ and HLA-DR in human T1DM.

The mechanisms by which the class II genes can influence susceptibility to, or protection from, T1DM are still the subject of discussion. Brown et al. *(133,134)* have characterized the structure of the crystallized HLA class II molecule. One hypothesis is that effective antigen-binding depends on the conformation of the antigen-binding site on the DQ dimer. The two critical residues, DQα 52 and DQβ 57 are located at opposite ends of the α-helices that form the antigen-binding site of the DQ molecule (*see* Fig. 3). It has been postulated that a substitution of an amino acid residue at these positions of the DQ molecule leads to conformational changes of the antigen-binding site and, consequently, to a modification of the affinity of the class II molecule for the "diabetogenic" peptide(s) *(22)*. In support for this hypothesis, it is known that in the DR molecule Asp-57 is involved in hydrogen- and salt-bonding with the antigenic peptide and the Arg-76 position of the α-chain, respectively *(130,131)*. Theoretically, modifications in the DRα Arg-76 residue would also alter the antigen-binding site. This is physiologically difficult to observe since the DRα-chain is not polymorphic.

It is noteworthy that studies of the regulatory regions of the genes encoding DQα- and DQβ-chains have shown that the level of transcription of these genes may also influence antigen binding. An increased level of production of a certain class II α-chain may increase the availability for dimerization *in trans* with the β-chain of the other haplotype *(135,136)*. Although the actual ratio of cis-encoded vs trans-encoded DQ heterodimers at the cell surface remains to be determined experimentally, it is possible that moderate differences in chain production translate into large functional differences with respect to antigen presentation and T-cell activation *(22)*. Studies by Demotz et al. *(137)* suggest that relatively few class II heterodimers need to be present at the surface of an antigen-presenting cell to efficiently crosslink the TCR and initiate a T-cell response. On this basis, it is easily understandable why the study of *IDDM1* must acknowledge the role of the T-cell and, more specifically, the role of particular TCRs in mediating disease.

T-CELL RECEPTOR CHARACTERISTICS AND SUSCEPTIBILITY TO T1DM

The TCR on a given peripheral T-cell is composed of separately encoded α- and β-chains that are disulfide linked. These dimers must form a molecular complex with the multichain CD3 complex to become functionally active at the cell surface. During the entire life of an individual, T-cells undergo a maturation process that occurs primarily in the thymus. During this process, precursor stem cells, initially from the fetal liver and then from bone marrow, enter the thymic *anlage,* where they are induced to rearrange their germline TCRα and TCRβ genes (*see* Fig. 6) *(138).* TCR gene rearrangements are essentially random, and most are nonproductive as a result of out-of-frame joints; however, these unsuccessful rearrangements are requisite for the expression of generally a single functional α/β TCR at the cell surface. Furthermore, the essentially random nature of these rearrangements among a large number of variable segments ensures an extremely large (10^{10}–10^{15}) repertoire of distinct antigen specificities present at the surface of the unselected thymocyte pool. Once a T-cell expresses a functional TCR at the cell surface, it is subject to either positive or negative selection events in the thymus *(139,140).* Both positive selection and negative selection depend on interactions among the TCR, MHC molecule, and antigenic self peptide. *Positive selection* occurs as thymic stromal cells bearing MHC molecules (containing self-peptide fragments) engage TCR molecules on the developing thymocytes and direct their continued maturation into functionally mature T-cells. T-cells with "useless" receptors (i.e., those that cannot bind with sufficient affinity to the MHC molecule) are not driven to mature and expand, and they eventually die. *Negative selection* refers to the poorly understood set of events that specifically eliminates or alternatively "anergizes" potentially autoreactive cells, thereby inducing "tolerance" to self (i.e., self-tolerance). During negative selection, factors such as affinity for self-antigen and antigen load likely influence the final outcome of cell death or clonal anergy. Thus, the peripheral T-cell repertoire of each person (including each individual of two monozygotic twins) is unique *(141)* and is a consequence of both the random generation of TCRs in the initial unselected thymocyte pool as well as of thymic positive and negative selection events.

Autoimmunity is thought to result from an imbalance between the two functionally opposite processes, *tolerance induction* and *immune responsiveness,* each dependent on the presence of class I and class II molecules with appropriate structures (dictated by the genes encoding them) that are able to present critical antigenic peptides. In genetically susceptible individuals, certain class II molecules may ineffectively present self peptides, thereby leading to inadequate negative selection of T-cell populations that could later become activated to manifest an autoimmune response. Nepom and Kwok explain the molecular basis of HLA-DQ associations with T1DM exactly on this basis *(142).* Paradoxically, some self peptides that normally negatively select T-cells are likely to lead to positive selection when the MHC molecule is, for example, the HLA-DQ3.2.

The HLA-DQ3.2 molecule is encoded by DQA1*0301 and DQB1*0302 genes, which are generally present on the most strongly T1DM-associated haplotype also encompassing HLA-DR4. Because of a characteristic structural motif for peptide binding, the HLA-DQ3.2 can be considered an intrinsically "unstable" MHC class II molecule. If in a

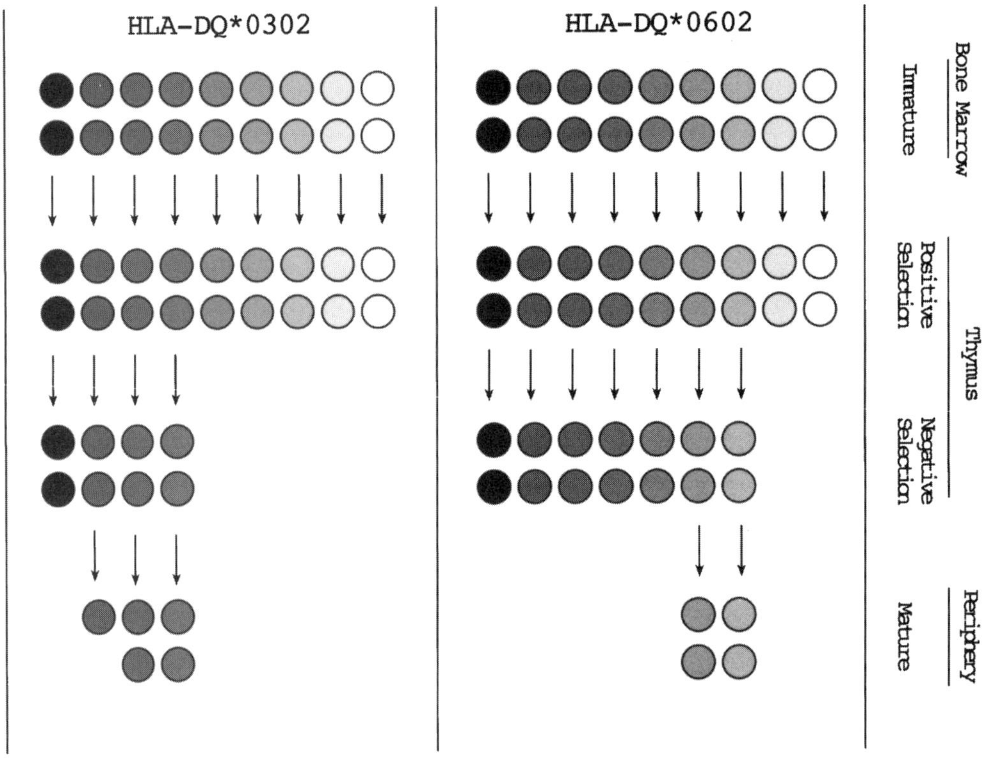

Fig. 7. Both positive and negative thymic selections contribute to form the repertoire of mature T-cells in the periphery from the precursors, or immature T-cells, originated in the bone marrow. Individuals carrying HLA-DQ alleles associated with resistance to the disease, like HLA-DQ*0602, will be able to negatively select in the thymus all the T-cells with an high affinity for peptides of the self (black dots), so that no autoreactive T-cells will be present in their peripheral blood and the chances to develop diabetes will be reduced. Individuals who have, instead, susceptibility alleles with low affinity for peptides of the self (e.g., HLA-DQ*03020) will negatively select less efficiently autoreactive T-cell clones that will then be present, even if in a relatively small number, among the peripheral T-cells. (Modified from ref. *142.*)

DQ3.2-positive individual, the T-cells that are negatively selected in the thymus are only those that recognize DQ3.2–peptide complexes in a "stable" high-affinity configuration, the result can easily be the release from the thymus of mature T-cells able to establish a potentially autoimmune repertoire in the periphery. Figure 7 illustrates these concepts.

Small structural changes, then, may result in large functional changes in the antigen-presenting capabilities of the class II molecules. One might conceive that the cells from a person who is heterozygous for both DQα and DQβ would contain all four chain combinations on their surface. Competition for binding the processed antigen could take place, with effective antigen binding dictated by the conformation of the antigen-binding site on each DQ dimer. As previously described, changes at either amino acid DQα-52 or DQβ-57, located at opposite ends of the α-helices that form the antigen-binding groove (*see* Fig. 3), could alter the configuration of the groove. Changes at both positions would likely inflict a great conformational effect on the molecule's antigen-presentation capability. Such conformational differences may be partially responsible for the observed hierarchy in the degree of susceptibility within the group of non-Asp-57 alleles and for the differences in the degree of protection afforded by each allele within the group of Asp-57 alleles. For example, the protective effect of the Asp-57 DQB1*0502 allele prevails over that of certain susceptible alleles, such as non-Asp-57 DQB1*0501. Conversely, the susceptible allele non-Asp-57 DQB1*0302 dominates over the protective effect of Asp-57 DQB1*0301.

Competition for antigen binding would also be influenced by the relative abundance of each form of heterodimer at the cell surface, which, in turn, is likely influenced by several factors: First, certain DQα- and DQβ-chains appear to be under structural constraints that limit the formation of dimers between them. For example, α-chains of the DQA1*0301 or DQA1*0501 alleles does not couple efficiently with the β-chain of the DQB1*0501 allele. Thus, persons who are heterozygous for these alleles would not be expected to readily form significant numbers of "hybrid" molecules between trans-encoded genes. Second, studies of the promoter regions of these genes suggest that the levels of transcription of the DQα- and DQβ-chain genes may differ among allelic variants *(136,143)*. These studies imply that a chain encoded by one gene may be synthesized in larger amounts than a chain encoded by the other allele, thereby increasing the probability of its participating in trans dimerization *(64)*.

Positive- and negative-selection events can also explain genetic resistance to T1DM. In many populations, the frequency of the DQB1*0602 allele is rarely found among patients with IDDM *(144,145)*. This suggests that this allele may play a protective role in the disease process. During thymic development, an unidentified diabetogenic peptide can preferentially bind to the DQB1*0602 molecule, and because of the relatively higher affinity and/or avidity it has with this than with other DQ molecules, it will form HLA-DQ molecule–antigenic peptide–TCR complexes more efficiently than other molecules. This could lead to negative selection and depletion of potentially self-peptide-reactive T-cells. Individuals with a typical DQB*0602 allele can then delete these potentially dangerous T-cells during thymic maturation and, therefore, are protected from developing diabetes (*see* Fig. 7). At present, carrying a "protective" DQB*0602 allele is considered as a criterion of exclusion for enrolling first-degree relatives of diabetic patients in clinical trials, such as the Diabetes Prevention Trial 1 (DPT-1), which is being carried out in the United States. This trial has been designed to prevent the progression to the clinical onset of T1DM in individuals considered at high risk for developing the disease *(146)*. However, this does not mean that carrying the DQB1*0602 allele confers 100% protection from developing the disease *(147,148)*. Our results suggest that prediabetics carrying the HLA haplotype DQA1*0102, DQB1*0602 have the tendency to be antibody negative for all islet autoantigens *(97)*. Seven percent of prediabetics in this study carried the HLA haplotype DQB1*0602, which confirms previous observations that the protective effect associated with DQB1*0602 is not absolute *(147,148)*. We found that 40% of prediabetics carrying the HLA haplotype DQA1*0102, DQB1*0602 were African-American.

THE INSULIN GENE REGION *(IDDM2)*

Investigation of the insulin gene *(INS)* region on chromosome 11p15 as a premier candidate for genetic association with T1DM began in the early 1980s (*see* Fig. 8) *(149–151)*. Insulin's central role in metabolism and blood glucose homeostasis and

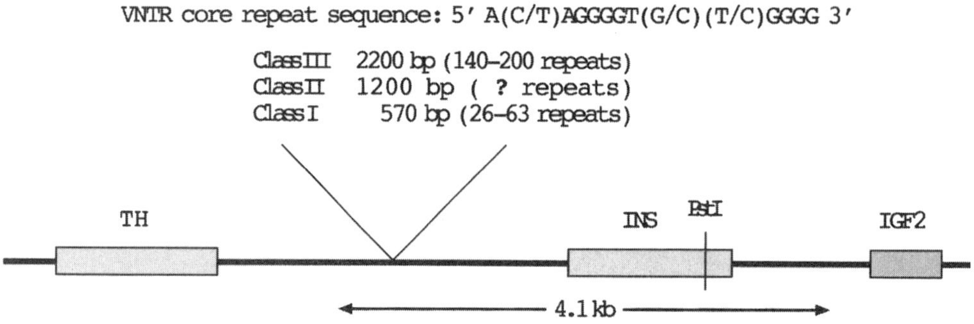

Fig. 8. The variable number of tandem repeats (VNTR) in the 5′ region of the insulin gene was grouped into three classes. The first with approx 40 repeats is called class I and the one with approx 160 repeats is class III; the number of repeats characteristic of class II genomes has not yet been formally determined. (Modified from ref. *51*.)

its unique distinction as the only known β-cell-specific antigen made it a likely front-runner to account for an inherited susceptibility to diabetes. However, early studies of the human insulin gene and its relation with T1DM, T2DM, and abnormal glucose regulation were inconclusive, presumably because of the relatively small sample sizes analyzed *(149–151)*. In 1991, Julier et al. provided evidence of genetic linkage for the insulin gene *(IDDM2)* with T1DM in a collection of multiplex families from France, the United States, and North Africa *(152)*. Subsequently, the investigations of Bain et al. have confirmed the evidence of linkage between *IDDM2* and type 1 diabetes *(153)*. Importantly, Bain et al. demonstrated linkage for *IDDM2* independent of the influence of HLA alleles (i.e., *IDDM1*) and the parental source of the *IDDM2* susceptibility allele.

Detailed sequence analysis of the insulin gene region identified a polymorphic locus, which consists of a VNTR, present within the 5′ regulatory region (promoter) adjacent to the coding sequence of the insulin gene. Each repeat element consists of a 14- to 15-bp DNA segment having the consensus nucleotide sequence A(C/T) AGGGGT(G/C)C(T/C/G)(G/A/T) (G/T/A)G(G/C/T) (*see* Fig. 8). The number of repeats within sequenced alleles ranges from 26 to >200, with 3 classes of alleles identified on the basis of overall size: class I, class II and class III. Class I *INS* VNTR alleles consist of 26–63 repeats, averaging 570 bp in length, and are associated with IDDM susceptibility. Class III alleles consist of 140–200 or more repeats and are considered to be protective from diabetes. In size, class III alleles are the largest variants, averaging over 2.2 kb in length. Finally, class II alleles (1.2 kb average length) are too rare in the populations studied to draw any conclusion about their association with IDDM susceptibility *(154)*.

Detailed analyses of the insulin region indicate the presence of a number of additional polymorphism outside the VNTR region that are in strong linkage disequilibrium with the VNTR itself, which then appears to be the primary association with T1DM susceptibility. Bennet et al. reported that a 698-VNTR class I subtype is negatively associated with disease susceptibility, in contrast to other class I alleles that confer susceptibility to disease *(154–156)*.

BIOLOGICAL SIGNIFICANCE OF THE VNTR REGION

A number of studies have suggested that the *INS* VNTR may have a biological role in the genetic regulation of insulin expression *(70,157,158)*. The proximity of this polymorphism to the *INS* transcriptional start site (<400 bp upstream) makes this an attractive hypothesis. Furthermore, an association between VNTR polymorphisms and human disease is not unprecedented. It has been suggested that the human *HRAS1* gene, which encodes the H-ras protooncogene and is associated with a genetic susceptibility to certain cancers, is under the allelic effects of a VNTR polymorphism that lies downstream of the gene *(159–161)*. Expansions of nucleotide triplet repeat minisatellites have also been implicated in numerous progressive neurological diseases such as myotonic dystrophy *(162)*. In vitro evidence suggests that these genetic elements may exert a regulatory effect by strengthening nucleosome formation, thereby altering local chromatin structure and, consequently, decreasing the efficiency of transcription from nearby genes *(162)*.

Nevertheless, the exact functional role of the *INS* variable number tandem repeat (VNTR) is still a subject of discussion *(163)* and debate in view of conflicting reports as to whether class I VNTR-containing promoter constructs induce are greater *(154,157)* or lesser *(158)* insulin gene expression in vitro. In two early reports *(154,157)*, it was asserted that class I-associated insulin expression (associated with diabetes susceptibility) was enhanced as compared with class III insulin gene expression, which is notably considered to be associated with protection from T1DM. In contrast, Kennedy et al. *(158)* have shown that class III VNTR reporter gene constructs had three time higher reporter gene expression than class I VNTR. Nonetheless, the results from Owerbach and Gabbay *(70)* do not support those of Kennedy et al. *(158)*. These controversial results raise the concept that methodological differences in conducting the experiments may account for some of these discrepancies. Presently, it remains to be determined how the variant insulin gene expression may influence T1DM susceptibility.

THE SEARCH FOR NOVEL NON-MHC SUSCEPTIBILITY GENES

Recent genomewide searches for T1DM susceptibility provided preliminary evidence for the existence of at least 18 loci associated with T1DM *(164)*. Because of the large number of markers tested, many of these putative regions suggestive of T1DM susceptibility linkage may have occurred by chance. Saturating the putative locus with many more informative markers is a must to demonstrate or rule out the existence of significant linkage. Further complicating the issue of suggestive linkage from genomewide scans is the broad range of selection criteria used for inclusion of families in the various datasets. Variations in the age of onset of T1DM can make the detection of linkage difficult. Confounding matters even more is the interaction of the various disease susceptibility loci that is the hallmark of polygenic diseases like T1DM, in that this interaction (additive, multiplicative, or epistatic) adds an additional level of difficulty in determining the significance of a logarithm of odds (LOD) score. Once suggestive linkage to a region has been determined, other powerful association-based tests that take advantage of linkage disequilibrium between a marker and the actual susceptibility alleles can be used to formally implicate a locus and a particular allele with susceptibility *(70)*.

The initial genome scan by Davies et al. *(164)* suggested the existence of 18 susceptibility loci. To date, suggestive linkage to 16 of those 18 susceptibility loci *(164)* (termed *IDDM,* followed by a number) does not necessarily imply the importance of that locus to susceptibility. The demonstration of significant linkage to some of these sites has been replicated in independent datasets, in some cases implicating a candidate gene. Linkage to other loci originally detected in the scan by Davies et al. awaits replication. It is important to note that some of the loci that showed suggestive, albeit weak, linkage in the scan by Davies et al. *(164)* could not be confirmed in other populations. This indicates the importance of replication in other datasets as well as the selection of a dense set of markers to cover as much of the genome as possible. Recent studies have revealed the genetic interaction of certain of these loci and their mode of interaction. For example, *IDDM1* (which is the class II HLA locus) and *IDDM2* (which is the VNTR upstream of the *INS* promoter) interact epistatically (i.e., the genes are functionally related, either in a biochemical or a physiological pathway), whereas *IDDM1* and *IDDM4* may act independently *(165).* In addition, *IDDM4* and *IDDM5* appear to have a greater frequency of shared alleles, identical-by-descent subgroups of datasets, which have HLA-DR3 in common. The linkage of *IDDM7* is stronger in subgroups lacking HLA-DR3 and, finally, *IDDM7* appears to show stronger evidence of linkage in subgroups homozygous for class I VNTR alleles at *IDDM2 (70).* All of these results will most likely depend on the nature of the population under study as there are already-established differences among populations in T1DM susceptibility at particular loci. The relative risk of haplotypes at *IDDM2* is dependent on the presence of HLA-DR4 in a French population *(152)* but not in American, Belgian, Finnish, or British datasets *(166).*

There is continuous debate, however, as to what criteria should be used when attempting to map non-HLA loci. Historically, in a monogenic disease, the generally accepted standard for significant linkage is considered to be a LOD score greater than 3 ($p < 10^{-4}$). Thomson *(167,168)* suggested a statistical level of $p = 0.001$ in considering presumable linkage in genomewide searches, followed by confirmation of the results in other populations to confirm linkage. Lander and Kruglyak *(45),* however, proposed more stringent criteria of a LOD score of 2.2, indicating suggestive linkage ($p < 7 \times 10^{-4}$) and a LOD score of 3.6 ($p < 2 \times 10^{-5}$) to achieve significant linkage. Even with a LOD score of 3.6, there is still a possibility of a false-positive rate of 5% in genomewide scans. Moreover, Lander and Kruglyak propose that further replication studies in different populations are necessary in order to verify significant linkage. Very few of the loci indicated in Table 2 will stand the criteria of Lander and Kruglyak for significant linkage. To circumvent this, some investigators propose that the HLA exerts a very powerful effect on overall susceptibility and, as a consequence, some loci will be missed although they may play some role in other biochemical or physiological pathways involved in susceptibility. Indeed, one means by which some loci were found has been to stratify based on the number of HLA alleles shared in sib-pair-based mapping approaches. This method was used to describe *IDDM13 (169).* Another approach stratifies based on the presence or absence of autoantibodies *(170).* To date, there has not been any rigorous statistical analysis on the validity of these stratifications, and although they may be justified, the recent failure to find linkage at all described loci except *IDDM1, IDDM2, IDDM5,* and *IDDM8* in more than 500 sib-pairs using stringent criteria (Polychronakos, personal communication) may, in part, be explained by the application of such stratifications.

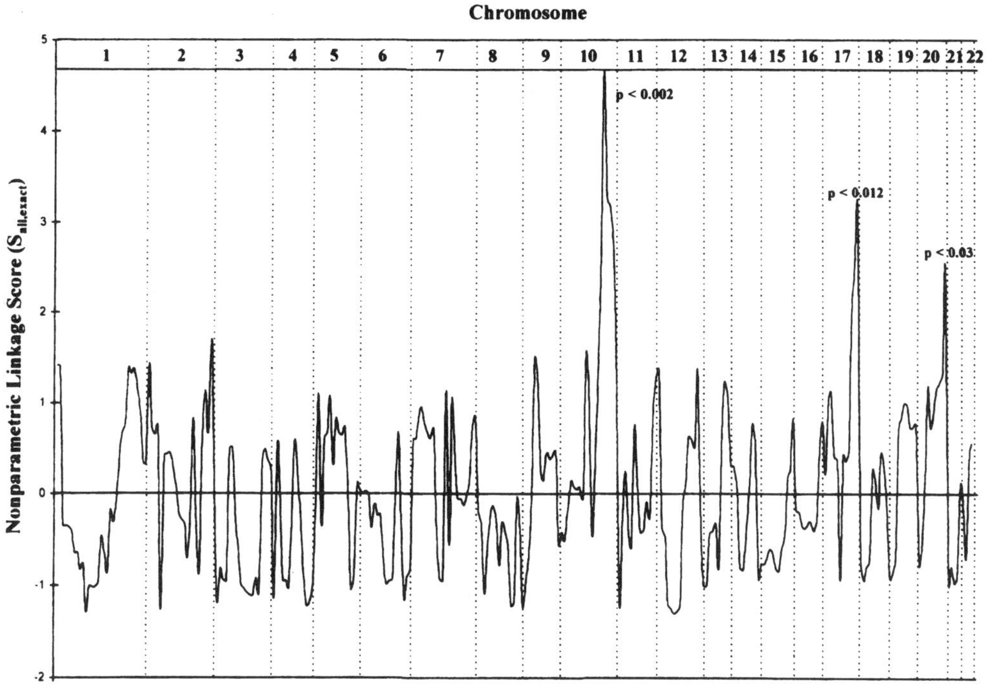

Fig. 9. Results of an initial genomewide (309 markers) multipoint NPL analysis using GENEHUNTER *(171)*. The maximum NPL value (0.002) corresponds to marker D10S1237 at chromosome 10q25. The evidence for linkage to this region was strengthened with the analysis of additional microsatellites and additional family members. (From ref. *46.*)

Finally, the last approach was to evaluate empirical power and efficiency of mapping complex disorders, such as autoimmune diabetes, studying large multiplex families from genetically and culturally homogeneous populations, such as a Bedouin family from Israel *(46)*. The extended pedigree of this multiplex Bedouin family included 248 individuals, along with 19 affected individuals in 3 generations. Results from genome scans for linkage indicate a predominant peak by nonparametric linkage (NPL) analysis that is seen for the long arm of chromosome 10 (10q25, *IDDM17*), with the maximum NPL occurring at D10S1237 ($p < 0.002$) (*see* Fig. 9). A high-resolution map of the candidate region on 10q was constructed using the Centre d'Etude du Polymorphisme Humain (CEPH) genotyping database and the Massachusetts Institute of Technology (MIT) physical mapping database to identify polymorphic markers and yeast artificial chromosome (YAC) clones *(46)*. With the higher density of markers, the evidence of linkage increased substantially ($p = 0.00004$) *(46)*. Furthermore, preliminary evidence indicates that the high-risk haplotype of *IDDM17* in the Bedouin Arab family may be present in as many as 5% of US families (Eisenbarth, personal communication).

In sum, genomewide searches are considered only an initial stage in discovering novel susceptibility genes in type 1 diabetes and in other polygenic diseases. First, linkage must be proven, which is not an easy task. Second, a large number of families from independent populations are required to confirm linkage and understanding the interactions of putative susceptibility genes.

A PATTERN IS ARISING: COLOCALIZATION OF AUTOIMMUNE DISEASE LOCI

Recently, it has been described that the position of provisional loci found in T1DM colocalize or overlap with loci found in different autoimmune/inflammatory diseases *(48,172)*. This is consistent with the hypothesis that, like the MHC, some of these provisional loci may involve common susceptibility genes or biochemical pathways that are central to normal immune function. Concannon et al. *(148)* identified a novel locus for T1DM (MLS=3.31) (Table 2) at human chromosome 1q at marker D1S1617. This locus colocalizes with loci for systemic lupus erythematosus (SLE) *(49)* and ankylosing spondylitis *(50)*. In human SLE, this locus is linked to high serum levels of antichromatin antibody, and in mouse SLE. This locus is linked to both anti-chromatin and anti-DNA antibody production *(173,174)*. This colocalization of suggestive genetic linkage for three autoimmune diseases suggests that genes at this locus may be involved in a pathway that might affect the quantitative regulation of antibody levels and that this may ultimately contribute to the development of the disease phenotype. Therefore, particular as yet undiscovered genes or pathways may contribute to immune dysregulation, a phenomenon detected in many different autoimmune diseases, possibly prior to the onset of overt clinical symptoms *(175)*.

Ten centimorgans is the approximate limit of resolution of a typical first-stage genomewide scan. For example, *IDDM2* found at 1lpl5.5 *(164)* is located at the exact position as loci for SLEk *(176)*, ankylosing spondylitis *(50)*, asthma *(177)*, and multiple sclerosis *(178)*. All four disease loci have been defined by the same polymorphic marker, D11S922, at the 0.323-cM position on human chromosome 11 *(179)*. A candidate gene at 1lpl5.5 is the insulin gene itself. VNTR polymorphisms in the 5′ end of the insulin gene have been associated and linked to IDDM *(180)*. One interpretation of this genetic linkage to insulin as a candidate gene is that there might be an involvement of an imprinted gene *(157,181–183)*, which may be under the same transcriptional effects of the VNTR as is the insulin gene. Colocalization of multiple autoimmune diseases at this location suggests that whatever the exact gene found at *IDDM2 (180)*, it may play a broader role in autoimmune development.

Although this general pattern of locus colocalization appears not to be found in human nonautoimmune disease *(172)*, it is possible that a pattern of colocalization of autoimmune disease may be the result of common biological pathways shared among related autoimmune/inflammatory abnormalities in coexisting human autoimmune disorders *(172)*.

CONCLUDING REMARKS

In T1DM, the application of genomewide scans has identified over 18 putative loci of statistical significance, but, for now, only linkage to HLA loci seems incontestable. Albeit much excitement has recently been generated by the results of genomewide scans, for many polygenic disorders, including T1DM, careful and rigorous replication as well as association studies in many populations must be conducted before any attempts are made by positional cloning or the candidate gene approach to identify potentially elusive sequence variations that could influence genetic susceptibility. One example of controversy in this field is a publication of studies with opposing results *(48,184,185)*.

It is noteworthy acknowledging that familial association of different autoimmune diseases in the same pedigree *(172),* association of different autoimmune disorders including T1DM in the same individual *(186,187),* and common clinical parameters of different autoimmune diseases *(6,188)* might share similar pathophysiologic mechanisms leading to autoimmunity. Colocalization and overlapping of candidate loci in autoimmune disease, such as T1DM, imply that common biological pathways may be involved in the immunopathogenesis of at least a subgroup of autoimmune diabetes and other clinically diversified autoimmune disorders. The latter example may resemble what occurs as a result of mutations of the autoimmune regulator gene *(AIRE) (189–191),* which forms the basis for genetic dysregulation in autoimmune polyendocrine syndrome type 1 (APS-I), a non-MHC-linked disorder that is also associated with autoimmune impairment of pancreatic β-cells.

REFERENCES

1. Eisenbarth GS. Type I diabetes mellitus: a chronic autoimmune disease. N Engl J Med 1986;314:1360–1368.
2. Rossini AA, Mordes JP, Handler ES. Speculation on the etiology of diabetes mellitus. Tumbler hypothesis. Diabetes 1988;37:257–261.
3. Bingley PJ, Christie MR, Bonifacio E, et al. Combined analysis of autoantibodies improves prediction of IDDM in islet cell antibody-positive relatives. Diabetes 1994;43:1304–1310.
4. Verge CF, Gianani R, Kawasaki E, et al. Prediction of type I diabetes mellitus in first degree relatives using a combination of insulin, glutamic acid decarboxylase and ICA512bdc/IA-2 autoantibodies. Diabetes 1996;45:926–933.
5. Pietropaolo M, Eisenbarth GS. Autoantibodies in human diabetes. Curr Dir Autoimmun 2001; 4:252–282.
6. Rose NR. Immunologic diagnosis of autoimmuity. In: Leffel, MS, Donnenberg, AD, Rose, NR, eds. Handbook of Immunology. CRC, New York, 1997, vol. 4, pp. 111–123.
7. Warram HH, Krolewski AS, Gottlieb MS, et al. Differences in risk of insulin-dependent diabetes in offspring of diabetic mothers and diabetic fathers. N Engl J Med 1984;311:149–152.
8. Warram JH, Rich SS, Krolewski AS. Epidemiology and genetics of diabetes mellitus. In: Kahn, CR Weir, GC, eds. Joslin's Diabetes Mellitus. Lea and Febiger, Philadelphia, 1994;13(12):201.
9. Wagener DK, Sacks JM, LaPorte RE, et al. The Pittsburgh study of insulin-dependent diabetes mellitus: risk for diabetes among relatives of IDDM. Diabetes 1982;31:136–144.
10. Bleich D, Polak M, Eisenbarth GS, et al. Decreased risk of type 1 diabetes in offspring of mothers who acquire diabetes during adrenarchy. Diabetes 1993;42:1433–1439.
11. Allen C, Palta M, D'Alessio DJ. Incidence and differences in urban–rural seasonal variation of type 1 (insulin-dependent) diabetes in Wisconsin. Diabetologia 1986;29:629–633.
12. Dorman JS, McCarthy BJ, O'Leary AL, et al. Risk factors for insulin-dependent diabetes. Diabetes in America, 2nd ed. National Institute of Diabetes and Digestive and Kidney Diseases, Washington, DC, 1995, pp. 165–177.
13. Warram JH, Krolewski AS, Kahn CR. Determinanats of IDDM and perinatal mortality in children of diabetic mothers. Diabetes 1988;37:1328–1334.
14. LaPorte RE, Matsushima M, Chang Y-F. Prevalence and incidence of insulin-dependent diabetes. Diabetes in America. 2nd ed. National Institute of Diabetes and Digestive and Kidney Diseases, Washington, DC, 1995, pp. 37–46.
15. Groop LC, Bottazzo GF, Doniach D. Islet cell antibodies identify latent type I diabetes in patients aged 35–75 years at diagnosis. Diabetes 1986;35:237–241.
16. Landin-Olsson M, Karlsson FA, Lernmark A, et al. Islet cell and thyrogastric antibodies in 633 consecutive 15- to 34-yr-old patients in the diabetes incidence study in Sweden. Diabetes 1992;41:1022–1027.
17. Rewers M, Hamman RF. Risk factors for non-insulin dependent diabetes. In: National Institute of Diabetes and Digestive and Kidney Diseases, ed. Diabetes in America, 2nd ed. National Institutes of Health, Washington, DC, 1995, Vol. 9, pp. 179–220.

18. Tuomi T, Groop LC, Zimmet PZ, et al. Antibodies to glutamic acid decarboxylase reveal latent autoimmune diabetes in adults with a non-insulin-dependent onset of diabetes. Diabetes 1993;42:359–362.
19. Zimmet PZ, Shaten BJ, Kuller LH, et al. Antibodies to glutamic acid decarboxylase and diabetes mellitus in the Multiple Risk Factor Intervention Trial. Am J Epidemiol 1994;140:683–690.
20. Turner R, Stratton I, Horton V, et al. UKPDS 25: autoantibodies to islet-cell cytoplasm and glutamic acid decarboxylase for prediction of insulin requirement in type 2 diabetes. Lancet 1997;350:1288–1293.
21. Morel PA, Dorman JS, Todd JA, et al. Aspartic acid at position 57 of the HLA-DQ beta chain protects against type I diabetes: a family study. Proc Natl Acad Sci USA 1988;85:8111–8115.
22. Trucco M. To be or not to be ASP 57, that is the question. Diabetes Care 1992;15:705–715.
23. Erlich HA, Bugawan TL, Scharf S, et al. HLA-DQβ sequence polymorphism and genetic susceptibility to IDDM. Diabetes 1990;39:96–103.
24. Horton V, Stratton I, Bottazzo GF, et al. Genetic heterogeneity of autoimmune diabetes: age of presentation in adults is influenced by HLA *DRB1* and *DQB1* genotypes (UKPDS 43). Diabetologia 1999;42:608–616.
25. Pietropaolo M, Barinas-Mitchell E, Pietropaolo SL, et al. Evidence of islet cell autoimmunity in elderly patients with Type 2 diabetes mellitus. Diabetes 2000;49:32–38.
26. Allen C, Palta M, D'Alessio DJ. Risk of diabetes in siblings and other relatives of IDDM subjects. Diabetes 1991;40:831–836.
27. Dahlquist G, Blom L, Tuvemo T, et al. The Swedish childhood diabetes study—results from a nine year case register and a one year case-referent study indicating that type 1 (insulin-dependent) diabetes mellitus is associated with both type 2 (non-insulin-dependent) diabetes mellitus and autoimmune disorders. Diabetologia 1989;32:2–6.
28. Dahlquist G, Blom L, Lonnberg G. The Swedish childhood diabetes study—a multivariate analysis of risk determinants for diabetes in different age groups. Diabetologia 1991;34:757–762.
29. Tuomilehto J, Lounamaa R, Tuomilehto-Wolf E, et al. Epidemiology of childhood diabetes mellitus in Finland—background of a nationwide study of type 1 (insulin-dependent) diabetes mellitus. Diabetologia 1992;35:70–76.
30. Tillil H, Kobberling J. Age-correlated empirical genetic risk estimates for first degree relatives of IDDM patients. Diabetes 1987;36:93–99.
31. Nepom GT. Class II antigens and disease susceptibility. Annu Rev Med 1995;46:17–25.
32. Vadheim CM, Rotter JI, Maclaren NK, et al. Preferential transmission of diabetic alleles within the HLA gene complex. N Engl J Med 1986;315:1314–1318.
33. Strominger JL. Biology of the human histocompatibility leukocyte antigen (HLA) system and a hypothesis regarding the generation of autoimmune disease. J Clin Invest 1986;77:1411–1415.
34. Lu SSS, Tun RYM, Hawa M, et al. Studies of diabetic twins. Diabetes Metab Rev 1991;7:223–238.
35. Dahlquist G. Environmental risk factors in human type I diabetes—an epidemiological perspective. Diabetes Metab Rev 1995;11:37–46.
36. Luppi P, Zanone MM, Hyoty H, et al. Restricted TCR Vβ gene expression and enterovirus infection in type 1 diabetes: a pilot study. Diabetologia 2000;43:1484–1497.
37. Dahl-Jorgensen K, Joner G, Hanssen KF. Relationship between cow's milk consumption and incidence of IDDM in childhood. Diabetes Care 1991;14:1081–1083.
38. Dahlquist G, Ivarsson S, Lindberg B, et al. Maternal enteroviral infection during pregnancy as a risk determinant for childhood insulin-dependent diabetes mellitus—a population based case-control study. Diabetes 1995;44:408–413.
39. Conrad B, Weidmann E, Trucco G, et al. Evidence for superantigen involvment in insulin-dependent diabetes mellitus etiology. Nature 1994;371:351–355.
40. Trucco M, LaPorte R. Exposure to superantigens as an immunogenetic explanation of type I diabetes mini-epidemics. J Pediatr Endocrinol 1995;8:3–10.
41. Bingley PJ, Gale EAM. Rising inidence of IDDM in Europe. Diabetes Care 1989;12:289–295.
42. Dorman JS, LaPorte RE, Tajima N, et al. Differential risk factors for death in insulin-dependent diabetic patients by duration of disease. Pediatr Adolesc Endocrinol 1986;15:289–299.
43. Lonnrot M, Korpela K, Knip M, et al. Enterovirus infection as a risk factor for beta-cell autoimmunity in a prospectively observed birth cohort: the Finnish Diabetes Prediction and Prevention Study. Diabetes 2000;49:1314–1318.
44. Conrad B, Trucco M. Superantigens as etiopathogenic factors in the development of insulin dependent diabetes mellitus. Diabetes Metab Rev 1995;10:309–338.

45. Lander ES, Kruglyak L. Genetic dissection of complex traits: guidelines for interpreting and reporting linkage results. Nat Genet 1995;11:241–247.
46. Verge CF, Vardi P, Babu S, et al. Evidence for oligogenic inheritance of Type 1 diabetes in a large Bedouin Arab family. J Clin Invest 1998;102:1569–1575.
47. Cucca F, Goy JV, Kawaguchi Y, et al. A male-female bias in type 1 diabetes and linkage to chromosome Xp in MHC HLA-DR3-positive patients. Nat Genet 1998;19:301–302.
48. Concannon P, Gogolin-Ewens KJ, Hinds DA, et al. A second-generation screen of the human genome for susceptibility to insulin-dependent diabetes mellitus. Nat Genet 1998;19:292–296.
49. Tsao BP, Cantor RM, Kalunian KC, et al. Evidence for linkage of a candidate chromosome 1 region to human systemic lupus erythematosus. J Clin Invest 1997;99:725–731.
50. Brown MA, Pile KD, Kennedy LG, et al. A genome-wide screen for susceptibility candidate loci in ankylosing spondylitis. Arthritis Rheum 1998;41:588–595.
51. Pietropaolo M, Trucco M. Major histocompatibility locus and other genes that determine the risk of development of type 1 diabetes mellitus. In: LeRoith D, Taylor SI, Olefsky JM, eds. Diabetes Mellitus. A Fundamental and Clinical Text. 2nd ed. Lippincott Williams & Wilkins, Philadelphia; 2000, pp. 399–410.
52. Friday RP, Trucco M, Pietropaolo M. Genetics of type 1 diabetes mellitus. Diabetes Nutr Metab 1999;12:3–26.
53. Serreze DV, Leiter EH. Genes and cellular requirements for autoimmune diabetes susceptibility in NOD mice. Curr Dir Autoimmun 2001;4:31–67.
54. Atkinson MA, Leiter EH. The NOD mouse model of type 1 diabetes: as good as it gets? Nat Med 1999;5:601–604.
55. Grenier DL, Handler ES, Nakano K, et al. Absence of the RT6 T cell subset in diabetes-prone BB/W rats. J Immunol 1986;136:148–151.
56. Powis SH, Mockridge I, Kelly A, et al. Polymorphism in a second ABC transporter gene located within the class II region of the human major histocompatibility complex. Proc Natl Acad Sci USA 1992;89(4):1463–1467.
57. Colonna M, Bresnahan M, Bahram S, et al. Alleleic variants of the human putative peptide transporter involved in antigen processing. Proc Natl Acad Sci USA 1992;89:3932–3936.
58. Germain RN. MHC-Dependent antigen processing and peptide presentation: providing ligands for T lymphocyte activation. Cell 1994;76:287–299.
59. Schwartz BD. The major histocompatibility complex and disease susceptibility. In: Bennett JC, Plum F, eds. Cecil Textbook of Medicine. 20th ed. WB Saunders, Philadelphia, 1996, pp. 1424–1432.
60. Klein J, Sato A. The HLA system. N Eng J Med 2000;11:782–786.
61. Degli Esposti MA, Leaver LA, Christiansen FT, et al. Ancestral haplotypes: conserved population MHC haplotypes. Hum Immunol 1992;34:242–252.
62. Zhang WJ, Degli Esposti MA, Cobain TJ, et al. Differences in gene copy number carried by different MHC ancestral haplotypes. J Exp Med 1990;171:2101–2114.
63. Termijtelen A, D'Amaro J, van Rood JJ, et al. Linkage disequilibrium in HLA cannot be explained by selective recombination. Tissue Antigens 1995;46:387–390.
64. Faas S, Trucco M. The genes influencing the susceptibility to IDDM in humans. J Endocrinol Invest 1994;17:477–495.
65. Tisch R, McDevitt H. Insulin-dependent diabetes mellitus. Cell 1996;85:294–297.
66. Pietropaolo M, Eisenbarth GS. Molecular targets of the autoimmunity of type I diabetes. In: Draznin B, LeRoith D, eds. Molecular Biology of Diabetes. Humana, Totowa, NJ, 1994, pp. 1–33.
67. Bingley PJ, for the ICARUS Group. Interaction of age, islet cell antibodies, insulin autoantibodies, and first-phase insulin response in predicting risk of progression to IDDM in ICA^+ relatives. The ICARUS Data Set. Diabetes 1996;45:1720–1728.
68. She J-X. Susceptibility to type I diabetes: HLA-DQ and DR revisited. Immunol Today 1996;17:323–329.
69. Aitman TJ, Todd JA. Molecular genetics of diabetes mellitus. Baillière's Clin Endocrinol Metab 1995;9:631–656.
70. Owerbach D, Gabbay KH. The search for IDDM susceptibility genes: the next generation. Diabetes 1996;45:544–551.
71. Lipes M, Eienbarth GS. Transgenic mouse models of type I Diabetes. Diabetes 1990;39:879–884.
72. Platz P, Jacobsen BK, Morling N, et al. HLA-D and HLA-DR antigens in genetic analysis of insulin-dependent diabetes mellitus. Diabetologia 1981;21:1108–1115.
73. Wolf E, Spencer KM, Cudworth AG. The genetic susceptibility to type I (insulin dependent) diabetes: analysis of the HLA-DR association. Diabetologia 1983;24:224–230.

74. Walker A, Cudworth AG. Type I (insulin-dependent) diabetic multiplex families: mode of genetic transmissions. Diabetes 1983;33:176–183.
75. Nerup JJ, Platz P, Anderson O, et al. HLA antigens and diabetes mellitus. Lancet 1974;2:864.
76. Cudworth AG, Woodrow JC. Genetic susceptibility in diabetes mellitus: analysis of the HLA association. Lancet 1976;2:846–850.
77. Barbosa J, Chern MM, Reinsmoen N, et al. HLA-Dw antigens in unrelated juvenile, insulin-dependent diabetics. Tissue Antigens 1979;14:426–430.
78. Sachs JA, Cudworth AG, Jaraquemada D, et al. Type I diabetes and the HLA-D locus. Diabetologia 1980;18:41–47.
79. Rudert WA, Trucco M. Rapid detection of sequence variation using polymers of specific digionucleotides. Nucleic Acid Res 1992;5:1146.
80. Faas SJ, Menon R, Braun ER, et al. Sequence-specific priming and exonuclease-released fluorescence detection of HLA-DQB1 alleles. Tissue Antigens 1996;48:97–112.
81. Menon R, Rudert WA, Braun ER, et al. Sequence-specific priming exonuclease-released fluorescence assay for a rapid and reliable HLA-A molecular typing. Mol Diagn 1997;2(2):99–111.
82. Todd JA, Bell JI, McDevitt HO. HLA-DQβ gene contributes to susceptibility and resistance to insulin-dependent diabetes mellitus. Nature 1987;329:509–604.
83. Khalil I, D'Auriol L, Gobet M, et al. A combination of HLA-DQ beta Asp 57-negative and HLA-DQ Arg 52 confers susceptibility to insulin-dependent diabetes mellitus. J Clin Invest 1990;85:1315–1319.
84. Lipton RB, Kocova M, LaPorte RE, et al. Autoimmunity and genetic factors contribute to the risk of insulin-dependent diabetes mellitus in families: islet cell antibodies and HLA DQ heterodimers. Am J Epidemiol 1992;136:503–512.
85. Gutierrez-Lopez MD, Bertera S, Chantres MT, et al. Susceptibility to type I diabetes in Spanish patients correlates quantitatively with expression of HLA-DQα Arg 52 and HLA-DQα non-Asp 57 alleles. Diabetologia 1992;35:583–588.
86. Erlich HA, Zeidler A, Chang J, et al. HLA class II alleles and susceptibility and resistance to insulin dependent diabetes mellitus in Mexican-American families. Nat Genet 1993;3:358–364.
87. Khalil I, Deschamps I, Lepage V, et al. Dose effect of cis- and trans-Encoded HLA-DQalpha/beta heterodimers in IDDM susceptibility. Diabetes 1992;41:378–384.
88. Dalton TA, Bennet JC. Autoimmune disease and the major histocompatibility complex: therapeutic implications. Am J Med 1992;92:183–188.
89. Owerbach D, Lernmark A, Platz P, et al. HLA-D region beta chain DNA endonuclease fragments differ between HLA-DR identical healthy and insulin dependent diabetic individuals. Nature 1983;303:813–817.
90. Cohen-Haguenaur O, Robbins E, Massart C, et al. A systematic study of HLA class II beta DNA restriction fragments in insulin-dependent diabetes mellitus. Proc Natl Acad Sci USA 1985;82:3335–3339.
91. Todd JA, Acha-Orbea H, Bell JI, et al. A molecular basis for MHC class II associated autoimmunity. Science 1988;240:1003–1009.
92. Sheehy MJ, Scharf SJ, Rowe JR, et al. A diabetes susceptible HLA haplotype is best defined by a combination of HLA-DR and DQ alleles. J Clin Invest 1989;83:830–835.
93. LaPorte RE, Fishbein HA, Drash AL, et al. The Pittsburgh IDDM registry. The incidence of IDDM in Allegheny County, PA. Diabetes 1981;30:279–284.
94. National Diabetes Data Group Classification and diagnosis of diabetes mellitus and other categories of glucose intolerance. Diabetes 1979;28:1039–1057.
95. Lipton RB, Atchison J, Dorman JS, et al. Genetic, immunological, and metabolic determinants of risk for type 1 diabetes mellitus in families. Diabet Med 1992;9:224–232.
96. The Expert Committee on the Diagnosis and Classification of Diabetes Mellitus. Report of the Expert Committee on the Diagnosis and Classification of Diabetes Mellitus. Diabetes Care 1997;20:1183–1197.
97. Pietropaolo M, Becker DJ, LaPorte RE, et al. Progression to insulin-requiring diabetes in seronegative prediabetic subjects: the role of two HLA-DQ high-risk haplotypes. Diabetologia 2002;45:66–76.
98. Thorsby E, Rønningen KS. Role of HLA genes in predisposition to develop insulin-dependent diabetes mellitus. Ann Med 1992;24:523–531.
99. Thorsby E, Ronningen KS. Particular HLA-DQ molecules play a dominant role in determining susceptibility or resistance to type I (insulin-dependent) diabetes mellitus. Diabetologia 1993;36:371–377.
100. Thorsby E. Invited anniversary review: HLA associated diseases. Hum Immunol 1997;53:1–11.
101. Cucca F, Muntoni F, Lampis R, et al. Combination of specific DRB1, DQA1, DQB1 haplotypes are associated with insulin-dependent diabetes mellitus in Sardinia. Hum Immunol 1993;37:85–94.

102. Kockum I, Wassmuth R, Holmberg E, et al. HLA-DQ primarily confers protection and HLA-DR susceptibility in type 1 (insulin-dependent) diabetes studied in population-based affected families and controls. Am J Hum Genet 1993;53:150–167.
103. Kockum I, Dahlquist G, Falorni A, et al. Genetic and immunological findings in patients with newly diagnosed insulin-dependent diabetes mellitus. Horm Metab Res 1996;28:344–347.
104. Cucca F, Lampis R, Frau F, et al. The distribution of DR4 haplotypes in Sardinia suggests a primary association of type 1 diabetes with DRB1 and DQB1 loci. Hum Immunol 1995;43:301–308.
105. Penny MA, Jenkins D, Mijovic CH, et al. Susceptibility to IDDM in a Chinese population: role of HLA class II alleles. Diabetes 1992;41:914–919.
106. Awata T, Kuzuya T, Matsuda A, et al. Genetic analysis of HLA class II alleles and susceptibility to type 1 (insulin-dependent) diabetes mellitus in Japanese subjects. Diabetologia 1992;35:419–424.
107. Huang HS, Peng JT, She JY, et al. HLA-Encoded susceptibility to insulin-dependent diabetes mellitus is determined by DR and DQ genes as well as their linkage disequilibrium in a Chinese population. Hum Immunol 1995;44:210–219.
108. Nepom GT, Erlich H. MHC class-II molecules and autoimmunity. Annu Rev Immunol 1991;9:493–525.
109. Tait BD, Drummond BP, Varney MD, et al. HLA-DRB1*0401 is associated with susceptibility to insulin-dependent diabetes mellitus independently of the DQB1 locus. Eur J Immunogenet 1995;22:289–297.
110. Yasunaga S, Kimura A, Hamaguchi H, et al. Different contribution of HLA-DR and DQ genes in susceptibility and resistance to insulin-dependent diabetes mellitus (IDDM). Tissue Antigens 1996;47:37–48.
111. Sanjeevi CB, Hook P, Landin-Olsson M, et al. DR4 subtypes and their molecular properties in a population-based study of Swedish childhood diabetes. Tissue Antigens 1996;47:275–283.
112. Awata T, Kuzuya T, Matsuda A, et al. High frequency of aspartic acid at position 57 of HLA-DQ β-chain in Japanese IDDM patients and non-diabetic subjects. Diabetes 1990;39:266–269.
113. Morales P, Martinez-Laso J, Martin-Villa JM, et al. High frequency of the HLA-DRB1*0405(Dw15)-DQw8 haplotype in Spaniards and its relationship to diabetes sus44eptibility. Hum Immunol 1991;32:170–175.
114. Van der Auwera B, Van Waeyenberge C, Schuit F, et al. DRB1*0403 protects against IDDM in Caucasians with the high-risk heterozygous DQA1*0301-DQB1*0302/DQA1*0501-DQB1*0201 genotype. Belgian Diabetes Registry. Diabetes 1995;44:527–530.
115. Noble JA, Valdes AM, Thomson G, et al. The HLA class II locus DPB1 can influence susceptibility to type 1 diabetes. Diabetes 2000;49:121–125.
116. Thomson G, Robinson WP, Kuhner MK, et al. Genetic heterogeneity, modes of inheritance, and risk estimates for a joint study of Caucasians with insulin-dependent diabetes mellitus. Am J Hum Genet 1988;43:799–816.
117. Thomson G, Robinson WP, Kuhner MK, et al. HLA and insulin gene associations with IDDM. Genet Epidemiol 1989;6:155–160.
118. Horn GT, Bugawan TL, Long CM, et al. Allelic sequence variation of the HLA-DQ loci: relationship to serology and to insulin-dependent diabetes mellitus susceptibility. Proc Natl Acad Sci USA 1988;85:6012–6016.
119. Baisch JM, Weeks T, Giles R, et al. Analysis of HLA-DQ genotypes and susceptibility in insulin-dependent diabetes mellitus. N Engl J Med 1990;322:1836–1841.
120. Sorrentino R, DeGrazia U, Buzzetti R, et al. An explanation for the neutral effect of DR2 on IDDM susceptibility in central Italy. Diabetes 1992;41:904–908.
121. Ronningen KS, Spurkland A, Iwe T, et al. Distribution of HLA-DRB1,-DQA1 and -DQB1 alleles and DQA1-DQB1 genotypes among Norwegian patients with insulin-dependent diabetes mellitus. Tissue Antigens 1991;37:105–111.
122. Ronningen KS, Spurkland A, Tait BD, et al. HLA class II associations in insulin-dependent diabetes mellitus among blacks, caucasoids, and Japanese. In: Tsuji K, Aizawa M, Sasazuki T, eds. HLA 1991: Proceedings of the 11th International Histocompatibility Workshop and Conference. Oxford University Press, Oxford, 1992, Vol. 1, pp. 713–722.
123. Zeliszewski D, Tiercy J, Boitard C, et al. Extensive study of DRbeta, DQalpha, and DQbeta gene polymorphism in 23 DR2-positive, insulin-dependent diabetes mellitus patients. Hum Immunol 1992;33:140–147.
124. Sanjeevi CB, Lybrand TP, DeWeese C, et al. Polymorphic amino acid variations in HLA-DQ are associated with systematic physical property changes and occurrence of IDDM. Diabetes 1995;44:125–131.

125. Kockum I, Sanjeevi CB, Eastman S, et al. Population analysis of protection by HLA-DR and DQ genes from insulin-dependent diabetes mellitus in Swedish children with insulin-dependent diabetes and controls. Eur J Immunogenet 1995;22:443–465.
126. Sanjeevi CB, DeWeese C, Landin-Olsson M, et al. Analysis of critical residues if HLA-DQ6 molecules in insulin-dependent diabetes mellitus. Tissue Antigens 1997;50:61–65.
127. Wen L, Wong FS, Tang J, et al. In vivo evidence for the contribution of human histocompatibility leukocyte antigen (HLA)-DQ molecules to the development of diabetes. J Exp Med 2000;191:97–104.
128. Miyazaki T, Uno M, Uehira M, et al. Direct evidence for the contribution of unique I-A^{NOD} to the development of insulitis in non-obese diabetic mice. Nature 1990;345:722–724.
129. Slattery RM, Kjer-Nielsen L, Allison J, et al. Prevention of diabetes in non-obese diabetic I-Ak transgenic mice. Nature 1990;345:724–726.
130. Lund T, O'Reilly L, Hutchings P, et al. Prevention of insulin-dependent diabetes mellitus in non-obese diabetic mice by transgenes encoding modified I-A beta chain or normal I-E alpha chain. Nature 1990;345:727–729.
131. Nishimoto H, Kikutani H, Yamamura K, et al. Prevention of autoimmune insulitis by expression of I-E molecules in NOD mice. Nature 1987;328:432–434.
132. Boitard C, Bendelac A, Richard MF, et al. Prevention of diabetes in nonobese diabetic mice by anti-I-A monoclonal antibodies: transfer of protection by splenic T cells. Proc Natl Acad Sci USA 1988;85:9719–9723.
133. Brown JH, Jardetzky T, Saper MA, et al. A hypothetical model of the foreign antigen binding site of class II histocompatibility molecules. Nature 1988;332:845–850.
134. Brown JH, Jardetzky TS, Gorga JC, et al. Three-dimensional structure of the human class II histocompatibility antigen HLA-DR1. Nature 1993;364:33–39.
135. Jardetzky TS, Brown JH, Gorga JC, et al. Three-dimensional structure of a human class II histocompatibility molecule complexed with superantigen. Nature 1994;368:711–718.
136. Turco E, Manfras BJ, Ge L, et al. The x boxes from promoters of HLA class II B genes at different loci do not compete for nuclear protein-specific binding. Immunogenetics 1990;32:117–128.
137. Demotz S, Grey HM, Sette A. The minimal number of class II MHC-antigen complexes needed for T cell activation. Science 1990;249:1028–1030.
138. Haars R, Kronenberg H, Gallaten WM, et al. Rearrangement and expression of T cell antigen receptor and γ-genes during thymic development. J Exp Med 1986;164:1–24.
139. von Boehmer H. Positive selection of lymphocytes. Cell 1994;76:219–228.
140. Nossal GJV. Negative selection of lymphocytes. Cell 1994;76:229–239.
141. Davey MP, Meyer MM, Bakke AC. T Cell receptor Vβ gene expression in monozygotic twins: discordance in CD8 subset and in disease states. J Immunol 1994;152:315–321.
142. Nepom GT, Kwok WT. Molecular basis for HLA-DQ association in IDDM. Diabetes 1998;47:1177–1184.
143. Anderson LC, Beaty JS, Nettles JW, et al. Allelic polymorphisms in transcriptional regulatory regions of HLA-DQB genes. J Exp Med 1991;173:181–192.
144. Carcassi C, Trucco G, Trucco M, et al. A new HLA-DR2 extended haplotype is involved in IDDM susceptibility. Hum Immunol 1991;31:159–164.
145. Pugliese A. Genetic protection from insulin-dependent diabetes mellitus. Diabetes Nutr Metab 1997;10:169–179.
146. DPT-1 Study Group The Diabetes Prevention Trial—Type 1 diabetes (DPT-1): implementation of screening and staging of relatives. Transplant Proc 1995;27:3377.
147. Pugliese A, Kawasaki E, Zeller M, et al. Sequence analysis of the diabetes-protective human leukocyte antigen-DQB1*0602 allele in unaffected, islet cell antibody-positive first degree relatives and in rare patients with type 1 diabetes. J Clin Endocrinol Metab 1999;84:1728–1728.
148. Greenbaum CJ, Schatz DA, Cuthbertson D, et al. Islet cell antibody-positive relatives with human leukocyte antigen DQA1*0102, DQB1*0602: identification by the Diabetes Prevention Trial-type 1. J Clin Endocrinol Metab 2000;85:1255–1260.
149. Bell GI, Karam JH, Rutter WJ. Polymorphic DNA region adjacent to the 5′ end of the human insulin gene. Proc Natl Acad Sci USA 1981;78:5759–5763.
150. Rotwein P, Chyn R, Chirgwin J, et al. Polymorphism in the 5′-flanking region of the human insulin gene and its possible relation to type II diabetes. Science 1981;213:1117–1120.
151. Owerbach D, Nerup J. Restriction fragment length polymorphism of the insulin gene in diabetes mellitus. Diabetes 1982;31:275–277.

152. Julier C, Hyer RN, Davies J, et al. Insulin-IGF2 region encodes a gene implicated in HLA-DR4-dependent diabetes susceptibility. Nature 1991;354:155–159.
153. Bain SC, Prins JB, Hearne CM, et al. Insulin gene region-encoded susceptibility to type 1 diabetes is not restricted to HLA-DR4-positive individuals. Nat Genet 1992;2:212–215.
154. Bennett ST, Lucassen AM, Gough SCL, et al. Susceptibility to human type 1 diabetes at IDDM2 is determined by tandem repeat variation at the insulin gene minisatellite locus. Nat Genet 1995;9:284–292.
155. Bennett ST, Wilson AJ, Cucca F, et al. *IDDM2-VNTR*-encoded susceptibility to type 1 diabetes: dominant protection and parental transmission of alleles of the insulin gene-linked minisatellite locus. J Autoimmun 1996;9:415–421.
156. Bennett ST, Wilson AJ, Esposito L, et al. Insulin VNTR allele-specific in type 1 diabetes depend on identity of untransmitted paternal allele. Nat Genet 1997;17:350–352.
157. Lucassen AM, Screaton GR, Julier C, et al. Regulation of insulin gene expression by the IDDM associated, insulin locus haplotype. Hum Mol Genet 1994;4:501–506.
158. Kennedy GC, German MS, Rutter WJ. The minisatellite in the diabetes susceptibility locus IDDM2 regulates insulin transcription. Nat Genet 1995;9:293–298.
159. Krontiris TG. Minisatellites and human disease. Science 1995;269:1682–1683.
160. Krontiris TG, Delvin B, Karp DD, et al. An association between the risk of cancer and mutation in the HRAS1 minisatellite locus. N Engl J Med 1993;329:517–523.
161. Kiaris H, Spandidos DA, Jones AS, et al. Mutations, expression and genomic instability of the H-ras proto-oncogene in squamous cell carcinomas of the head and neck. Br J Cancer 1995;72:123–128.
162. Wang YH, Griffith J. Expanded CTG triplet block from the myotonic dystrophy gene create the strongest known nucleosome positioning elements. Nat Genet 1995;25:570–573.
163. McGinnis RE, Spielman RS. Insulin expression: is *VNTR* allele 698 really anomalous? Nat Genet 1995;10:378–380.
164. Davies JL, Kawaguchi Y, Bennett ST, et al. A genome-wide search for human type I diabetes susceptibility genes. Nature 1994;371:130–136.
165. Cordell HJ, Todd JA, Bennett ST, et al. Two-locus maximum lod score analysis of a multifactorial trait: joint consideration of *IDDM2* and *IDDM4* with *IDDM1* in type I diabetes. Am J Hum Genet 1995;57:920–934.
166. Todd JA. Genetic analysis of type 1 diabetes using whole genome approaches. Proc Natl Acad Sci USA 1995;92:8560–8565.
167. Thomson G. Identifying complex disease genes: progress and paradigms. Nat Genet 1994;8:108–110.
168. Thomson G. Strategies involved in mapping diabetes genes: an overview. Diabetes Rev 1997;5:106–115.
169. Morahan G, Huang D, Tait BD, et al. Markers on distal chromosome 2q linked to insulin-dependent diabetes mellitus. Science 1996;272:1811–1813.
170. Van der Auwera BJ, Vanderwalle CL, Schuit F. et al. CTL-4 gene polymorphism confers susceptibility to insulin-dependent diabetes mellitus (IDDM) independently from age and from other genetic or immune disease markers. The Belgian Diabetes Registry. Clin Exp Immunol 1997;110:98–103.
171. Kruglyak L, Daly M, Reeve-Daly MP, et al. Parametric and nonparametric linkage analysis: a unified multipoint approach. Am J Hum Genet 1996;58:1347–1363.
172. Becker KG, Simon RM, Bailey-Wilson JE, et al. Clustering on non-major histocompatibility complex susceptibility candidate loci in human autoimmune diseases. Proc Natl Acad Sci USA 1998;95:8879–8894.
173. Morel L, Rudofsky UH, Longmate JA, et al. Polygenic control of susceptibility to murine systemic lupus erythematosus. Immunity 1995;1:219–229.
174. Kono DH, Burlingame RW, Owens DG, et al. Lupus susceptibility loci in New Zealand mice. Proc Natl Acad Sci USA 1994;91:19,168–19,172.
175. Gottlieb PA, Eisenbarth GS. Diagnosis and treatment of pre-insulin dependent diabetes. Annu Rev Med 1998;49:391–405.
176. Gaffney PM, Kearns GM, Shark KB, et al. A genome-wide search for susceptibility genes in human systemic lupus erythematosus sib-pair families. Proc Natl Acad Sci USA 1998;95:14,875–14,879.
177. Daniels SE, Bhattacharrya S, James A, et al. A genome-wide search for quantitative trait loci underlying asthma. Nature 1996;383:247–250.
178. Haines JL, Ter-Minassian M, Bazyk A, et al. A complete genome screen for multiple sclerosis underscores a role for the major histocompatibility complex. Nat Genet 1996;13:469–471.
179. Collins A, Frezal J, Teague J, et al. A metric map of humans: 23,500 loci in 850 bands. Proc Natl Acad Sci USA 1998;93:14,771–14,775.

180. She J-X, Marron MP. Genetic susceptibility factors in type 1 diabetes: linkage, disequilibrium and functional analyses. Curr Opin Immunol 1998;114:370–376.
181. Lucassen AM, Julier C, Beressi JP, et al. Susceptibility to insulin dependent diabetes maps to a 4.1 kb segment of DNA spanning the insulin gene and associated VNTR. Nat Genet 1993;4:305–310.
182. Halminen M, Veijola R, Reijonen H, et al. Effect of polymorphism in the insulin gene region on IDDM susceptibility and insulin secretion. Eur J Clin Invest 1996;26:847–852.
183. Vafiadis P, Bennett ST, Todd JA, et al. Divergence between genetic determinants of IGF2 transcription levels in leukocytes and of IDDM2-encoded susceptibility to type 1 diabetes. J Clin Endocrinol Metab 1998;83:2933–2939.
184. Mein CA, Esposito L, Dunn MG, et al. A search for type 1 diabetes susceptibility genes in families from the United Kingdom. Nat Genet 1998;19:297–300.
185. Lernmark Å, Ott J. Sometimes it's hot, sometimes it's not. Nat Genet 1998;19:213–214.
186. Sattar MA, Al-Sughyer AA, Siboo R. Coexistence of rheumatoid arthritis, ankylosing spondylitis and dermatomyositis in a patient with diabetes mellitus and the associated linked HLA antigens. Br J Rheumatol 1988;27:146–149.
187. Yamato E, Ikegami H, Kawaguchi Y, et al. Insulin-dependent diabetes mellitus associated with autoimmune thyroiditis and rheumatoid arthritis. Am J Med Sci 1997;313:64–66.
188. Rose NR. Autoimmune disease—tracing the shared threads. Hosp Pract 1997;32:147–154.
189. Aaltonen J, Horelli-Kuitunen N, Fan J-B, et al. High-resolution physical and transcriptional mapping of the autoimmune polyendocrinopathy–candidiasis–ectodermal dystrophy locus on chromosome 21q22.3. Genome Res 1997;7:820–829.
190. The Finnish–German APECED Consortium. An autoimmune disease, APECED, caused by mutations in a novel gene featuring two PHD-type zinc-finger domains. Nat Genet 1997;17:399–403.
191. Nagamine K, Peterson P, Scott HS, et al. Positional cloning of the APECED gene. Nat Genet 1997;17:393–398.
192. Luppi P, Rossiello MR, Faas S, Trucco M. Genetic background and environment contribute synergistically to the onset of autoimmune diseases. J Mol Med 1995;73:381–393.
193. Rosner G, Martell J, Trucco M. Hematopoietic Stem Cell Therapy. Churchill Livingstone, Philadelphia, 2000, pp. 233–251.
194. Serreze DV, Leiter EH. Genes and cellular requirements for autoimmune diabetes susceptibility in NOD mice. In: von Herrath H, ed. Molecular Pathology of Insulin Dependent Diabetes Mellitus. Karger, New York, 2001, pp. 31–67.
195. Nepom GT. Class II antigens and disease susceptibility. Annu Rev Med 1995;46:17–25.

3 Prediction and Prevention of Type 1 Diabetes

Aristides K. Maniatis, MD *and*
George S. Eisenbarth, MD, PhD

CONTENTS

PREDICTION OF TYPE 1A DIABETES

Introduction

At present, the prediction of type 1 diabetes is not a major clinical issue outside of trials for diabetes prevention. Patients, especially children, usually present acutely with diabetes with a dramatic history of polyuria, polydipsia, and weight loss. Despite what in retrospect is almost always a clear-cut clinical history of diabetes, a significant number of children have a delay in diagnosis, which increases the risk of severe metabolic decompensation with diabetic ketoacidosis (DKA), cerebral edema, and death. In Colorado for instance, with a population of four million, approx 1 child dies at the onset of type 1 diabetes every 2 yr. Overall in the United States, DKA occurs in 25–50% of children with new-onset diabetes, and symptomatic cerebral edema occurs in approx 1% of DKA episodes. Of those patients with clinically apparent cerebral edema, between 40% and 90% die *(1)*.

In an attempt to identify risk factors for cerebral edema, a multicenter study evaluated several laboratory value parameters on hospital admission and different therapeutic regimens. It revealed that hypocarbia and treatment with bicarbonate were the two independent variables that placed patients at highest risk for cerebral edema *(1)*. Perhaps the greatest risk factor for poor outcomes, however, is the misdiagnosis or delay in diagnosis once the child is seen by a health care provider. Therefore, for acutely ill children, one should have a very low threshold for obtaining a urine and finger-stick glucose, two simple rapid tests that can rule out diabetes.

From: *Contemporary Endocrinology: Type 1 Diabetes: Etiology and Treatment*
Edited by: M. A. Sperling © Humana Press Inc., Totowa, NJ

Despite the usual acute dramatic presentation of diabetes, there is now considerable evidence that type 1 diabetes (particularly the common immune form of type 1 diabetes termed type 1A diabetes) is a chronic autoimmune disorder *(2,3)*. In studies of relatives of patients with type 1A diabetes and recent studies of children from the general population, anti-islet autoantibodies usually precede the development of diabetes by years *(4–9)*. There may be some children with acute development of autoimmunity and rapid progression to diabetes, but discovering such children in prospective studies will require considerable effort, as it appears that they are rare. There are a number of reports of acute development of type 1 diabetes ascribed to acute viral infections *(10)*. It is likely that these reports may represent viral infections occurring in individuals who expressed anti-islet autoantibodies years prior to the acute infection. A recent report from Japan described several individuals with likely a form of type 1B diabetes, who, despite marked hyperglycemia, had normal HbA1c levels, suggesting a truly acute development of diabetes *(11)*. These individuals also had elevated pancreatic serum enzymes and pancreatitis but not islet inflammation. In the United States, with a much higher incidence of type 1 diabetes compared to Japan, it is rare to find individuals presenting with diabetes with normal HbA1c and it is likely that the great majority have had hyperglycemia for months prior to diagnosis.

Stages in the Development of Type 1A Diabetes

One can divide the development of type 1A diabetes into a series of stages, beginning with genetic susceptibility and ending with essentially complete destruction of all islet β-cells (*see* Fig. 1). At the end of the process, individuals are truly insulin dependent, but during earlier phases of the disease, glucose metabolism is normal, becomes impaired, and even at the onset of diabetes, a significant amount of insulin is produced. The amount of insulin produced endogenously is determined by measuring C-peptide, the peptide cleaved from proinsulin, because C-peptide is not contained within the exogenous insulin used for therapy. Some individuals will produce C-peptide for more than 5 yr after the onset of type 1A diabetes, but the great majority become C-peptide negative (usually defined as less than 1–2 pmol/L of C-peptide following standard meal stimulation) within several years. Overall, children have a more rapid course of loss of C-peptide. Between 5% and 20% of adults thought to have type 2 diabetes have a slowly progressive form of type 1A diabetes *(12,13)*. These adults produce significant C-peptide for several years after diabetes onset and can be treated with oral hypoglycemic agents. One term for such adults is LADA, or latent autoimmune diabetes of adults *(14,15)*. These adults usually express anti-islet autoantibodies and this has led to their recent recognition.

Although Fig. 1 aids in conceptualizing the development of type 1 diabetes, the disease process, in fact, is more complex, and both genetic and environmental factors may act to modify disease progression during any of the stages *(3)*.

Genetic Risk

Clinical

Approximately 1/300 children in the United Sates develop type 1A diabetes throughout their life, with a reported incidence of approx 15/100,000. Finland has the highest incidence, approaching 50/100,000 *(16)*, and Japan has one of the lowest (approx 1/100,000 in children). The incidence appears to be increasing worldwide and recent

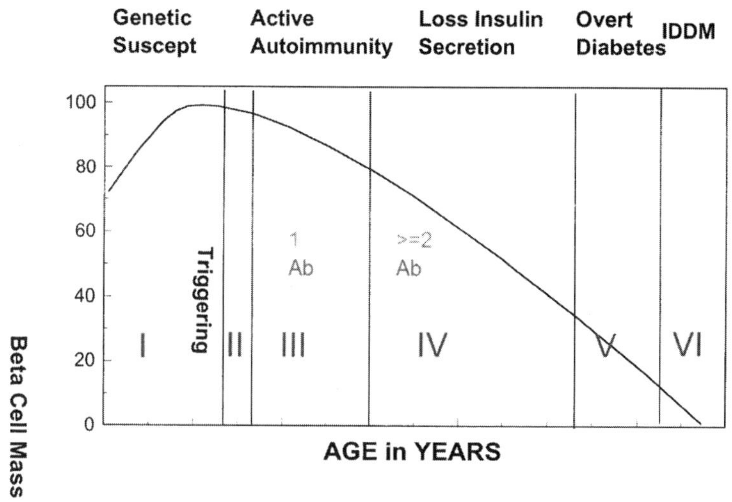

Fig. 1. Hypothetical stages in the development of type 1A diabetes. IDDM, insulin-dependent diabetes mellitus. (Modified from ref. *2*.)

data from Colorado suggest that the incidence has increased to 25/100,000 *(17,18)*. The etiology of the increasing incidence is not defined, but it suggests environmental change (either decreasing protective factors or increasing "triggering" factors). First-degree relatives of patients with type 1A diabetes have a risk of approx 5%, including siblings, offspring, and parents. The risk of type 1A diabetes of an offspring of a mother with diabetes is less than for a father with type 1A diabetes *(19)*, and siblings appear to have a risk for early childhood anti-islet autoimmunity and diabetes approximately twice that of offspring *(20)*. Dizygotic twins have a risk similar to siblings, and monozygotic twins have a "lifetime" risk of approx 50% *(21)*. As illustrated in Fig. 2, initially discordant monozygotic twins of patients with type 1A diabetes can progress to diabetes decades after the onset of diabetes in their proband twin. In addition, there appears to be genetic heterogeneity in eventual concordance, with twin mates whose twin developed diabetes after age 25 having a relatively low risk of progression to diabetes *(21)*. Despite the high risk to relatives, it must be realized that between 85% and 90% of children developing type 1A diabetes do not have a relative with the disease.

In addition to a family history of diabetes predicting an increased risk, diabetes is also associated with other autoimmune diseases. Two of the most dramatic syndromes associated with diabetes begin in neonates or very young children, and mutations underlying autoimmunity have been defined. These syndromes are termed "autoimmune polyendocrine syndrome type I" (APS-1) *(22)* and "X-linked polyendocrinopathy, immune dysfunction, and diarrhea" (XPID) *(23)*. Approximately 18% of patients with the autosomal mutations of the autoimmune regulator *(AIRE)* gene underlying the APS-I syndrome develop type 1A diabetes, in addition to their mucocutaneous candidiasis, Addison's disease, and/or hypoparathyroidism *(24)*. The XPID syndrome presents with fatal overwhelming neonatal autoimmune disease, and it is suggested that such children might benefit from bone marrow transplantation *(23)*.

Much more common associations with type 1A diabetes include celiac disease *(25–27)*, thyroid autoimmunity, Addison's disease (often as part of APS-II) *(28)*, myasthenia gravis, and pernicious anemia. For example, 1/20 children with type 1A

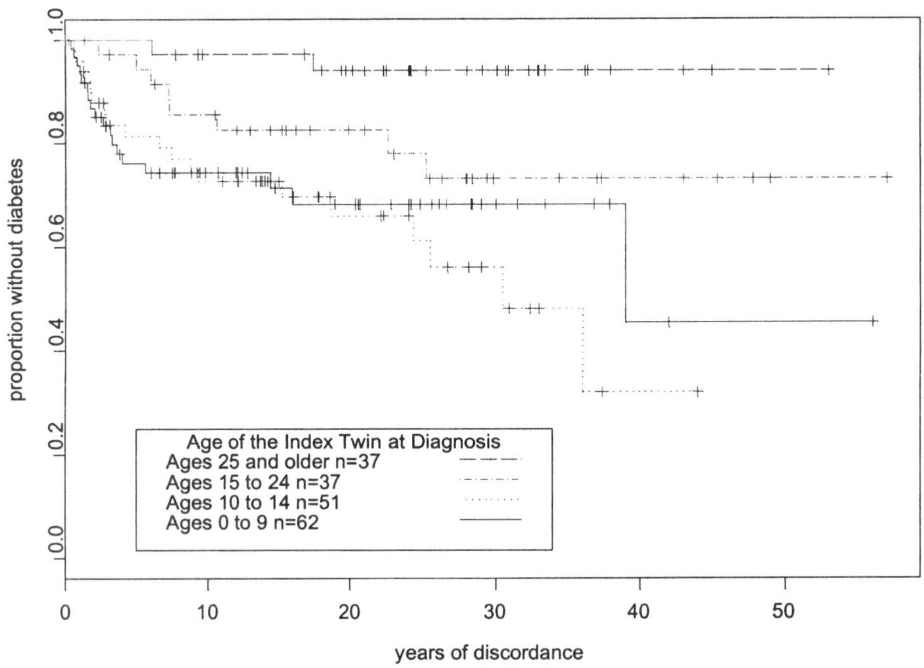

Fig. 2. Progression to diabetes of initially discordant monozygotic twins of patients with type 1A diabetes, subdivided by the age of diabetes onset of the proband twin. (From ref. *21.*)

diabetes have celiac disease. Approximately 1/10 express antitransglutaminase autoantibodies, and half of these (thus, 1/20) have celiac disease on biopsy *(27,29)*. Most of these children are asymptomatic. In addition, relatives of patients with type 1A diabetes also have an increased frequency of nondiagnosed celiac disease *(27)*. Thyroid autoimmunity is usually screened for with determination of thyroid-stimulating hormone (TSH) levels. Addison's disease probably occurs in approx 1/200 individuals with type 1A diabetes compared to 1/20,000 in the general population. The presence of 21-hydroxylase autoantibodies suggests the need for prospective evaluation of adrenal function *(28,30)*.

Laboratory-Defined Genetic Risk

At present, the best-defined genetic markers for common forms of type 1A diabetes are alleles of genes within the major histocompatibility complex (MHC) on the sixth chromosome *(31–33)*. There are more than 100 genes within the complex, but the genes providing prognostic information are predominantly DRβ, DQα, and DQβ. Each allele of each of these genes is now defined at the nucleotide level and is given a specific number (e.g., DRB1*0301). The first two numbers usually refer to older serologic typing and the last two numbers specify a specific sequence. The genes of the complex are in close genetic proximity. Thus, they are linked when inherited (because crossing over between genes within a family is rare) and are in linkage dysequilibrium (alleles of different genes are nonrandomly associated with each other on the same chromosome in the population). Therefore, one can define alleles of a single gene, a group of alleles of different genes on the same chromosome (a haplotype), or, what is most important in determining

Table 1
Diabetes Risk by HLA DQ and DR Haplotypes

	DRB1	*DQA1*	*DQB1*
High risk	0401 (0405,0402) (DR4)	0301	0302
	0301 (DR3)	0501	0201
	0801	0401	0402
Moderate risk	0401 (0405,0402)	0301	0301
	0401 (0405,0402)	0301	0303
	0403	0301	0302
	0101	0101	0501
	1601	0102	0502
Low risk	1101	0501	0301
Protective	1501 (DR2)	0102	0602
	0701	0201	0303
	1401	0101	0503

diabetes risk, the genotype of an individual (namely all of the alleles on an individual's two sixth chromosomes). For example, an individual with the two DQ haplotypes, DQA1*0501, DQB1*0201 (DR3 associated) and DQA1*0301, DQB1*0302 (DR4 associated) have the highest risk for type 1 diabetes. As each allele codes for a specific molecule and all the combinations of these molecules are possible, such individuals will have four different DQ molecules (DQA*0501/DQB1*0201, DQA1*0301 DQB1*0302) on the surface of their antigen-presenting cells, as expected, but also DQA1*0501/DQB1*0302 and DQA1*0301/DQB1*0201. Individuals of African descent have a haplotype with DQA1*0301/DQB1*0201 on the same chromosome and, as expected, it confers high risk. In addition to risk, some human leukocyte antigen (HLA) DQ molecules are associated with protection from type 1A diabetes. The DQA1*0102/DQB1*0602 haplotype is present in approx 20% of most populations but in less than 1% of children developing type 1A diabetes *(34)*. Protection appears to be dominant over susceptibility *(35)*. Patients with DQA1*0102/DQB1*0602 and diabetes may have unusual variants of diabetes (e.g., type 2 diabetes in children) or may be currently unexplained exceptions. Another remarkably protective DQ haplotype is DQA1*0201/DQB1*0303, but this haplotype is relatively uncommon.

DR alleles also influence diabetes risk. DRB1*1401 is reported to provide dominant protection similar to DQA1*0102/DQB1*0602, although, again, it is relatively uncommon *(36)*. The DR4 allele, DRB1*0403, when associated with DQA1*0301/DQB1*0302 decreases the risk associated with the DQB1*0302. There is no simple "rule" for diabetes risk, and Table 1 summarizes a series of haplotype-associated risks. The observation that aspartic acid at position 57 of the DQ molecule is associated with protection from type 1A diabetes has too many exceptions to be useful (e.g., DQA1*0401/DQB1*0402 and DQA1*0301/DQB1*0401 are both high risk).

At present, the genetic risk associated with HLA alleles is primarily utilized in research studies. A few centers in Europe, the United States, and Canada have begun epidemiologic studies in which thousands of children are HLA typed at birth, the risk of diabetes (and often celiac disease) is determined, and individuals are followed for the development of anti-islet autoantibodies and diabetes *(37,38)*. A child with the highest-risk HLA genotype for type 1 diabetes from the general population has a risk of approx 5% of developing diabetes and will comprise approx 40% of all children developing type 1A diabetes. In contrast, a child with the same HLA DR and DQ alleles who is the offspring of a patient with type 1A diabetes has a risk of approx 20% *(39)*, and a sibling has a risk exceeding 40% of activating anti-islet autoimmunity. This extremely high risk for relatives explains the participation of relatives in most of the trials for the prevention of diabetes.

Alleles of genes within the MHC appear to account for approximately half of the familial aggregation of type 1A diabetes. It is likely that such DR and DQ alleles direct autoimmunity to certain target organs. For instance, although DQA1*0102/DQB1*0602 protects from type 1A diabetes, it is associated with high risk for multiple sclerosis. A major effort is underway to identify additional genetic risk factors. It is clear that variation of a nucleotide tandem repeat sequence 5′ of the insulin gene contributes to diabetes risk *(40–42)*. The group of alleles with the largest number of repeats provides protection from diabetes, and these alleles appear to account for a little less than 10% of the familial aggregation in Western countries. Of note, the tandem repeat associated with diabetes protection is associated with greater thymic insulin messenger RNA *(43)*.

Autoantibody Expression/T-Cell Assays

More than 90% of children presenting with type 1A diabetes express one of three anti-islet autoantibodies (autoantibodies reacting with insulin [IAA], an islet enzyme termed glutamic acid decarboxylase 65 [GAD65], or a molecule of unknown function termed ICA512 [or IA-2]) *(4)*. These autoantibodies are typically present years prior to the development of diabetes. A relatively simple rule relates most of our current knowledge for prediction of diabetes, namely expression of two or more of the above autoantibodies is associated with a high risk of progression to diabetes (*see* Fig. 3) *(4,44,45)*. Expression of a single anti-islet autoantibody is associated with a risk of approx 20%, whereas most individuals (but not all) expressing multiple anti-islet autoantibodies progress to diabetes over the next 5–10 yr. Insulin autoantibodies appear to be unique in that they are usually the first autoantibody to appear in the youngest children developing type 1A diabetes *(46)*, and a high level of the autoantibody correlates with a more rapid progression to diabetes. For adults developing type 1A diabetes, GAD65 autoantibodies provide the highest sensitivity.

Although autoantibody testing has rapidly improved, the technology is relatively young, and when being applied to individuals, there are important caveats, as listed in Table 2. We currently do not utilize the cytoplasmic islet cell autoantibody test in that it has proven difficult to standardize, and when such antibodies are present in the absence of what are termed "biochemical" autoantibodies, diabetes risk is low. Insulin antibodies are induced by insulin therapy, even with human insulin; thus, several weeks postinsulin therapy, one may be measuring induced antibodies. Autoantibodies are not always static and they disappear in a few children who progress to diabetes prior to the onset of diabetes. One should not rely upon a single determination of autoantibodies. The presence of antibodies at more than one time-point has a much greater clinical relevance.

Although we have concentrated on autoantibodies, it is likely that (comparable to animal models of type 1A diabetes) the T-lymphocytes destroy islet β-cells *(47,48)*, and

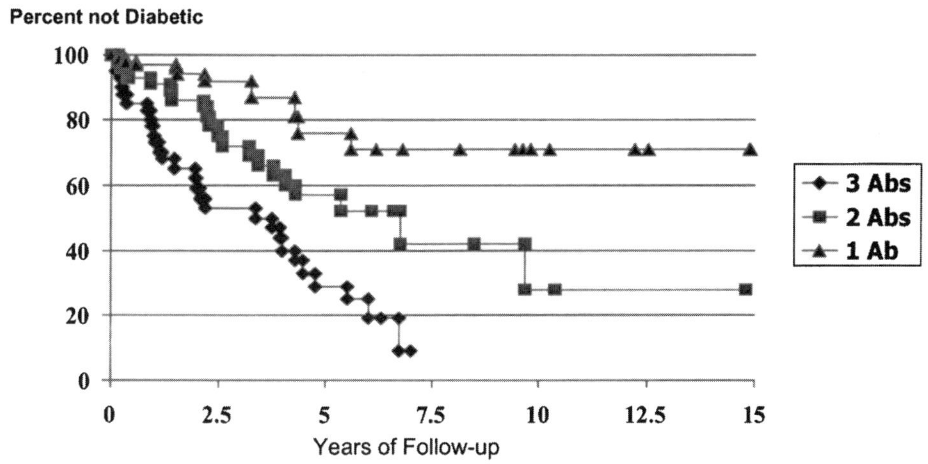

3 Ab n =	41	17	8	1		
2 Abs n =	44	27	15	4	2	1
1 Abs n =	93	23	14	10	6	4

Fig. 3. "Combinatorial" prediction of type 1 diabetes. (From ref. *4*.)

Table 2
Caveats of Autoantibody Testing

- Cytoplasmic islet cell antigen (ICA) assay is difficult to standardize.
- Radio-binding assays rather than enzyme-linked immunosorbent assay (ELISA) should be utilized.
- Laboratories differ in sensitivity and specificity: specificity should be set at >99%.
- Insulin antibodies develop after insulin therapy.
- Transient antibodies may occur and appear to have little prognostic significance.
- Young prediabetic children have high frequency of IAA, whereas prediabetic adults have a high frequency of GAD65.

autoantibodies are of marginal pathogenic significance in humans. Their lack of pathogenesis is suggested by the absence of diabetes in infants born to mothers expressing anti-islet autoantibodies. At present, assays for autoreactive T-lymphocytes are in their infancy, and a recent T-cell workshop suggested that proliferation assays were not sufficient to distinguish autoreactive T-cells associated with diabetes *(49)*. Two new techniques that are being applied offer some optimism, namely quantitation of individual T-cells producing cytokines (enzyme-linked immuno spot [ELISPOT]) *(50)* and analysis of T-cells with MHC complexed with peptides (termed "tetramer analysis") *(51,52)*.

Metabolic Progression

The great majority of individuals developing type 1A diabetes lose the ability to secrete insulin following intravenous glucose months to years prior to the onset of diabetes *(53–59)*. The test is usually performed with the infusion of 0.5 g/kg of glucose over several minutes, with determination of fasting insulin and insulin at 1 and 3 min after glucose infusion. The Islet Cell Antibody Register User Study (ICARUS) testing has been widely adopted *(59)*.

Loss of first-phase insulin secretion upon intravenous glucose tolerance testing (IVGTT) can precede abnormalities of glucose tolerance. For any given expression of anti-islet autoantibodies, loss of first-phase insulin secretion is associated with an earlier progression to overt diabetes. The test itself has a number of caveats. In very young children, a first-test effect has been observed, with almost absent first-phase secretion *(60)*. Children younger than 8 yr have lower first-phase secretion compared to teenagers and adults, and percentiles by age groups have been calculated. Finally, the diagnosis of type 1A diabetes relies upon fasting glucose or glucose on an oral glucose tolerance test, and individuals can have both type 1A and insulin resistance usually associated with type 2 diabetes.

PREVENTION OF TYPE 1A DIABETES

Introduction

In general, the prevention of a disease process requires that certain underlying criteria be met. First, there must be an accurate means of identifying subjects at risk for developing the disease (or an extremely safe intervention such as vaccination) and, second, there must be some intervention that can modulate the disease process. Prediction of type 1 diabetes was discussed in the previous section, and the latter is the focus of this subsequent section. The prevention of type 1 diabetes can theoretically be implemented with three different strategies: a primary, secondary, or tertiary approach. The primary prevention strategy involves initiation of an intervention before the onset of autoimmunity. This involves the identification of modulating or precipitating factors in the disease process and intervening in subjects at genetic risk that have no evidence of β-cell damage. The secondary prevention strategy would delay or suppress continued β-cell destruction in subjects with evidence of autoimmunity, but who are still euglycemic. The tertiary prevention strategy would focus on subjects after the onset of clinical diabetes. The goals of this last strategy would be to induce a prolonged remission, allow for potential β-cell regeneration, and/or preserve residual β-cell function in the hopes of delaying the complication triad of retinopathy, nephropathy, or neuropathy *(61,62)*.

Primary Prevention

To date, there is only one primary prevention trial, the Trial to Reduce IDDM in the Genetically at Risk (TRIGR) from Finland *(38)*. The hypothesis of TRIGR is that avoidance of cow's milk protein in the first 6–8 mo of life can prevent subsequent diabetes. The premise was based on early epidemiologic data from Norway and Sweden that reported that the duration of breast-feeding was inversely proportional to the risk of developing diabetes *(63)*. Other Finnish studies of sibling pairs revealed that the siblings with diabetes had higher levels of cow's milk protein antibodies than their age- and HLA-matched sibling pair, and they hypothesized that high levels of IgG anti-bovine serum albumin (BSA) were an independent risk factor for the development of type 1 diabetes, serving as an environmental trigger *(64–66)*. Diet experiments in the nonobese diabetic (NOD) mouse using a casein hydrolysate formula (which contains no large proteins or BSA) were promising, revealing a marked decreased incidence of autoimmune diabetes in the test diet cohort *(67)*. The hypothesized mechanism is that antibodies to BSA crossreact (via molecular mimicry) with a β-cell membrane protein (p69), which is also induced in islet cells by interferon (IFN)-γ. Gut permeability to cow's milk protein early in life could allow for immune sensitization, and a subsequent viral infection producing IFN-γ would induce an increase in p69 expression and expose the β-cells to transient immune-mediated destruction *(63)*. The TRIGR study has enrolled infants that have both a first-degree relative with diabetes and a high-risk HLA type to be randomized into either a casein hydrolysate formula or a cow's milk-based formula, with the primary end points being age of diabetes onset and incidence of diabetes by age 10 yr. The results of this trial are still pending.

Some studies, however, have found no association of cow's milk exposure and β-cell autoimmunity, the precursor to clinical type 1 diabetes. The Diabetes Autoimmunity Study in the Young (DAISY) from Denver, Colorado screened 253 children with a first-degree relative with type 1 diabetes for evidence of β-cell autoimmunity, defined as elevated levels of insulin, GAD, or ICA512 (IA-2) autoantibodies. There was no association between the early exposure of cow's milk protein or other dietary protein (cereal, fruit, vegetable, or meat) and the development of β-cell autoimmunity *(68)*. These results were later independently confirmed with the Australian BabyDIAB trial of 317 infants with a first-degree relative with type 1 diabetes and the German BabyDIAB trial. The study prospectively examined infants from birth to 29 mo of age for the effect of both breast-feeding and the introduction of cow's milk protein on the development of β-cell autoimmunity. Analyses were performed on cohorts based on the number of autoantibodies that they developed: none, one transiently detected, one permanently detected, or greater than two autoantibodies detected. There were no significant differences in these cohorts in terms of duration of breast-feeding or introduction of cow's milk protein, thereby leading to the investigators' conclusion that there is no association between cow's milk protein and the development of islet autoimmunity *(69)*.

In addition to early infant diet, other environment risk determinants have been implicated in the potential pathogenesis of type 1 diabetes, including enteroviral infections and vaccine administration. These determinants may serve as immune triggers or disease modulators, but, to date, no large trials are focusing on these agents for primary intervention studies *(70–75)*. At present, only congenital rubella infection is clearly associated with risk for type 1A diabetes *(76–78)*.

Secondary Prevention

Several trials have adopted the secondary prevention approach to delay or prevent the continued β-cell destruction in subjects that are currently euglycemic. In general, two separate agents are being studied in these trials: nicotinamide and insulin.

Nicotinamide

The rationale for using nicotinamide in intervention trials is based on animal models (both the NOD mouse and the Bio-Breeding [BB] rat) that nicotinamide prolongs remission, preserves β-cell function, and may prevent immune-mediated diabetes *(79,80)*. Its suitability for human trials has been tested, and nicotinamide was found not to alter insulin secretion or glucose kinetics *(81)*. The proposed mechanism of nicotinamide is the suppression of the poly(ADP-ribose)polymerase (PARP) enzyme, which both controls early steps of apoptosis and is involved in MHC class II gene expression *(82,83)*.

An early German nicotinamide intervention trial, Deutsche Nicotinamide Intervention Study (DENIS), was terminated in 1997, because it was unlikely to have the statistical power specified in the hypothesis to detect an 80% reduction in the incidence of type 1 diabetes from 30% to 6%, with a power of 90%. The negative results of the study, however, cannot exclude the possibility of a weaker (less than 80%) risk reduction *(84)*. A controversial population-based study of several thousand New Zealand school children revealed a 56% protective effect of nicotinamide after an average follow-up of 7.1 yr, but the lack of randomization and unorthodox study design place the relevance of these results in question *(85)*.

Currently, the European Nicotinamide Diabetes Intervention Trial (ENDIT) is testing whether it is possible to decrease the incidence of type 1 diabetes by 40% (i.e., from 35% down to 20%) over 5 yr in ICA-positive (≥20 JDF units) first-degree relatives. It is a large (over 500 subjects) international, multicenter, randomized, double-blind control trial using a slow-release nicotinamide preparation. Results reported orally in 2002 were negative. A potential concern about the ENDIT study is the relationship between the serum peak concentration and the biologically effective concentration, because it has been estimated that the current dosing will lead to only a 50% inhibition of PARP activity *(61,79)*.

Insulin

The second agent used in intervention trials is insulin. For several years, it has been shown in animal models (BB rat and NOD mouse) that subcutaneous insulin is effective in preventing insulitis and delaying the onset of diabetes *(86–88)*. There is a strong correlation between the titer of IAA and the development of diabetes, particularly among younger children. Normally, insulin is not present on the surface of β-cells, but following injury or intense β-cell activity, it may be presented as an antigen on the β-cells, leading to immune-mediated destruction. Therefore, administration of exogenous insulin may lead to "β-cell rest" and protection of the islet cells *(89)*. A pilot study from Boston, Massachusetts in 1993 followed high-risk individuals, with the treatment cohort receiving low-dose subcutaneous daily insulin with 5-d courses of intravenous insulin every 9 mo for 2.3–3.3 yr. Of those declining treatment, all (7/7) developed diabetes, whereas of the treatment group, only 1/5 developed diabetes, a statistically significant difference *(90)*. The large-scale, multicenter intervention study, the Diabetes Prevention Trial-1 (DPT-1), was initiated in 1994. The DPT-1 has two arms, based on estimated risk of developing type 1 diabetes in the subsequent 5 yr. Estimations of risk are based on ICA titers, first-phase insulin response, and the lack of a known protective HLA allele. The high-risk group (>50% risk) receives low-dose parenteral insulin injections twice daily and an annual 4-d insulin infusion. They are matched to an untreated, but closely monitored, group. The second arm includes the intermediate risk group (25–50% risk). They receive daily oral insulin vs placebo in a double-blind study design. To date, over 90,000 relatives have been screened, with 339 in the high-risk arm and more than 300 in the intermediate-risk arm. In the design of the trial, low-doses of insulin were intentionally chosen to minimize the risk of hypoglycemia. A potential criticism of the DPT-1, however, is that these insulin doses may not be enough for the immune-modulating protective effect as observed in the animal models. Results of the parenteral portion of the trial presented by Dr. Skyler at the American Diabetes Association meeting in 2001 indicate that parenteral insulin did not slow progression to diabetes. The predictors utilized, however, well-identified progressors to type 1 diabetes, and an ancillary study of biochemical autoantibodies suggests the importance of GAD65 and ICA512 autoantibodies for the design of future prevention trials. The results of the oral insulin trial should be available in 2 yr.

Tertiary Prevention

The goal of tertiary prevention strategies is to induce a prolonged remission, allow for potential β-cell regeneration, and/or preserve residual β-cell function, after the clinical onset of insulin deficiency. Trials using this approach have been largely unsuccessful. Early studies of immunosuppressive agents (such as cyclosporin) revealed that while administered, they prevented further loss of C-peptide secretion, resulting in improved metabolic function. Upon discontinuation, however, the protective effect diminished *(91–94)*. Given the rather severe toxicity profile of these agents (particularly renal toxicity), the high risk-to-benefit ratio has currently made immunosuppressive therapy not an option for diabetes prevention. A meta-analysis of nicotinamide used in conjunction with insulin for the treatment of individuals with new-onset type 1 diabetes has shown preservation of residual β-cell function *(95)*, although other studies have failed to show promising results *(96,97)*. For the moment, intervention trials for nicotinamide are largely focusing on secondary prevention.

A large number of new agents successfully preventing type 1A diabetes in animal models are entering clinical trials. As reviewed by Atkinson and Leiter *(98)*, more than 100 different therapies prevent type 1 diabetes in the NOD mouse model and it is likely that disease prevention may be too "easy" in this model. The BB rat model is more demanding, but suffers from the presence of a T-cell lymphopenia autosomal recessive mutation that is likely to limit successful immunomodulation. Nevertheless, the existence of these models has stimulated development of agents for type 1A diabetes prevention. Probably the most exciting pathway goes under the rubric of "immunologic vaccination." Antigens or peptides of autoantigens can be administered to the NOD mouse and prevent the development of diabetes. The three major molecules studied have been insulin, GAD, and a heat-shock protein. Biotechnology companies are bringing all three molecules to clinical trials, usually in new-onset diabetes patients, where the goal is the preservation of C-peptide. We have been particularly interested in insulin and a peptide of insulin, namely amino acids 9–23 of the insulin B chain. When Daniel and Wegmann *(99)* administered this peptide to NOD mice, 90% of the diabetes could be prevented with a single injection. An altered peptide ligand of this peptide (replacing 2 of the 15 amino acids with alanine) has been developed and is in clinical trials. Not only do NOD mice have T-cells reacting with this peptide, but a recent report indicates similar reactivity in humans. In general, administration of such peptides for prevention of diabetes is thought to be associated with generation of T-lymphocytes (e.g., Th2) that respond to the peptide but produce protective cytokines that block the T-cell destruction of β-cells *(100)*.

CONCLUSION

It is now possible to predict type 1A diabetes in humans with reasonable accuracy. In fact, the Immunology of Diabetes Society has issued a position statement outlining recommendations on the prediction of type 1A diabetes *(9)*. Prevention of diabetes is possible in animal models, and a major effort is underway to carry these observations from the "bench" into the clinic in order to make prevention in humans a reality. The National Institutes of Health is about to establish a trial network to pioneer trials of preventive therapies, and this effort will be critically dependent on multicenter collaboration and support by physicians through the United States and Canada; currently over 20 centers are proposed for the network. With our limited knowledge at this time, one cannot be sure of the exact time line for diabetes prevention, but with the continued research efforts and new trials underway, the time line is likely shortening day by day.

ACKNOWLEDGMENTS

Research supported by grants from the National Institutes of Health DK32083,DK55969,DK32493, an Autoimmunity Center of Excellence grant AI46374, a Diabetes Endocrine Research Center grant P30 DK57516; AM was supported by NIH fellowship T32 AI50248, and Clinical Research Center grants (Children's Hospital MO1RR00069, University Hospital MO1RR00051), the Juvenile Diabetes Research Foundation International, the American Diabetes Association Mentor based fellowship grant, and the Children's Diabetes Foundation.

REFERENCES

1. Glaser N, Barnett P, McCaslin I, Nelson D, Trainor J, Louie J, et al. Risk factors for cerebral edema in children with diabetic ketoacidosis. N Engl J Med 2001;344:264–269.
2. Eisenbarth GS. Type I diabetes mellitus. A chronic autoimmune disease. N Engl J Med 1986;314:1360–1368.
3. Atkinson MA, Eisenbarth GS. Type 1 diabetes: new perspectives on disease pathogenesis and treatment. Lancet 2001;358:221–229.
4. Verge CF, Gianani R, Kawasaki E, Yu L, Pietropaolo M, Jackson RA, et al. Prediction of type I diabetes in first-degree relatives using a combination of insulin, GAD, and ICA512bdc/IA-2 autoantibodies. Diabetes 1996;45:926–933.
5. Bingley PJ, Bonifacio E, Williams AJK, Genovese S, Bottazzo GF, Gale EAM. Prediction of IDDM in the general population: strategies based on combinations of autoantibody markers. Diabetes 1997;46:1701–1710.
6. Kimpimaki T, Kulmala P, Savola K, Vahasalo P, Reijonen H, Ilonen J, et al. Disease-associated autoantibodies as surrogate markers of type 1 diabetes in young children at increased genetic risk. Childhood Diabetes in Finland Study Group. J Clin Endocrinol Metab 2000;85:1126–1132.
7. Schenker M, Hummel M, Ferber K, Walter M, Keller E, Albert ED, et al. Early expression and high prevalence of islet autoantibodies for DR3/4 heterozygous and DR4/4 homozygous offspring of parents with type I diabetes: the German BABYDIAB study. Diabetologia 1999;42:671–677.
8. Maclaren N, Lan M, Coutant R, Schatz D, Silverstein J, Muir A, et al. Only multiple autoantibodies to islet cells (ICA), insulin, GAD65, IA-2 and IA-2beta predict immune-mediated (type 1) diabetes in relatives. J Autoimmun 1999;12:279–287.
9. Bingley PJ, Bonifacio E, Ziegler AG, Schatz D, Atkinson M, Eisenbarth GS. Proposed guidelines on screening for risk of type 1 diabetes. Diabetes Care 2001;24:398.
10. Rewers M, Norris JM. Epidemiology of type I diabetes. In: Eisenbarth GS, Lafferty KJ, eds. Type I Diabetes: Molecular, Cellular, and Clinical Immunology. Oxford University Press, New York, 1996, pp. 172–208.
11. Imagawa A, Hanafusa T, Miyagawa J, Matsuzawa Y. A novel subtype of type 1 diabetes mellitus characterized by a rapid onset and an absence of diabetes- related antibodies. Osaka IDDM Study Group. N Engl J Med 2000;342:301–307.
12. Turner R, Stratton I, Horton V, Manley S, Zimmet P, Mackay IR, et al. UKPDS 25: autoantibodies to islet-cell cytoplasm and glutamic acid decarboxylase for prediction of insulin requirement in type 2 diabetes. UK Prospective Diabetes Study Group. Lancet 1997;350:1288–1293.
13. Horton V, Stratton I, Bottazzo GF, Shattock M, Mackay I, Zimmet P, et al. Genetic heterogeneity of autoimmune diabetes: age of presentation in adults is influenced by HLA DRB1 and DQB1 genotypes (UKPDS 43). UK Prospective Diabetes Study (UKPDS) Group. Diabetologia 1999;42:608–616.
14. Zimmet PZ, Tuomi T, Mackay IR, Rowley MJ, Knowles W, Cohen M, et al. Latent autoimmune diabetes mellitus in adults (LADA): the role of antibodies to glutamic acid decarboxylase in diagnosis and prediction of insulin dependency. Diabet Med 1994;11:299–303.
15. Carlsson A, Sundkvist G, Groop L, Tuomi T. Insulin and glucagon secretion in patients with slowly progressing autoimmune diabetes (LADA). J Clin Endocrinol Metab 2000;85(1):76–80.

16. Tuomilehto J, Karvonen M, Pitkaniemi J, Virtala E, Kohtamaki K, Toivanen L, et al. Record-high incidence of type I (insulin-dependent) diabetes mellitus in Finnish children. The Finnish Childhood Type I Diabetes Registry Group. Diabetologia 1999;42:655–660.
17. Diabetes Epidemiology Research International Group. Secular trends in incidence of childhood IDDM in 10 countries. Diabetes 1998;39:858–864.
18. Feltbower RG, McKinney PA, Bodansky HJ. Rising incidence of childhood diabetes is seen at all ages and in urban and rural settings in Yorkshire, United Kingdom. [letter]. Diabetologia 2000;43:682–684.
19. El-Hashimy M, Angelico MC, Martin BC, Krolewski AS, Warram JH. Factors modifying the risk of IDDM in offspring of an IDDM parent. Diabetes 1995;44:295–299.
20. Eisenbarth GS, Elsey C, Yu L, Rewers M. Infantile anti-islet autoimmunity: DAISY study. Diabetes 1998;47:A210 (abstract).
21. Redondo MJ, Yu L, Hawa M, Mackenzie T, Pyke DA, Eisenbarth GS, et al. Heterogenity of type 1 diabetes: analysis of monozygotic twins in Great Britain and the United States. Diabetologia 2001;44:354–362.
22. Eisenbarth GS, Gottlieb P. Immunoendocrinopathy syndromes. In: Larsen PR, Kronenberg H, Melmed S, Polonsky KS, eds. Williams Textbook of Endocrinology, 10th ed. WB Saunders, Philadelphia, 2003, pp. 47–60.
23. Patel D. Escape from tolerance in the human X-linked autoimmunity-allergic disregulation syndrome and the Scurfy mouse. J Clin Invest 2001;107:155–157.
24. Perheentupa J, Miettinen A. Autoimmune polyendocrinopathy–candidiasis–ectodermal dystrophy. In: Eisenbarth GS, ed. Endocrine and Organ Specific Autoimmunity. Landes Bioscience, Georgetown, TX, 1999, pp. 19–40.
25. Bao F, Yu L, Babu S, Wang T, Hoffenberg EJ, Rewers M, et al. One third of HLA DQ2 homozygous patients with type 1 diabetes express celiac disease associated transglutaminase autoantibodies. J Autoimmun 1999;13:143–148.
26. Bao F, Rewers M, Scott F, Eisenbarth GS. Celiac disease. In: Eisenbarth GS, ed. Endocrine and Organ Specific Autoimmunity. Landes, Bioscience, Georgetown, TX, 1999, pp. 85–96.
27. Hummel M, Bonifacio E, Stern M, Dittler J, Schimmel A, Ziegler AG. Development of celiac disease-associated antibodies in offspring of parents with type I diabetes. Diabetologia 2000;43:1005–1011.
28. Yu L, Brewer KW, Gates S, Wang T, Babu S, Gottlieb PA, et al. DRB1*04 and DQ alleles: expression of 21-hydroxylase autoantibodies and risk of progression to Addison's disease. J Clin Endocrinol Metab 1999;84:328–335.
29. Hoffenberg EJ, Bao F, Eisenbarth GS, Uhlhorn C, Hass JE, Sokol RJ, et al. Silent celiac disease in American children at genetic risk. J Pediatr Gastroenterol Nutr 2000;31:S65 (abstract).
30. Falorni A, Laureti S, Nikoshkov A, Picchio ML, Hallengren B, Vandewalle CL, et al. 21-Hydroxylase autoantibodies in adult patients with endocrine autoimmune diseases are highly specific for Addison's disease. Belgian Diabetes Registry. Clin Exp Immunol 1997;107:341–346.
31. Nepom GT. Immunogenetics and IDDM. Diabetes Rev 1993;1:93–103.
32. Todd JA. From genome to aetiology in a multifactorial disease, type 1 diabetes. Bioessays 1999;21:164–174.
33. Bach J-F. Insulin-dependent diabetes mellitus as an autoimmune disease. Endocr Rev 1994;15: 516–542.
34. Baisch JM, Weeks T, Giles R, Hoover M, Stastny P, Capra JD. Analysis of HLA-DQ genotypes and susceptibility in insulin- dependent diabetes mellitus. N Engl J Med 1990;322:1836–1841.
35. Pugliese A, Kawasaki E, Zeller M, Yu L, Babu S, Solimena M, et al. Sequence analysis of the diabetes-protective human leukocyte antigen-DQB1*0602 allele in unaffected, islet cell antibody-positive first degree relatives and in rare patients with type 1 diabetes. J Clin Endocrinol Metab 1999;84:1722–1728.
36. Redondo MJ, Kawasaki E, Mulgrew CL, Noble J, Erlich H, Freed J, et al. DRB1*1401: A class II allele being as protective as DQB1*0602. Diabetes 1999;48:813–813 (abstract).
37. Rewers M, Bugawan TL, Norris JM, Blair A, Beaty B, Hoffman M, et al. Newborn screening for HLA markers associated with IDDM: diabetes autoimmunity study in the young (DAISY). Diabetologia 1996;39:807–812.
38. Paronen J, Knip M, Savilahti E, Virtanen SM, Ilonen J, Akerblom HK, et al. Effect of cow's milk exposure and maternal type 1 diabetes on cellular and humoral immunization to dietary insulin in infants at genetic risk for type 1 diabetes. Finnish Trial to Reduce IDDM in the Genetically at Risk Study Group. Diabetes 2000;49:1657–1665.

39. Ziegler A-G, Hummel M, Schenker M, Bonifacio E. Autoantibody appearance and risk for development of childhood diabetes in offspring of parents with type 1 diabetes. The 2-year analysis of the German BABYDIAB study. Diabetes 1999;48:460–468.
40. Bell GI, Horita S, Karam JH. A polymorphic locus near the human insulin gene is associated with insulin-dependent diabetes mellitus. Diabetes 1984;33:176–183.
41. Bennett ST, Wilson AJ, Cucca F, Nerup J, Pociot F, McKinney PA, et al. *IDDM2-VNTR*-encoded susceptibility to type 1 diabetes: dominant protection and parental transmission of alleles of the insulin gene-linked minisatellite locus. J Autoimmun 1996;9:415–421.
42. Vafiadis P, Bennett ST, Todd JA, Nadeau J, Grabs R, Goodyer CG, et al. Insulin expression in human thymus is modulated by INS VNTR alleles at the IDDM2 locus. Nat Genet 1997;15:289–292.
43. Pugliese A, Zeller M, Fernandez A, Zalcberg LJ, Bartlett RJ, Ricordi C, et al. The insulin gene is transcribed in the human thymus and transcription levels correlate with allelic variation at the INS VNTR-IDDM2 susceptibility locus for type I diabetes. Nat Genet 1997;15:293–297.
44. Füchtenbusch M, Ferber K, Standl E, Ziegler A-G, et al. Prediction of type I diabetes postpartum in patients with gestational diabetes mellitus by combined islet cell autoantibody screening: A prospective multicenter study. Diabetes 1997;46:1459–1467.
45. Bingley PJ, Christie MR, Bonifacio E, Bonfanti R, Shattock M, Fonte M-T, et al. Combined analysis of autoantibodies improves prediction of IDDM in islet cell antibody-positive relatives. Diabetes 1994;43:1304–1310.
46. Yu L, Robles DT, Abiru N, Kaur P, Rewers M, Kelemen K, et al. Early expression of anti-insulin autoantibodies of man and the NOD mouse: evidence for early determination of subsequent diabetes. Proc Natl Acad Sci USA 2000;97:1701–1706.
47. Suri A, Katz JD. Dissecting the role of CD4+ T cells in autoimmune diabetes through the use of TCR transgenic mice. Immunol Rev 1999;169:55–65.
48. Wong FS, Janeway CAJ. The role of CD4 vs. CD8 T cells in IDDM. J Autoimmun 1999;13:290–295.
49. Roep BO, Atkinson MA, Van Endert PM, Gottlieb PA, Wilson SB, Sachs JA. Autoreactive T cell responses in insulin-dependent (type 1) diabetes mellitus. Report of the First International Workshop for Standardization of T cell assays. J Autoimmun 1999;13:267–282.
50. Alleva DG, Crowe PD, Jin L, Kwok WW, Ling N, Gottschalk M, et al. A disease-associated cellular immune response in type 1 diabetics to an immunodominant epitope of insulin. J Clin Invest 2001;107:173–180.
51. Wong FS, Karttunen J, Dumont C, Wen L, Visintin I, Pilip IM, et al. Identification of an MHC class I-restricted autoantigen in type 1 diabetes by screening an organ-specific cDNA library. Nat Med 1999;5:1026–1031.
52. Reichstetter S, Ettinger RA, Liu AW, Gebe JA, Nepom GT, Kwok WW. Distinct T cell interactions with HLA class II tetramers characterize a spectrum of TCR affinities in the human antigen-specific T cell response. J Immunol 2000;165:6994–6998.
53. Srikanta S, Ganda OP, Eisenbarth GS, Soeldner JS. Islet cell antibodies and beta cell function in monozygotic triplets and twins initially discordant for type I diabetes mellitus. N Engl J Med 1983;308:322–325.
54. Srikanta S, Ganda OP, Gleason RE, Jackson RA, Soeldner JS, Eisenbarth GS. Pre-type I diabetes. Linear loss of beta cell response to intravenous glucose. Diabetes 1984;33:717–720.
55. Chase HP, Cuthbertson DD, Dolan LM, et al. First phase insulin release (FPIR) during the intravenous glucose tolerance test (IV-GTT) as a risk factor for type 1 diabetes. J Pediatr 2001;138:244–249.
56. Colman PG, McNair P, Steele C, Gellert S, Tait B, Honeyman M, et al. Linear decline in insulin production prior to development of type 1 diabetes—a reality. Diabetes 2000;49:A36–A36 (abstract).
57. Böhmer KP, Kolb H, Kuglin B, Zielasek J, Hübinger A, Lampeter EF, et al. Linear loss of insulin secretory capacity during the last six months preceding IDDM. Diabetes Care 1994;17:138–141.
58. Wagner R, Genovese S, Bosi E, Becker F, Bingley PJ, Bonifacio E, et al. Slow metabolic deterioration towards diabetes in islet cell antibody positive patients with autoimmune polyendocrine disease. Diabetologia 1994;37:365–371.
59. Bingley PJ. Interactions of age, islet cell antibodies, insulin autoantibodies, and first-phase insulin response in predicting risk of progression to IDDM in ICA+ relatives: the ICARUS data set. Diabetes 1996;45:1720–1728.
60. Allen HF, Jeffers BW, Klingensmith GJ, Chase HP. First-phase insulin release in normal children. J Pediatr 1993;123:733–738.
61. Knip M. Prediction and prevention of type 1 diabetes. Acta Paediatr 1998;425(Suppl):54–62.

62. Rosenbloom AL, Schatz DA, Krischer JP, Skyler JS, Becker DJ, LaPorte RE, et al. Therapeutic controversy: prevention and treatment of diabetes in children. J Clin Endocrinol Metab 2000;85:494–522.
63. Akerblom HK, Savilahti E, Saukkonen TT, Paganus A, Virtanen SM, Teramo K, et al. The case for elimination of cow's milk in early infancy in the prevention of type 1 diabetes: the Finnish experience. Diabetes Metab Rev 1993;9:269–278.
64. Saukkonen T, Virtanen SM, Karppinen M, Reijonen H, Ilonen J, Räsänen L, et al. Significance of cow's milk protein antibodies as risk factor for childhood IDDM: interactions with dietary cow's milk intake and HLA-DQB1 genotype. Diabetologia 1998;41:72–78.
65. Vaarala O, Knip M, Paronen J, Hamalainen AM, Muona P, Vaatainen M, et al. Cow's milk formula feeding induces primary immunization to insulin in infants at genetic risk for type 1 diabetes. Diabetes 1999;48:1389–1394.
66. Virtanen SM, Hypponen E, Laara E, Vahasalo P, Kulmala P, Savola K, et al. Cow's milk consumption, disease-associated autoantibodies and type 1 diabetes mellitus: a follow-up study in siblings of diabetic children. Childhood Diabetes in Finland Study Group. Diabet Med 1998;15:730–738.
67. Karges W, Hammond-McKibben D, Cheung RK, Visconti M, Shibuya N, Kemp D, et al. Immunological aspects of nutritional diabetes prevention in NOD mice. Diabetes 1997;46:557–564.
68. Norris JM, Beaty B, Klingensmith G, Yu L, Hoffman M, Chase HP, et al. Lack of association between early exposure to cow's milk protein and β-cell autoimmunity: Diabetes Autoimmunity Study in the Young (DAISY). JAMA 1996;276:609–614.
69. Couper JJ, Steele C, Beresford S, Powell T, McCaul K, Pollard A, et al. Lack of association between duration of breast-feeding or introduction of cow's milk and development of islet autoimmunity. Diabetes 1999;48:2145–2149.
70. Chehadeh W, Weill J, Vantyghem MC, Alm G, Lefebvre J, Wattre P, et al. Increased level of interferon-alpha in blood of patients with insulin-dependent diabetes mellitus: relationship with coxsackievirus B infection. J Infect Dis 2000;181:1929–1939.
71. Honeyman MC, Coulson BS, Stone NL, Gellert SA, Goldwater PN, Steele CE, et al. Association between rotavirus infection and pancreatic islet autoimmunity in children at risk of developing type 1 diabetes. Diabetes 2000;49:1319–1324.
72. Juhela S, Hyoty H, Roivainen M, Harkonen T, Putto-Laurila A, Simell O, et al. T-Cell responses to enterovirus antigens in children with type 1 diabetes. Diabetes 2000;49:1308–1313.
73. Lonnrot M, Korpela K, Knip M, Ilonen J, Simell O, Korhonen S, et al. Enterovirus infection as a risk factor for beta-cell autoimmunity in a prospectively observed birth cohort: the Finnish Diabetes Prediction and Prevention Study. Diabetes 2000;49:1314–1318.
74. Abiru N, Yu L, Redondo MJ, Eisenbarth GS. Modification of the environment is NOT the most efficient way to prevent type 1 diabetes. Diabetes Technol Ther 2000;2:609–616.
75. Dahlquist G. Environmental risk factors in human type 1 diabetes—an epidemiological perspective. Diabetes Metab Rev 1998;11:37–46.
76. Rubenstein P. The HLA system in congenital rubella patients with and without diabetes. Diabetes 1982;31:1088–1091.
77. Lindberg B, Ahlfors K, Carlsson A, Ericsson UB, Landin-Olsson M, Lernmark A, et al. Previous exposure to measles, mumps, and rubella—but not vaccination during adolescence—correlates to the prevalence of pancreatic and thyroid autoantibodies. Pediatrics 1999;104:e12.
78. Schopfer K, Matter L, Flueler U, Werder E. Diabetes mellitus, endocrine autoantibodies and prenatal rubella infection. Lancet 1982;2:159.
79. Gale EA. Theory and practice of nicotinamide trials in pre-type 1 diabetes. J Pediatr Endocrinol Metab 1996;9:375–379.
80. O'Brien BA, Harmon BV, Cameron DP, Allan DJ. Nicotinamide prevents the development of diabetes in the cyclophosphamide-induced NOD mouse model by reducing beta-cell apoptosis. J Pathol 2000;191:86–92.
81. Bingley PJ, Caldas G, Bonfanti R, Gale EAM. Nicotinamide and insulin secretion in normal subjects. Diabetologia 1993;36:675–677.
82. Kolb H, Burkart V. Nicotinamide in type 1 diabetes. Mechanism of action revisited. Diabetes Care 1999;22(Suppl 2):B16–B20.
83. Gale EA. Molecular mechanisms of beta-cell destruction in IDDM: the role of nicotinamide. Horm Res 1996;45(Suppl 1):39–43.
84. Lampeter EF, Klinghammer A, Scherbaum WA, Heinze E, Haastert B, Giani G, et al. An attempt to prevent type 1 diabetes. Diabetes 1998;47:980–984.

85. Elliott RB, Pilcher CC, Fergusson DM, Stewart AW. A population-based strategy to prevent insulin-dependent diabetes using nicotinamide. J Pediatr Endocrinol Methods 1996;9:501–509.
86. Muir A, Luchetta R, Song H-Y, Peck A, Krischer J, Maclaren N. Insulin immunization protects NOD mice from diabetes. Autoimmunity 1993;15:58 (abstract).
87. Daniel D, Wegmann DR. Protection of nonobese diabetic mice from diabetes by intranasal or subcutaneous administration of insulin peptide B-(9–23). Proc Natl Acad Sci USA 1996;93:956–960.
88. Hancock WW, Polansky M, Zhang J, Blogg N, Weiner HL. Suppression of insulitis in non-obese diabetic (NOD) mice by oral insulin administration is associated with selective expression of interleukin-4 and -10, transforming growth factor-beta, and prostaglandin-E. Am J Pathol 1995;147:1193–1199.
89. Sperling MA. Aspects of the etiology, prediction, and prevention of insulin-dependent diabetes mellitus in childhood. Pediatr Clin North Am 1997;44:269–284.
90. Keller RJ, Eisenbarth GS, Jackson RA. Insulin prophylaxis in individuals at high risk of type I diabetes. Lancet 1993;341:927–928.
91. Assan R, Feutren G, Debray-Sachs M, Quiniou-Debrie M, Laborie C, Thomas G, et al. Metabolic and immunological effects of cyclosporine in recently diagnosed type I diabetes mellitus. Lancet 1985;1:67–71.
92. Carel J-C, Boitard C, Eisenbarth G, Bach J, Bougnères P. Cyclosporine delays but does not prevent clinical onset in glucose intolerant pre-type I diabetic children. J Autoimmun 1996;9:739–745.
93. Martin S, Schernthaner G, Nerup J, Gries FA, Koivisto VA, Dupre J, et al. Follow-up of cyclosporin A treatment in type I (insulin-dependent) diabetes mellitus: lack of long-term effects. Diabetologia 1991;34:429–434.
94. Dupre J, Stiller CR, Gent M, Donner A, Von Graffenried B, Heinrichs D, et al. Clinical trials of cyclosporin in IDDM. Diabetes Care 1988;11:37–44.
95. Pozzilli P, Browne PD, Kolb H. Meta-analysis of nicotinamide treatment in patients with recent-onset IDDM. The Nicotinamide Trialists. Diabetes Care 1996;19:1357–1363.
96. Vidal J, Fernandez-Balsells M, Sesmilo G, Aguilera E, Casamitjana R, Gomis R, et al. Effects of nicotinamide and intravenous insulin therapy in newly diagnosed type 1 diabetes. Diabetes Care 2000;23:360–364.
97. Pozzilli P, Visalli N, Signore A, Baroni MG, Buzzetti R, Cavallo MG, et al. Double blind trial of nicotinamide in recent-onset IDDM (the IMDIAB III study). Diabetologia 1995;38:848–852.
98. Atkinson M, Leiter E. The NOD mouse model of type 1 diabetes: as good as it gets? Nat Med 1999;5:601–604.
99. Daniel D, Wegmann DR. Protection of nonobese diabetic mice from diabetes by intranasal or subcutaneous administration of insulin peptide B-(9–23). Proc Natl Acad Sci USA 1996;93:956–960.
100. Homann D, Holz A, Bot A, Coon B, Wolfe T, Petersen J, et al. Autoreactive CD4+ T cells protect from autoimmune diabetes via bystander suppression using the IL-4/Stat6 pathway. Immunity 1999;11:463–472.

4 Molecular Biology of β-Cell Destruction by Autoimmune Processes

Åke Lernmark, MD *and*
Choon Hee Chung, MD, PhD

CONTENTS

INTRODUCTION

The development of type 1 diabetes is closely related to the disappearance of β-cells from the islets of Langerhans. Loss of β-cells was already documented in the beginning of the last century when patients died from diabetes prior to the discovery of insulin. As pointed out by Gepts *(1),* authors also described inflammatory cells in the islets of Langerhans, but it was not until the post-insulin-discovery era that the inflammatory lesion was referred to as insulitis *(2).* The rediscovery of insulitis combined with rigorous morphometric analyses of β-cell loss by Gepts *(1)* was crucial to emerging views that, in fact, insulin-dependent diabetes mellitus was an autoimmune disease. Further analyses by Gepts and LaCompte *(3)* suggested that the islet inflammatory lesion in patients with short duration had surprising features of chronic rather than acute inflammatory appearance. Later, quantitative analyses showed that the loss of β-cells were substantial not only in the pancreas of long-term but also in patients with short-term diabetes *(4,5).* Loss of β-cells may be rapid, to the extent that immune markers such as autoantibodies to islet cell antigens have not yet formed or slow as exemplified by numerous individuals reported to be islet cell autoantibody positive for more than a decade before their clinical onset of type 1 diabetes *(6).* Further studies are needed before we fully understand and are able to stage the pathogenesis of type 1 diabetes as reflected by autoimmune destruction of pancreatic β-cells. The autoimmune process may begin when pancreatic β-cell autoantigens are no longer recognized by the

From: *Contemporary Endocrinology: Type 1 Diabetes: Etiology and Treatment*
Edited by: M. A. Sperling © Humana Press Inc., Totowa, NJ

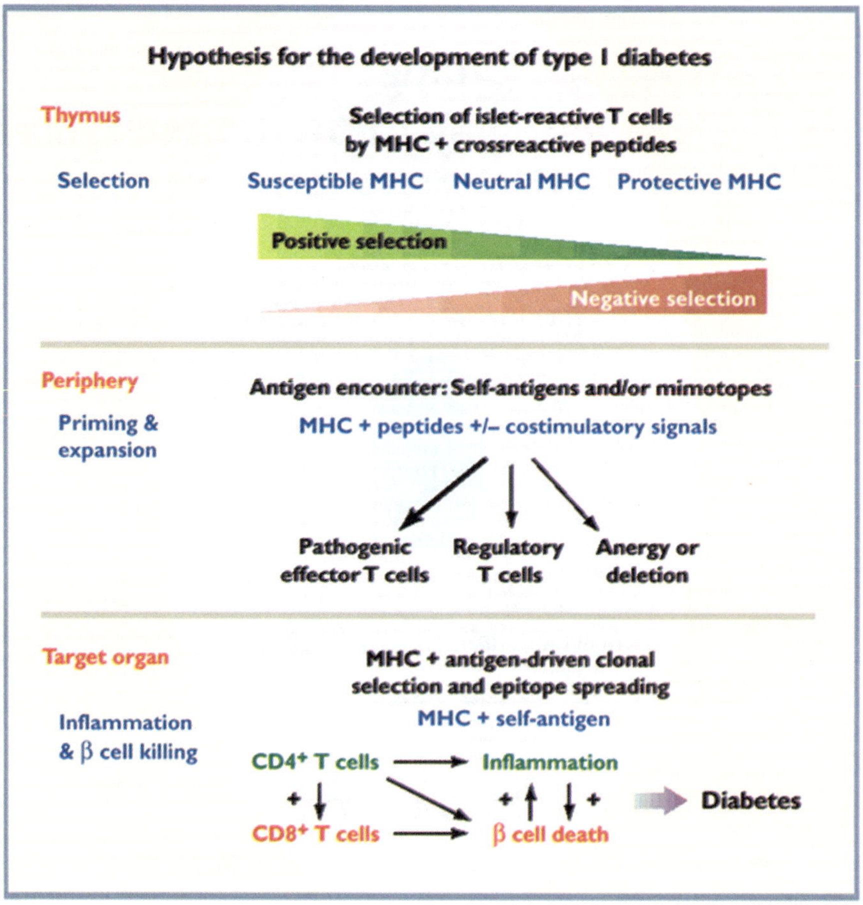

Fig. 1. Immunological aspects of β cell loss in type 1 diabetes. MHC, major histocompatibility complex. (Reproduced with permission from ref. *150*.)

immune system as self but rather as non-self (Fig. 1). During this process of emerging autoimmunity, it may be possible to detect autoantibodies and perhaps autoreactive lymphocytes as potentially useful indicators of β-cell autoimmunity.

It is often suggested that β-cell destruction is attributed directly to an autoimmune process in most patients who develop type 1 diabetes. Although there are alternative mechanisms, it is noteworthy that more than 90% of type 1 diabetes patients at the time of clinical diagnosis have autoantibodies against one or several β-cell-specific autoantigens *(7,8)*. It is similarly remarkable that almost 90% of children developing type 1 diabetes are positive for the human leukocyte antigen (HLA) haplotypes DQA1*0301-B1*0302, DQA1*0501-B1*02, or both *(7,9)*]. The strong association with distinct HLA class II factors also supports the notion that type 1 diabetes is an autoimmune disease and supports the concept that autoreactivity with several autoantigens such as glutamic acid decarboxylase (GAD65), IA-2, and insulin will be important to both cell-mediated and humoral immune abnormalities. Why are autoantibodies (Ab) such as GAD 65Ab, IA-2Ab, and insulin autoantibodies (IAAs) produced in type 1 diabetes? The immune response to these and other candidate β-cell autoantigens is likely to be initiated by antigen-presenting cells

(Fig. 1). The recognition of the antigens as non-self needs to be clarified and it remains to be determined whether thymic selection or the homology to an exogenous antigen is important to initiate an immune response to the autoantigen *(10)*. It cannot be excluded that a peptide of an exogenous antigen may bind to HLA class II molecules, resulting in an antigenic shift to an autoantigen. Misrecognition of the trimolecular complex of HLA and peptide may stimulate helper T-cells that assist B-lymphocytes to make autoantibodies, which, in turn, crossreact with an autoantigen.

What is the initial antigen? This question has been difficult to answer in humans. Numerous studies in the spontaneously diabetic (nonobese diabetic [NOD]) mouse have attempted to identify autoantigens recognized prior to insulitis and diabetes *(11,12)*. These investigations suggested that GAD65 was an early target and that the reactivity of both T-cells and antibodies were spreading to other antigens during the course of the disease. A recent report *(13)* using antisense oligonucleotide of GAD65 prevented the development of diabetes in the NOD mouse. These and other authors therefore suggested that GAD65 is a major autoantigen in NOD diabetes. They also suggested that an initial immune response to GAD65 is associated with insulitis and β-cell destruction in this animal. Several other reports indicate that autoantibodies may be formed as an immune reaction secondary to the destruction of pancreatic β-cells.

An important aspect of islet inflammation is to identify which cell from the immune system appears first in the islet to initiate or perhaps maintain an immune response directed against the β-cells. This question may be moot if it can be demonstrated that β-cell destruction is a primary event and that the initial immune response occurs in the lymph nodes draining the pancreas. Regardless of the location, the initial presentation of an antigen will most likely be carried out by an antigen-presenting cell (APC), such as a macrophage or dendritic cell. Although a popularized hypotheses for some time *(14)*, data could not be generated to support the hypothesis that β-cells are their own APCs. Rather, studies of human *(5,15)* and animal pancreas *(16)* suggest that macrophages engulfing β-cell granules may have been the source of major histocompatibility complex (MHC) class II antigen and islet-hormone-positive cells.

When an exogenous virus invades and replicates in the islet cells, macrophages appear and are most likely involved in the phagocytosis of damaged and lysed cells. Macrophages and dendritic cells are detectable, often before lymphocyte-dominated insulitis, in human *(5,17,18)*, NOD mouse *(19)*, and Bio-Breeding (BB) rat *(20–23)* pancreas. In humans, HLA class II molecules bind peptides generated by antigen processing and the peptide is finally presented in a trimolecular complex on the cell surface. The trimolecular complex is recognized by the T-cell receptor (TCR) on CD4+ T-cells at the same time as the macrophage or dendritic cell produces cytokines such as interleukin (IL)-12. This cytokine stimulates CD4+ T-cells to primarily produce IL-2 and interferon (IFN)-γ, which are referred to as Th1 cytokines. CD4+ T-cells of the Th1 type tend to support cell-mediated immune reactions. The APCs may also induce CD4+ T-cells to produce IL-4 and IL-10. These cytokines are referred to as Th2 cytokines because they are important in promoting humoral immune responses. The cytokines released by Th1 cells may activate cytotoxic T-cells (CD8+) as well as macrophages. Activated macrophages may release free radicals and cytokines such as IL-1, tumor necrosis factor (TNF)-α and IFN-γ, which may in themselves have direct deleterious effects on the β-cells.

Cytotoxic CD8+ T-cells are activated with help from CD4+ helper T-cells. CD8+ cytotoxic T-cell TCRs recognize peptides presented on HLA class I molecules on the target cells, including β-cells. This is important because endogenous autoantigen peptides such as those generated from GAD65 are readily presented on HLA class I molecules. A cytotoxic CD8+ T-cell is, therefore, able to deliver a killer signal to the target β-cell with remarkable precision. It is important to note in this regard that the antigen recognized by the immune system does not have to be expressed on the β-cell surface. A CD8+ T-cell with a TCR that recognizes a GAD65 peptide presented by an HLA class I molecule on the β-cell surface is sufficient for killing.

The autoantibody response is also dependent on help from CD4+ T-cells. CD4+ T-cells express CD40 ligand (CD154), which recognize the CD40 receptor on the B-lymphocyte surface to stimulate antibody production. The autoimmune response in type 1 diabetes is, therefore, similar to most other organ-specific autoimmune disorders in that both T-cells and autoantibody-producing B-cells are involved in the immune abnormalities associated with, as well as predicting, the disease *(24)*. The molecular biology of β-cell destruction is therefore both diverse and complicated and the detailed mechanisms are yet poorly understood. The immune abnormalities may, in fact, involve phenomena associated with both the innate as well as the aquired immune system. At the time of clinical diagnosis of type 1 diabetes, about 80% of the β-cells have been specifically destroyed. We will briefly review the many pathways that may contribute to this specific end point that is causing lifelong dependence of daily insulin injections. The readers are also referred to several recent reviews on the etiology and pathogenesis of type 1 diabetes *(8,25–27)*.

ISLET CELL AUTOANTIGENS

GAD

There are two isoforms of GAD (GAD65 and GAD67) and these are encoded by different genes (*see* Table 1). GAD65 is encoded by a gene on chromosome 10, and GAD67 by a gene on chromosome 2 *(28,29)*. The GAD65 molecule consists of 585 amino acids, whereas GAD67 consists of 594 amino acids. There is about 65% overall amino acid homology between the two GAD isoforms, with greatest diversity at the N-terminus. GAD65 is expressed mostly in the brain and in islet cells, although expression in other tissues has also been reported. GAD67 is expressed mostly in the brain, but some expression in non-β islet cells, testes, and ovary is also evident. GAD65 is more predominant in the pancreatic β-cells in humans, whereas GAD67, but not GAD65, seems to be more highly expressed in mouse pancreatic islets. The claim that GAD65 is an initiating antigen in NOD mouse diabetes *(11,12)* is inconsistent with the difficulty to clearly demonstrate that mouse β-cells are expressing GAD65 *(30)*. In contrast to the NOD mouse and BB rat diabetes, GAD65Ab detected in standardized radioligand binding assays *(24,31,32)* are readily detected in type 1 diabetes both before and at the clinical onset of type 1 diabetes. The GAD65 autoantibodies appear heterogeneous and it is of interest that some GAD65Abs predict type 1 diabetes better than others.

Two major regions in the middle and C-terminal parts of the GAD65 molecule appear to be involved in forming the autoantibody binding sites *(33–35)*. The C-terminal end of amino acids from position 451 to 570 is important, as well as the amino acids in the middle of the sequence (amino acids from about 240 to 360). The C-terminal and middle part of GAD65 form a conformational autoantibody epitope that seems to be highly predictive of type 1 diabetes *(35)*. Autoantibody binding to GAD65 does not appear to be

Table 1
Major Autoantigens in Type 1 Diabetes

	GAD 65	*IA-2*	*Insulin*
Amino acid length	585	974	51
Molecular weight (Da)	65,000	106,000	6,000
Cell type	Neuroendocrine	Neuroendocrine	Pancreatic islets
Intracellular location	Secretory vesicles	Secretory vesicles	Secretory vesicles
Function	Converts glutamic acid to gamma-aminobutyric acid (GABA): inhibitory neurotransmitter	Enzymatically inactive member of protein tyrosine phosphatase (PTP) family	Insulin receptor ligand

dependent on the region between amino acids 361 and 436, which contains the pyridoxal phosphate-binding site that defines the active site of the GAD enzyme. This observation is consistent with reports that GAD65Ab in patients with type 1 diabetes does not affect GAD enzyme activity. A small proportion (10–20%) of type 1 diabetes sera contain antibodies reactive with GAD67, but this is believed to be the result of crossreactivity of a subpopulation of GAD65Ab that reacts with both GAD isoforms *(36)*. Prediction of type 1 diabetes may be improved by analyzing the epitope specificity of GAD65 autoantibodies *(35,37,38)*. Further improvement of the positive predictive value may come from the analysis of autoantibody subtypes and isotypes *(39,40)*.

Human islets seem predominantly to express GAD65 and, interestingly, the expression is primarily restricted to the β-cells. GAD67 is also expressed at a much reduced level in the β-cells, but is detectable in the non-β-cell population. In rat cells, GAD65 is also predominantly in the β-cells, but is detected in α-cells as well *(41)*. Taken together, it is possible, at least in humans, that GAD65 may be able to direct an immune response to the pancreatic β-cells. Because GAD65 is expressed intracellularly and not on the cell surface, it is likely that a β-cell-specific immune attack will be carried out by CD8+ cytotoxic T-cells (CTL), rather than by GAD65 autoantibodies. Class I-restricted and either GAD65- *(42)* or insulin *(43)*-specific CTLs have been described in type 1 diabetes. It is critical to determine the role of GAD65 in the cell-mediated immune response to the β-cells and the subsequent autoantibody response that is currently used to predict type 1 diabetes.

IA-2

IA-2 is a single-chain protein consisting of 979 amino acids with a molecular weight of about 106 kDa (*see* Table 1). The antigen has a short transmembrane section almost in the middle of the sequence (amino acids 577–600). The IA-2 antigen is expressed in secretory granules not only in β-cells but also in other endocrine cells *(44,45)*. An IA-2 isoform, IA-2 β or phogrin, has also been described *(46)*; however, most IA-2Ab-positive subjects react with IA-2 and measurements of phogrin antibodies do not markedly increase prediction of type 1 diabetes *(47)*. IA-2Ab are more frequently detected in young patients (under 15 yr of age) with shorter disease duration. It has been suggested that the appearance of IA-2Ab is a marker of ensuing type 1 diabetes *(48,49)*. The autoantibody epitopes associated with risk for type 1 diabetes are located between the transmembrane sequence and the C-terminus *(47)* peptides and epitope mapping. T-cell lines have been derived from diabetic patients representing amino acids 831–850 and 841–860 of IA-2 *(50)*. The overlapping portion may represent an immunodominant region of the molecule. Another study reported a nearby dominant epitope, VIVMLT-PLVEDGVKQC (amino acids 805–820), which elicited the highest T-cell responses in all at-risk relatives *(51)*. This epitope has 56% identity and 100% similarity over nine amino acids with a sequence in VP7, a major immunogenic protein of human rotavirus. Both the IA-2 and the virus peptide bound to HLA DRB1*0401. This dominant IA-2 epitope peptide also had 45–75% identity and 64–88% similarity over 8–14 amino acids to sequences in Dengue, cytomegalovirus, measles, hepatitis C, canine distemper viruses, and the bacterium *Haemophilus influenzae*. Three other IA-2 epitope peptides were 71–100% similar over 7–12 amino acids to herpes-, rhino-, hanta-, and flaviviruses. Two others were 80–82% similar over 10–11 amino acids to sequences in milk, wheat, and bean proteins. These detailed studies are important to test whether activation of CD4+ T-cells can be mediated by rotavirus and other viruses, as well as dietary proteins. Activation may either provoke or worsen β-cell autoimmunity through molecular mimicry with IA-2 and thereby increase the risk for type 1 diabetes *(52)*.

Cytotoxic CD8+ T-lymphocytes (CTL) were detected against the IA-2 amino acid 797–805 peptide and restricted by HLA-A2 *(53)*. Although IA-2 peptide-specific CTL were detected in patients, as well as in nonaffected controls, the data suggest that it is now possible to generate IA-2-specific T-cells for further studies of the role of this autoantigen in the process of β-cell destruction in type 1 diabetes. It will be of particular importance to identify CTLs as able to kill human β-cells, and the question would be one of how many of these cells can reproducibly be found in the peripheral blood. Future directions may include the identification of such cells not only in blood samples from susceptible individuals but perhaps also in the pancreas, using high-resolution imaging techniques. IA-2 peptide-dependent and HLA class I-restricted CD8+ CTLs may be of particular importance to β-cell destruction because in some first-degree relatives to type 1 diabetes subjects, AI-2Ab seem to mark a rapid onset of type 1 diabetes *(54)*.

Insulin

Insulin or proinsulin is a truly islet-cell-specific autoantigen. The insulin gene on human chromosome 11 is predominantly expressed in the pancreatic β-cell (*see* Table 1). However, studies in humans indicate that the insulin gene may also be expressed in the thymus with possible implications for induction of immune tolerance *(55,56)*. IAAs were first described in 1983 *(57)*, and although recent standardization workshops have yet to identify a reliable and reproducible assay system *(31)*, most data suggest that IAAs are primarly associated with type 1 diabetes in children *(58–62)*. The IAAs appear to react with a conformation-dependent epitope *(63)*, perhaps explaining the failure to detect disease-associated IAAs by enzyme-linked immunosorbent assay (ELISA) or similar tests *(64)*. An improved IAA assay was recently reported *(65)* and IAAs combined with either GAD65Ab, IA-2Ab, or both, predict type 1 diabetes in first-degree relatives *(66,67)* and in the general population *(68)*. Because only some insulin is expressed on the β-cell surface *(69)*, it is unclear to what extent conformation-dependent IAAs observed in children with new onset type 1 diabetes *(70)* could contribute to the mechanism of β-cell killing.

Although it has been notoriously difficult to generate CD4+ or CD8+ T-cells restricted by insulin peptides and type 1 diabetes-associated HLA *(71)*, recent studies in mice expressing human class II molecules show promising results toward the isolation of insulin-specific T-cell clones *(72,73)*. Furthermore, using X-ray crystallography, the three-dimensional structure of DQ8 complexed with an immunodominant peptide from insulin has been determined *(74)*. It was suggested that the similarity of the DQ8, DQ2, and I-A(g7) peptide-binding pockets indicates that diabetes may be caused by the same antigen-presentation event(s) in humans and NOD mice.

Diabetes may be generated in mice following manipulation to break tolerance combined with immunization with the insulin B9-23 peptide *(75)*. Similar mechanisms need to be studied in humans to determine the possible importance of an anti-insulin immune response in β-cell destruction. The role of insulin in CTL killing of β-cells requires the expression of insulin peptides on HLA class I molecules. It is well known that HLA class I is expressed on the surface of β-cells *(76)* and that insulitis is associated with an increased expression of these molecules *(77,78)*. Novel techniques such as HLA tetramers *(79)* may prove useful in identifying T-cells that have TCRs recognizing specific insulin peptides on either CD4+ or CD8+ T-cells. It will be important to identify HLA class I-restricted and insulin peptide-dependent CTLs that are able to kill human β-cells and uncover the possible role of such cells in β-cell destruction.

Other Antigens

A number of other proteins have been reported to be related to autoimmune diabetes. These candidate autoantigens have been reviewed elsewhere *(7,80)*. Using recombinant antigens labeled by in vitro transcription/translation *(81)* in the radioligand assay proved useful for GAD65Ab *(81,82)*. However, subsequently standardized *(31,32)* assays have indicated that autoantibodies against these autoantigens do not show significant diagnostic sensitivity, specificity, and predictive value for type 1 diabetes *(83)*. The possible role in β-cell destruction of islet cell candidate autoantigens such as 69 kDa (ICA69) *(84)*, carboxypeptidase H *(85)*, ganglioside GM2-1 *(86)*, imogen 38 *(87)*, peripherin *(88)*, heat-shock proteins *(89)*, CD38 *(90)*, glima 38 *(91)*, and yet to be isolated autoantigens and peptides that are reported to stimulate T-cell proliferation in vitro *(87,92,93)* remains to be determined. Although the appearance of autoantibodies to these autoantigens does not seem to contribute to type 1 diabetes risk, it cannot be excluded that these and other autoantigens may contribute to CTL-mediated β-cell destruction. There is a lack of knowledge on the importance of heterogeneity in type 1 diabetes, which is exemplified by the fact that HLA association is much dependent on age *(94–96)* and ethnic background *(97)*.

HETEROGENEITY OF HUMAN TYPE 1 DIABETES

Diabetes mellitus is classified based on clinical criteria into type 1 and type 2 diabetes *(98)*. Recently, a growing number of monogenic diabetes disorders have been identified *(98)*. Type 1 diabetes develops acutely. Ketoacidosis and coma develop unless insulin is administered. Type 2 diabetes develops mostly as a result of insulin resistance associated with obesity and β-cell dysfunction and occurs insidiously, and most patients are successfully controlled by diet, exercise, or oral hypoglycemic agents. It is well known that recommendations for diabetes classification do not apply to all ethnic groups *(98)*. The heterogeneity of autoimmune diabetes development is

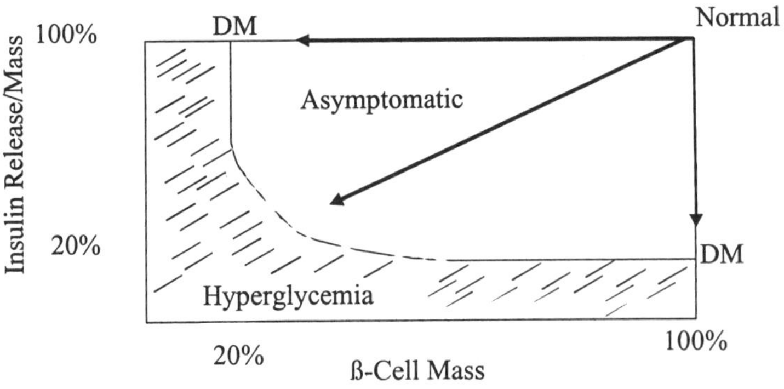

Fig. 2. Development of diabetes (DM) is illustrated to be a function of insulin release/mass and β-cell mass. Diabetes may develop if all islets are removed or if the β-cell function is completely inhibited. Different diabetes phenotypes may be dependent of a combination of the two parameters. This illustration was created by Dr. Daniel L. Cook.

illustrated in Fig. 2. Diabetes will appear as a function of loss of β-cell mass and loss of β-cell function. Different clinical phenotypes may develop, dependent on the combination of loss of β-cell mass and loss of function. Loss of function is envisaged when the islets of Langerhans are infiltrated by macrophages that are releasing cytokines that inhibit β-cell function but do not kill the cells. A different severity of inflammation may lead to variable degree of β-cell inhibition and resulting hyperglycemia. In addition, the degree of insulin resistance is also critical *(99)*. Some subjects may encounter a severe loss of β-cells but, despite this, may not develop diabetes because of their high insulin sensitivity *(100)*. The relationship between insulin resistance and β-cell function is illustrated in Fig. 3. Other subjects may develop diabetes at modest β-cell loss because they are highly insulin resistant. Therefore, it is not surprising that type 1 diabetes or autoimmune diabetes is associated with a large number of different phenotypes, as illustrated next.

In addition to the typical autoimmune type 1 diabetes patients, there are patients with insidious onset and insulin dependency who are classified with slowly progressive type 1 diabetes *(101,102)*. There are no diagnostic criteria established for these patients. Other patients classified with type 2 diabetes may, in fact, have latent autoimmune diabetes in adult (LADA) (for a recent review, *see* ref. *103*), also referred to as slowly progressive insulin-dependent diabetes mellitus [or SPIDDM *(102)*] or type 1,5 diabetes *(104)* because they have islet cell antibodies (ICAs) or GAD65Ab. It is noted that the overall autoantibody frequency in type 2 patients varies between 6% and 10% *(105)*. However, the positive predictive value that a GAD65Ab positive type 2 diabetes patient will be treated with insulin within 5 yr is 100% *(106,107)*. The corresponding prevalence of GAD65Ab among other ethnic groups has been reported to be 7.5% among Japanese *(108)*, 12% among Caucasians in Scandinavia *(109)*, and 10% in the United Kingdom *(105)*, but only 2.8% in northern Italy *(110)* or 3–4% in Korean type 2 patients *(111)*. The degree of β-cell destruction and insulitis in these patients remains to be clarified. To complicate the heterogeneity of autoimmune diabetes even further, it has also been found that patients with diabetes may develop GAD65 autoantibodies after the clinical diagnosis *(112)*. It is speculated that the progressive β-cell loss in

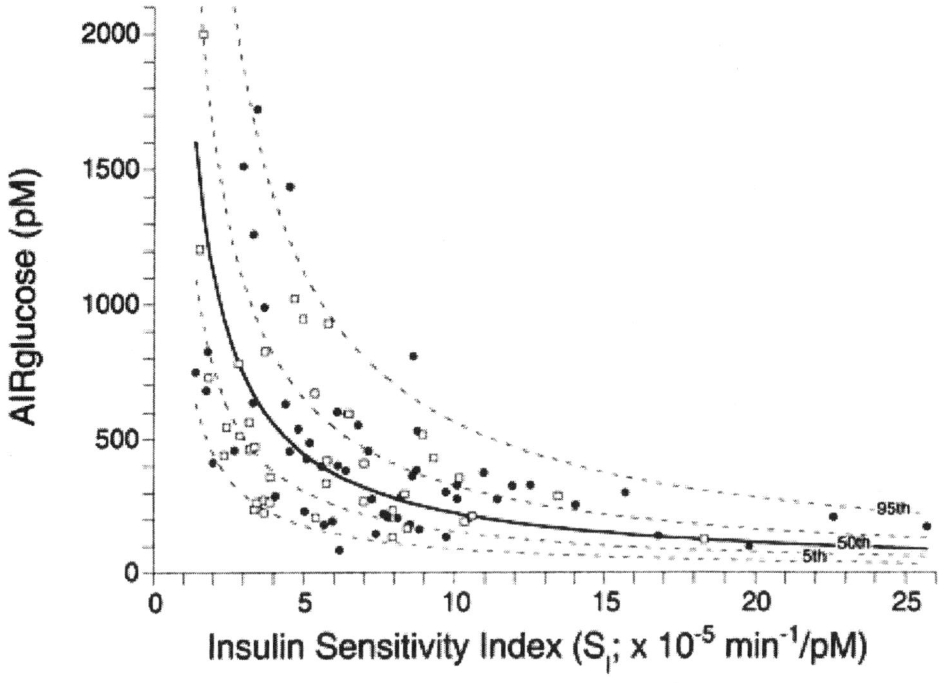

Fig. 3. Relationship between insulin sensitivity and β-cell function quantified as the first-phase insulin response (AIRglucose) in 93 (55 males and 38 females) apparently healthy, nondiabetic subjects under the age of 45 yr. The cohort demonstrates a broad range of insulin sensitivity and β-cell function. The solid line depicts the best-fit relationship (50th percentile) and the broken lines represent the 5th, 25th, 75th, and 95th percentiles. The relationship is best described by a hyperbolic function so that any change in insulin sensitivity is balanced by a reciprocal and proportionate change in β-cell function. Patients at risk for developing type 1 diabetes may vary in clinical onset, dependent on the combination of insulin sensitivity and residual β-cell function. (Copyright © 1993 American Diabetes Association. From Diabetes, Vol. 42, 1993; 1663–1672. Reprinted with permission from the American Diabetes Association.)

these patients is slow and that the presence of GAD65Ab marks a slow, but progressive, immune-mediated β-cell killing.

In contrast to these patients masquerading as type 2 diabetic patients, an acute onset of type 1 diabetes is also reported *(113)*. These patients have lower glycosylated hemoglobin values, diminished urinary excretion of C peptide, a more severe metabolic disorder with ketoacidosis, as well as higher serum pancreatic enzyme concentrations, compared to type 1 patients with a less dramatic onset. GAD65, IA-2, and IAAs were negative, but immunohistologic studies of pancreatic biopsy specimens from three patients revealed T-lymphocyte-predominant infiltrates in the exocrine pancreas but no insulitis. Some patients with idiopathic type 1 diabetes have an apparent nonautoimmune disease characterized by the absence of insulitis and of diabetes-related antibodies, a remarkably abrupt onset, and high serum pancreatic enzyme concentrations. Diabetes may, therefore, develop in association with a spectrum of variable β-cell loss and sometimes the marker is present without symptoms of diabetes.

In first-degree relatives of patients with type 1 diabetes who have antibodies to islet antigens, such as insulin, GAD65, or IA-2, the risk of diabetes increases with the number of antibodies *(24,66)*. However, diabetes does not develop in all antibody-positive relatives. In long-term prospective studies, many such relatives have remained normoglycemic despite the presence of both ICAs and a reduced ability to secrete insulin *(6)*. The overall frequency of first-degree relatives who have one or several islet cell autoantibodies is 5–8%; however, few from all of these subjects go on to develop type 1 diabetes. It is unclear to what extent autoantibody-positive subjects have lost β-cells and to what extent they have insulitis.

Novel autoantibody screening methods permit screening the general population for islet cell autoantibodies to predict disease *(24)*. Screening of newborn children and follow-up of children at risk for type 1 diabetes confirm that islet cell autoantibodies predict disease *(34,114–116)*. The possible correlation between the antibody markers and degree of β-cell destruction remains to be determined. Although there seems to be a considerable risk for infants to develop type 1 diabetes if they are positive for more than one antibody, the situation in adults appears to be different. In screening subjects who had been subjected to a health survey, GAD65Ab were found more often among subjects with impaired glucose tolerance or undiagnosed diabetes *(117)*. In addition, in two independent observations, GAD65Ab-positive subjects had an increased body mass index (BMI) compared to matched autoantibody negative subjects *(117,118)*. These data suggest that similar to type 2 diabetes, the metabolic burden of obesity and insulin resistance could precipitate postpubertal clinical onset in subjects with slowly progressive autoimmune diabetes. It is still unclear how much β-cell destruction as well as regeneration is present in such individuals because none had developed diabetes at follow-up 9 yr later *(119)*.

In conclusion, the type 1 diabetes phenotype is highly heterogeneous. The symptoms at the time of clinical onset vary with age and ethnicity. Acute-onset type 1 diabetes with a minimum of immune-related phenomena may occur at any age and may be associated with exocrine dysfunction. The majority of patients develop type 1 diabetes in association with one or several islet autoantibodies that predict the disease. Slow progressive type 1 diabetes is most often characterized by autoimmunity against the pancreatic islet β-cells. The experience in analyzing type 2 diabetes patients for islet cell autoantibodies has demonstrated that GAD65Ab is the best predictive marker for loss of residual β-cell function and development of insulin dependency. The inconstant type 1 diabetes phenotype at the time of clinical diagnosis may be the result of different degrees of insulitis in combination with variable insulin sensitivity.

CLINICAL STUDIES: INSULITIS

Type 1 diabetes mellitus is characterized by infiltration of the islets of Langerhans by mononuclear cells *(1)*. The phenotype of mononuclear cells accumulating in pancreatic islets in type 1 diabetes is variable *(18,26,120,121)*. The number of pancreatic specimens obtained at onset is very limited, as are studies by biopsies *(121)*. Taken together, monocytes/macrophages are identified among other mononuclear cell types in islet infiltrates. V beta 8-positive T-cells were identified in one study *(120)*, but T-cells expressing other V beta T-cell receptors were also reported. The vascular endothelium of the islets and many small vessels near the islets showed expression of the intercellular adhesion molecule-1. Other studies have reported the presence of both T- and B-lymphocytes and deposits of immunoglobulin *(14)*, suggesting that close to the time of clinical diagnosis, the insulitis observed is chronic rather than acute. Several hypotheses have been suggested to explain the loss of β-cells. The majority of these hypotheses are difficult to test in humans. Therefore, inference is most often made from studies in laboratory animals. As a combination of animal and human insulitis, there are a number of mechanisms for potential β-cell death that are worth considering.

Apoptosis as a Mechanism of β-Cell Death

Apoptosis or programmed cell death is an integral part of tissue homeostasis and apoptotic cells are rapidly cleared from tissues by scavenger macrophages or by immature dendritic cells to prevent inappropriate inflammatory responses. Apoptosis refers to the morphological features of programmed cell death, which is a normal process contributing to tissue turnover during development and in the adult. Traditionally, apoptosis is not expected to be associated with a subsequent immune response. Cells that undergo apoptosis are characterized by shrinkage, nuclear condensation, membrane blebbing, and membrane changes that eventually lead to phagocytosis of the affected cell. The possible role of apoptosis in type 1 diabetes pathogenesis has recently been reviewed *(122,123)*. The following signaling pathways have been implied in apoptosis: the Fas system, stress-activated protein kinases, serine/threonine kinases, the Ras signaling pathway, protein kinase C, calcium signaling pathways, ceramide, cAMP, and free radicals. There are two gene families that are particularly important in the control of apoptosis: the genes encoding the IL-1β-converting enzyme (ICE) family of cystein proteases (caspases) and those related to the proto-oncogene bcl-2. The inducible form of nitric oxide synthase is induced by IL-1β or IL-1β combined with IFN-γ in isolated human islets *(123,124)*. Consequently, nitric oxide (NO) is formed. NO contributes to both β-cell necrosis and to apoptosis. Most data suggest that the main mode of cell death induced by cytokines in human β-cells is apoptosis. Rodent islet cells appear more sensitive to cytokine-induced apoptosis and necrosis. The antioxidant defense mechanisms may be more developed in human islets, and both glucose oxidation and ATP production seem to be maintained. It has been proposed that the apoptotic program after the death signal delivered by cytokines is maintained in human islets. Unfortunately, only in vitro observations support the possible role of any one of these pathways of apoptosis in islet cell function. Although the role of apoptotic signals after human islet isolation have identified inhibition of the stress-activated protein kinase pathways as important to islet cell survival following islet isolation for transplantation *(125)*, it remains to be clarified if apoptosis is increased in human insulitis. It is critical that pancreatic specimens from humans at risk or at the time of clinical diagnosis *(126)* are carefully evaluated for markers of apoptosis, necrosis, or both, because it cannot be excluded that drugs in the future might be targeted toward pathways of apoptosis.

Death by Marcophages, T-Cells, or B-Cells

Insulitis is associated with the specific killing of β-cells. The β-cell specificity in type 1 diabetes-related cell killing is remarkable because glucagon, somatostatin, and pancreatic polypeptide (PP) cells appear unaffected by the autoimmune attack *(4,5)*. Insulitis may be less frequent in older patients, occurring in 6 out of 12 patients with clinical onset between 14 and 21 yr and in 1 out of 6 patients with clinical onset between 21 and 30 yr *(127,128)*. The presence of damaged or degenerated β-cells can attract and activate macrophages whose secreting products can affect healthy surrounding β-cells *(129)*. In one patient with acute onset, there where virtually no islets with infiltrating lymphocytes but numerous islets were infiltrated by macrophages *(5)*. Complete loss of β-cells preferentially seems to occur in patients with clinical onset under the age of 7 and the depletion was completed within the first year of clinical disease (for a review of the literature, *see* ref. *5*). Other features observed in the pancreas of patients who died close to the clinical onset include that insulitis primarily occurs in islets containing insulin-positive cells *(127)*. This is interpreted as a sign for T-cell migration to β-cell-specific antigens. Immunostaining of biopsied pancreatic islets from patients with type 1 diabetes reveals that most of the infiltrating lymphocytes are CD8+ T-cells and a few are CD4+ helper T-cells *(121,130)*. However, in pancreas with insulitis, not all islets with β-cells are infiltrated by lymphocytes; in fact, only a minority of their islets showed signs of insulitis. Patients at an older age at onset showed fewer islets with lymphocytic infiltration. In patients with clinical onset over the age of 21 yr, insulitis has been reported as a rare phenomenon *(26)*. The descriptive analysis of pancreatic islets at the time of clinical diagnosis of type 1 diabetes does not explain the mechanisms by which β-cells are killed and we have not learned much since the rediscovery of insulitis by Gepts in 1965 *(1)*.

In How Many Ways Can the β-Cells Get Killed?

Killing by Virus

Since Yoon et al. *(131)* isolated coxsackie B4 virus from the pancreas of a patient with type 1 diabetes, various viruses have been studied to examine their diabetogenic potential and to what extent viruses represent an environmental factor that contributes to the disease. The viral infection seems to be able to indirectly activate autoreactive T-cells that, in turn, can generate initial pancreatic tissue damage. Damaged β-cells release previously ignored self antigens that may activate an autoimmune process, rapidly promoting the generation of insulitis and, eventually, overt diabetes by immune-mediated β-cell killing. Viral infections could trigger type 1 diabetes through several mechanisms; for example, (1) sequence similarities between islet-cell GAD65 and coxsackie virus could cause immune attack against coxsackie virus to also target the beta cells, (2) enteroviral infections could sustain autoimmunity until a final "hit" results in β-cell destruction following lysis of the cells, (3) acute or chronic enteroviral infections of peri-insular tissue could lead to β-cell destruction from an abundance of free radicals *(132)*, or (4) rapid replication of virus in β-cells may cause β-cell lysis, clearance of debris by lymphatic drainage to pancreatic lymph nodes where antigen presentation takes place, resulting in an autoimmune reaction to beta cell antigens *(133)*. The relationship between coxsackie B virus infection and GAD65 autoimmunity has recently received the most attention. The sequence homology of an amino acid peptide between human GAD65 and the coxsackie virus p2-C protein provides the support of specific molecular mimicry *(10,134)*. IA-2 is another molecular target of pancreatic islet autoimmunity in immune-mediated type 1 diabetes. The epitope spanning 805–820 amino acid was found to have 56% identity and 100% similarity over 9 amino acid with a sequence in VP7, a major immunogenic protein of human rotavirus *(51,52)*. The role of virus antigen molecular mimicry in disease association and in the generation of insulitis remains to be clarified. It is also not clarified whether infection by one of the many viruses implicated in type 1 diabetes initiates or enhances the disease process.

Killing by T-Cells

Antigen-specific T-cell activation results in the differentiation of naive CD4+ Th cells into Th1 and Th2 clones based on their pattern of cytokine production and effector functions. Th1 cells produce IL-2 and IFN-γ and promote cell-mediated responses and delayed-type hypersensitivity reactions. Th2 cells produce IL-4, IL-5, IL-10, and IL-13 and stimulate humoral immunity. It is speculated that the progression of type 1 diabetes from insulitis to overt diabetes may be controlled by Th1 rather than Th2 cells because human islets are primarily infiltrated by CD8+ T-cells. It has, therefore, been suggested that Th1 cytokines promote, whereas Th2 cytokines protect from the onset and progression of type 1 diabetes. However, this appear to be a serious oversimplification because in some cases Th2 cells and their cytokines may accelerate β-cell destruction. Although nothing is known in humans, the Th2-induced component of anti-β-cell immunity appeared to be mediated by local production of IL-10, but not IL-4, and accelerated the autoimmune destruction of β islets *(135)*. Th2 cytokines, in particular IL-10, may promote necrosis through occlusion of the microvasculature, thereby reducing the viability of the larger islets. Th2 cytokines promote peri-insulitis and frank insulitis by enhancing major histocompatibility complex class II expression, thereby stimulating the accumulation of macrophages and B-cells *(136)*.

It is evident that Th1 cells are not the sole mediators of islet β-cell destruction, that Th2 cells are not inhibitory or benign, as was previously suggested, because they are capable of inducing islet β-cell destruction, and that both Th1 and Th2 cytokines appear to cooperate in driving β-cell destruction. Th1-driven attacks are more rapid and aggressive and are sustained for a longer time period. This suggested that Th2-mediated attacks are responsible for an early phase of type 1 diabetes, whereas Th1-driven responses are responsible for the persistent and sustained attacks. Th1 lesions comprised focally confined insulitis consisting primarily of CD8+ and CD4+ T-cells, and islet β-cells die by apoptosis, thereby sparing surrounding exocrine tissue. In contrast, Th2 lesions were more dispersed and consisted primarily of macrophages, with a notable scarcity of T-cells and β-cells die by necrosis. Also, there is an accumulation of fibroblasts and the generation of extensive extracellular matrix and adipose tissue in Th2 lesions, which subsequently leads to tissue necrosis *(137)*. The above represents speculations primarly based on animal studies. Studies in humans are required to dissect the mechanisms by which T-cells may kill β-cells. It is hypothesized that future immunotherapy must take into consideration the delicate balance between Th1 and Th2 cells during distinct phases of insulitis and type 1 diabetes development.

Killing by Mediators

Mediators of β-cell destruction include factors secreted from CD8 T-cell granules (e.g., perforin and granzymes), T-cell surface molecules (e.g., Fas-L, TNF, and other TNF family members), as well as secreted cytokines (e.g., TNF, IFN-γ). All of these mediators are known to induce DNA fragmentation and the morphological changes of apoptosis through complex signaling cascades that involve the activation of cystein proteases or caspases *(138)*. It was investigated whether or not the Fas-FasL system was involved in insulitis. Pancreas biopsy specimens showed insulitis in 6/13 of recent-onset patients. In these six patients, Fas was expressed in both the islets and infiltrating cells but not in either cell type in the seven other patients without insulitis. Double immunostaining revealed that FasL-positive cells was primarily CD8+ but could also be found on macrophages and CD4+ cells. It was speculated that Fas on β-cells may interact with FasL on infiltrating cells to trigger apoptotic β-cell death in inflamed islets *(139)*.

PRECLINICAL STUDIES

Animal Studies

The availability of BB rats and NOD mice has greatly enhanced our understanding of the possible pathogenic mechanisms involved in immune-mediated type 1 diabetes. The human immune response is, however, different from that of the rodents and preclinical trials may not always be applicable to humans. For example, macrophages play an essential role in initiating animal insulitis: They are the first infiltrating cells and an immune intervention directed against macrophages prevent diabetes development. Several inflammatory mediators produced by macrophages may cause islet β-cell destruction in murine insulin-dependent diabetes, but as indicated earlier, human β-cells appear more resistant to cytokine-induced apoptosis or necrosis.

The balance of subsets of CD4+ T-cells, including T-helper 1 (Th1) and T-helper 2 (Th2), is also speculated to be involved in β-cell killing. More mRNA for Th1 cytokines and less for Th2 cytokines are produced by lymphocytes infiltrating the pancreatic islets in female NOD mice that are diabetes-prone, whereas more mRNA for Th2 cytokines and less for Th1 cytokines in male NOD mice as produced. Oral administration of insulin, in particular the immunodominant B chain, was associated with progressive reduction in β-cell destruction in NOD mice concomitant with decreased expression of Th1 cytokines and a corresponding increase in Th2 cytokine expression *(138)*. Apoptosis was most frequent in the insulin-negative islet area comprised of mononuclear cell infiltrate and was localized to CD8+ T-cells. The rarity of detectable apoptotic β-cells in spontaneous prediabetic mice with pronounced insulitis and reduced insulin-positive islet areas most likely reflects the rapid clearance of apoptotic β-cells *(138)*. It was reported that β-cell apoptosis was present at 3 wk of age before the appearance of T-cells in NOD islets and it also has been observed before the appearance of insulitis in transgenic mouse models of accelerated diabetes *(140)*.

CD4+ T-cells that are responsive to GAD and are diabetogenic in NOD mice *(141)* as well as GAD65 peptide restricted CD8+ T-cells have been isolated in mice *(142)* and also found in humans *(42)*. GAD has a region of similarity to the coxsackie virus P-2C protein. T-cells in humans that may respond in a viral infection could crossreact with this endogenous autoantigen *(143)*. It was shown that infection with coxsackie B4 virus accelerated mouse diabetes *(144)*. It was suggested that diabetes following viral infection in the TCR-transgenic mice occurs more in response to bystander activation of inflammatory cells than by molecular mimicry.

Several transgenic models have been developed in NOD mice in order to attempt to further clarify the role of GAD in diabetes. Mutation of GAD was used because it was not presumed to affect immunoreactivity and previous attempts to generate transgenic mice had failed. This was thought perhaps to be the result of toxicity of widespread expression of functional GAD. Another transgenic model expressed GAD65 on the RIP-7 promotor, such that the GAD65 was expressed at high levels in the pancreatic islets *(145)*. Two lines were generated, one of which expressing higher levels of

GAD65 was protected from diabetes. In another model, an antisense construct was used to prevent the expression of both GAD65 and GAD67. In these mice, the spontaneous development of diabetes was also inhibited *(13)*. It is unclear whether the protection from diabetes is solely the result of the immunologic effects of suppression of GAD65 and GAD67.

Within the islets of NOD mice, there are CD4+ T-cells that recognize insulin *(146)*. The immunodominant peptide consists of amino acids 9–23 of the B chain, and when cloned, these cells are capable of causing diabetes on adoptive transfer *(147)*. In analyzing pathogenic CD8+ T-cells in the NOD mice, highly diabetogenic CD8+ T-cell clones were found to recognize a peptide consisting of amino acids 15–23 of the B chain of insulin *(148)*. Thus, the insulin B chain is an important target for both pathogenic CD4+ and CD8+ T-cells as well as insulin autoantibodies *(62)* in the NOD mice.

In Vitro Studies

Apoptotic cells can induce immune responses. In vitro culture of apoptotic cells with dendritic cells resulted in the presentation of antigen and stimulation of both MHC class I-restricted CD8+ T-cells and MHC class II-restricted CD4+ T-cells. Macrophages were also able to present antigen from apoptotic cells and activate CD8+ T-cells. Incubation of apoptotic cells with peritoneal macrophages resulted in greater secretion of proinflammatory (Th1) cytokines when compared with incubation with nonapoptotic cells *(149)*. Other studies have shown that dual labeling of terminal dUTP nick end-labeling (TUNEL)-positive cells and either β-cells or infiltrating T-cells revealed that a minority of apoptotic cells were β-cells and the majority were infiltrating cells *(138)*. In vitro systems may, therefore, not fully reflect insulitis and the β-cell killing that takes place in vivo. The numerous studies on isolated islets exposed to TNF-α, IL-1β, and oxygen radicals, especially nitric oxide, are reviewed elsewhere *(122,123,142)*. Although of theoretical interest and important to understand mechanisms of cell death, in general, and β-cell, in particular, the reality is that our understanding of human β-cell killing of importance to type 1 diabetes is rudimentary.

CONCLUSIONS

The molecular mechanisms of β-cell killing associated with the development of human type 1 diabetes are largely unknown. The islets of Langerhans are often but not always infiltrated with immune system cells, primarily CD8+ T-cells, CD4+ T-cells, and macrophages at the time of clinical onset. Insulitis may be more severe and more common in the young at age at onset. Little is known about cell infiltration in subjects at risk for developing type 1 diabetes, such as being positive for GAD65, IA-2, or insulin autoantibodies. There is a major gap in knowledge about whether the molecular mechanism of β-cell destruction involves β-cell autoantigen-specific CD8+ T-cells, CD4+ T-cell, or macrophage-induced cytokine-mediated apoptosis or necrosis or a combination of these factors. The exquisite β-cell specificity may be best explained by cell-mediated, perhaps even antibody-mediated cytotoxicity directed against β-cell specific antigens such as GAD65, IA-2, or insulin. Numerous preclinical and in vitro investigations support a possible role of these mechanism, but the major lack of studies in humans hampers progress toward clinical trials to prevent or inhibit β-cell destruction associated with the development of type 1 diabetes.

ACKNOWLEDGMENTS

Studies in the authors' laboratory were supported in part by the National Institutes of Health (grants DK26190, AI42380, DK53004, DK17047), the Juvenile Diabetes Research Foundation International, and the American Diabetes Association.

REFERENCES

1. Gepts W. Pathologic anatomy of the pancreas in juvenile diabetes mellitus. Diabetes 1965;14:619–633.
2. von Meyenburg H. Über "insulitis" bei diabetes. Schweitz Med Wochenschr 1940;21:554–561.
3. Gepts W, LaCompte PM. The pancreatic islets in diabetes. Am J Med 1981;70:105–115.
4. Rahier J, Goebbels RM, Henquin JC. Cellular composition of the human diabetic pancreas. Diabetologia 1983;24:366–371.
5. Lernmark Å, Klöppel G, Stenger D, Vathanaprida C, Fält K, Landin-Olsson M, et al. Heterogeneity of human islet pathology in newly diagnosed childhood insulin-dependent diabetes mellitus. Macrophage infiltrations and expression of HLA-DQ and glutamic acid decarboxylase. Virchows Archiv 1995;425:631–640.
6. Greenbaum CJ, Sears KL, Kahn SE, Palmer JP. Relationship of beta-cell function and autoantibodies to progression and nonprogression of subclinical type 1 diabetes—follow-up of the Seattle Family Study. Diabetes 1999;48:170–175.
7. Schranz D, Lernmark Å. Immunology in diabetes: an update. Diabetes Metab Rev 1998;14:3–29.
8. Gottlieb PA, Eisenbarth GS. Diagnosis and treatment of pre-insulin dependent diabetes. Annu Rev Med 1998;49:391–405.
9. Thomson G. An overview of the genetic analysis of complex diseases, with reference to type 1 diabetes. Best Pract Res Clin Endocrinol Metab 2001;15:265–277.
10. Kukreja A, Maclaren NK. Current cases in which epitope mimicry is considered as a component cause of autoimmune disease: immune-mediated (type 1) diabetes. Cell Mol Life Sci 2000;57:534–541.
11. Kaufman DL, Clare-Salzler M, Tian J, Forsthuber T, Ting GSP, Robinson P, et al. Spontaneous loss of T-cell tolerance to glutamic acid decarboxylase in murine insulin-dependent diabetes. Nature 1993;366:69–72.
12. Tisch R, Yang X-D, Singer SM, Liblau RS, Fugger, L, McDevitt HO. Immune response to glutamic acid decarboxylase correlates with insulitis in non-obese diabetic mice. Nature 1993;366:72–75.
13. Yoon JW, Yoon CS, Lim HW, Huang QQ, Kang Y, Pyun KH, et al. Control of autoimmune diabetes in NOD mice by GAD expression or suppression in beta cells. [see comments]. Science 1999;284:1183–1187.
14. Bottazzo GF, Dean BM, McNally JM, MacKay EH, Swift PGF, Gamble DR. *In situ* characterization of autoimmune phenomena and expression of HLA molecules in the pancreas in diabetic insulitis. N Engl J Med 1985;313:353–360.
15. Huang X, Yuan J, Goddard A, Foulis A, James R, Lernmark Å, et al. Interferon expression in the pancreata of patients with type 1 diabetes. Diabetes 1995;44:658–664.
16. In't Veld PA, Pipeleers DG. *In situ* analysis of pancreatic islets in rats developing diabetes: appearance of nonendocrine cells with surface MHC class II antigens and cytoplasmic insulin immunoreactivity. J Clin Invest 1988;82:1123–1128.
17. Hanafusa T, Miyazaki A, Miyagawa J. Examination of islets in the pancreas biopsy specimens from newly diagnosed type 1 (insulin-dependent) diabetic patients. Diabetologia 1990;33:105–111.
18. Foulis AK, McGill M, Farquharson A. Insulitis in type 1 (insulin-dependent) diabetes mellitus in man—macrophages, lymphocytes, and interferon-λ containing cells. J Pathol 1991;165:97–103.
19. Lee KU, Amano K, Yoon JW. Evidence for initial involvement of macrophage in development of insulitis in NOD mice. Diabetes 1998;37:989–991.
20. Voorbij HAM, Jeucken PHM, Kabel PJ, Haan MD, Drexhage HA. Dendritic cells and scavenger macrophages in pancreatic islets of prediabetic BB rats. Diabetes 1989;38:1623–1629.
21. Hanenberg H, Kolb-Bachofen V, Kantwerk-Funke G, Kolb H. Macrophage infiltration precedes and is a prerequisite for lymphocytic insulitis in pancreatic islets of pre-diabetic BB rats. Diabetologia 1989;32:126–134.
22. Lee KU, Kim MK, Amano K, Pak CY, Jaworski MA, Mehta JG, et al. Preferential infiltration of macrophages during early stages of insulitis in diabetes-prone BB rats. Diabetes 1988;37:1053–1058.

23. Bieg S, Simonson W, Ellefsen K, Lernmark A. Rel B is an early marker of autoimmune islet inflammation in the biobreeding (BB) rat. Pancreas 2000;20:47–54.
24. Notkins AL, Lernmark A. Autoimmune type 1 diabetes: resolved and unresolved issues. J Clin Invest 2001;108:1247–1252.
25. Bach J-F. Insulin-dependent diabetes mellitus as an autoimmune disease. Endocrine Rev 1994;15:516–542.
26. Pipeleers D, Ling Z. Pancreatic beta cells in insulin-dependent diabetes. Diabetes Metab Rev 1992;8:209–227.
27. Eizirik DL, Sandler S, Palmer JP. Repair of pancreatic beta-cells. A relevant phenomenon in early IDDM? Diabetes 1993;42:1383–1391.
28. Karlsen AE, Hagopian WA, Grubin CE, Dube S, Disteche CM, Adler DA, et al. Cloning and primary structure of a human islet isoform of glutamic acid decarboxylase from chromosome 10. Proc Natl Acad Sci USA 1991;88:8337–8341.
29. Bu D-F, Erlander MG, Hitz BC, Tillakaratne NJK, Kaufman DL, Wanger-McPherson CB, et al. Two human glutamate decarboxylases, 65-kDa GAD and 67-kDa GAD, are each encoded by a single gene. Proc Natl Acad Sci USA 1992;89:2115–2119.
30. Kim J, Richter W, Aanstoot H-J, Shi Y, Fu Q, Rajotte R, et al. Differential expression of GAD65 and GAD67 in human, rat, and mouse pancreatic islets. Diabetes 1993;42:1799–1808.
31. Verge CF, Stenger D, Bonifacio E, Colman PG, Pilcher C, Bingley PJ, et al. Combined use of autoantibodies (IA-2 autoantibody, GAD autoantibody, insulin autoantibody, cytoplasmic islet cell antibodies) in type 1 diabetes: Combinatorial Islet Autoantibody Workshop. Diabetes 1998;47:1857–1866.
32. Mire-Sluis AR, Das RG, Lernmark Å. The World Health Organization International Collaborative Study for Islet Cell Antibodies. Diabetologia 2000;43:1282–1292.
33. Kim J, Namchuck M, Bugawan T, Fu Q, Jaffe M, Shi Y, et al. Higher autoantibody levels and recognition of a linear NH2-terminal epitope in the autoantigen GAD65, distinguish Stiff–Man syndrome from insulin-dependent diabetes mellitus. J Exp Med 1994;180:595–606.
34. Bonifacio E, Lampasona V, Bernasconi L, Ziegler AG. Maturation of the humoral autoimmune response to epitopes of GAD in preclinical childhood type 1 diabetes. Diabetes 2000;49:202–208.
35. Hampe CS, Hammerle LP, Bekris L, Ortqvist E, Kockum I, Rolandsson O, et al. Recognition of glutamic acid decarboxylase (GAD) by autoantibodies from different GAD antibody-positive phenotypes. J Clin Endocrinol Metab 2000;85:4671–4679.
36. Falorni A, Örtqvist E, Persson B, Lernmark Å. Radioimmunoassays for glutamic acid decarboxylase (GAD65) and GAD65 autoantibodies using ^{35}S or ^{3}H recombinant human ligands. J Immunol Methods 1995;186:89–99.
37. Falorni A, Ackefors M, Carlberg C, Daniels T, Persson B, Robertson J, et al. Diagnostic sensitivity of immunodominant epitopes of glutamic acid decarboxylase (GAD65) autoantibodies epitopes in childhood IDDM. Diabetologia 1996;39:1091–1098.
38. Falorni A, Gambelunghe G, Forini F, Kassi G, Cosentino A, Candeloro P, et al. Autoantibody recognition of COOH-terminal epitopes of GAD65 marks the risk for insulin requirement in adult-onset diabetes mellitus. J Clin Endocrinol Metab 2000;85:309–316.
39. Petersen JS, Kulmala P, Clausen JT, Knip M, Dyrberg T. Progression to type 1 diabetes is associated with a change in the immunoglobulin isotype profile of autoantibodies to glutamic acid decarboxylase (GAD65). Clin Immunol 1999;90:276–281.
40. Hawa MI, Fava D, Medici F, Deng YJ, Notkins AL, De Mattia G, et al. Antibodies to IA-2 and GAD65 in type 1 and type 2 diabetes: isotype restriction and polyclonality. Diabetes Care 2000;23:228–233.
41. Karlsen AE, Hagopian WA, Petersen JS, Boel E, Dyrberg T, Grubin CE, et al. Recombinant glutamic acid decarboxylase representing a single isoform expressed in human islets detects IDDM associated 64K autoantibodies. Diabetes 1992;41:1355–1359.
42. Panina-Bordignon P, Lang R, van Endert PM, Benazzi E, Felix AM, Pastore RM, et al. Cytotoxic T cells specific for glutamic acid decarboxylase in autoimmune diabetes. J Exp Med 1995;181:1923–1927.
43. Kimura K, Kawamura T, Kadotani S, Inada H, Niihira S, Yamano T. Peptide-specific cytotoxicity of T lymphocytes against glutamic acid decarboxylase and insulin in type 1 diabetes mellitus. Diabetes Res Clin Pract 2001;51:173–179.
44. Lan MS, Lu J, Goto Y, Notkins AL. Molecular cloning and identification of a receptor-type protein tyrosine phosphatase, IA-2, from human insulinoma. DNA Cell Biol 1994;13:505–514.

45. Solimena M, Dirkx R Jr, Hermel JM, Pleasic WS, Shapiro JA, Caron L, et al. ICA 512, an autoantigen of type I diabetes, is an intrinsic membrane protein of neurosecretory granules. EMBO J 1996;15:2102–2114.
46. Wasmeier C, Hutton JC. Molecular cloning of phogrin, a protein-tyrosine phosphatase homologue localized to insulin secretory granule membranes. J Biol Chem 1996;271:18,161–18,170.
47. Kawasaki E, Yu L, Rewers MJ, Hutton JC, Eisenbarth GS. Definition of multiple ICA512/phogrin autoantibody epitopes and detection of intramolecular epitope spreading in relatives of patients with type 1 diabetes. Diabetes 1998;47:733–742.
48. LaGasse J, Jelinek L, Sexson S, LoftonDay C, Breininger J, Sheppard P, et al. An islet-cell protein tyrosine phosphatase is a likely precursor to the 37-kDa autoantigen in type 1 diabetes: Human and macaque sequences, tissue distribution, unique and shared epitopes, and predictive autoantibodies. Mol Med 1997;3:163–173.
49. Savola K, Bonifacio E, Sabbah E, Kulmala P, Vahasalo P, Karjalainen J, et al. IA-2 antibodies—a sensitive marker of IDDM with clinical onset in childhood and adolescence. Diabetologia 1998;41:424–429.
50. Hawkes CJ, Schloot NC, Marks J, Willemen SJ, Drijfhout JW, Mayer EK, et al. T-cell lines reactive to an immunodominant epitope of the tyrosine phosphatase-like autoantigen IA-2 in type 1 diabetes. Diabetes 2000;49:356–366.
51. Honeyman MC, Stone NL, Harrison LC. T-Cell epitopes in type 1 diabetes autoantigen tyrosine phosphatase IA-2: potential for mimicry with rotavirus and other environmental agents. Mol Med 1998;4:231–239.
52. Honeyman MC, Coulson BS, Stone NL, BGellert SA, Goldwater PN, Steele CE, et al. Association between rotavirus infection and pancreatic islet autoimmunity in children at risk of developing type 1 diabetes. Diabetes 2000;49:1319–1324.
53. Takahashi A, Tsujihata M, Yokota A, Yamaguchi Y, Ueda Y, Akazawa S, et al. A new method of detection of islet cell antibodies (ICA) using peroxidase-labeled protein A, and incidence of ICA in type 1 (insulin-dependent) diabetes. Diabetologia 1986;29:378–382.
54. Gorus FK, Goubert P, Semakula C, Vandewalle CL, DeSchepper J, Scheen A, et al. IA-2-autoantibodies complement GAD(65)-autoantibodies in new-onset IDDM patients and help predict impending diabetes in their siblings. Diabetologia 1997;40:95–99.
55. Pugliese A, Zeller M, Fernandez JA, Zalcberg LJ, Bartlett RJ, Riocordi C, et al. The insulin gene transcribed in the human thymus and transcription level correlate with allelic variation at the INS VNTR-IDDM2 susceptibility locus for type 1 diabetes. Nat Genet 1997;15:293–297.
56. Vafiadis P, Bennett ST, Todd JA, Nadeau J, Grabs R, Goodyer CG, et al. Insulin expression in human thymus is modulated by INS VNTR alleles at the IDDM2 locus. Nat Genet 1997;15:289–292.
57. Palmer JP, Asplin CM, Clemons P, Lyen K, Tatpati O, Raghu PK, et al. Insulin antibodies in insulin-dependent diabetics before insulin treatment. Science 1983;222:1337–1339.
58. Vardi P, Ziegler AG, Matthews, JH, Diub S, Keller RJ, Ricker AT, et al. Concentration of insulin autoantibodies at onset of type I diabetes: inverse log-linear correlation with age. Diabetes Care 1988;9:736–739.
59. Landin-Olsson M, Palmer JP, Lernmark Å, Blom L, Sundkvist G, Nyström L, et al. Predictive value of islet cell and insulin autoantibodies for type 1 (insulin-dependent) diabetes mellitus in a population-based study of newly-diagnosed diabetic and matched control children. Diabetologia 1992;35:1068–1073.
60. Gorus FK, Vandewalle CL, Dorchy H, Van Crombrugge P, Schuit FC, Pipeleers DG, et al. Influence of age on the associations among insulin autoantibodies, islet cell antibodies, and HLA DQA1*0301-DQB1*0302 and siblings of patients with type 1 (insulin-dependent) diabetes mellitus. J Clin Endo Metab 1994;78:1172–1178.
61. Komulainen J, Kulmala P, Savola K, Lounamaa R, Ilonen J, Reijonen H, et al. Clinical, autoimmune, and genetic characteristics of very young children with type 1 diabetes. Diabetes Care 1999;22:1950–1955.
62. Yu L, Robles DT, Abiru N, Kaur P, Rewers M, Kelemen K, et al. Early expression of antiinsulin autoantibodies of humans and the NOD mouse: evidence for early determination of subsequent diabetes. Proc Natl Acad Sci USA 2000;97:1701–1706.
63. Castano L, Ziegler A, Ziegler R, Shoelson S, Eisenbarth GS. Characterization of insulin autoantibodies in relatives of patients with insulin-dependent diabetes mellitus. Diabetes 1993;42:1202–1209.
64. Greenbaum CJ, Palmer JP, Kuglin B, Kolb H. Insulin autoantibodies measured by radioimmunoassay methodology are more related to insulin-dependent diabetes mellitus than those measured by

enzyme-linked immunosorbent assay: results of the Fourth International Workshop on the Standardization of Insulin Autoantibody Measurement. J Clin Endcrinol Metab 1992;74:1040–1044.
65. Williams AJK, Bingley PJ, Bonifacio E, Palmer JP, Gale EAM. A novel micro-assay for insulin autoantibodies. J Autoimmun 1997;10:473–478.
66. Verge CF, Gianani R, Kawasaki E, Yu L, Pietropaolo M, Jackson RA, et al. Prediction of type I diabetes in first-degree relatives using a combination of insulin, GAD, and ICA512bdc/IA-2 autoantibodies. Diabetes 1996;45:926–933.
67. Komulainen J, Knip M, Sabbah E, Vahasalo P, Lounamaa R, Akerblom HK, et al. Autoimmune and clinical characteristics of type I diabetes in children with different genetic risk loads defined by HLA-DQB1 alleles. Clin Sci (Colch) 1998;94:263–269.
68. Bingley PJ, Bonifacio E, Williams AJK, Genovese S, Bottazzo GF, Gale EAM. Prediction of IDDM in the general population: strategies based on combinations of autoantibody markers. Diabetes 1997;46:1701–1710.
69. Aguilar-Diosdado M, Parkinson D, Corbett J, Kwon G, Marshall C, Gikngerich R, et al. Potential autoantigens in IDDM. Expression of carbox-peptidase-H and insulin but not GAD on the beta-cell surface. Diabetes 1994;43:418–425.
70. Brooks-Worrell BM, Nielson D, Palmer JP. Insulin autoantibodies and insulin antibodies have similar binding characteristics. Proc Assoc Am Physicians 1999;111:92–96.
71. Peakman M, Tree TI, Endl J, van Endert P, Atkinson MA, Roep BO. Characterization of preparations of GAD65, proinsulin, and the islet tyrosine phosphatase IA-2 for use in detection of autoreactive T-cells in type 1 diabetes: report of phase II of the Second International Immunology of Diabetes Society Workshop for Standardization of T-cell Assays in Type 1 Diabetes. Diabetes 2001;50:1749–1754.
72. Wen L, Wong FS, Burkly L, Altieri M, Mamalaki C, Kioussis D, et al. Induction of insulitis by glutamic acid decarboxylase peptide-specific and HLA-DQ8-restricted CD4(+) T cells from human DQ transgenic mice. J Clin Invest 1998;102:947–957.
73. Congia M, Patel S, Cope AP, De Virgiliis S, Sonderstrup G. T cell epitopes of insulin defined in HLA-DR4 transgenic mice are derived from preproinsulin and proinsulin. Proc Natl Acad Sci USA 1998;95:3833–3838.
74. Lee KH, Wucherpfennig KW, Wiley DC. Structure of human insulin peptide-HLA-DQ8 complex and susceptibility to type 1 diabetes. Nat Immunol 2001;2:501–507.
75. Abiru N, Yu L, Miao D, Maniatis AK, Liu E, Moriyama H, et al. Transient insulin autoantibody expression independent of development of diabetes: comparison of NOD and NOR strains. J Autoimmun 2001;17:1–6.
76. Baekkeskov S, Kanatsuna T, Klareskog L, Nielsen DA, Peterson PA, Rubenstein AH, et al. Expression of major histocompatibility antigens on pancreatic islet cells. Proc Natl Acad Sci USA 1981;78:6456–6460.
77. Campbell IL, Oxbrow L, West J, Harrison LC. Regulation of MHC protein expression in pancreatic β-cells by interferon-λ and tumour necrosis factor-α. Mol Endocrinol 1988;2:101–107.
78. Foulis AK, Farquharson MA, Hardman R. Aberrant expression of class II major histocompatibility complex molecules by B cells and hyperexpression of class I major histocompatibility complex molecules by insulin containing islets in type 1 (insulin-dependent) diabetes mellitus. Diabetologia 1987;30:333–343.
79. Novak EJ, Liu AW, Nepom GT, Kwok WW. MHC class II tetramers identify peptide-specific human CD4(+) T cells proliferating in response to influenza A antigen. J Clin Invest 1999;104:R63–R67.
80. Atkinson M, Kaufman D, Newman D, Tobin A, Maclaren N. Islet cell cytoplasmic autoantibody reactivity to glutamate decarboxylase in insulin-dependent diabetes. J Clin Invest 1993;91:350–356.
81. Grubin CE, Daniels T, Toivola B, Landin-Olsson M, Hagopian WA, Li L, et al. A novel radioligand binding assay to determine diagnostic accuracy of isoform-specific glutamic acid decarboxylase antibodies in childhood IDDM. Diabetologia 1994;37:344–350.
82. Petersen JS, Hejnaes KR, Moody A, Karlsen AE, Marshall MO, Hoier-Madsen M, et al. Detection of GAD65 antibodies in diabetes and other autoimmune diseases using a simple radioligand assay. Diabetes 1994;43:459–465.
83. Lampasona V, Ferrari M, Bosi E, Pastore MR, Bingley PJ, Bonifacio E. Sera from patients with IDDM and healthy individuals have antibodies to ICA69 on Western blots but do not immunoprecipitate liquid phase antigen. J Autoimmun 1994;7:665–674.
84. Pietropaolo M, Castano L, Babu S, Buelow R, Kuo Y-LS, Martin S, et al. Islet cell autoantigen 69KDa (ICA69): molecular cloning and characterization of a novel diabetes-associated autoantigen. J Clin Invest 1993;92:359–371.

85. Castano L, Russo E, Zhou L, Lipes M, Eisenbarth G. Identification and cloning of a granule autoantigen (carboxypeptidase-H) associated with type 1 diabetes. J Clin Endocrinol Metab 1991;73:1197–1201.
86. Dotta F, Previti M, Lenti L, Dionisi S, Casetta B, D'Erme M, et al. GM2-1 pancreatic islet ganglioside: identification and characterization of a novel islet-specific molecule. Diabetologia 1995;38:1117–1121.
87. Arden SD, Roep BO, Neophytou PI, Usac EF, Duinkerken G, de Vries RRP, et al. Imogen 38: a novel 38-kD islet mitochondrial autoantigen recognized by T cells from a newly diagnosed type 1 diabetic patient. J Clin Invest 1996;97:551–561.
88. Boitard C, Villa MC, Becourt C, Gia HP, Huc C, Sempe P, et al. Peripherin: an islet antigen that is cross-reactive with nonobese diabetic mouse class II gene products. Proc Natl Acad Sci USA 1992;89:172–176.
89. Ozawa Y, Kasuga A, Nomaguchi H, Maruyama T, Kasatani T, Shimada A, et al. Detection of autoantibodies to the pancreatic islet heat shock protein 60 in insulin-dependent diabetes mellitus. J Autoimmun 1996;9:517–524.
90. Pupilli C, Giannini S, Marchetti P, Lupi R, Antonelli A, Malavasi F, et al. Autoantibodies to CD38 (ADP-ribosyl cyclase/cyclic ADP-ribose hydrolase) in Caucasian patients with diabetes: effects on insulin release from human islets. Diabetes 1999;48:2309–2315.
91. Aanstot HJ, Kang SM, Kim J, Lindsay LA, Roll U, Knip M, et al. Identification and characterization of glima 38, a glycosylated islet cell membrane antigen, which together with GAD(65) and IA2 marks the early phases of autoimmune response in type 1 diabetes. J Clin Invest 1996;97:2772–2783.
92. Geluk A, vanMeijgaarden KE, Schloot NC, Drijfhout JW, Ottenhoff THM, Roep BO. HLA-DR binding analysis of peptides from islet antigens in IDDM. Diabetes 1998;47:1594–1601.
93. Roep BO, Kallan AA, Hazenbos WLW, Bruining GJ, Bailyes EM, Arden SD, et al. T-Cell reactivity to 38 kD insulin- secretory-granule protein in patients with recent-onset type 1 diabetes. Lancet 1991;337:1439–1441.
94. Graham J, Kockum I, Sanjeevi CB, Landin-Olsson M, Nystrom L, Sundkvist G, et al. Negative association between type 1 diabetes and HLA DQB1*0602-DQA1*0102 is attenuated with age at onset. Swedish Childhood Diabetes Study Group. Eur J Immunogenet 1999;26:117–127.
95. Robert J-J, Deschamps I, Chevenne D, Roger M, Mogenet A, Boitard C. Relationship between first-phase insulin secretion and age, HLA, islet cell antibody status, and development of type 1 diabetes in 220 juvenile first-degree relatives of diabetic patients. Diabetes Care 1991;14:718–723.
96. Caillat-Zucman A, Garchon H-J, Timsit J, Assan R, Boitard C, Idriss D-S, et al. Age-dependent HLA genetic heterogeneity of type 1 insulin-dependent diabetes mellitus. J Clin Invest 1992;90:2242–2250.
97. Thorsby E, Rønningen KS. Particular HLA-DQ molecules play a dominant role in determining susceptibility or resistance to type 1 (insulin-dependent) diabetes mellitus. Diabetologia 1993;36:371–377.
98. The Expert Committee on the Diagnosis and Classification of Diabetes Mellitus. Report of the expert committee on the diagnosis and classification of diabetes mellitus. Diabetes 1997;20:1183–1194.
99. Kahn SE, Prigeon RL, McCulloch DK, Boyko EJ, Bergman RN, Schwartz MW, et al. Quantification of the relationship between insulin sensitivity and beta-cell function in human subjects. Evidence for a hyperbolic function. Diabetes 1993;42:1663–1672.
100. Kahn SE. Clinical review 135: the importance of beta-cell failure in the development and progression of type 2 diabetes. J Clin Endocrinol Metab 2001;86:4047–4058.
101. Tuomi T, Zimmet P, Rowley MJ, Min HK, Vichayanrat A, Lee HK, et al. Differing frequency of autoantibodies to glutamic acid decarboxylase among Koreans, Thais, and Australians with diabetes mellitus. Clin Immunol Immunopathol 1995;74:202–206.
102. Kobayashi T, Tamemoto K, Nakanishi K, Kato N, Okubo M, Kajio H, et al. Immunogenetic and clinical characterization of slowly progressive IDDM. Diabetes Care 1993;16:780–788.
103. Pozzilli P, Di Mario U. Autoimmune diabetes not requiring insulin at diagnosis (latent autoimmune diabetes of the adult): definition, characterization, and potential prevention. Diabetes Care 2001;24:1460–1467.
104. Juneja R, Hirsch IB, Naik RG, Brooks-Worrell BM, Greenbaum CJ, Palmer JP. Islet cell antibodies and glutamic acid decarboxylase antibodies, but not the clinical phenotype, help to identify type 1(1/2) diabetes in patients presenting with type 2 diabetes. Metabolism 2001;50:1008–1013.
105. Turner R, Stratton I, Horton V, Manley S, Zimmet P, Mackay IR, et al. UKPDS 25: autoantibodies to islet-cell cytoplasm and glutamic acid decarboxylase for prediction of insulin requirement in type 2 diabetes. UK Prospective Diabetes Study Group. Lancet 1997;350:1288–1293.
106. Hagopian WA, Karlsen AE, Gottsater A, Landin-Olsson M, Grubin CE, Sundkvist G, et al. Quantitative assay using recombinant human islet glutamic acid decarboxylase (GAD-64) showed 64K autoantibody positivity at onset predicts diabetes type. J Clin Invest 1993;91:368–374.

107. Törn C, Landin-Olsson M, Ostman J, Schersten B, Arnqvist H, Blohme G, et al. Glutamic acid decarboxylase antibodies (GADA) is the most important factor for prediction of insulin therapy within 3 years in young adult diabetic patients not classified as type 1 diabetes on clinical grounds. Diabetes Metab Res Rev 2000;16:442–447.
108. Kasuga A, Maruyama T, Ozawa Y, Takei I, Falorni A, Lernmark Å, et al. Antibody to the Mr 65,000 isoform of glutamic acid decarboxylase are detected in non-insulin-dependent diabetes in Japanese. J Autoimmun 1996;9:105–111.
109. Tuomi T, Groop LC, Zimmet PZ, Rowley MJ, Knowles W, Mackay IR. Antibodies to glutamic acid decarboxylase reveal latent autoimmune diabetes mellitus in adults with a non-insulin-dependent onset of disease. Diabetes 1993;42:359–362.
110. Bosi EP, Garancini MP, Poggiali F, Bonifacio E, Gallus G. Low prevalence of islet autoimmunity in adult diabetes and low predictive value of islet autoantibodies in the general adult population of northern Italy. Diabetologia 1999;42:840–844.
111. Park Y, Lee H, Takino H, Abiru N, Kawasaki E, Eisenbarth GS. Evaluation of the efficacy of the combination of multiple autoantibodies to islet-specific antigens in Korean type 1 diabetic patients. Acta Diabetol 2001;38:51–56.
112. Landin-Olsson M, Arnqvist HJ, Blohme G, Littorin B, Lithner F, Nystrom L, et al. Appearance of islet cell autoantibodies after clinical diagnosis of diabetes mellitus. Autoimmunity 1999;29:57–63.
113. Imagawa A, Hanafusa T, Miyagawa J, Matsuzawa Y. A novel subtype of type 1 diabetes mellitus characterized by a rapid onset and an absence of diabetes-related antibodies. Osaka IDDM Study Group. [see comments]. N Engl J Med 2000;342:301–307.
114. Norris JM, Beaty B, Klingensmith G, Yu L, Hoffman M, Chase HP, et al. Lack of association between early exposure to cow's milk protein and beta-cell autoimmunity. Diabetes Autoimmunity Study in the Young (DAISY). JAMA 1996;276:609–614.
115. Ilonen J, Simell O, Knip M, Akerblom HK. Screening for genetic IDDM risk and prevention trials in infancy. Diabetes Metab Rev 1998;14:188–189.
116. Kimpimaki T, Kupila A, Hamalainen AM, Kukko M, Kulmala P, Savola K, et al. The first signs of beta-cell autoimmunity appear in infancy in genetically susceptible children from the general population: the Finnish Type 1 Diabetes Prediction and Prevention Study. J Clin Endocrinol Metab 2001;86:4782–4788.
117. Rolandsson O, Hägg E, Hampe C, Sullivan EP, Nilsson M, Jansson G, et al. Levels of glutamate decarboxylase (GAD65) and tyrosine phosphatase-like protein (IA-2) autoantibodies in the general population are related to glucose intolerance and body mass index. Diabetologia 1999;42:555–559.
118. Weets I, Van Autreve J, Van der Auwera BJ, Schuit FC, Du Caju MV, Decochez K, et al. Male-to-female excess in diabetes diagnosed in early adulthood is not specific for the immune-mediated form nor is it HLA-DQ restricted: possible relation to increased body mass index. Diabetologia 2001;44:40–47.
119. Rolandsson O, Hägg E, Nilsson M, Hallmans G, Lernmark Å. Prediction of diabetes by screening with body mass index, oral glucose tolerance test (OGT) and islet cell autoantibodies in a regional population. J Intern Med 2001;249:279–288.
120. Hänninen A, Jalkanen S, Salmi M, Toikkanen S, Nikolakaros G, Simell O. Macrophages, T cell receptor usage, and endothelial cell activation in the pancreas at the onset of insulin-dependent diabetes mellitus. J Clin Invest 1992;90:1901–1910.
121. Itoh N, Hanafusa T, Miyazaki A, Miyagawa J-I, Yamagata K, Yamamoto K, et al. Mononuclear cell infiltration and its relation to the expression of major histocompatibility complex antigens and adhesion molecules in pancreas biopsy specimens from newly diagnosed insulin-dependent diabetes mellitus patients. J Clin Invest 1993;92:2313–2322.
122. Mauricio D, Mandrup-Poulsen T. Apoptosis and the pathogenesis of IDDM: a question of life and death. Diabetes 1998;47:1537–1543.
123. Eizirik DL, Darville MI. Beta-cell apoptosis and defense mechanisms: lessons from type 1 diabetes. Diabetes 2001;50(Suppl. 1):S64–S69.
124. Eizirik DL, Strandell E, Sandler S. Culture of mouse pancreatic islets in different glucose concentrations modifies B cell sensitivity to streptozotocin. Diabetologia 1988;31:168–174.
125. Paraskevas S, Aikin R, Maysinger D, Lakey JR, Cavanagh TJ, Agapitos D, et al. Modulation of JNK and p38 stress activated protein kinases in isolated islets of Langerhans: insulin as an autocrine survival signal. Ann Surg 2001;233:124–133.
126. Conrad B, Weidmann E, Tucco G, Rudert WA, Behboo R, Ricordi CR, et al. Evidence for superantigen involvement in insulin-dependent diabetes mellitus aetiology. Nature 1994;371:351–355.

127. Foulis AK, Stewart JA. The pancreas in recent-onset type 1 (insulin-dependent) diabetes mellitus: insulin content of islets, insulitis and associated changes in the exocrine acinar tissue. Diabetologia 1984;26:456–461.
128. Foulis AK, Liddle CN, Farquharson MA, Richmond JA, Weir RS. The histopathology of the pancreas in type I (insulin-dependent) diabetes mellitus: a 25-year review of deaths in patients under 20 years of age in the United Kingdom. Diabetologia 1986;29:267–274.
129. Kolb-Bachofen V, Kolb H. A role for macrophages in the pathogenesis of type 1 diabetes. Autoimmunity 1989;3:145–155.
130. Imagawa A, Hanafusa T, Tamura S, Moriwaki M, Itoh N, Yamamoto K, et al. Pancreatic biopsy as a procedure for detecting in situ autoimmune phenomena in type 1 diabetes: close correlation between serological markers and histological evidence of cellular autoimmunity. Diabetes 2001;50:1269–1273.
131. Yoon J-W, Austin M, Onodera T, Notkins AL. Isolation of a virus from the pancreas of a child with diabetic ketoacidosis. N Engl J Med 1975;300:1174–1179.
132. Wendorf MA. Diabetes and enterovirus autoimmunity in glacial Europe. Med Hypotheses 1999;52:423–429.
133. Hoglund P, Mintern J, Waltzinger C, Heath W, Benoist C, Mathis D. Initiation of autoimmune diabetes by developmentally regulated presentation of islet cell antigens in the pancreatic lymph nodes. J Exp Med 1999;189:331–339.
134. Hou J, Said C, Franchi D, Dockstader P, Chatterjee NK. Antibodies to glutamic acid decarboxylase and P2-C peptides in sera from Coxsackie virus B4-infected mice and IDDM patients. Diabetes 1994;43:1260–1266.
135. Balasa B, Van Gunst K, Jung N, Balakrishna D, Santamaria P, Hanafusa T, et al. Islet-specific expression of IL-10 promotes diabetes in nonobese diabetic mice independent of Fas, perforin, TNF receptor- 1, and TNF receptor-2 molecules. J Immunol 2000;165:2841–2849.
136. Almawi WY, Tamim H, Azar ST. Clinical review 103: T helper type 1 and 2 cytokines mediate the onset and progression of type I (insulin-dependent) diabetes. J Clin Endocrinol Metab 1999;84:1497–1502.
137. Azar ST, Tamim H, Beyhum HN, Habbal MZ, Almawi WY. Type I (insulin-dependent) diabetes is a Th1- and Th2-mediated autoimmune disease. Clin Diagn Lab Immunol 1999;6:306–310.
138. Augstein P, Stephens LA, Allison J, Elefanty AG, Ekberg M, Kay TW, et al. Beta-cell apoptosis in an accelerated model of autoimmune diabetes. Mol Med 1998;4:495–501.
139. Moriwaki M, Itoh N, Miyagawa J, Yamamoto K, Imagawa A, Yamagata K, et al. Fas and Fas ligand expression in inflamed islets in pancreas sections of patients with recent-onset type I diabetes mellitus. Diabetologia 1999;42:1332–1340.
140. O'Brien BA, Harmon BV, Cameron DP, Allan DJ. Apoptosis is the mode of beta-cell death responsible for the development of IDDM in the nonobese diabetic (NOD) mouse. Diabetes 1997;46:750–757.
141 Zekzer D, Wong FS, Ayalon O, Millet I, Altieri M, Shintani S, et al. GAD-reactive CD4+ Th1 cells induce diabetes in NOD/SCID mice. J Clin Invest 1998;101:68–73.
142. Quinn A, McInerney MF, Sercarz EE. MHC class I-restricted determinants on the glutamic acid decarboxylase 65 molecule induce spontaneous CTL activity. J Immunol 2001;167:1748–1757.
143. Atkinson MA, Bowman MA, Campbell L, Darrow BL, Kaufman DL, Maclaren NK. Cellular immunity to a determinant common to glutamate decarboxylase and coxsackie virus in insulin-dependent diabetes. J Clin Invest 1994;94:2125–2129.
144. Horwitz MS, Bradley LM, Harbertson J, Krahl T, Lee J, Sarvetnick N. Diabetes induced by coxsackie virus: initiation by bystander damage and not molecular mimicry. Nat Med 1998;4:781–785.
145. Bridgett M, Cetkovic-Cvrlje M, O'Rourke R, Shi Y, Narayanswami S, Lambert J, et al. Differential protection in two transgenic lines of NOD/Lt mice hyperexpressing the autoantigen GAD65 in pancreatic beta-cells. Diabetes 1998;47:1848–1856.
146. Daniel D, Gill RG, Schloot N, Wegmann D. Epitope specificity, cytokine production profile and diabetogenic activity of insulin-specific T cell clones isolated from NOD mice. Eur J Immunol 1995;25:1056–1062.
147. Daniel D, Wegmann DR. Protection of nonobese diabetic mice from diabetes by intranasal or subcutaneous administration of insulin peptide B-(9–23). Proc Natl Acad Sci USA 1996;93:956–960.
148. Wong FS, Karttunen J, Dumont C, Wen L, Visintin I, Pilip IM, et al. Identification of an MHC class I-restricted autoantigen in type 1 diabetes by screening an organ-specific cDNA library. Nat Med 1999;5:1026–1031.
149. Uchimura E, Kodaira T, Kurosaka K, Yang D, Watanabe N, Kobayashi Y. Interaction of phagocytes with apoptotic cells leads to production of pro-inflammatory cytokines. Biochem Biophys Res Commun 1997;239:799–803.
150. Wucherpfennig KW, Eisenbarth GS. Type 1 diabetes. Nat Immunol 2001;2:767–768.

5

Type 1 Diabetes in Autoimmune Syndromes

Tiinamaija Tuomi, MD, PhD and Jaakko Perheentupa, MD, PhD

CONTENTS

INTRODUCTION

Two fundamentally different autoimmune polyendocrine syndromes (APSs) are generally recognized, and type 1 diabetes mellitus is common in both (*see* Table 1). APS type 1 (APS-1) or autoimmune polyendocrinopathy–candidiasis–ectodermal dystrophy (APECED) is an autosomal recessive disease. It can often be diagnosed by clinical criteria (presence of mucocutaneous candidiasis and/or hypoparathyroidism, which do not occur in APS-2) or by DNA analysis. The definition of APS type 2 has varied. One common definition of APS-2 sets the presence of adrenocortical insufficiency (AI) as a criterion *(1–3),* and the combination of AI with autoimmune thyroid disease (AITD) or type 1 diabetes mellitus has also been called the Schmidt or Carpenter syndrome. With that limitation of APS-2, combinations of AITD with components other than AI are called APS3. Remaining combinations, like type 1 diabetes with myasthenia gravis or sarcoidosis, have been named APS4. However, there is no solid basis for such separations other than of APS-1 from the rest. Thus, according to the widest definition, which we subscribe to, various combinations of at least one autoimmune endocrine disease with at least one other autoimmune disorder (endocrine or nonendocrine) are collectively called APS-2 *(4).* Obviously, APS-2 thus defined is much more common than the Schmidt syndrome. It includes all combinations of type 1 diabetes mellitus with any other autoimmune disease, save combinations including

From: *Contemporary Endocrinology: Type 1 Diabetes: Etiology and Treatment*
Edited by: M. A. Sperling © Humana Press Inc., Totowa, NJ

Table 1
Comparison of Types 1 and 2 of Autoimmune Polyendocrine Syndrome (APS)

	APS-I	*APS-II*
Inheritance	Recessive autoimmune regulator *(AIRE)* gene in chromosome 21q22.3	Polygenic
Appearance	Infancy to adulthood; highest in childhood	Childhood to adulthood; highest in early adulthood
Mucocutaneous candidiasis	Eventually most patients, even all	None
Hypoparathyroidism	Eventually most patients	None
Adrenocortical insufficiency	Eventually most patients	<50%
Type 1 diabetes mellitus	Common	≈50%
Graves' disease	None or very rare	Common
Hashimoto's thyroiditis	None	Common
Hypothyroidism	Common	Common
Gonadal failure	Eventually most females; eventually common in males	Less common
Keratopathy	Common	None
B_{12} vitamin malabsorption	Common	Rare
Hepatitis	Common	Rare
Steatorrhea	Common	Celiac disease occurs
Alopecia	Common	Common
Vitiligo	Common	Common

Note: Because new component diseases tend to develop with age, exact prevalence figures for disease components give definite information only when given for specific age groups.

hypoparathyroidism and/or mucocutaneous candidiasis. The component endocrine disorders are not known to be different in pathogenesis, pathology, or clinical picture when occurring as components of an APS compared with when occurring alone. Therapy is an exception, as changes in the sufficiency of one hormone (e.g., appearance of deficiency or institution of substitution for it) may affect the sufficiency, endogenous or by replacement, of another hormone *(vide infra).*

When an endocrine disease appears in a previously endocrinologically healthy subject, it is usually not possible to predict whether an APS is to develop. As an exception, nonendocrine autoimmune components such as alopecia and vitiligo, or, in APECED, ectodermal hallmarks *(vide infra),* may be present before the first endocrine component and may allow recognition of the syndrome at appearance of the first endocrine component.

IMMUNOLOGY

Most of the autoimmune endocrine disorders appear initially as infiltration of the gland by lymphocytes and macrophages. This may lead to destruction and atrophy of the gland with deficiency of its hormone. Sometimes, it halts or even reverses at a stage of relative hypofunction. This has been documented for thyroiditis *(5)* and adrenalitis *(6),* and may be true for insulitis *(7,8).* The destructive process is presumed to be T-cell mediated. Commonly, antibodies to certain antigens of the gland appear in blood, most frequently antibodies against intracellular enzymes. The role of such autoantibodies remains unclear, but they are important as diagnostic messengers from an autoimmune process and appear commonly before clinical hormone deficiency.

Exceptions to this uncertainty of antibody role are some antibodies against membrane receptors, like the α-chain of the acetylcholine receptor in myasthenia gravis and the thyrotropin receptor in AITD. Antibodies to thyrotropin receptor can act as either agonists causing Graves' hyperthyroidism or blockers causing hypothyroidism. The net effect depends on their relative activities. Other important thyroid autoantigens are microsomal thyroid peroxidase and thyroglobulin. Thyroid autoimmunity, defined by the presence of any thyroid antibody, is much more common than clinical AITD and does not always herald the development of hypothyroidism. Part of this difference may be a result of the slowness of the destructive process. Agents inhibiting thyroid hormone synthesis, such as lithium and amiodarone, may turn subclinical hypothyroidism into manifest disease.

The most common antiadrenocortical antibodies are directed against 21-hydroxylase (P450c21). Although positivity for them does not always predict AI, AI is almost always preceded by their appearance in blood. Anti-P450c21 antibodies are equivalent to antiadrenal antibodies demonstrated by indirect immunofluorescence *(9,10)*. Of the other enzymes of adrenal steroid hormone synthesis, cholesterol side-chain cleavage enzyme (P450scc), 3-β hydroxysteroid dehydrogenase (3β HSD) and 17-α-hydroxylase (P450c17) are also present in the ovarian granulosa and theca cells and the testicular Leydig cells *(11–16)*. Circulating antibodies against them predict the development of premature ovarian failure *(17)*. Sera positive by immunofluorescence against those steroid-producing cells contain antibodies specific for P450scc, P450c17, and/or (rarely) 3β HSD *(15)*.

Diabetes-related autoantibodies are discussed elsewhere in this book. No antiparathyroid autoantibodies are recognized. Autoantibodies against the calcium sensing receptor have been reported in hypoparathyroidism *(18)*, but this finding has not been confirmed. They were not found in a large series of Finnish patients with hypoparathyroidism of APECED (Spiegel and Perheentupa, unpublished).

Patients with parietal cell atrophy or autoimmune vitamin B_{12} malabsorption (pernicious anemia) have autoantibodies against the intrinsic factor or the gastric H^+/K^+-ATPase. The latter is the specific antigen for the parietal cell antibody detected by indirect immunofluorescence *(19,20)*. In the chronic autoimmune hepatitis of APS-1, P450 1A2 may be a specific hepatic autoantigen *(22–23)*.

In alopecia, immunoreactivity has been observed against differentiating keratinocytes in hair follicles *(24)*. Antibodies against tyrosine hydroxylase correlated with the presence of alopecia in patients with APS-1 *(25–26)*, and antibodies against transcription factors SOX9 and SOX10 correlated with the presence of vitiligo in various patients *(27)*. Antibodies against tryptophan hydroxylase of intestinal mucosa correlate with intestinal dysfunction in patients with APS-1 *(28)*.

APS-1, AUTOIMMUNE POLYENDOCRINOPATHY–CANDIDIASIS–ECTODERMAL DYSTROPHY

There are two known autosomal recessive autoimmune diseases: autoimmune lymphoproliferation syndrome *(29)* and APECED, which is the more common one. The clinical hallmarks of APECED are mucocutaneous candidiasis and hypoparathyroidism, but neither of these is always present (*see* Table 2). Although rare, APECED

Table 2
Prevalences (%) of the Common Components of APECED at Various Ages, Estimated[a] from Finnish Series of 89 Patients

	Age (yr)							
Component	*1*	*2*	*5*	*10*	*15*	*20*	*30*	*40*
Hypoparathyroidism	0	6	33	64	78	84	85	86
Addison's disease	0	0	8	39	63	71	77	79
Diabetes mellitus	0	0	2	3	6	10	14	23
Hypothyroidism	0	0	0.6	1.5	2.4	5	11	18
Ovarian atrophy[b]					39	57	64	72
Male hypogonadism						9	18	26
Pernicious anemia[c]	0	0	0	2	10	17	20	31
Hepatitis[d]	1	2	4	11	15	17	17	17
Candidiasis	24	41	63	79	93	95		100
Keratopathy[e]	0	4	9	16	21	22	22	22
Alopecia	0	0	4	15	29	34	40	40
Vitiligo	0.5	1	2	8	15	19	22	26

[a] Estimated from the observed incidence rates at the age intervals, assuming that all the patients live until the age of 40 yr.
[b] Primary amenorrhea in 52%, secondary in 48%.
[c] Includes patients without clinical disease but with circulating antibodies against parietal cells and/or intrinsic factor receptor in (2 of 21).
[d] Includes three patients who died of fulminant hepatitis.
[e] Six (32%) of the patients developed blindness (5) or severely impaired vision (1).
Source: Unpublished data from J. Perheentupa.

seems to occur in most populations. Three populations have an exceptionally high prevalence: Iranian Jews (estimated at 1 : 9,000) *(30),* the Sardinians (1 : 14,000) *(31),* and the Finns (1 : 25,000).

Genetics

APECED is an autosomal recessive disease caused by mutations in the autoimmune regulator *(AIRE)* gene on chromosome 21q22.3 *(43,46). AIRE* contains 14 exons. It is mainly expressed in subsets of epithelial and monocyte lineage cells in thymus medulla, in rare cells in lymph node paracortex and medulla, spleen, and fetal liver, and in very few blood leukocytes. These all are antigen-presenting cells. Wider expression is disputed, but it has been reported also in the respiratory system, central nervous system, endocrine glands, urinary system, and genitals *(32).* Human and mouse *AIRE* promoters include conserved sites for several transcription factors, which are thymus-specific or important in hematopoesis *(33).*

The Aire protein consists of 545 amino acids. At its amino terminal is a highly conserved ASS domain necessary for subnuclear targeting and dimerization, which appears to be essential for its transcription activating action *(34).* Sp100, AIRE-1, NucP41/75, and DEAF-1/suppressin (SAND) domain is needed for DNA binding; two plant homeodomain type Zn fingers presumably serve protein–protein interaction, and two nuclear localization signals and four LXXLL motifs act in nuclear receptor binding. Human and mouse Aire proteins are 71% identical *(33,35).* They exist in nucleoplasmic granules and, occasionally, along the cytoplasmic microtubular cytoskeleton

(36,37). The protein is an activator of gene transcription *(38)*, but its exact physiological role is unknown. It may be involved in the determination of thymic stromal organization and, thus, in the induction of self-tolerance *(39,40)*.

To date, some 35 mutations of *AIRE* have been described in patients with APECED, most of them in four mutational hotspots *(34,41–45)*. Many are either missense mutations in the ASS region, presumably preventing the dimerization, or nonsense mutations leading to truncation of the protein. The internationally most common mutation, C889T, covers almost 90% of the Finnish APECED genes *(46)*. It leads to a deletion of both Zn fingers and most of the SAND domain. The second most common mutation *(34,46)*, predominant in the United States *(41)* and the United Kingdom *(44)*, is a 13 nucleotide deletion, which leads to a protein lacking the C-terminal third. The predominant Sardinian mutant protein *(31)* consists only of the N-terminal fourth. All of the reported Iranian Jewish patients are homozygous for a missense mutation in a single nucleotide, which disrupts the dimerization domain *(34)*. In approx 10% of the *AIRE* genes of clinically ascertained patients, identification of a mutation has failed *(34)*. These may be mutations of the promoter region or the introns.

Determinants of the wide variability of the APECED phenotype *(vide infra)* are mostly unknown. The Iranian Jewish patients have been reported to have much less candidiasis and adrenocortical insufficiency than other patients *(30)*, which could depend on their unique mutation. Otherwise, only the prevalence of candidiasis seems to depend on the nature of the mutation *(34a)*. The HLA appears to be a determinant of the prevalence of Addison's disease, alopecia, and diabetes; there are no gender-specific differences *(34a)*.

Clinical Picture

APECED is a multicomponent disease (*see* Table 2) with a widely variable clinical picture *(2,47–50)*. Its most common components are mucocutaneous candidiasis, hypoparathyroidism, and adrenocortical insufficiency, but more than 10 other components may occur. The following description is mainly based on our experience with 89 Finnish patients (45 males and 44 females) (Perheentupa J, unpublished).

Endocrine Components

Hypoparathyroidism appeared from the second year to the fifth decade, with peak incidence at 2–11 yr. Its prevalence gradually reaches 86% (*see* Table 2). It remained the only endocrinopathy in 20% of our patients at the age 20 yr and in 18% at 30 yr. Adrenocortical insufficiency appeared from the fourth year to the fifth decade, with peak incidence at 4–12 yr. Its prevalence reaches 79% (*see* Table 2). It remained the only endocrinopathy in 8% of our patients at the age of 20 yr and 11% at 30 yr. Deficiencies of cortisol and aldosterone could appear even 5 yr apart. Diabetes mellitus appeared at the age of 4–58 yr, with the highest incidences in the second, fourth, and fifth decades (for details, *see* a subsequent subsection). Hypogonadism develops eventually in more than two-thirds of female patients and in one-third of males. It was the result of autoimmune gonadal atrophy in all except one male patient, who had gonadotropin deficiency. Male infertility resulting from antisperm antibodies is also on record *(51)*. Hypothyroidism rises eventually to the incidence of 18%. Pernicious anemia developed in 21 patients by 6.1–48 yr of age, with peak incidence at around 15 yr. Its prevalence appears to reach one-third by the age of 40 yr.

Other pituitary hormone deficiencies also occur, mostly singly. Growth hormone deficiency developed in four (4%) of our patients (in one patient together with ACTH deficiency), and several others are on record *(45,49,52).* Three patients have been reported with central diabetes insipidus *(49,53)* and two patients with ACTH deficiency *(54).*

Other Autoimmune Components

Alopecia developed in 29 (33%) of our patients by the age of 2.5–30 yr, being the first or part of the initial manifestation in two. It was universal in 24 patients (27%). Vitiligo of a highly variable extent appeared in 19 patients (21%) by the age of 1.7–47 yr. In a few patients, the spots have faded, but in most, they grew with time.

Gastrointestinal disorders are common. Autoimmune hepatitis is the most dangerous of all the common components of APECED *(47,55).* It developed at the ages of 0.7–16.8 in 14 patients. Of them, three died of fulminant hepatitis within 2 mo, despite intensive therapy. Six other patients had clearly elevated serum levels of alanine aminotransferase that subsided without immunosuppressive medication. Cholelithiasis may occur *(56).*

Keratopathy of the eyes may be a serious problem, which calls for intensive local medication with glucocorticoid and, often, antimicrobials. Of our patients, 19 (21%) developed keratopathy at the ages of 1.0–16 yr. Five of them became blind, and a sixth has only 30% of normal visual acuity. The early symptoms are intense photophobia, blepharospasm, and lacrimation. In nine (10%) patients, keratopathy was the first or part of the initial manifestation of APECED or the first after oral candidiasis. Other less common eye manifestations include recurring irodocyclitis, optic atrophy, retinal detachment, and severe dry eye *(57).*

Sjögren's syndrome was reported in 12% of a series of 41 patients and scleroderma in 1 patient *(49).* One of our patients (patient Sf, *see* Fig. 1) died of complications of rapidly advancing rheumatoid arthritis. Eight (9%) of our pediatric patients, as well as one reported previously *(49),* experienced a flashing rash over several months, which often was associated with peaks of fever. Several cases of autoimmune hemolytic anemia are on the record *(49),* including one of ours. Patients with acquired splenic atrophy have been reported *(49,56,58).* Interstitial nephritis developed in six (7%) of our patients; two of them needed kidney transplantation.

Nonautoimmune Components

Candidiasis involves the mouth first, appearing in the mildest cases as intermittent soreness of mouth corners (angular cheilosis). It tends to remain unnoticed; hence, the prevalence figures at early ages are probably erroneously low. More severe forms include an acute inflammation of most of the oral mucosa, hyperplastic chronic candidiasis with thick white coating of the tongue, and atrophic disease with scant coatings and a scarred thin mucosa with leukoplakia-like areas *(59).* This chronic condition is carcinogenic; four of our patients developed epithelial carcinoma of the oral mucosa at the age of 27–45 yr and three of them died of it. Hence, candidiasis should be carefully followed and suppressed by good dental care and oral hygiene and local and systemic antimycotics. Candidal esophagitis is painful and may cause strictures, and intestinal mucosal candidiasis may manifest as abdominal pain, meteorism, and diarrhea. The infection may spread to the skin of the face and hands and to the nails. Candidal vulvovaginitis often develops in postpubertal female patients. The peak incidence of candidiasis is over the first year of life. In some patients, it appears late, and in our series, the prevalence of 100%, intermittent cases included, was not reached until in the fifth decade of life (*see* Table 2).

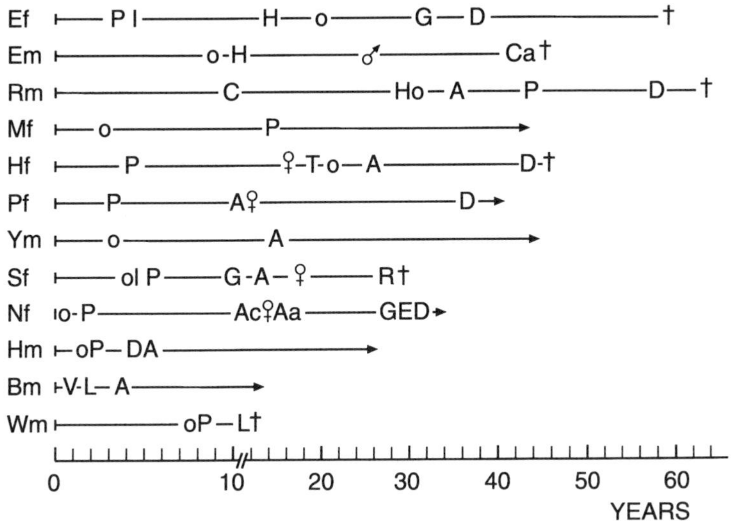

Fig. 1. Disease histories of six Finnish female (f) and six male (m) patients with APECED, illustrating the wide variation of the clinical course. The lines start at birth, and end at death (+) or arrowhead indicating age at latest follow-up. The age at the appearance of the component disease is indicated by symbols for the component diseases: A, adrenocortical insufficiency, Ac, cortisol deficiency, Aa, aldosterone deficiency; C, cornea—keratopathy; Ca, oral carcinoma; D, diabetes mellitus; E, exocrine pancreatic insufficiency; G, pernicious anemia ; H, hair—alopecia; I, intestine—steatorrhea; L, liver—hepatitis; o, oral candidiasis; P, parathyroid—hypoparathyroidism; R, rheumatoid arthritis; T, thyroid—hypothyroidism; V, vasculitis; ♂ or ♀ for hypogonadism.

Ectodermal dystrophy's most frequent component is enamel hypoplasia of permanent teeth *(59,60),* which affects three-fourths of our patients *(47).* Pitted nail dystrophy is present in half of the patients and tympanic membrane calcium salt deposits in a third of the patients.

Fourteen of our patients (16%) had prolonged periods of watery or fatty diarrhea. Specific diagnosis was reached only in a few of them. Most of the patients with watery diarrhea had hypoparathyroidism and they experienced periods of diarrhea and hypocalcemia. Of note, one patient's intractable diarrhea and therapy-resistant hypocalcemia responded to high-dose intravenous methylprednisolone and maintenance oral methotrexate *(61).* Atrophy of the exocrine pancreas with diabetes developed in another patient (patient Nf, *see* Fig. 1). Two other such cases are on record *(45,62);* in one of them, fat excretion responded to immunosuppressive medication *(45).* The chronic diarrhea of a 12-yr-old patient of ours was caused by defective bile acid reabsorption and controlled with cholestyramine therapy. Intestinal lymphangiectasia was reported as a cause of diarrhea in one patient *(63).*

Individual Variation

The clinical picture also varies very widely in aspects other than age at appearance of the individual disease components. In our series, the total number of component diseases varies from 2 to 10 (median 4), and the number of endocrine components from 1 to 5 (median 2). The classic triad of candidiasis, hypoparathyroidism, and adrenal insufficiency was present in 50% of the patients at the age of 20 yr and in 55% at 30 yr.

The frequency is lower (40%) at 40 yr because of exclusion of some patients because of death.

The components to appear first or as part of the initial clinical picture were candidiasis in 54%, hypoparathyroidism in 31%, adrenal insufficiency in 6%, keratopathy in 7%, chronic diarrhea in 7%, alopecia in 2%, flashing rash with fever in 2%, hepatitis in 1%, and vitiligo in 1%. Of the endocrinopathies, the first one was hypoparathyroidism alone in 64%, then adrenal insufficiency alone in 27%, hypoparathyroidism and adrenal insufficiency together in 6%, growth hormone deficiency in 1%, and hypothyroidism in 1%.

Diagnostics

The criterion of firm clinical diagnosis of APECED is the presence of at least two of the following: chronic or recurring mucocutaneous candidiasis, hypoparathyroidism, and adrenocortical insufficiency (or antiadrenal or 21-hydroxylase autoantibodies). If a sibling fulfills this criterion, one of any of the autoimmune or clear ectodermal components of APECED suffices for the diagnosis. The two-of-the-three criteria became fulfilled within the first 5 yr of life in only 22% of our patients, in the next 5-yr period in another 45%, in the second decade of life in 22%, in the third in 4.5%, and only later in 2%. It was not fulfilled by the time of his death from consequences of APECED at the age of 45 yr in one patient; his diagnosis depended on his sister's diagnosis (patient Em, *see* Fig. 1). Thus, the criterion gives no false-positive diagnoses, but false-negatives are common, especially at a young age. Hence, for appropriate clinical diagnostics, knowledge of the other disease components should be utilized. When a person under the age of 50 yr has developed a disease that belongs to the components of APECED, the patient should be checked for the ectodermal, oral, and ophthalmic components. If two components of APECED are present without any other definite explanation, the patient should be followed for development of further components or a search for *AIRE* mutations should be considered. Mutation diagnosis is available from several specialized laboratories internationally. The relatively large number of mutations and the fact that many others remain unrecognized cause problems in the mutation approach to the diagnosis. Hence, APECED cannot be excluded. Even in Finland, routine search is only available for the three most common mutations.

Patients with the diagnosis of APECED should receive written information about the possibility and symptoms of further disease components with instructions on where to turn in case they appear. Later, it is necessary to check repeatedly that the patient has adopted this information. The patient should be followed at least one or two times annually for signs of new components and thorough anamnestic details and physical examination including search for oral candidiasis, search for antibodies, and determination of serum levels of calcium, inorganic phosphate, sodium, potassium, alanine aminotransferase, corticotropin, thyrotropin and gonadotropins, plasma renin activity, and blood glycohemoglobin, as appropriate in the patient's situation of the disease.

Diabetes in Association with APECED

The prevalence of type 1 diabetes in our Finnish patients with APECED is 18% (*see* Table 2), in contrast to 0.5% in the background population. Lower frequencies of 2–4% have been reported for patients from the United States and Italy *(2,49)*, but the difference could be merely the result of patient selection (e.g., with respect to age). Of our 16 patients with diabetes, 14 were clinically considered to have type 1 diabetes. The

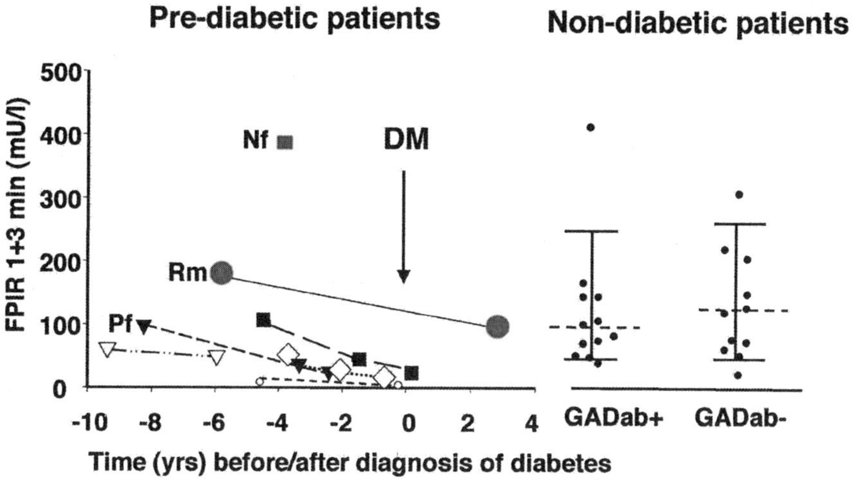

Fig. 2. The first-phase insulin response (sum of 1- and 3-min insulin concentration) to intravenous glucose tolerance test in APECED patients, who developed diabetes during the follow-up (prediabetic patients), and in GADab-positive and GADab-negative patients still nondiabetic at the last visit. Nf, Rm, and Pf refer to case reports in the text as well as Fig. 1. The *x*-axis depicts time before or after the diagnosis of diabetes (DM) at time 0. The vertical and horizontal bars depict the mean and 95% confidence intervals for the nondiabetic groups.

two others are discussed. The age at diagnosis of type 1 diabetes was 4–45 yr (median: 19.4), 6 of the 14 patients were above 20 yr. The male-to-female ratio was 1.3 : 1 and there was no obvious association between the presence of type 1 diabetes and any of the other disease components.

Patient Nf (Figs. 1 and 2) developed persistent watery diarrhea at 27 yr of age and lost 7 kg (lowest body mass index: 17.39 kg/m^2). A low fecal elastase 1 (8 µg/g) and high fatty acid excretion (159 mmol/d) confirmed the diagnosis of severe exocrine pancreatic insufficiency. Her bowel function normalized with enzyme supplementation. Four years later, she was diagnosed with diabetes, and treatment was initiated with multiple daily insulin injections. She was negative for GAD antibodies (GADab) from age 6 to 25 yr, but had a marginally positive sample at 32 yr, 1 yr after the diagnosis of diabetes; antibodies to islet cell antigens (ICAs), IA2 (IA2ab), and insulin (IAAs) were negative. The etiology of the pancreatic insufficiency is unclear; two patients with APECED and exocrine pancreatic insufficiency preceding diabetes have been described, one of them ICA positive *(46,62)*.

Patient Rm, with an unusually late appearance of APECED (Figs. 1 and 2), became hypertensive at the age of 40–50 yr. His HbA1c level was constantly >6% at 59 yr and 7% a year later; his body mass index was normal (24.7 kg/m^2). However, he was well controlled with diet treatment (HbA1c: 7.2%; fasting serum glucose: 5.3 mmol/L; C-peptide: 0.64 nmol/L) until his sudden death at the age of 63 yr. The cause of death is unclear, but he had had syncopes during his last year and had received a pacemaker for sick sinus syndrome. He was negative for GADab, ICA, IA2ab, and IAA. Clinically, this patient had type 2 diabetes.

Of our patients with APECED and diabetes, 73% were positive for GADab, 55% for ICA, and 36% for IA2ab and IAA before or at the time of diagnosis of diabetes *(7,64)*.

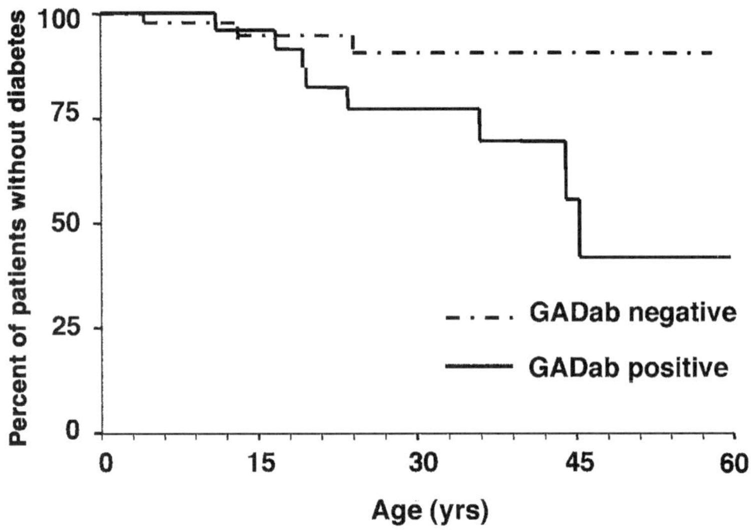

Fig. 3. The frequency of APECED patients without diabetes according to age and whether they had GADab.

These figures are compatible with what has been published for classical type 1 diabetes in this age group. Surprisingly, GADab, especially, also occurred frequently in the nondiabetic patients with APECED, of whom 41% had GADab and 28% ICA in 1995 *(7)*. However, 5 yr later, two of the antibody-positive subjects had developed diabetes and the frequency of "false-positive" antibodies had fallen to 36% for GADab, 23% for ICA, and 4% for IA2ab *(64)*. Evidently, the presence of GADab is associated with the development of diabetes, although not in all cases (*see* Fig. 3). Subclinical insulitis, which might not progress to clinical diabetes in all cases, is very difficult to investigate. Both the fasting C-peptide concentration (0.5 ± 0.24 vs 1.03 ± 0.49 nmol/L) and the first-phase insulin response to intravenous glucose (75.6 ± 37.9 vs 166.4 ± 112.7 mU/L) were lower for GADab+ than the GADab– group *(7)* in our nondiabetic patients. Although two of these patients, who since developed diabetes, had very low first-phase insulin response to an intravenous glucose test during a few years before the diagnosis of diabetes, some of the nondiabetic individuals, irrespective of antibody status, also have similarly low insulin responses (*see* Fig. 2). The puzzling fact that they have not developed diabetes or that some of the diabetic patients had very low insulin response for years before developing diabetes is most likely explained with extreme insulin sensitivity.

Patient Pf (Figs. 1 and 2) had very low first-phase insulin response to intravenous glucose for several years before the diagnosis of type 1 diabetes at the age of 36 yr. At that time, she was nonsymptomatic and had a low body mass index of 17.2 kg/m^2. Her fasting blood glucose was 7.7 mmol/L. One month later, her fasting blood glucose levels were greater than 10 mmol/L, HbA1c was 9.1%, and fasting C-peptide was 0.32 nmol/L. She was initially on lispro insulin at meals, and 2 yr later commenced on neutral protamine Hagedorn (NPH) insulin twice daily. She was strongly positive for GADab since 13 yr of age and for ICA since 19 yr, but she was negative for IAA and IA2ab.

Although the GADab-positive patients have a lower median first-phase insulin response, their difference from the GADab-negative patients is not statistically significant, in contrast to Tuomi et al. *(7),* after the exclusion of the patients who later developed diabetes. The groups may be too small and heterogeneous (for age, body mass index, insulin sensitivity) for adequate comparison, or the intravenous glucose test may be too insensitive to reveal small differences in insulin secretion. In a sensitive test for maximal insulin secretory capacity (i.e., stimulation with both supranormal glucose concentration and arginine), nondiabetic GADab+ patients with autoimmune thyroiditis had lower maximal insulin response than GADab– matched patients with thyroiditis *(8).* With the same test, GADab+ type 2 diabetic patients had a reduced maximal insulin secretory capacity compared with GADab– patients shortly after diagnosis, when there was no difference in either the glycemic control or the fasting C-peptide levels between the groups *(65).* These data support the association between GADab positivity and subclinical β-cell insufficiency. However, a third possibility is that there really is no difference between the GADab-positive and GADab-negative patients with APECED, except shortly before the diabetic stage. Of note, the insulin secretions in APECED patients have not been compared with non-APECED control subjects. Thus, pancreatic autoimmune processes different from those commonly seen in type 1 diabetes that lead to relative insulin deficiency could be operative in most patients with APECED. Patient Nf is a possible example.

The human leukocyte antigen (HLA) genes do not seem to determine the development of diabetes in APECED. The DRB1, DQA1, and DQB1 risk genotypes, which generally confer susceptibility to type 1 diabetes, were not associated with type 1 diabetes in the Finnish patients with APECED *(7).* However, the protective HLA-haplotype DR15-DQA1*0102-DQB1*0602 may protect from diabetes even in APECED, as none of the diabetic patients, in contrast to 27% of the nondiabetic patients, had this haplotype (one-tailed $p = 0.047$) *(34a,64).*

APS-2

All combinations of adrenocortical insufficiency, thyroid disease (Graves' disease, goitrous or atrophic thyroiditis), type 1 diabetes, celiac disease, hypogonadism, pernicious anemia (vitamin B_{12} malabsorption), vitiligo, alopecia, myasthenia gravis, and the collagen vascular diseases, which include at least one of the said endocrine diseases but exclude hypoparathyroidism and mucocutaneous candidiasis, are collectively called APS type 2. The co-occurrence of these diseases is presumably the result of a common genetic background. No exact incidence or prevalence figures are available, and they would probably vary with the population concerned. APS-2 is more common than APS-1, with a general prevalence of at least 1 per 10,000. Females are affected two to four times more often than men. The highest incidence of the components is in the third to the fifth decade of life, but a substantial number of patients develop the first component disease, usually type 1 diabetes, already in the first and second decade (*see* Fig. 4).

Common Genetic Basis for Type 1 Diabetes and Other Autoimmune Diseases?

The familial clustering of different autoimmune diseases suggests that the same susceptibility gene variants are either causative or permissive for the development of these diseases. The genetics of type 1 diabetes is reviewed elsewhere in this book. This review includes only those genetic associations that have been reported to be shared between type

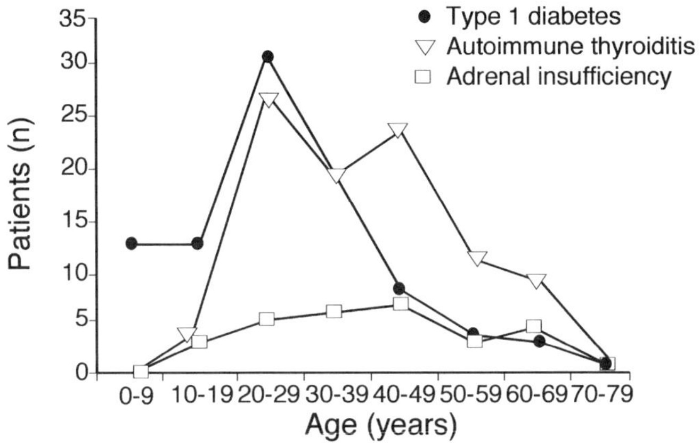

Fig. 4. Age at manifestation of type 1 diabetes, adrenocortical insufficiency, and autoimmune thyroid disease in a series of 151 patients with autoimmune polyendocrine syndrome type 2. (From ref. *66*, with permission.)

1 diabetes and the other disease components. All autoimmune diseases, except APECED and the autoimmune lymphoproliferation syndrome, are considered to be polygenic and multifactorial in origin, and a causal role has not been proven for any candidate gene.

Genes coding for HLAs are associated with most known autoimmune diseases. Because of the strong linkage disequilibrium in the short arm of chromosome 6, it has not been possible to pinpoint a single gene in this gene-rich segment as the real culprit. It is also possible that the region harbors more than one gene of interest. The heterozygous genotype DRB1*0404, DQA1*0301, DQB1*0302 with DRB1*0301, DQA1*0501, DQB1*0201 seems to give a major risk for type 1 diabetes and adrenal insufficiency. It seems that of all DR4 alleles associated with diabetes, only DRB1*0404 increases the risk for adrenal insufficiency *(4)*. DR3 and especially the associated DQA1*0501, DQB1*02 are also associated with celiac disease, Graves' disease, Hashimoto's thyroiditis, myasthenia gravis, and Sjogren's syndrome. On the other hand, DR2-DQA1*0102,DQB1*0602 protects, even in the presence of antibodies, from adrenal insufficiency and type 1 diabetes *(4,67–70)*.

Interestingly, type 1 diabetes, Graves' thyrotoxicosis, adrenal insufficiency, celiac disease and primary biliary cirrhosis have all also been associated with certain variants of the gene on chromosome 2q33 coding for the cytotoxic T-lymphocyte (cell surface) antigen-4 (CTLA-4) *(71–73)*. This molecule is a key negative regulator of T-cell function. Hashimoto's thyroiditis (HT) is also associated with both HLA genes and CTLA4, but the associations are less clear *(70)*. A third locus (IDDM6), associated with type 1 diabetes, Graves' disease, rheumatoid arthritis, and systemic lupus erythematosus, lies in the long arm of chromosome 18 *(74)*.

Clinical Picture

The disease combinations within the definition of APS-2 change with the age of the patient population. Also, the population's genetic background may modify the clinical phenotype of this polygenic disease. Exact information about the clinical picture and course is meager. Only a recent report from Germany *(66)* is based on our present definition of APS-2 and gives some longitudinal data.

Table 3
Prevalence (%) of the Main Component Diseases in a Series of 151 Patients (114 Females) of All Ages with APS-2

Component disease	*Prevalence*
Autoimmune thyroid disease, total	66
Graves' disease	33
Hashimoto's thyroiditis	33
Type 1 diabetes mellitus	61
Adrenocortical insufficiency	19
Hypogonadism	5
Pernicious anemia	5
Vitiligo	20
Alopecia	6

Note: These include all patients with diagnosis of APS-2 among the total of 15,000 patients seen at the Endocrine Clinic, University Hospital Mainz over the years 1992–1996. No age-specific figures are available of patients diagnosed according to the present criteria.

Source: ref. *66,* with permission.

Diabetes appears to be the most prevalent of the single-component diseases (*see* Table 3). Graves' and Hashimoto's diseases are equally common, and the joint prevalence of thyroid disease exceeds the prevalence of diabetes. Diabetes was significantly more common in males and thyroid disease in females. The mean age of manifestation was 27 yr for diabetes and between 36 and 40 yr for the other components (*see* Fig. 4). Diabetes was also the first component to appear in 48% of the individual patients, followed by 19% for Graves' disease, 17% for Hashimoto's disease, and 15% for adrenocortical insufficiency. Only diabetes showed a gender difference with respect to the order of appearance; it was the first in 65% of the males, in contrast to 43% of the females.

Of combinations of the component diseases, diabetes with thyroid disease was the most common, occurring in 33%. The second, diabetes with adrenal insufficiency, made up 15%, followed by diabetes with vitiligo (10%), thyroid disease with vitiligo (10%), and diabetes with adrenal insufficiency (3%). The combination of diabetes, adrenal insufficiency and thyroid disease, traditionally called the Schmidt or Carpenter syndrome, accounted for only 3%.

Autoimmune Thyroid Disease (AITD) in Patients with Type 1 Diabetes

Hypothyroid or hyperthyroid AITD has been observed in 10–24% of patients with type 1 diabetes *(75–78)*. Also, postpartum thyroiditis may occur in 22% of diabetic mothers compared with 5% of nondiabetic mothers *(79)*. In the majority of cases, the diagnosis of diabetes precedes that of hypothyroidism and either succeeds or coincides with hyperthyroidism *(80)*. Thus, the prevalence of AITD depends on the age of the diabetic patient group at the time of study. Accordingly, 4.8% of juvenile-onset patients studied before age 18 *(77)* and 15% of those studied at a mean age of 42 yr *(76)* had HT. Graves' disease has been reported in 9.3% of patients with type 1 diabetes *(76)*.

In addition, between 5% and 25% of type 1 diabetic patients without clinical thyroid disease have antibodies to thyroid microsomal antigens (TMAb) or thyroid peroxidase (TPOAb) *(75–79,81–86)*. In addition to differences in the antibody assays, the large variation in antibody frequencies reflects differences in patient selection and whether thyroid function was actually studied or not. In three population-based studies of newly diagnosed patients with type 1 diabetes, TMAb or TPOAb were found in 5–8% of Swedish patients under 35 yr at diagnosis, and in 10–11% of Finnish and Australian patients under 15 yr at diagnosis *(82–85)*. Antibody positivity was more common in Caucasoid than in African-American patients *(81)*. Thyroid antibodies occur more frequently in women than in men, both in patients with diabetes and in nondiabetic subjects *(81,87)*. Of note, the prevalence of both hypothyroidism and thyrogastric antibodies in the background population increases with age, and increased thyrotropin levels (>5 μU/L) were found in 13.6% of women and 5.7% of men over 60 yr *(81,88)*. TMAb were observed in 6.3% of 18- to 24-yr-old women compared with 9.2% of those aged 65–74 yr; the respective figures for men were 0.9% and 2.3% *(87)*. It seems that young diabetic patients have these antibodies as frequently as the background geriatric population.

The predictive value of thyroid antibody positivity for the development of AITD during one's lifetime is not known. However, in a large series studied in the United States, 38% of TMSAb+ patients developed hypothyroidism after the diagnosis of type 1 diabetes and two to four additional patients per year have developed hypothyroidism during the follow-up *(80,81)*. Although patients with type 1 diabetes diagnosed at an older age more often have thyrogastric antibodies than those diagnosed before age 15, seroconversion to positive after the development of diabetes is uncommon *(81)*.

Pernicious Anemia in Patients with Type 1 Diabetes

Pernicious anemia (PA) is considered to occur frequently in association with type 1 diabetes, but epidemiologic studies, including clinical characterization of patients, are few. Of 200 patients with insulin-dependent diabetes, 4% had PA defined by an abnormal Schilling test and decreased serum cobalamin concentration; in addition, 3% had latent PA with abnormal Schilling test but normal cobalamin concentration. Twenty-seven percent of all patients, including all patients with clinical or latent PA, had antibodies to parietal cells *(89)*. The increased frequency of antibodies to parietal cells (PCA) or to H^+K^+-ATPase among type 1 diabetic patients has been confirmed in several studies. In general, gastric antibodies are found in 3–27% of patients *(75,81–84,86,89)*, with higher frequencies in patients diagnosed with type 1 diabetes at an older age than in those diagnosed before age 15 *(81–83)*. Seroconversion to positive after the development of diabetes is considered to be uncommon *(81)*. An increased prevalence of PCA in females than in males has been reported in some studies *(81)* but not in others *(86)*, and there seems to be no difference between Caucasians and African-Americans in the United States *(81)*. The prevalence of gastric antibodies increases with age in both diabetic *(81)* and nondiabetic subjects, and the prevalence in the general population reaches 9.6% in the eighth decade *(20)*. Of 54 PCA-positive patients, 14 (26%) had latent or clinical PA *(89)*, which compares well with a Belgian study showing hypergastrinemia in 27% of PCA-positive type 1 diabetic patients compared with 7% of PCA-negative patients. Clinical PA was found in 10.5% compared with 0.5%, respectively *(86)*.

Celiac Disease in Patients with Type 1 Diabetes

The prevalence of celiac disease (CD) in the general population is estimated at about 0.3%. As CD is often symptomless (silent CD), its recognized prevalence depends on how actively antibody tests or small-bowel biopsies are carried out, as well as the extent of exposure to gluten *(90)*. CD is considered to be rare in the absence of IgA antibodies (or IgG in case of patients with IgA deficiency) to gliadin (AGA), reticulin (ARA), endomysium (EMA), or the specific antigen tissue transglutaminase (tTGA) *(91)*. However, the true diagnostic value of these antibodies for silent CD is unknown, as small-bowel biopsies have not been performed in large unselected patient cohorts.

Celiac disease is 4–20 times more prevalent in patients with type 1 diabetes (1.3–6%) *(92–100)* than in the general population. As explained here, the true prevalence could be even higher. However, no CD was found in the absence of AGA in the only reported study that included biopsies of all newly diagnosed patients without preselection (for) by antibody positivity *(92)*. The prevalence of CD-associated antibodies varies between 2.6% and 11.6% among patients with type 1 diabetes who are not on a gluten-free diet *(75,92,94–102)*. High antibody levels are considered to be more specific for CD *(98)*.

Adrenal Insufficiency in Patients with Type 1 Diabetes

Although rare, adrenal insufficiency (AI) is about 50 times more common in patients with type 1 diabetes (0.12–0.5%) than in the general population (93–117 per million) *(103,104)*. Antibodies to adrenal cortex (AA) or 21-hydroxylase (21-OHA) are present in 0.2–2.3% of type 1 diabetic patients *(7,67,84,86,105–108)*. In a study on 8840 adult patients with organ-specific autoimmune disease, 50% of patients with AA progressed to impaired adrenal function (decreased response to intravenous ACTH) *(107)*. It is not clear whether the predictive value of the antibodies is associated with the age of the subject. Fewer adult (36%) than juvenile (90%) patients developed impaired adrenal function, but no distinction was made between APS-1 and APS-2 *(106,107)*. In most cases, the diagnosis of IDDM preceded that of AI *(66,109)*; the latency time from the AA-positive test may be as long as 7 yr *(107)*.

Development of Type 1 Diabetes in Patients with Other Autoimmune Diseases

Islet cell antigens were originally discovered in patients with miscellaneous organ-specific autoimmune disorders *(110)* and later demonstrated in 6% of patients with clinical or serologic evidence of endocrine autoimmunity. Since then, ICAs have been observed in 14%, GADab in 14–21%, and IA2ab in 4% of patients with APS-2 *(111,112)*. The predictive value of these antibodies for diabetes is unclear in APS-2. Most studies have pooled patients with different clinical combinations of autoimmune diseases together with antibody-positive patients without clinical evidence of endocrine dysfunction. However, only 14% of 186 ICA+ subjects with clinical and/or serological evidence of endocrine autoimmunity developed type 1 diabetes during a mean follow-up of 4.8 ± 3.2 yr *(113,114)*. Another study found 3.6% of 3042 patients with 1 or more autoimmune diseases to be ICA+; 40% of those persistently ICA+ compared with 2.7% of ICA– patients developed diabetes during a mean follow-up of 1.7 yr *(115)*.

ICAs and GADab in patients with APS or Stiff–Man syndrome (SMS) have been suggested to have different specificity than antibodies from patients with type 1 diabetes only *(116–119)* and to be less predictive for diabetes. Also, only sera from patients with APS-1 or SMS inhibited the enzymatic activity of GAD *(120),* and antibodies to GAD67 in addition to GAD65ab are present mainly in patients with APS *(7,111).* However, all of these findings could reflect the fact that polyendocrine patients often have higher concentrations of GADab, which augments the detection of minor antibody reactivities (i.e., those to linear and aminoterminal epitopes, GAD67, or those affecting enzymatic activity) *(7,121,122).*

Among adult Swedish patients with Graves' disease, 4.3% had type 1 diabetes *(123).* There are no such prevalence data on HT. ICAs and GADab occur in 1.4–2.5% and 1.8–13%, respectively, of patients with AITD *(123–126).* The predictive value of diabetes-related antibody positivity is unclear. During a 2-yr follow-up, 2 of 16 (12.5%) GADab+ and 9 of 431 (2.0%) GADab– Swedish patients with HT developed diabetes *(8).*

Of patients with CD, 0.8–8.4% have type 1 diabetes *(127–129).* The prevalence of diabetes may be associated with age at onset of CD: In a large study on Italian patients, 0.8% of those under 2 yr compared with 6.6% of those over 10 yr had diabetes (125). ICAs were found in 6.6% and GADab in 3% of CD patients before initiation of a gluten-free diet. Interestingly, all seroconverted to antibody negative on diet *(129).* Of Australian patients with PA, 1.6–4% had type 1 diabetes *(89,130),* whereas no data exist on the presence of diabetes-related autoantibodies in this patient group. Of Danish patients with autoimmune adrenal insufficiency, 18% had type 1 diabetes *(109),* but in northern Italy and Norway, this prevalence was only 1.2–3% *(131,132).* In addition, 5.6–8.5% of the nondiabetic patients have diabetes-related antibodies *(131–133),* but their predictive value is not known.

Who Should Be Screened?

Ideally, all patients diagnosed with type 1 diabetes should be screened for thyroid, celiac, adrenal, and gastric antibodies at the time of diagnosis. The subjects positive for any antibody should then be tested for the function of the respective gland (thyroid hormone levels and thyroid-stimulating hormone, gastroscopy, ACTH test and plasma renin concentration, serum cobalamin). Antibody testing is obviously dependent on the availability of the test and its cost. However, at least all patients with a tendency toward hypoglycemia, diarrhea, or weight loss should be tested for thyroid function, CD, and adrenal insufficiency. Also, all patients with anemia or neuropathy should be tested for cobalamin concentration.

To screen for the development of diabetes, once-a-year blood glucose testing is probably sufficient for patients with any single autoimmune endocrine disease as well as for patients with vitiligo and alopecia. For patients with two or more autoimmune components, screening for GADab might help in selecting those patients at risk for diabetes. They should be given information about symptoms of the condition and then receive regular follow-up.

EFFECT OF CO-OCCURRING DISEASES ON GLYCEMIC CONTROL AND TREATMENT OF DIABETES

Hyperthyroidism leads to insulin resistance and increased insulin doses to control hyperglycemia. This should be taken into account when thyrostatic therapy is commenced for a diabetic patient, and the insulin doses should be adequately reduced to avoid hypoglycemia when euthyroidism is reached. On the other hand, hypothyroidism in a diabetic patient is often diagnosed after an increased frequency of hypoglycemia. Treatment of hypothyroidism will lead to an increased demand for insulin. Hypocortisolism can cause hypoglycemia both in diabetic and nondiabetic subjects. Patients with type 1 diabetes are particularly sensitive to changes in cortisone levels and usually need hydrocortisone substitution divided in at least three daily doses or supplementation with a longer-acting preparation (e.g., prednisone) to avoid nocturnal hypoglycemia. Untreated CD can lead to malabsorption and hypoglycemia. Correction of hypothyroidism may provoke an Addisonian crisis in patients with subclinical adrenal insufficiency.

REFERENCES

1. Betterle C, Volpato MJ, Greggio NA, Presotto F. Type 2 polyglandular autoimmune disease. J Pediatr Endocrinol Metab 1996;9:113–123.
2. Neufeld M, Maclaren N, Blizzard RM. Two types of autoimmune Addison's disease associated with different polyglandular autoimmune syndromes. Medicine 1981;60:355–362.
3. Trence DL, Morley JE, Handwerger BS. Polyglandular autoimmune syndrome. Am J Med 1984;77:107–116.
4. Redondo MJ, Eisenbarth GS. Autoimmune polyendocrine syndrome type II. In: Eisenbarth GS, ed. Molecular Mechanisms of Endocrine and Organ Specific Autoimmunity. Landes, Austin, TX, 1999, pp. 44–61.
5. Maenpaa J, Raatikka M, Rasanen J, Taskinen J, Wager O. Natural course of juvenile autoimmune thyroiditis.J Pediatr 1985;107:898–904.
6. De Bellis A, Bizarro A, Rossi R, et al. Remission of subclinical adrenocortical failure in subjects with adrenal autoantibodies. J Clin Endocrinol Metab 1993;76:1002–1007.
7. Tuomi T, Bjorses P, Falorni A, et al. Antibodies to glutamic acid decarboxylase and insulin-dependent diabetes in patients with autoimmune polyendocrine syndrome type I. J Clin Endocrinol Metab 1996;81:1488–1494.
8. Lethagen AL, Ericsson UB, Hallengren B, Groop L, Tuomi T. GADab positivity is associated with an impaired insulin response to glucose and arginine in nondiabetic patients with autoimmune thyroiditis. J Clin Endocrinol Metab 2002;87(3):1177–1183.
9. Bednarek J, Furmaniak J, Wedlock N. Steroid 21-hydroxylase is a major autoantigen in idopathic Addison's disease. FEBS Lett 1992;309:51–55.
10. Winqvist O, Karlsson FA, Kampe O. 21-hydroxylase, a major autoantigen in idiopathic Addison's disease. Lancet 1992;339:1559–1562.
11. Uibo R, Aavik E, Peterson P, et al. Autoantibodies to cytochrome P450 enzymes P450scc, P450c17, and P450c21 in autoimmune polyglandular disease types I and II and isolated Addison's disease. J Clin Endocrinol Metab 1994;78:223–328.
12. Uibo R, Perheentupa J, Ovod V, Krohn KJE. Characterization of adrenal autoantigens recognized by sera from patients with autoimmune polyglandular syndrome (APS) type I. J Autoimmun 1994;7:399–411.
13. Winqvist O, Gustafsson J, Rorsman F, Karlsson FA, Kempe O. Two different cytochrome P450 enzymes are the adrenal antigens in autoimmune polyendocrine syndrome type I and Addison's disease. J Clin Invest 1993;92:2377–2385.
14. Winqvist O, Gebre-Medhin G, Gustafsson J, et al. Identification of the main gonadal autoantigens in patients with adrenal insufficiency and associated ovarian failure. J Clin Endocrinol Metab 1995;80:1717–1723.
15. Arif S, Vallian S, Farzaneh F, et al. Identification of 3 β-hydroxysteroid dehydrogenase as a novel target of steroid cell autoantibodies: association of autoantibodies with endocrine autoimmune disease. J Clin Endocrinol Metab 1996;81:4439–4445.
16. Krohn K, Uibo R, Aavik E, Peterson P, Savilahti K. Identification by molecular cloning of an autoantigen associated with Addison's disease as steroid 17 alpha-hydroxylase. Lancet 1992;339:770–773.
17. Ahonen P, Miettinen A, Perheentupa J. Adrenal and steroidal cell antibodies in patients with autoimmune polyglandular disease type I and risk of adrenocortical and ovarian failure. J Clin Endocrinol Metab 1987;64:494–500.
18. Li Y, Song Y, Rais N, et al. Autoantibodies to the extracellular domain of the calcium sensing receptor in patients with acquired hypoparathyroidism. J Clin Invest 1996;97:910–914.

19. Burman P, Mardh S, Norberg, Karlsson FA. Parietal cell antibodies in pernicious anemia inhibit H+, K+-adenosine triphosphatase, the proton pump of the stomach. Gastroenterology 1989;96:1434–1438.
20. Toh BH, van Driel IR, Gleeson PA. Pernicious anemia. N Engl J Med 1997;337:1441–1448.
21. Manns MP, Griffin KJ, Quattrochi L, et al. Identification of cytochrome P450IA2 as a human autoantigen. Arch Biochem Biophys 1990;280:229–232.
22. Clemente MG, Obermayer-Straub P, Meloni A, et al. Cytochrome P450 1A2 is a hepatic autoantigen in autoimmune polyglandular syndrome type 1. J Clin Endocrinol Metab 1997;82:1353–1361.
23. Obermayer-Straub P, Perheentupa J, Braun S, et al. Hepatic auto-antigens in patients with autoimmune polyendocrinopathy–candidiasis–ectodermal dystrophy. Gastroenterology 2001;121:668–677.
24. Hedstrand H, Perheentupa J, Ekwall O, et al. Antibodies against hair follicles are associated with alopecia totalis in autoimmune polyendocrine syndrome type I. J Invest Dermatol 1999;113:1054–1058.
25. Hedstrand H, Ekwall O, Haavik J, et al. Identification of tyrosine hydroxylase as an autoantigen in autoimmune polyendocrine syndrome type 1. Biochem Biophys Res Commun 2000;267:456–461.
26. Song Y-H, Conner E, Li Y, Zorovich B, Balducci P, Maclaren NL. The role of tyrosinase in autoimmune vitiligo. Lancet 1994;344:1049–1052.
27. Hedstrand H, Ekwall O, Olsson MJ, et al. The transcription factors SOX9 and SOX10 are melanocyte autoantigens related to vitiligo in autoimmune polyendocrine syndrome type I. J Biol Chem 2001;276:35, 390–35, 395.
28. Ekwall O, Hedstrand H, Grimelius L, et al. Identification of tryptophan hydroxylase as an intestinal autoantigen. Lancet 1998;352:279–283.
29. Canale VC, Smith CH. Chronic lymphadenopathy simulating malignant lymphoma. J Pediatr 1967;70:891–899.
30. Zlotogora J, Shapiro MS. Polyglandular autoimmune syndrome type I among Iranian Jews. J Med Genet 1992;29:824–826.
31. Rosatelli MC, Meloni A, Meloni A, et al. A common mutation in Sardinian autoimmune polyendocrinopathy–candidasis–ectodermal dystrophy patients. Hum Genet 1998;103:428–434.
32. Halonen M, Pelto-Huikko M, Eskelin P, Peltonen L, Ulmanen I, Kolmer M. Subcellular location and expression pattern of autoimmune regulator (Aire), the mouse orthologue of human gene defective in autoimmune polyendocrinopathy candidiasis ectodermal dystrophy. J Histochem Cytochem 2001;49:197–208.
33. Mittaz L, Rossier C, Heino M, et al. Isolation and characterization of the mouse Aire gene. Biochem Biophys Res Commun 1999;255:483–490.
34. Bjorses P, Halonen M, Palvimo JJ, et al. Mutations in the AIRE gene: effects on subcellular location and transactivation function of the autoimmune polyendocrinopathy–candidiasis–ectodermal dystrophy protein. Am J Hum Genet 2000;66:378–392.
34a. Halonen M, Eskelin P, Myhre, A-G, et al. AIRE mutations and human leukocyte antigen genotypes as determinants of the Autoimmune Polyendocrinopathy-Candidiasis-Ectodermal Dystrophy phenotype. J Clin End Metab 2002;87:2568–2574.
35. Blechschmidt K, Schweiger M, Wertz K, et al. The mouse *Aire* gene: comparative genomic sequencing, gene organization, and expression. Genome Res 1999;9:158–166.
36. Bjorses P, Pelto-Huikko M, Kaukonen J, Aaltonen J, Peltonen L, Ulmanen I. Localization of the APECED protein in distinct nuclear structures. Hum Mol Genet 1999;8:259–266.
37. Rinderle C, Christensen HM, Schweiger S, Lehrach H, Yaspo ML. AIRE encodes a nuclear protein co-localizing with cytoskeletal filaments: altered sub-cellular distribution of mutants lacking the PHD zinc fingers. Hum Mol Genet 1999;8:277–290.
38. Pitkanen J, Doucas V, Sternsdorf T, et al. The autoimmune regulator protein has transcriptional transactivating properties and interacts with the common coactivator CREB-binding protein. J Biol Chem 2000;275:16,802–16,809.
39. Zuklys S, Balciunaite G, Agarwal A, Fasler-Kan E, Palmer E, Hollander GA. Normal thymic architecture and negative selection are associated with *Aire* expression, the gene defective in autoimmune polyendocrinopathy–candidiasis–ectodermal dystrophy (APECED). J Immunol 2000;165:1976–1983.
40. Heino M, Peterson P, Kudoh J, et al. Autoimmune regulator is expressed in the cells regulating immune tolerance in thymus medulla. Biochem Biophys Res Commun 1999;257:821–825.
41. Heino M, Scott HS, Chen Q, et al. Mutation analyses of North American APS-1 patients. Hum Mutat 1999;13:69–74.
42. Scott HS, Heino M, Peterson P, et al. Common mutations in autoimmune polyendocrinopathy–candidiasis–ectodermal dystrophy patients of different origins. Mol Endocrinol 1998;12:1112–1119.

43. Nagamine K, Peterson P, Scott HS, et al. Positional cloning of the APECED gene. Nat Genet 1997;17:393–398.
44. Pearce SH, Cheetham T, Imrie H, et al. A common and recurrent 13-bp deletion in the autoimmune regulator gene in British kindreds with autoimmune polyendocrinopathy type 1. Am J Hum Genet 1998;63:1675–1684.
45. Ward L, Paquette J, Seidman E, et al. Severe autoimmune polyendocrinopathy–candidiasis–ectodermal dystrophy in an adolescent girl with a novel *AIRE* mutation: response to immunosuppressive therapy. J Clin Endocrinol Metab 1999;84:844–852.
46. The Finnish–German APECED Consortium. An Autoimmune disease, APECED, caused by mutations in a novel gene featuring two PHD-type zinc-finger domains. Nat Genet 1997;17:399–403.
47. Ahonen P, Myllarniemi S, Sipil I, Perheentupa J. Clinical variation of autoimmune polyendocrinopathy–candidiasis–ectodermal dystrophy (APECED) in a series of 68 patients. N Engl J Med 1990;322:1829–1836.
48. Perheentupa J. Autoimmune endocrinopathy–candidiasis–ectodermal dystrophy (APECED). Horm Metab Res 1996;28:353–356.
49. Betterle C, Greggio NA, Volpato MJ. Autoimmune polyglandular syndrome type I. J Clin Endocrinol Metab 1998;83:1049–1055.
50. Perheentupa J, Miettinen A. Autoimmune polyendocrine syndrome type I. In: Eisenbarth GS, ed. Molecular Mechanisms of Endocrine and Organ Specific Autoimmunity: Landes, Austin, TX, 1999, pp. 19–40.
51. Tsatsoulis A, Shalet SM. Antisperm antibodies in the polyglandular autoimmune syndrome type I: response to cyclical steroid therapy. Clin Endocrinol 1991;35:299–303.
52. Franzese A, Valerio G, Di Mario S, Iannucci MP, Bloise A, Tenore A. Growth hormone insufficiency in a girl with the autoimmune polyendocrinopathy–candidiasis–ectodermal dystrophy. J Endocrinol Invest 1999;22:66–69.
53. Scherbaum WA, Wass JAH, Besser GM, Bottazo GF, Doniach D. Autoimmune cranial diabetes insipidus: its association with other endocrine diseases and with histiocytosis X. Clin Endocrinol 1986;25:411–420.
54. Arvanitakis C, Knouss RF. Selective hypopituitarism. Impaired cell-mediated immunity and chronic mucocutaneous candidiasis. JAMA 1973;225(12):1492–1495.
55. Michele TM, Fleckenstein J, Sprignoli AR, Thuluvath PJ. Chronic active hepatitis in the type I polyglandular autoimmune syndrome. Postgrad Med J 1994;70:128–131.
56. Friedman TC, Thomas PM, Fleischer TA, Feuillan P, Parker RI, Cassorla F. Frequent occurrence of asplenism and cholelithiasis in patients with autoimmune polyendocrine disease type I. Am J Med 1991;91:625–630.
57. Merenmies L, Tarkkanen A. Chronic bilateral keratitis in autoimmune polyendocrinopathy–candidiasis–ectodermal dystrophy. Acta Ophthalmol Scand 2000;78:532–535.
58. Parker RI, O'Shea P, Forman EN. Acquired splenic atrophy in a sibship with the autoimmune polyendocrinopathy–candidiasis syndrome. J Pediatr 1990;117:591–593.
59. Myllarniemi S, Perheentupa J. Oral findings in the autoimmune polyendocrinopathy–candidiasis syndrome and other forms of hypoparathyroidism. Oral Surg 1978;45:721–729.
60. Lukinmaa P-L, Waltimo J, Pirinen S. Microanatomy of the dental enamel in autoimmune polyendocrinopathy–candidiasisis–ectodermal dystrophy: report of three cases. J Craniofac Genet Dev Biol 1996;16:174–181.
61. Padeh S, Theodor R, Jonas A, Passwell JH. Severe malabsorption in autoimmune polyendocrinopathy–candidosis–ectodermal dystrophy syndrome successfully treated with immunosuppression. Arch Dis Child 1997;76:532–534.
62. Sciré G, Magliocca FM, Cianfarani S, Scalamandrè A, Petrozza V, Bonamico M. Autoimmune polyendocrine candidiasis syndrome with associated chronic diarrhea caused by intestinal infection and pancreas insufficiency. J Pediatr Gastroenterol Nutr 1991;13:224–227.
63. Bereket A, Lowenheim M, Blethen SL, Kane P, Ichyama AJ. Intestinal lymphangiectasia in a patient with autoimmune polyglandular disease type I and steatorrhea. J Clin Endocrinol Metab 1995;80:933–935.
64. Gylling M, Tuomi T, Bjorses P, et al. Beta-cell antibodies, human leukocyte antigen II alleles, and type 1 diabetes in autoimmune polyendocrinopathy–candidiasis–ectodermal dystrophy. J Clin Endocrinol Metab 2000;85(12):4434–4440.
65. Carlsson L, Sundkvist G, Groop L, Tuomi T. Insulin and glucagon secretion in patients with slowly progressing autoimmune diabetes (LADA). J Clin Endocrinol Metab 2000;85:76–80.

66. Förster G, Krummenauer F, Kuhn I, Beyer J, Kahaly G. Das polyglandul re autoimmunsyndrom Typ II: epidemiologie und manifesationsformen. Dtsch Med Wochenschr 1999;124:1476–1481.
67. Yu L, Brewer W, Gates S, et al. DRB1*04 and DQ alleles: expression of 21-hydroxylase autoantibodies and risk of progression to Addison's disease. J Clin Endocrinol Metab 1999;84:328–335.
68. Gough SCL. The genetics of Graves' disease. Endocrinol Metab Clin North Am 2000;29(2):255–266.
69. Trier JS. Celiac sprue. N Engl J Med 1991;325:1709–1719.
70. Barbesino G, Chiovato L. The genetics of Hashimoto's disease. Endocrinol Metab Clin North Am 2000;29(2):357–374.
71. Badenhoop K. CTLA4 variants in type 1 diabetes: some stirrups serve better backing endocrine autoimmunity. Clin Endocrinol 2000;52(2):139–140.
72. Djilali-Saiah I, Larger E, Harfouch-Hammoud E, et al. No major role for the CTLA-4 gene in the association of autoimmune thyroid disease with IDDM. Diabetes 1998;47(1):125–127.
73. Agarwal K, Jones DEJ, Daly AK, et al. CTLA-4 gene polymorphism confers susceptibility to primary biliary cirrhosis. J Hepatol 2000;32(4):538–541.
74. Vaidya B, Imrie H, Perros P, et al. Evidence for a new Graves' disease susceptibility locus at chromosome 18q21. Am J Hum Genet 2000;66(5):1710–1714.
75. Kontiainen S, Schlenzka A, Koskimies S, Rilva A, Maenpaa J. Autoantibodies and autoimmune diseases in young diabetics. Diabetes Res 1990;13:151–156.
76. McCanlies E, O'Leary LA, Foley TP, et al. Hashimoto's thyroiditis and insulin-dependent diabetes mellitus: differences among individuals with and without abnormal thyroid function. J Clin Endocrinol Metab 1998;83:1548–1551.
77. Hansen D, Bennedbaek FN, Hansen LK, Hoier-Madsen M, Jacobsen BB, Hegedus L. Thyroid function, morphology and autoimmunity in young patients with insulin-dependent diabetes mellitus. Eur J Endocrinol 1999;140:512–518.
78. Rattarasarn C, Diosdado MA, Ortego J, et al. Thyroid autoantibodies in Thai type 1 diabetic patients: clinical significance and their relationship with glutamic acid decarboxylase antibodies. Diabetes Res Clin Pract 2000;49:107–111.
79. Gerstein HC. Incidence of postpartum thyroid dysfunction in patients with type 1 diabetes mellitus. Ann Intern Med 1993;118(6):419–423.
80. Riley W, Maclaren NK, Lezotte DC, Spillar RP, Rosenbloom AL. Thyroid autoimmunity in insulin-dependent diabetes mellitus: the case for routine screening. J Pediatr 1981;98(3):350–354.
81. Maclaren NK, Riley WJ. Thyroid, gastric, and adrenal autoimmunities associated with insulin-dependent diabetes mellitus. Diabetes Care 1985;8(Suppl 1):34–38.
82. Landin-Olsson M, Karlsson A, Dahlquist G, Blom L, Lernmark A, Sundkvist G. Islet cell and other organ-specific autoantibodies in all children developing type 1 (insulin-dependent) diabetes mellitus in Sweden during one year and in matched control children. Diabetologia 1989;32:387–395.
83. Landin-Olsson M, Karlsson FA, Lernmark A, Sundkvist G. Islet cell and thyrogastric antibodies in 633 consecutive 15- to 34-yr-old patients in the diabetes incidence study in Sweden. Diabetes 1992;41:1022–1027.
84. Vahasalo P, Petays T, Knip M, et al. Relation between antibodies to islet cell antigens, other autoantigens and cow's milk proteins in diabetic children and unaffected siblings at the clinical manifestation of IDDM. Autoimmunity 1996;23:165–174.
85. Verge CF, Howard NJ, Rowley MJ, et al. Anti-glutamate decarboxylase and other antibodies at the onset of childhood IDDM: a population-based study. Diabetologia 1994;37:1113–1120.
86. De Block CE, De Leeuw IH, Van Gaal LF. High prevalence of manifestations of gastric autoimmunity in parietal cell antibody-positive type 1 (insulin-dependent) diabetic patients. The Belgian Diabetes Registry. J Clin Endocrinol Metab 1999;84:4062–4067.
87. Tunbridge WMG, Evered DC, Hall R, et al. The spectrum of thyroid disease in a community: the Whickham survey. Clin Endocrinol 1977;7:481–493.
88. Sawin CT, Castelli WP, Hershman JM, McNamara P, Bacharach P. The aging thyroid. Thyroid deficiency in the Framingham Study. Arch Intern Med 1985;145(8):1386–1388.
89. Ungar B, Stocks AE, Martin FI, Whittingham S, Mackay IR. Intrinsic-factor antibody, parietal-cell antibody, and latent pernicious anemia in diabetes mellitus. Lancet 1968;2(7565):415–418.
90. Cronin CC, Shananan F. Insulin-dependent diabetes mellitus and coeliac disease. Lancet 1997;349(9058):1096–1097.
91. Dieterich W, Ehnis T, Bauer M, et al. Identification of tissue transglutaminase as the autoantigen in celiac disease. Nat Med 1997;3(7):797–801.

92. Savilahti E, Simell O, Koskimies S, Rilva A, Akerblom HK. Celiac disease in insulin-dependent diabetes mellitus. J Pediatr 1986;108(5):690–693.
93. Collin P, Salmi J, Hallstrom O, et al. High frequency of coeliac disease in adult patients with type-I diabetes. Scand J Gastroenterol 1989;24(1):81–84.
94. Barera G, Bianchi C, Calisti L, et al. Screening of diabetic children for coeliac disease with antigliadin antibodies and HLA typing. Arch Dis Child 1991;66(4):491–494.
95. Seissler J, Schott M, Boms S, et al. Autoantibodies to human tissue transglutaminase identify silent coeliac disease in type I diabetes. Diabetologia 1999;42:1440–1441.
96. Saukkonen T, Savilahti E, Reijonen H, et al. Coeliac disease: frequent occurrence after clinical onset of insulin-dependent diabetes mellitus. Childhood Diabetes in Finland Study Group. Diabet Med 1996;13(5):464–470.
97. Sjoberg K, Eriksson KF, Bredberg A, Wassmuth R, Eriksson S. Screening for coeliac disease in adult insulin-dependent diabetes mellitus. J Intern Med 1998;243(5):133–140.
98. Bao F, Yu L, Babu S, et al. One third of HLA DQ2 homozygous patients with type 1 diabetes express celiac disease-associated transglutaminase autoantibodies. J Autoimmun 1999;13(1):143–148.
99. Carlsson AK, Axelsson IE, Borulf SK, et al. Prevalence of IgA-antiendomysium and IgA-antigliadin autoantibodies at diagnosis of insulin-dependent diabetes mellitus in Swedish children and adolescents. Pediatrics 1999;103(6):1248–1252.
100. Kordonouri O, Dieterich W, D S, et al. Autoantibodies to tissue transglutaminase are sensitive serological parameters for detecting silent coeliac disease in patients with type 1 diabetes mellitus. Diabet Med 2000;17:441–444.
101. Lampasona V, Bonfanti R, Bazzigaluppi E, et al. Antibodies to tissue transglutaminase C in type I diabetes. Diabetologia 1999;42(10):1195–1198.
102. Agardh D, Nilsson A, Tuomi T, et al. Tissue transglutaminase autoantibodies associated with HLA-DQB1*02 predict silent coeliac disease at diagnosis of childhood type I diabetes mellitus. Pediatr Endocrinol 2001;2:58–65.
103. Willis AC, Vince FP. The prevalence of Addison's disease in Coventry, UK. Postgrad Med J 1997;73(859):286–288.
104. Laureti S, Vecchi L, Santeusanio F, Falorni A. Is the prevalence of Addison's disease underestimated? J Clin Endocrinol Metab 1999;84(5):1762.
105. Nerup J. Addison's disease—serological studies. Acta Endocrinol 1974;76(1):42–58.
106. Betterle C, Volpatao M, Rees Smith B, et al. Adrenal cortex and steroid 21-hydroxylase autoantibodies in children with organ-specific autoimmune diseases: II. Markers of high progression to clinical Addison's disease. J Clin Endocrinol Metab 1997;82:939–942.
107. Betterle C, Volpatao M, Rees Smith B, et al. Adrenal cortex and steroid 21-hydroxylase autoantibodies in adults with organ-specific autoimmune diseases: I. Markers of low progression to clinical Addison's disease. J Clin Endocrinol Metab 1997;82:932–938.
108. Falorni A, Laureti S, Nikoshkov A, et al. 21-Hydroxylase autoantibodies in adult patients with endocrine autoimmune diseases are highly specific for Addison's disease. Clin Exp Immunol 1997;107:341–346.
109. Nerup J. Addison's disease—clinical studies. A report of 108 cases. Acta Endocrinol 1974;76(1): 127–141.
110. Bottazzo GF, Florin-Christensen A, Doniach D. Islet-cell antibodies in diabetes mellitus with autoimmune polyendocrine deficiencies. Lancet 1974;2:1279–1283.
111. Seissler J, S B, Yassin N, et al. Association between antibodies to MR 67,000 isoform of glutamate decarboxylase (GAD) and type 1 (insulin-dependent) diabetes mellitus with coexisting autoimmune polyendocrine syndrome type II. Autoimmunity 1995;19(4):231–238.
112. Morgenthaler NG, Seissler J, Achenbach P, et al. Antibodies to the tyrosine phosphatase-like protein IA-2 are highly associated with IDDM, but not with autoimmune endocrine diseases or stiff man syndrome. Autoimmunity 1997;25(4):203–211.
113. Bosi E, Becker F, Bonifacio E, et al. Progression to type 1 diabetes in autoimmune endocrine patients with islet cell antibodies. Diabetes 1991;40:977–984.
114. Wagner R, Genovese S, Bosi E, et al. Slow metabolic deterioration towards diabetes in islet cell antibody positive patients with autoimmune polyendocrine disease. Diabetologia 1994;37(4):365–371.
115. Betterle C, Presotto F, Magrin L, et al. The natural history of pre-type 1 (insulin-dependent) diabetes mellitus in patients with autoimmune endocrine diseases. Diabetologia 1994;37:95–103.

116. Genovese S, Bonifacio E, McNally JM, et al. Distinct cytoplasmic islet cell antibodies with different risks for type 1 (insulin-dependent) diabetes mellitus. Diabetologia 1992;35:385–388.
117. Butler MH, Solimena M, Dirk R Jr, Hayday A, DeCamilli P. Identification of a dominant epitope of glutamic acid decarboxylase (GAD-65) recognized by autoantibodies in Stiff–Man syndrome. J Exp Med 1993;178:2097–2106.
118. Kim J, Namchuk M, Bugawan T, et al. Higher autoantibody levels and recognition of a linear NH2-terminal epitope in the autoantigen GAD65 distinguish Stiff–Man–syndrome from insulin-dependent diabetes mellitus. J Exp Med 1994;180:595–606.
119. Powers AC, Bavik K, Tremble J, Daw K, Scherbaum WA, Banga JP. Comparative analysis of epitope recognition of glutamic acid decarboxylase (GAD) by autoantibodies from different autoimmune disorders. Clin Exp Immunol 1999;118(3):349–356.
120. Bjork E, Velloso LA, Kampe O, Karlsson FA. GAD autoantibodies in IDDM, Stiff–Man syndrome, and autoimmune polyendocrine syndrome type I recognize different epitopes. Diabetes 1994;43(1):161–165.
121. Tuomi T, Rowley MJ, Knowles W, et al. Autoantigenic properties of native and denatured glutamic acid decarboxylase: evidence for a conformational epitope. J Immunol Immunopathol 1994;71:53–59.
122. Sohnlein P, Muller M, Syren K, et al. Epitope spreading and a varying but not disease-specific GAD65 antibody response in type 1 diabetes. Diabetologia 2000;43:210–217.
123. Hallengren B, Falorni A, Landin-Olsson M, Lernmark A, Papadopoulos KI, Sundkvist G. Islet cell and glutamic acid decarboxylase antibodies in hyperthyroid patients: at diagnosis and following treatment. J Intern Med 1996;293:63–68.
124. Kawasaki E, Abiru N, et al. Autoantibodies to glutamic acid decarboxylase in patients with autoimmune thyroid disease: relation to competitive insulin autoantibodies. J Autoimmun 1995;8:633–643.
125. Pietropaolo M, Peakman M, et al. Combined analysis of GAD65 and ICA512(IA-2) autoantibodies in organ and non-organ-specific autoimmune diseases confers high specificity for insulin-dependent diabetes mellitus. J Autoimmun 1998;11(1):1–10.
126. Yamaguchi Y, Chikuba N, et al. Islet cell antibodies in patients with autoimmune thyroid disease. Diabetes 1991;40(3):319–322.
127. Collin P, Reunala T, Pukkala E, Laippala P, Keyrilainen O, Pasternack A. Coeliac disease—associated disorders and survival. Gut 1994;35(9):1215–1218.
128. Volta U, De Franceschi L, Molinaro N, Tetta C, Bianchi FB. Organ-specific autoantibodies in coeliac disease: do they represent an epiphenomenon or the expression of associated autoimmune disorders? Ital J Gastroenterol Hepatol 1997;29(1):18–21.
129. Ventura A, Magazzu G, Greco L. Duration of exposure to gluten and risk for autoimmune disorders in patients with celiac disease. Gastroenterology 1999;117:297–303.
130. Davis RE, McCann VJ, Stanton KG. Type 1 diabetes and latent pernicious anemia. Med J Aust 1992;156:160–162.
131. Zelissen PMJ, Bast EJEG, Croughs RJM. Associated autoimmunity in Addison's disease. J Autoimmun 1995;8:121–130.
132. Soderbergh A, Winqvist O, Norheim I, et al. Adrenal autoantibodies and organ-specific autoimmunity in patients with Addison's disease. Clin Endocr 1996;45:453–460.
133. Laureti S, Aubourg P, Calcinaro F, et al. Etiological diagnosis of primary adrenal insufficiency using an original flowchart of immune and biochemical markers. J Clin Endocrinol Metab 1998;83(9):3163–3168.

6 The Metabolic Basis of Insulin Secretion

Nicolai M. Doliba, PhD, DSci
and Franz M. Matschinsky, MD

Contents

INTRODUCTION

All vertebrates use insulin-producing pancreatic β-cells to achieve fuel homeostasis *(1)*. These cells are able to measure the nutrient levels of the blood on a moment-to-moment basis and secrete insulin at rates that are exactly appropriate for the maintenance of optimal fuel levels. Therefore, the levels of circulating nutrients such as glucose, fatty acids, and amino acids are precisely controlled in mammals during fasting and feeding alike. The role of the pancreatic β-cells in fuel homeostasis is thus analogous to that of the thermostat in heating and cooling systems *(2,3)*.

The feedback loop of fuel homeostasis is completed by the insulin receptors in liver, muscle, and adipose tissue that control fuel removal from the blood and, of course, by the regulated parameters of glucose, amino acids, and fatty acids. In humans in the resting conditions, these nutrient levels are approx 5 m*M* for glucose, approx 3.5 m*M* for the physiological mixture of 20 amino acids, and approx 0.3 m*M* for fatty acids. These levels refer to the postabsorptive situation, 8–12 h after a mixed meal containing carbohydrates, fats, and proteins. It is the role of the β-cell to maintain glucose levels at a "set point" of around 5 m*M*. The level of a regulated parameter (e.g., glucose) that triggers a regulatory function, in this case the activation of insulin secretion, is defined as threshold. The

From: *Contemporary Endocrinology: Type 1 Diabetes: Etiology and Treatment*
Edited by: M. A. Sperling © Humana Press Inc., Totowa, NJ

threshold for glucose-stimulated insulin secretion coincides physiologically with the set point of around 5 m*M*. The glucose threshold is a very important parameter of β-cell physiology, because most other β-cell fuel secretagogues and neuroendocrine agents may modify the glucose threshold for stimulation of hormone secretion.

The amount of insulin secreted by β-cells is markedly influenced by the insulin responsiveness of the major target tissues of the hormone: muscle, adipocytes, and liver. In insulin-resistant states such as obesity or in the early stages of non-insulin-dependent diabetes mellitus (NIDDM), a compensatory increase in insulin secretion is observed. This compensatory response can involve both an increase in islet β-cell mass and a lowering of the threshold for glucose-stimulated insulin secretion. The latter change results in higher rates of insulin secretion at glucose concentrations lower than the normal stimulatory threshold. Increased β-cell mass and lowered glucose threshold may then increase the basal level of insulin in the blood (i.e., the insulin levels at fasting glucose levels).

It is the purpose of this chapter to present an outline of the current understanding of the biochemical and molecular mechanisms involved in nutrient-stimulated insulin secretion. The present chapter contains a concise version of our previous reviews on this topic, including some verbatim excerpts *(2–6)*. Some illustrative primary experimental data are also presented.

GENERAL PRINCIPLES OF NUTRIENT SENSING

The biochemical engineering of the pancreatic β-cells uniquely equips them to operate as the body's fuelstat. They respond to a representative sampling of small monomeric fuel molecules such as glucose or fatty acids, rather than to large polymeric macromolecules such as glycogen or triglycerides. All of the relevant nutrients are stimulators of insulin secretion; inhibitory nutrient molecules do not seem to exist, although several hormones such as somatostatin or catecholamines can serve an inhibitory role. The group of physiological nutrients includes monosaccharides such as glucose, several L-amino acids such as glutamine, alanine, or leucine, long-chain fatty acids such as palmitate or oleate, or ketone bodies such as β-hydroxybutryate or acetoacetate. It is noteworthy that most blood-borne metabolic intermediates or end products do not function as physiological β-cell stimulants or inhibitors. This includes acetone, lactate, pyruvate, glycerol, citrate, urea, uric acid, and ammonia.

In metabolic stimulus sensing as exemplified by the islet β-cell, intermediary metabolism integrates the input from multiple fuel molecules to generate specific intermediates known as coupling factors that link fuel metabolism with hormone secretion. In addition, other ligands, often peptide hormones, bind to specific receptors to trigger a cascade of events that lead to a desired metabolic or biochemical response, as exemplified by glucagon-stimulated activation of catabolic processes via generation of the second-messenger cAMP. In the islet β-cell, both types of signaling systems are operative and converge to influence distal aspects of the signaling process. For example, glucose-stimulated insulin secretion is potentiated by glucagonlike peptide-1, which binds to a receptor related to the glucagon receptor, and by neurotransmitters such as acetylcholine, which transduce their signals via muscarinic receptors *(6)*. Interestingly, these receptor-mediated signaling ligands are ineffective as insulin secretagogues in the absence of a significant threshold rate of glucose metabolism.

In view of the primacy of glucose as a β-cell secretagogue, it will come as no surprise that our understanding of stimulus/secretion coupling events for glucose are much more advanced than for other metabolic fuels. The following section will, therefore, focus on biochemical and molecular factors that translate increases in circulating glucose concentrations into increases in insulin secretion. We will, however, also attempt to summarize what is known about β-cell responses to fuels other than glucose, with particular emphasis on amino acids and fatty acids.

THE GLUCOSE SENSING SYSTEM: A BASIC MODEL

Blood glucose is the most effective physiological fuel stimulus of insulin secretion *(3)*. When the level of blood glucose increases, hormone secretion is enhanced with a characteristic dependency on the blood glucose level. A consensus minimal model delineating the manifold roles of glucose in insulin secretion by the β-cell has been developed. Those mechanisms are summarized schematically in Fig. 1, modified from a previous review *(4)*.

Glucose stimulates insulin secretion by entry into β-cells and further metabolism that generates coupling factors rather than by binding to cell surface receptors. Entry of glucose into the β-cell is achieved by Na^+-independent facilitated glucose transporters with a capacity markedly higher than the β-cell glycolytic rate. The Na^+-independent glucose transporters constitute a gene family known as glucose transporter (GLUTs 1–5) *(7)*. GLUT-2 has a K_m for glucose and capacity for glucose transport higher than other members of the family and is the isoform that is primarily expressed in rodent islets under basal conditions *(8,9)*. Human islets also express GLUT-2, but at lower levels than rodent islets *(10,11)*. Human islets, at least after isolation from cadaver pancreata, also express significant levels of the low-K_m glucose transporters GLUT-1 and GLUT-3, whereas these transporters are either low or absent in normal rodent islets in vivo *(10)*. This suggests that the capacity of transmembraneous transport is more important for β-cell function than the molecular and kinetic characteristics. Upon entry of glucose into β-cells, the sugar is metabolized (phosphorylated to glucose-6-P by glucokinase) to serve as a stimulus of insulin secretion, and glucokinase is the pacemaker of glycolysis and the glucose-induced respiratory response of the β-cell. Glucokinase, also known as hexokinase IV, contributes more than 90% of the glucose-phosphorylating capacity in this cell type. Glucokinase is a member of a gene family (the hexokinases) and differs from other members in several functional aspects. Glucokinase explains the hexose specificity (glucose>mannose>fructose as pathway substrates) and the anomeric discrimination (α-anomers of glucose and mannose are preferred). Glucokinase has an $S_{0.5}$ for glucose of about 8 m*M*, sigmoidal substrate dependency (indicated by a Hill coefficient of 1.7), and, unlike hexokinases I and II, is not allosterically inhibited by the product of its reaction, glucose-6-P *(12,13)*. Its K_m for its other substrate, Mg ATP^{2-}, is about 0.4 m*M*, meaning that the enzyme operates at near saturation in β-cells, where adenosine triphosphate (ATP) levels average approx 2.5 m*M*. Glucose transport capacity exceeds glucokinase (in rodent islets cells) by about 100-fold, which is consistent with the pacemaker role of this enzyme as a glucose sensor system. However, glucose transport of β-cells was shown to be greatly reduced in animals with diabetes mellitus of different etiology *(14)*. The glucokinase glucose sensor paradigm has received a strong boost from the discovery of glucokinase mutations in patients with the maturity-onset diabetes of the young (MODY)-2 syndrome *(15)*. Close to 150 such mutations have been discovered. Thus, β-cells are equipped with specialized

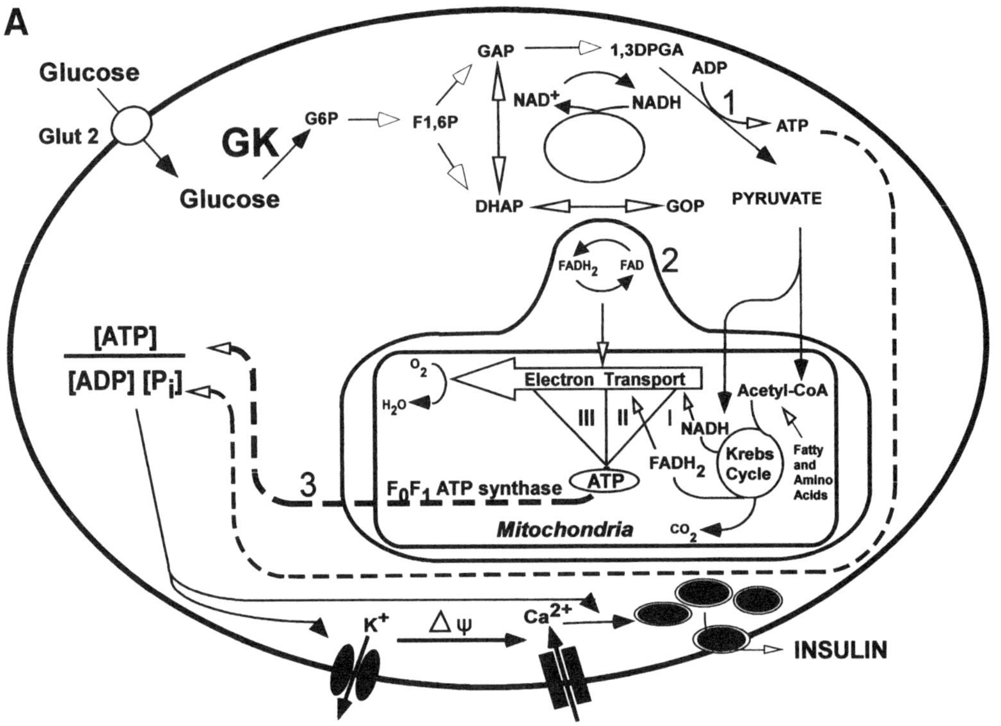

Fig. 1. Metabolic signaling in pancreatic β-cells. Four aspects of stimulus secretion coupling in pancreatic β-cells are highlighted. **Panel A** depicts the role of adenine nucleotides as metabolic coupling factors in glucose-stimulated insulin release. Three sites for energy generation are highlighted: Site 1 is at the lower part of the glycolytic pathway generating two ATP net for every glucose molecule; site 2 is related to the transfer of cytosolic reducing equivalents to mitochondria via hydrogen shuttles; and site 3 refers to ATP generation by the citric acid cycle. Electron transport and oxidative phosphorylation are quantitatively more pre-eminent for total ATP production of the cell. A critical role of glycolytic and hydrogen shuttle-dependent ATP for glucose-induced insulin release is, however, possible. The potassium channel and different steps in exocytosis are the targets of this signaling chain. **Panel B** addresses the putative role of lipid-related metabolic coupling factors. Citrate and, secondarily, malonyl-CoA are such examples of mitochondrial coupling factors. Acetyl-CoA carboxylase may be controlled by 5′AMP-dependent proteinkinase, a critical sensor of the cellular P-potential. Protein kinase C and processes in exocytosis are hypothetical targets of this signaling pathway. **Panel C** illustrates the role of transdeamination in amino acid (AA) metabolism of β-cells. AA enter the β-cells and are funneled into intermediary metabolism through transdeamination involving transaminases (TAs) and glutamate dehydrogenase (GDH). Leucine serves as unique allosteric activator of GDH. Leucine is also catabolized to acetyl-CoA and may serve as proxy for a protein load. *(Figure continues on next two pages.)*

B

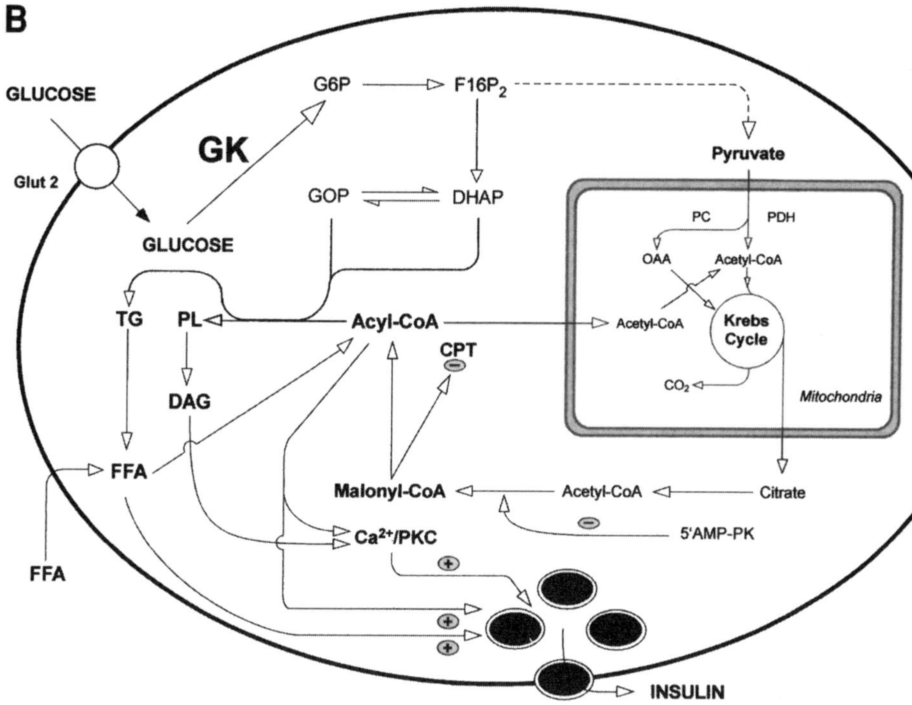
GLUCOSE
Glut 2
GLUCOSE
GK
G6P
F16P$_2$
GOP
DHAP
Pyruvate
PC
PDH
OAA
Acetyl-CoA
Acetyl-CoA
Krebs Cycle
CO_2
Mitochondria
TG
PL
Acyl-CoA
CPT
DAG
FFA
FFA
Malonyl-CoA
Acetyl-CoA
Citrate
5'AMP-PK
Ca^{2+}/PKC
INSULIN

C

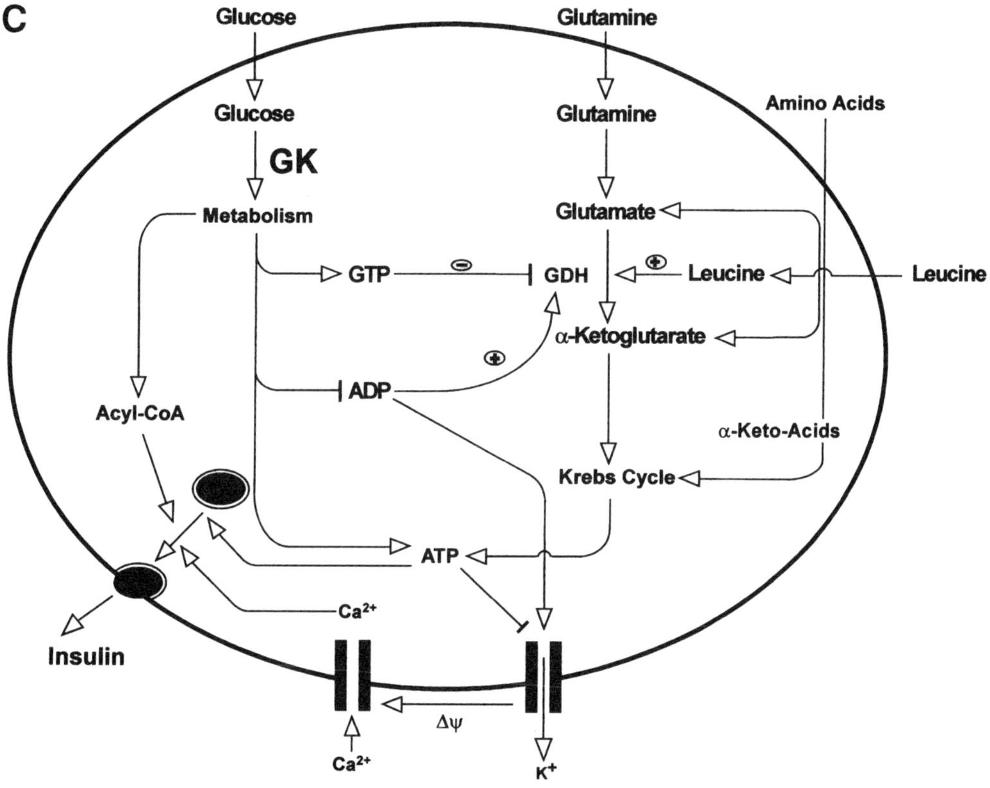
Glucose
Glutamine
Glucose
Glutamine
Amino Acids
GK
Metabolism
Glutamate
GTP
GDH
Leucine
Leucine
α-Ketoglutarate
ADP
Acyl-CoA
α-Keto-Acids
Krebs Cycle
ATP
Ca^{2+}
Insulin
Δψ
Ca^{2+}
K$^+$

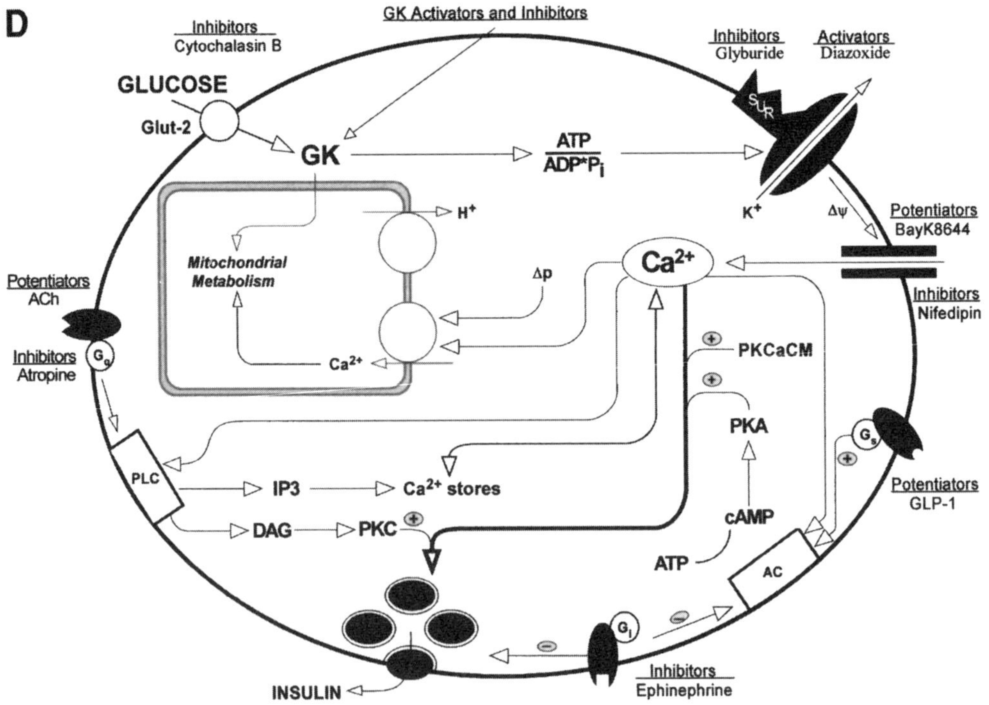

Fig. 1. *(continued)* **Panel D** illustrates the complexities of neuroendocrine regulation and drug actions in fuel-stimulated insulin release. Neural and endocrine factors may act by modifying rather than by initiating intracellular signaling pathways involved in substrate-controlled insulin release. Glucose activates the adenylate cyclase-protein kinase A (AC-PKA), phospholipase C-protein kinase C (PLC-PKC) and PKCaCM signaling pathways, all depending on cytosolic Ca^{2+} levels. The effect of glucose on cytosolic Ca^{2+} is thus critical for the understanding of this interconnected activation process. For example, the glucose-induced rise of cAMP is Ca^{2+} dependent, as is the glucose-induced elevation of DAG and IP_3. Acetycholine and glucagon-like peptide (GLP-1) are striking examples. They greatly augment the cAMP, IP_3 and DAG responses but are not able to initiate insulin release in the absence of fuel, most importantly glucose, because the substrate increase of the P-potential is an absolute requirement for initiation of secretion. The following abbreviations are used: AC, adenylate cyclase; AMP-PK, 5′AMP-dependent protein kinase; Ca^{2+}/PKC, protein kinase C; CPT-I, carnitine palmityl-CoA transferase type I; DAG, diacylglyceride; $\Delta\psi$, cell membrane potential; Δp, mitochondrial proton motive force, a function of ΔpH and $\Delta\psi$ across the mitochondrial membrane; DHAP, dihydroxyacetone-phosphate; 1,3 DPGA, 1,3 glycerate bisphosphate; $F1,6P_2$, fructose 1,6-bisphosphate; FFA, free fatty acids; GAP, glyceraldehyde-3-phosphate; Gi, Gq, and Gs, trimeric G-proteins; GK, glucokinase; Glut-2, glucose transporter type 2; G6P, glucose-6-phosphate; GOP, α-glycero-phosphate; IP_3, inositol triphosphate; OAA, oxalacetate; PC, pyruvate carboxylase; PDH, pyruvate dehydrogenase complex; PKCaCM, calcium/calmodulin-dependent protein kinase; PL, phospholipids; SUR, sulfonyl urea receptor; TG, triglycerides. (Updated version of Fig. 1 of ref. *4*.)

proteins that mediate glucose transport and phosphorylation, and these proteins have kinetic features that could allow them to regulate glucose metabolism in response to changes in the external glucose concentration.

Importantly, the capacity of β-cells for glucose phosphorylation is, by far, the lowest of all enzymatic steps of glycolysis *(12)*. At physiological glucose concentrations, most of the glucose-6-P produced in the glucokinase reaction efficiently flows into glycolysis, with little storage in the form of glycogen or entry into the pentose monophosphate shunt. Normal β-cells appear to lack classical glucose-6-phosphatase (G-6-Pase) *(16,17)*. They also do not contain a prominent enzymatic apparatus for glycogen metabolism. P-Fructokinase is the next potential regulatory step, as is universally true for glycolysis. Fructose-2,6-P_2 appears to be quantitatively unimportant as a P-fructokinase activator. Fructose-6-phosphate as the substrate and fructose-1,6-P_2 as the product of the enzyme are powerful allosteric activators of P-fructokinase, overriding feedback inhibition by ATP and other intermediates. The glycolytic intermediate pool from fructose-1,6-P_2 to P-enolpyruvate is in equilibrium, and pyruvate is generated at a rate determined by fructose-1,6-P_2, P-enolpyruvate, and ADP levels. Its rate of production keeps pace with glucose phosphorylation.

An important coupling factor produced by glucose metabolism in the β-cells is ATP (*see* Fig. 1A). ATP can be produced by three different mechanisms in the β-cells. First, it is considered that a large fraction of the NADH produced in the glyceraldehyde phosphate dehydrogenase reaction can be transferred to the mitochondria for entry into the electron-transport chain via the α-glycero-P and aspartate/malate shuttles. In keeping with this idea, the activity level of the mitochondrial glycero-P dehydrogenase is higher in islets than in most other cell types in which it has been measured (with brown fat an exception) *(18)*. Second, ATP is generated in the phosphoglycerate kinase and pyruvate kinase reactions of glycolysis. Finally, ATP can be produced in mitochondria from oxidation of pyruvate. Electron transport from NADH or reduced flavin adenine dinucleotide ($FADH_2$) to cytochrome-*c* appears to be in equilibrium, and the level of cytochrome-*c*, in turn, determines the actual rate of cytochrome-*c* oxidase *(19)*. Electron transport is coupled to proton pumping across the mitochondrial membrane, and the proton motive force thus generated (ΔpH and Δψ) results in ATP synthesis *(20,21)*. Complex V, or the F_0F_1 ATPase, thus plays a central role in metabolic coupling. Metabolism of each glucose molecule in the glycolytic stretch increases ATP generation by six to eight molecules (including glycolytic ATP and depending on the relative contribution of the shuttles). Less than half of pyruvate generated from glucose is then oxidized to CO_2 and H_2O *(12)*. Further, a very small fraction of pyruvate is reduced to lactate in β-cells, as a result of relatively low levels of lactate dehydrogenase *(18,22,23)* and, as it seems, more importantly, reflecting the high capacity of cytosolic glycero-P dehydrogenase to regenerate NAD^+. Thus, a significant fraction of the pyruvate may leave the cell as such or in the form of alanine or, alternatively, could serve an anaplerotic function, allowing the production of cytosolic byproducts of mitochondrial metabolism such as malonyl CoA *(24–26)*. Pyruvate carboxylation to oxalacetate by mitochondrial pyruvate carboxylase is a critical first step in this process. The enhanced provision of glycolytic NADH and of pyruvate leads to an increase in β-cell respiration of 30–50% in response to stimulatory glucose levels *(22)*. Thus, a critical feature of the minimal model is that the rate of β-cell glucose metabolism is precisely governed by the external glucose concentration and so is the rate of ATP production.

Another intriguing and important issue that will be dealt with is the relevance of the interplay among glucose, lipid, and amino acid metabolism in the regulation of insulin secretion. The long-chain acyl-CoA hypothesis of stimulus–secretion coupling holds that part of the signal for insulin secretion that is generated by glucose catabolism is the production of cytosolic malonyl-CoA, which is derived from citrate produced in the tricarboxylic acid (TCA) cycle *(3,24,26–29)*. Malonyl-CoA, in addition to being the proximal precursor of fatty acid biosynthesis, is an important regulatory molecule. An increase in its levels causes inhibition of the mitochondrial enzyme carnitine palmitoyltransferase I (CPT-I), which regulates entry of long-chain acyl-CoAs into the mitochondria for oxidation *(30)*. Thus, increases in malonyl-CoA secondary to increased glucose metabolism cause diversion of long-chain acetyl-CoA (LC-CoA) from oxidation to esterification pathways, and it has been proposed that increases in the levels of cytosolic LC-CoA esters are a signal transduction intermediate in glucose-stimulated insulin secretion *(28,29,31)*. Feasible sites at which increased LC-CoA could influence insulin secretion include conversion to bioactive metabolites such as diacylglycerol or inositol trisphosphate (IP3), contribution to plasma membrane or secretory granule membrane lipid turnover, or direct acylation of proteins involved in secretory granule trafficking.

As the glucose level rises and metabolism increases, there is a concomitant increase of the phosphate potential (ATP/ADP × Pi) of the β-cell that signals glucose abundance. The increased ATP/ADP × Pi stimulates insulin secretion by influencing two distinct processes. First, the conductance of adenine nucleotide-sensitive K^+ channels (K_{ATP} channels) is regulated by the cytosolic ATP and ADP levels, with ATP^{4-} serving as an inhibitor and $MgADP^-$ as an activator of the channel *(32–36)*. Thus, as the ATP/ADP × Pi is increased, the open-state probability of these channels is decreased and the plasma membrane of the β-cell becomes depolarized. Membrane depolarization opens voltage-sensitive Ca^{2+} channels with a critical threshold of about –50 mV, which causes the cytosolic Ca^{2+} to rise *(36)*. The threshold potential of voltage-sensitive Ca^{2+} channels is the most plausible regulatory feature or factor that governs the sharply defined threshold of the β-cell for glucose-stimulated insulin secretion. This glucose-regulated mechanism for increasing cellular Ca^{2+} levels is modified by the effects of potentiators of glucose that act via generation of cAMP or activation of phospholipases C (as summarized in Fig. 1C).

The increased phosphate potential also stimulates insulin secretion by enhancing the efficacy of critical steps of exocytosis. This became clear from experiments of Henquin and co-workers who incubated islets with diazoxide and 30 m*M* K^+ to render K_{ATP} channels insensitive to regulation by cellular adenine nucleotides *(37)*. Under these conditions, glucose was still capable of stimulating insulin secretion, albeit not as effectively as in islets with normally functioning channels. The interpretation of these results is that the P-potential directly influences exocytosis of insulin containing secretory granules, possibly at the level of providing energy for the movement of granules to the cell surface, fusion with the plasma membrane, and extrusion of the granular content.

Biochemical events that mediate insulin secretion distal to the glucose-induced increases in the phosphate potential and intracellular Ca^{2+} are not well understood. Potentially relevant is the activation of two types of protein kinase: protein kinase C (PKC) and Ca^{2+}–calmodulin-dependent protein kinase (PKCaCM), during exposure of islets to stimulatory glucose. In fresh rat islets, there is strong evidence that glucose causes translocation of PKC and resultant phosphorylation of one of its substrates, myristoylated alanine-rich C kinase substrate (MARCKS) *(38,39)*. The activation of PKC is secondary to enhanced glycolytic flux and to the concomitant increases in intracellular Ca^{2+}, because mannoheptulose, an inhibitor of glucose phosphorylation, or nitrendipine, an inhibitor of voltage-gated Ca^{2+} channels, blocks the response. MARCKS is a calmodulin-binding protein, and its phosphorylation by PKC reduces its affinity for its binding partner. This, in concert with the large increase in intracellular Ca^{2+} induced by glucose, likely serves to activate PKCaCM. In vitro studies have demonstrated that phosphorylation of several proteins in islet cell extracts occurs in a Ca^{2+}- and calmodulin-dependent fashion. Although it has been speculated that the role of PKCaCM or other Ca^{2+}–calmodulin-regulated kinases such as myosin light-chain kinase may be to phosphorylate cytoskeletal or secretory granule proteins, thereby effecting movement of granules within cells and exocytosis, definitive evidence for such a process and detailed mechanistic explanations are lacking.

The basic model of glucose-stimulated insulin secretion may thus be summarized as follows. An increase in circulating glucose concentration is "sensed" by the β-cell via a proportional increase in metabolic rate. Both glucose transport and glucokinase participate in this translation of glucose concentration into insulin secretion via the regulation of the entry of glucose into glycolysis, with a dominant role being played by glucokinase, as discussed. The activation of glycolysis increases the phosphate potential (ATP/ADP + Pi) by the generation of ATP at three sites: (1) the distal portion of glycolysis, (2) shuttling of reducing equivalents into the mitochondria and activation of the electron-transport chain and oxidative phosphorylation, and (3) pyruvate oxidation. The increase in ATP/(ADP + Pi) causes inhibition of K_{ATP} channels, because ATP^{4-} is an inhibitor and $MgADP^{-}$ is an activator, resulting in membrane depolarization and Ca^{2+} influx. The rise in intracellular Ca^{2+} triggers insulin secretion by the combination of the mechanisms discussed earlier or possibly by as yet undiscovered pathways. Involvement of the cAMP-PKA pathway is particularly important. Marked potentiation of nutrient stimulation of insulin secretion is also achieved by activation of β-cell neurotransmitter and hormone receptors, but as it seems only in the presence of glucose. Potentiation of substrate-induced insulin release by vagal acetylcholine and enteric hormones such as glucagon-like peptide (GLP-1) and glucose-dependent insulinotropic polypeptide (GIP) are physiological events associated with ingestion, digestion, and absorption of a meal and must, therefore, be considered to fully appreciate regulation of insulin secretion in whole animals. The mechanisms by which nutrient and hormonal effectors interact with the basic glucose stimulatory processes as outlined in Fig. 1 are discussed in later sections of the chapter and experimental data that support this model are presented in the following section.

EXPERIMENTAL ILLUSTRATIONS OF THE BASIC MODEL

As has been reviewed in an earlier section, stimulus secretion coupling in pancreatic β-cells stimulated by glucose and amino acids (AA) is mediated by metabolic coupling factors that are generated by energized mitochondria of the secretory cells. To assess the mechanisms by which different nutrients stimulate insulin release from pancreatic β-cells, we employed nuclear magnetic resonance (NMR) technology, respirometry and biochemical analysis to study the metabolic events that occurred in continuously superfused rodent islets and mouse β-HC9 cells during hormone release. Islets were layered between cytodex beads suitable for perifusion in bulk. Figure 2 presents the dynamics of insulin and glucagon release (A) and O_2 consumption (B) in response to stimulation with glucose and amino acids. Oxygen consumption increased as anticipated with increasing levels of glucose and insulin release increased approx 12-fold to 20-fold when glucose reached maximal level of 30 m*M*. High glucose suppressed and amino acids increased glucagon release. The experiment illustrates the physiologically important point that islets do not sustain continued increase insulin release when stimulated with an amino acid mixture (AAM) alone. However, the AAM maintains a significant insulin release in the presence of low (3 m*M*) or high (30 m*M*) glucose. It is noteworthy

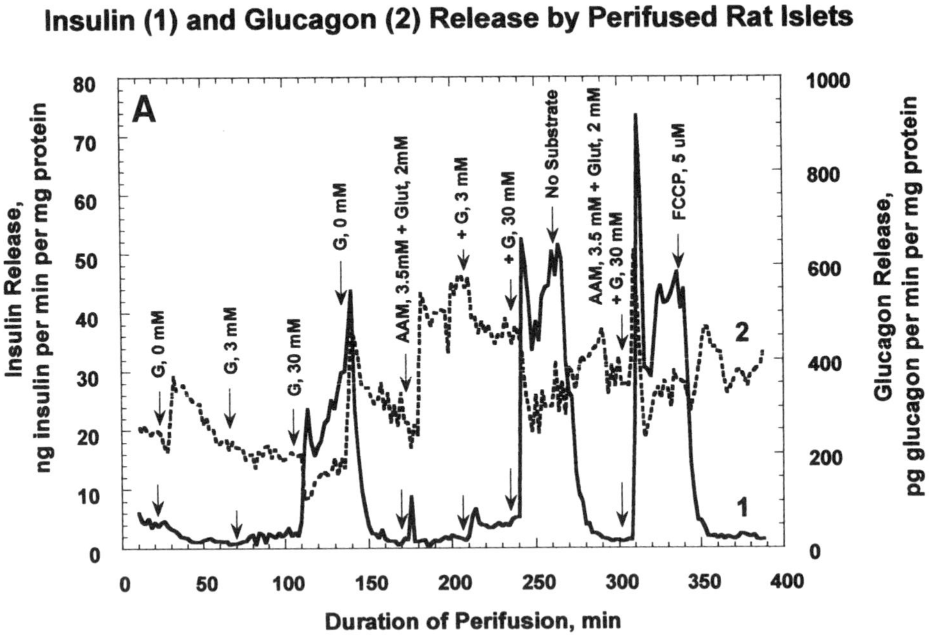

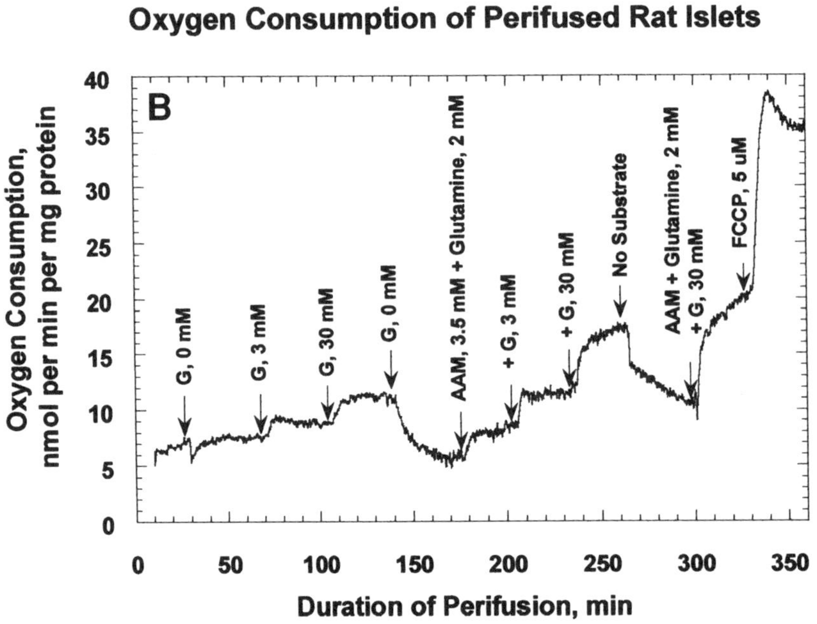

Fig. 2. Secretory and metabolic responses of isolated pancreatic islets. **Panels A** and **B** show insulin, glucagon release and O_2 consumption upon stimulation with glucose and amino acids. Cultured rat islets (4–5 d at 10 m*M* glucose) were layered between cytodex beads, resulting in a 1 × 2-cm columnar arrangement allowing perifusion at a rate of approx 2 mL/min. Clark oxygen electrodes were used to measure the arteriovenous (AV) difference of O_2 to calculate the respiratory rate. Samples from outflow were collected every 2 min to measure insulin and glucagon content. The conditions were changed as indicated in the panels.

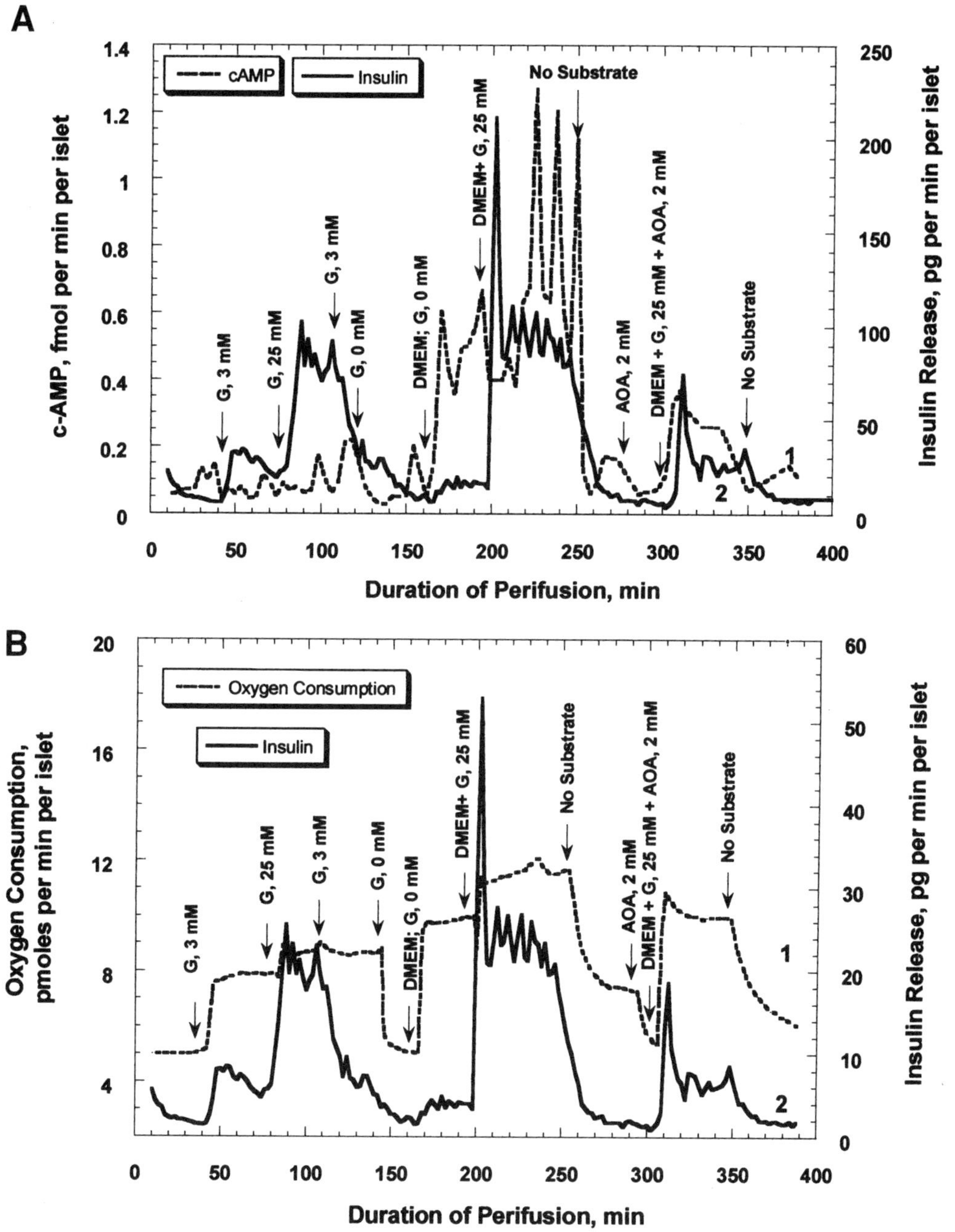

Fig. 3. Simultaneous measurement of cAMP and insulin release (**A**) and oxygen consumption (**B**) in perifused rat islets. The cAMP was measured by radioimmunoassay *(41)* using the Biotrak cAMP[^{125}I] assay system from Amersham Pharmacia Biotech. Oxygen consumption was recorded polarographically with a Clark electrodes.

that 3 and 30 m*M* glucose in the presence of AAM increased V_{O_2} even further. The uncoupler of respiration and oxidative phosphorylation carbonyl cyanide p-(trifluoromethoxy)phenylhydrazone (FCCP) (5 μ*M*) blocked insulin release, as expected, but surprisingly did not affect glucagon release. This puzzling finding needs to be explored.

Oxygen consumption was markedly increased after addition of FCCP, indicating the strong coupling between islet respiration and oxidative phosphorylation. These data demonstrate the critical role of energy metabolism in fuel-stimulated insulin release.

As amply documented in the literature, cAMP serves as a potentiator of the secretory process and may actually play a permissive role in nutrient-induced insulin release. Specifically, cAMP modifies the operation of voltage-dependent calcium channels and promotes Ca^{2+} influx in a clonal pancreatic β-cell line (HIT T-15) *(40)*. The involvement of cAMP is illustrated in Fig. 3, which presents results of the continuous measurement of cAMP, insulin release (*see* Fig. 3A) and oxygen consumption (*see* Fig. 3B) of perifused islets during nutrient-stimulated insulin release. Cyclic-AMP release was significantly elevated only during perifusion with Dulbecco's modified Eagle's medium (DMEM), which contains high amino acid levels. However, it is remarkable that a 12-fold increase in cAMP release and a twofold increase in oxygen consumption were not sufficient to cause a more than marginal increase of insulin release from perifused islets. Further addition of 25 m*M* glucose produced a burst of insulin and cAMP release with oscillatory changes and a further increase in islet oxygen consumption. This demonstrates that many biochemical requirements (i.e., an increase P-potential, availability of potentiators like cAMP, and factors yet to be discovered) have to be met for initiation and maintenance of insulin exocytosis. Aminoxyacetate (AOA), an inhibitor of transaminases, markedly decreased insulin and cAMP release caused by the powerful combined action of DMEM and 25 m*M* glucose in perifused islets, suggesting a critical need for transamination reactions (e.g., in the malate/aspartate shuttle) for fuel-based stimulus-secretion coupling in pancreatic β-cells. The detailed biochemical study of pancreatic islets is limited because of scarcity of material and cellular heterogeneity of pancreatic islets. Therefore, large batches of tumor-derived cultured pancreatic βHC9-cells were used for respiratory and NMR studies. In this case, cells were incorporated in agarose beads, to maintain them in a stable environment and prevent them from escaping from the superfusion system. A glucose concentration as low as 0.5 m*M* when introduced into a fuel-free medium caused an increase in oxygen consumption (*see* Fig. 4). Further stepwise increments of glucose concentration elevated respiration. In contrast, insulin release was unchanged until the glucose concentration reached a threshold of about 4.5 m*M*, illustrating a critical feature of β-cell biology. The respiratory response was reversible upon glucose removal from the perfusate. Hutton and Malaisse *(42)* had shown with isolated islets that the minimal concentration at which glucose evoked respiratory changes was approx 3 m*M*, which corresponded closely to the threshold for increased insulin biosynthesis, ^{86}Rb net uptake, or ^{45}Ca net uptake, but was about 2 m*M* lower than that required to stimulate insulin release. The studies on βHC9 cells indicate that glucose at very low concentrations provoked an immediate increase in islets respiration. The difference may be partly the result of the tumorous nature of the βHC9 cells. The discrepancy needs to be resolved by carefully re-examining this issue with modern methods.

In order to investigate β-cell bioenergetics in depth, noninvasive NMR technology was used in studies of phosphorus metabolism, which became feasible with large batches of agarose embedded βHC9 cells. Figure 5 presents selected ^{31}P-NMR spectra of superfused βHC9 cells with low (3 m*M*) and high (30 m*M*) glucose alone and in the presence of AAM. Each spectrum clearly displays the resonances of P_i, PCr, and ATP (γ, α and β) peaks. Continuous monitoring (every 5 min) of phosphorus metabolites (*see* Fig. 6A) and insulin release (*see* Fig. 6B) demonstrates that increasing the glucose concentration from 3 to 30 m*M* leads to a marked increase in phosphorylation potential

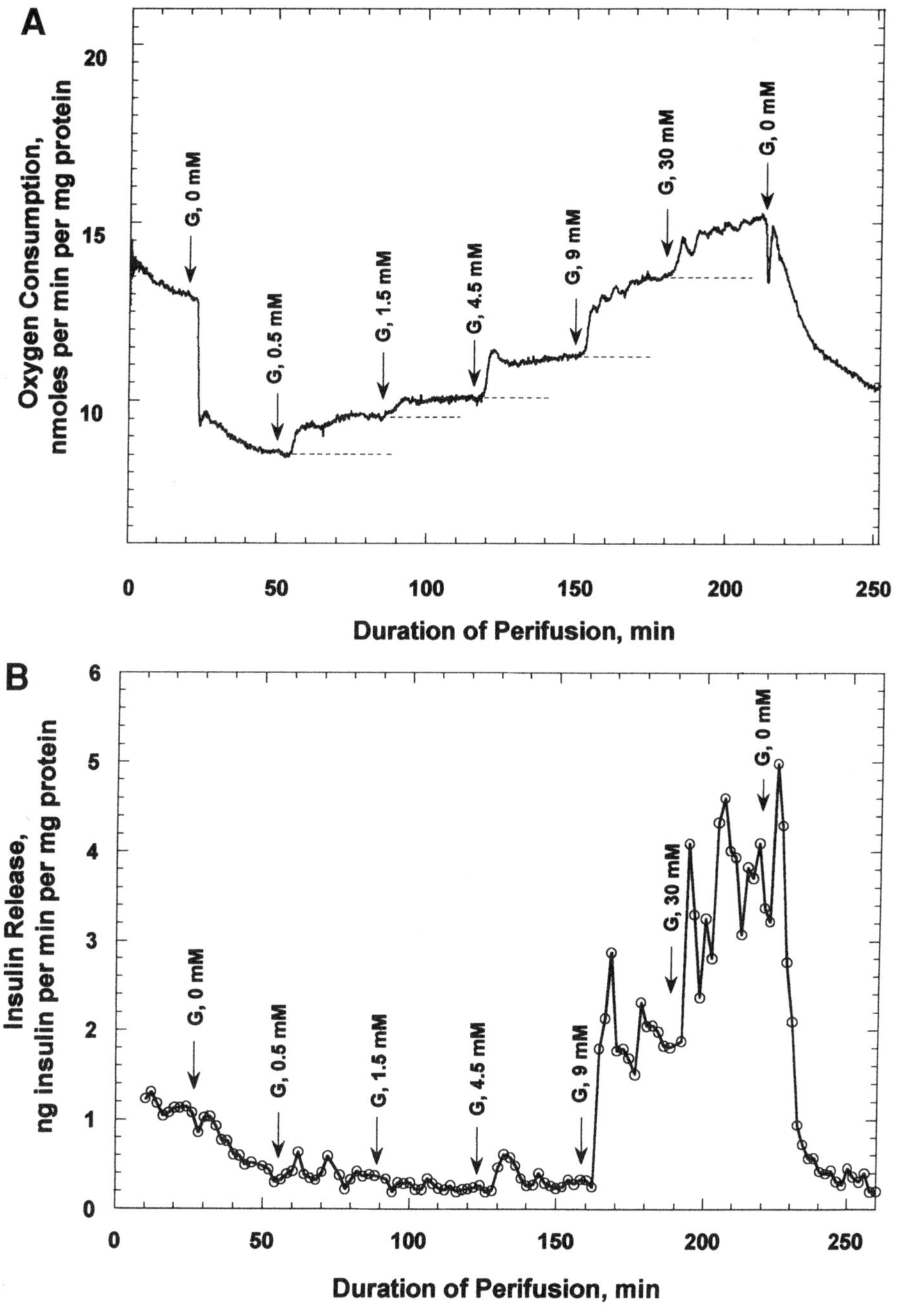

Fig. 4. Oxygen consumption (**A**) and insulin release (**B**) in perifused βHC9 cells exposed to stepwise increases in perfusate glucose. Tumor-derived cultured pancreatic βHC9-cells were used. Cells were incorporated in agarose beads 800–1000 μm in diameter. O_2 consumption was measured polarographically.

as evidenced by increased PCr and decreased P_i peak areas (*see* Fig. 6). It is remarkable that the ATP level as indicated by the β-peak of the nucleotide remains constant. At the same time, insulin release increased 15- to 20-fold. After removal of secretagogues, the PCr decreased and P_i increased and, again, the ATP level remained

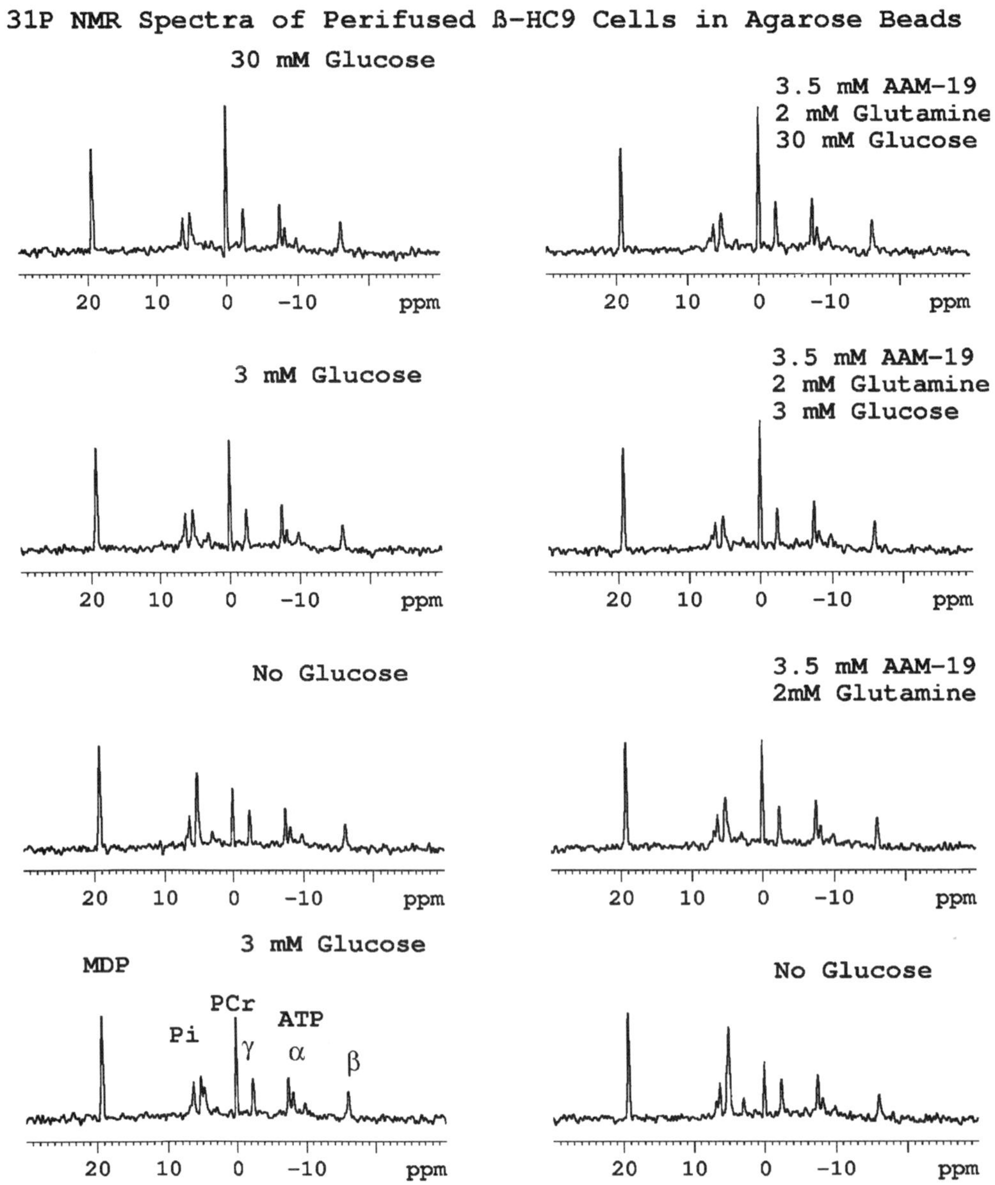

Fig. 5. ^{31}P-NMR spectra of superfused βHC9 cells during exposure to low (3 m*M*) and high (30 m*M*) glucose concentration in nutrient-free medium and in the presence of a physiological mixture of amino acids. Cultured cells were supplemented with 25 m*M* creatine 48 h before the experiment to augment the P-creatine peak, a sensitive indicator of the P-potential. Beads containing cells were placed in a 10-mm-diameter glass NMR tube and maintained in place by a filter. Each NMR sample contained approx 1.5 mL of the beads (approx 20 mg of cell protein). The ^{31}P-NMR measurements were performed with an Avance DMX-400 Spectrometer at 162 MHz. Each exposure lasted 30 min and each ^{31}P-NMR spectrum (acquired in 5-min periods [5000 transients]) represents the last spectrum of each intervention. Peak assignments are indicated as follows: MDP = methylene diphosphonate standard; P_i = inorganic phosphate; PCr = phosphocreatine; ATP = adenosine triphosphate (γ, α, β).

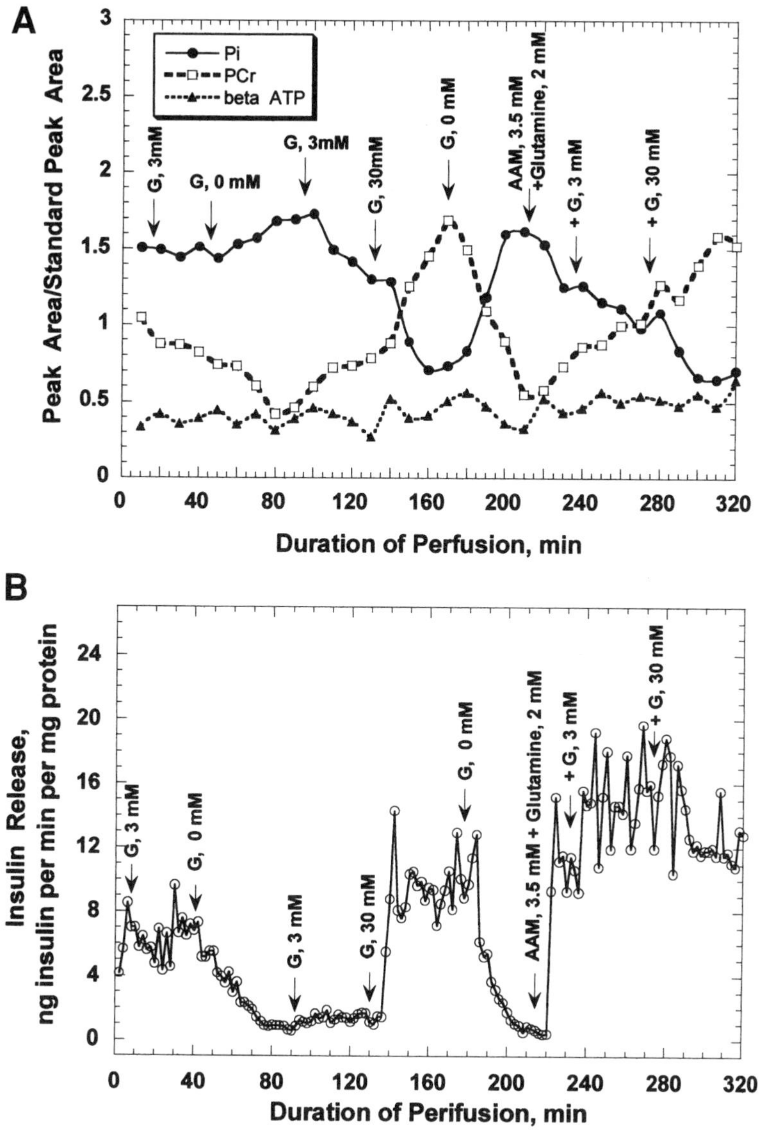

Fig. 6. ^{31}P-NMR allows the continuous measurement of changes in phosphorylation potential during insulin release. Superfused βHC9 cells are monitored during exposure to high glucose and physiological concentrations of amino acids. ^{31}P-NMR spectra were acquired consecutively in 5-min periods.

unchanged. Exposure of βHC9 cells to 3.5 m*M* of an AAM led to marked increase in phosphorylation potential (P-potential) as evidenced by increased PCr and decreased P_i peak areas of ^{31}P-NMR spectra of superfused βHC9 cells. High glucose (30 m*M*) in the presence of AAM further increased the P-potential of βHC9 cells. Insulin release was elevated during stimulation with AAM and increased further with additional low glucose. High glucose decreased insulin release slightly, possibly as a result of the inhibition of glutamate dehydrogenase, an essential step for amino acid metabolism. It seems likely that inhibition of the ATP-sensitive K^+ channels and thus depolarization of the β-cell membrane during glucose-stimulated insulin release is the result of changes in free

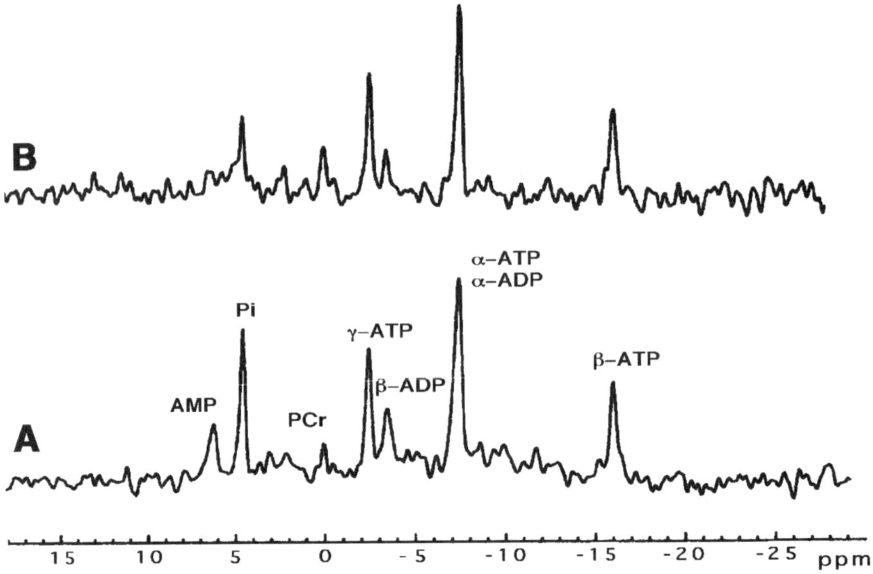

Fig. 7. ^{31}P-NMR spectra of superfused mitochondria from βTC3 (**A**) and βHC9 (**B**) cells. Mitochondria were incorporated into agarose beads (i.e., 7 mg mitochondrial protein per experiment). Mitochondria were continuously superfused with oxygenated buffer containing pyruvate (0.5 m*M*) plus malate (0.5 m*M*) and 0.6 m*M* ADP. Peak assignments are indicated as follows: AMP, adenosine monophosphate; P_i, inorganic phosphate; PCr, phosphocreatine; ATP, adenosine triphosphate (α, β); ADP, adenosine diphosphate (α, β).

ADP rather than free ATP, as demonstrated in these experiments. The effective level of ATP that inhibits the channel in patch-clamping studies was found to vary with half-maximal inhibition occurring at concentrations between 15 and 200 μ*M (43).* Because free ATP concentrations in the β-cell are in the millimolar range, two explanations have been advanced to explain why the ATP-sensitive K^+ channels are not closed at the ambient concentrations of ATP found in the β-cell: ADP^{3-} may compete with ATP^{4-} for binding to the channels, and increases in the K_i of ATP or $MgADP^-$ may serve as an activator *per se.* The latter explanation is more plausible.

To better understand the role of β-cell mitochondria in stimulus–secretion coupling, direct studies of isolated mitochondria of βHC9 and βTC3 cells were initiated using noninvasive ^{31}P- and ^{13}C-NMR spectroscopy. As an example, Fig. 7 presents ^{31}P-NMR spectra of superfused mitochondria from βTC3 (*see* Fig. 7A) and βHC9 (*see* Fig. 7B) cells oxidizing pyruvate plus malate in the presence of 0.6 m*M* ADP. This method allows a clear resolution of free ATP (γ and β) and ADP (β) signals. Isolated β-cell mitochondria embedded in agarose beads are remarkably stable (no decrease in ATP production is seen for more than 7 h). During this time, they may be subjected to various interventions illustrating the unique potential of the approach.

FATTY ACIDS AS INSULIN SECRETAGOGUES

Fatty acids trigger secretion of insulin in a glucose-dependent manner *(3,44).* Fatty acids serve as an important endogenous fuel of islet tissue incubated with low glucose or in the absence of glucose. The possibility has been considered that a high level of fatty acids may inhibit the glucokinase glucose sensor because acyl-CoA, the first metabolite in fatty acid catabolism, is a very potent inhibitor of this enzyme *(3)*. However, this inhibition is competitive with glucose and is therefore significant only when glucose levels are less than 5 m*M*. It is also not clear whether free levels of acyl-CoA are ever high enough for a fuel effect to take place. If the glucose level is high (approx 7.5 m*M*), as seen after a mixed meal, fatty acids can stimulate insulin release. On the other hand, fatty acid oxidation is effectively blocked by high glucose (i.e., by about 75%). This is probably the result of the accumulation of malonyl-CoA *(28,29,45)*. The increase in malonyl-CoA, acting via its capacity to inhibit CPT-I *(30)*, results in inhibition of fatty acid oxidation, increased *de novo* lipid synthesis, and a rise in diacylglycerol content. Vara and Tamirit-Rodriquez *(46,47)* noted that the insulin secretagogues glucose and leucine share the ability to divert fatty acids from the oxidation pathway into esterification products. Note, however, oral superphysiological levels of leucine are needed. It has been also shown that the starvation-induced blunting of glucose-stimulated insulin secretion (GSIS) in perifused rat islets and in the perfused rat pancreas *(48–50)* could be largely offset by addition of 2-bromostearate (2-BrS), an inhibitor of CPT-I. Thus, alterations of the transferase activity or significant changes of its malonyl-CoA sensitivity could greatly modify this regulatory switch. Because it is hypothesized that increases in the levels of malonyl-CoA and cytosolic LC-CoA esters are signal transduction intermediates in glucose-stimulated insulin secretion and may serve as critical factors in β-cell function, such a change could be physiologically or pathologically relevant. This concept has come to be known as the "long-chain acyl-CoA hypothesis" *(24,28,29)*. Possible sites at which increased LC-CoA could influence insulin secretion include conversion to bioactive metabolites such as diacylglycerol or inositol trisphosphate (IP_3), contribution to plasma membrane or secretory granule membrane lipid turnover, or direct acylation of proteins involved in secretory granule trafficking. Although the proposed mechanisms are plausible, direct evidence for any of these actions of lipids on insulin secretion has not been provided to date.

Consistent with an important role of β-cell lipids in glucose sensing, lowering of circulating fatty acids via administration of nicotinic acid or adenovirus-induced hyperleptinemia completely abrogates insulin secretion in response to glucose, amino acids, or sulfonylureas *(51,52)*. These experimental manipulations may lower lipid stores in β-cells, but full secretory function can be restored by provision of fatty acids to the pancreas of such animals. However, in contrast to the positive acute effects of lipids on islet function, long-term exposure to hyperlipidemic conditions results in a condition that has been characterized as "lipotoxicity," wherein lipid overstorage is thought to lead to the syndrome of β-cell dysfunction associated with insulin-resistant and diabetic states, including β-cell hyperplasia, basal hyperinsulinemia, and loss of glucose responsiveness *(53)*. Exposure of islets to palmitic acid for 1 h reduced glucose-stimulated proinsulin biosynthesis in a dose-dependent manner *(54)*. Sprague–Dawley rats fed a diet with 40% fat for 3 wk were glucose intolerant, and in vitro insulin secretion at high glucose was only increased 8.5-fold over basal, compared with 28-fold in control rats *(55)*. Decreased insulin release was associated with a twofold increase of islet uncoupling protein-2 mRNA (UCP-2) expression. UCP-2 catalyzes a mitochondrial inner-membrane H^+ leak that bypasses ATP synthase, thereby reducing cellular ATP content *(55)*. It is extrapolated that UPC-2 induction may deenergize β-cell mitochondria, an effect yet to be proven.

A new study using molecular and pharmacological tools suggests that the LC-CoA hypothesis may require re-evaluation *(56)*. Recombinant adenovirus containing the cDNA-encoding malonyl-CoA decarboxylase (AdCMV-MCD), an enzyme that decarboxylates malonyl CoA to acetyl-CoA, was employed in this approach. Treatment of INS-1 cells with AdCMV-MCD prevented the normal glucose-induced rise in malonyl-CoA levels, such that its concentration in AdCMV-MCD-treated cells at 20 m*M* glucose was lower than control cells at 3 m*M* glucose. That the normal link between glucose and lipid metabolism had been significantly disrupted by this approach was shown by the fact that in the presence of 20 m*M* glucose, AdCMV-MCD-treated cells were less effective at suppressing [1- ^{14}C] palmitate oxidation, and incorporated 43% less labeled palmitate and 50% less labeled glucose into cellular lipids than controls. In spite of the large metabolic changes caused by expression of malonyl-CoA decarboxylase (MCD), insulin secretion in response to glucose was unaltered relative to controls. On the other hand, treatment of INS-1 cells or fresh rat islets of Langerhans with triacsin C, an inhibitor of LC-CoA synthetase caused potent attenuation of palmitate oxidation and glucose or palmitate incorporation into cellular lipids in both INS-1 cells and fresh rat islets, but had no effect on glucose-stimulated insulin secretion in either group. Thus, neither overexpression of MCD nor treatment with triacsin C had any effect on the rate of glucose usage in the β-cell preparations. Based on these data, the authors concluded that there is no direct correlation between the extent to which lipids are directed toward oxidative or esterification pathways and insulin secretion. However, there is evidence that whereas triacsin C is almost completely effective in blocking triglyceride and phospholipid synthesis from glycerol, incorporation of oleate or arachidonate into phospholipids was less impaired *(56)*. Similarly, it has been observed that triacsin C inhibits conversion of [1-^{14}C] palmitate into triglycerides by more than 90%, whereas incorporation of the same substrate into phospholipids is reduced by 50% *(56)*. Thus, although the effects of MCD expression or triacsin C treatment on lipid fluxes in the cited studies were large, they were not complete, and it remains possible that the residual flux of substrate into specific esterification or biosynthetic pathways is sufficient for the maintenance of glucose responsiveness. Note also that complete depletion of islet triglycerides by experimental hyperleptinemia results in abrogation of fuel-mediated insulin secretion in rats *(57)*, apparently indicating that at least a minimal pool of lipids must be present in β-cells in order for normal fuel sensing to take place.

Based on these results, the following modification of the LC-CoA hypothesis was suggested *(4)*. Because the normal link between glucose and lipid metabolism can be markedly disrupted with no effect on glucose usage or insulin secretion, attention is refocused on a coupling factor produced as an immediate byproduct of the glycolytic and mitochondrial pathways. The data are consistent with the tenants of the basic model highlighted in Fig. 1A, in which a primary signal is the glucose-driven increase in ATP to ADP ratio, leading to inhibition of ATP-sensitive K^+ channels and influx of extracellular Ca^{2+}. The abrogation of glucose-stimulated insulin secretion by lipid depletion may then be explained by the absence of essential modulators of secretory granule trafficking and/or exocytosis. Examples of distal sites at which lipids may be acting include generation of signaling molecules such as diacylglycerol or IP_3, or via contribution to secretory granule or plasma membrane turnover. That lipids are acting at a distal rather than a proximal site is supported by the finding that lipid-depleted islets not only fail to respond to glucose but also show no response to arginine, leucine, or the sulfonylurea glibenclamide *(58)*. The mechanism by which fatty acids exert these important modulatory effects on insulin secretion remains to be established. Finally, it should be underlined that the data do not discount the possibility that the malonyl CoA/CPT-I metabolic signaling network may play important roles in long-term processes related to insulin secretion (i.e., β-cell growth, apoptosis, regulation of important metabolic genes, and toxic effects related to chronic exposure of β-cells to high concentrations of fatty acids, a phenomenon termed "lipotoxicity") *(24–27,53)*.

Recent data by Sugden et al. *(59)* suggest that the pyruvate dehydrogenase complex (PDC) may occupy a pivotal position in coordinate fuel utilization governing the contribution of glucose and fatty acids as metabolic fuels. Active PDC permits glucose oxidation and allows the formation of mitochondrially derived intermediates (e.g., malonyl-CoA and citrate) that reflect fuel abundance. Fatty acids oxidation suppresses the PDC activity. PDC inactivation by phosphorylation is catalyzed by pyruvate dehydrogenase kinases (PDKs 1–4). The hypothesis was developed *(59)* that PDK4 is a "lipid status"-responsive PDK isoform facilitating fatty acids oxidation and signaling through citrate formation. Thus, substrate interactions at the level of gene transcription may extend glucose–fatty acids interactions over a longer time period.

AMINO ACID AS INSULIN SECRETAGOGUES

The amino acids that are derived from the protein meals, infusion of physiological amino acid mixtures, or certain individual amino acids have been shown to stimulate insulin release in humans *(60,61)*. Amino acids are glucose-dependent secretory stimuli. Unlike glucose, they cannot by themselves cause insulin secretion from normal β-cells *(3)*. These nutrients can only act as insulin secretagogues when the level of glucose is higher than 4–5 m*M* *(61–64)*. This makes physiological sense, because it allows them to be mobilized from muscle and adipose tissue during starvation, when blood glucose levels are low. In this circumstance, insulin secretion ceases and glucose levels are then maintained by hepatic gluconeogenesis, which produces glucose from specific amino acids and lipid-derived glycerol. The changes of blood sugar levels markedly influence the responsiveness of the β-cells to individual amino acids. For example, hypoglycemia reduces insulin release to amino acid mixtures and most individual amino acids. However, chronic hypoglycemia in man greatly sensitizes the pancreatic β-cell to leucine when administered in high pharmacological dosages *(61)*. A plausible explanation for these results is that amino acids are potent fuel stimulants of β-cells that activate metabolic signaling pathways, fundamentally similar to those discussed earlier for glucose but with characteristics that are special and unique for individual members of this nutrient class. Amino acids can be assumed to be transported into the β-cell by several transporters that are well characterized in other tissues and probably present in β-cells. Most of them are then likely to be transaminated by a family of pyridoxal-P-dependent enzymes that transfer the amino group to α-ketoglutarate to form glutamate *(65)*. The carbon skeletons of the amino acids are converted to pyruvate, acetyl-CoA, α-ketoglutarate, succinyl-CoA, fumarate, and oxaloacetate and provide substrates for the citric acid cycle. Glutamate serves as the predominant final product of the transamination reactions and is oxidatively deaminated by glutamate dehydrogenase. This process is termed transdeamination. Studies with the isolated perfused rat pancreas and with isolated perifused rat islets have supported this view and have demonstrated, in addition, that physiological amino acid mixtures and even pharmacological concentrations of individual amino acids require the presence of permissive levels of glucose (i.e., 2.5–5.0 m*M*) to be effective β-cell stimulants *(64)*. However, in view of the in vivo findings in man, it should not be surprising that leucine is an exception *(66,67)*. When the isolated perfused pancreas or isolated islets are fuel deprived, most importantly when they are maintained in the absence of glucose, even if only for a period of 2 h or less, they are highly responsive to leucine at supraphysiological levels (10–20 m*M*). The findings with leucine as a secretagogue both in man and in a variety of experimental systems using rodent islet tissue were explained by a twofold action of leucine on β-cell metabolism and, consequently, insulin release *(68–75)*. First, leucine may enter β-cell intermediary metabolism by the classical process of transamination and may thus act similar to other metabolic substrate stimuli. In this process, α-ketoglutarate serves as the predominant acceptor of the amino group to form glutamate, and the other product, α-ketoisocaproate (KIC), is thought to be oxidized by branched chain α-ketoacid dehydrogenase (BCKDH) to yield acetoacetate and acetyl-CoA. To complete the process of transdeamination, the product glutamate is reoxidized to α-ketoglutarate. Further catabolism of α-ketoglutarate results in the generation of GTP potentially important for signal transduction. Acetoacetate and actyl-CoA metabolism may result in the production of additional reducing equivalents and energy production. Second, leucine is also an effective allosteric activator of glutamate dehydrogenase (GDH), which generates α-ketoglutarate, NH_3 and NAD(P)H. Leucine thus accelerates its own breakdown by removing glutamate and generating α-ketoglutarate.

In the normal pancreatic β-cell, the critical reaction of transdeamination, catalyzed by GDH, appears to be very strongly inhibited so that oxidation of glutamate is relatively slow. Thus, little ATP and malonyl-CoA would be generated from amino acids, explaining the lack of the response when amino acids are present in the absence of glucose. The activity of the GDH is tightly controlled by the energy potential of the cell *(76)*. It is strongly inhibited by GTP, which is a downstream product and is probably in equilibrium with the phosphate potential ATP/(ADP × Pi). It is also activated by ADP, such that the GTP/ADP ratio of the mitochondria is a critical determinant of the enzyme's rate *(77)*. The stimulation of insulin release by amino acids in the presence of glucose may be the result of enhanced production of pyruvate, α-ketoglutarate, and oxalacetate that would result from even a small increase in glucose metabolism. These metabolites can act as acceptors for the transamination reaction and should, therefore, enhance the degradation of amino acids, allowing them to potentiate the stimulatory effect of glucose.

It is difficult to quantify the relative contributions of these two actions of leucine for the stimulation of insulin secretion. However, activation of GDH by the amino acid is probably sufficient to stimulate the β-cells, given a permissively high glutamate supply. This conclusion is based on the stimulatory effect of the nonmetabolized leucine analog 2-amino-bicyclo-norbonane carboxylic acid (BCH) *(69,70)*, which shares with leucine the GDH activating capacity and, therefore, its ability to stimulate insulin release. These results show that enhanced metabolism of the mitochondrial substrate glutamate is sufficient to cause insulin secretion.

We speculate here that the enzyme is very strongly inhibited at basal conditions but that it may be activated by at least two distinct pathways. First, GDH may be sensitized to its activator by β-cell fuel depletion, because of hypoglycemia, for example, as seen in insulinoma cases. As discussed earlier, patients with an insulinoma are leucine hypersensitive. It can be surmised that the GTP/ADP ratio of β-cells is low in this situation and that less leucine is required to overcome the block. The other pathway may be operative following a protein meal. Protein feeding results in elevated serum levels of the branched-chain amino acids and of glutamine and alanine, whereas neither the blood sugar nor the other amino acids change substantially *(61,62)*. Glutamine, converted by β-cell glutaminase to glutamate, could increase the substrate level for GDH, whereas the branched-chain amino acids leucine, isoleucine, and valine could activate GDH and also serve as substrates for transamination, thus diverting and lowering α-ketoglutarate (a known inhibitor of GDH) *(78)*.

The precision of this control mechanism is illustrated by a recently discovered syndrome of familial hyperinsulinemia associated with mild hyperammonemia *(79,80)*. Patients with this syndrome present with fasting hypoglycemia characterized by inappropriately low β-hydroxybutyrate and free fatty acid levels and an unexpectedly large glycemic response to an injection of glucagon. The patients also have moderately elevated plasma ammonia levels unaffected by protein feeding or restriction. Treatment with diazoxide, which opens K_{ATP} channels and prevents insulin secretion, reliably improves the hypoglycemia. The underlying defect was speculated to involve a site that is common to the regulation of amino acid metabolism of both pancreatic β-cells and hepatocytes and was subsequently shown to be the result of mutations of GDH that interfere with the inhibition of the enzyme by GTP *(80)*. The syndrome is thus best described as persistent GDH-linked hyperinsulinemic hypoglycemia in infancy (PHHI-GDH). The findings in these patients suggest that the β-cell GDH needs to be maintained in a low-activity state and that a high GTP/ADP ratio may accomplish that. It appears that the activation of β-cell GDH by lowering of blood glucose or by fuel depletion in general results physiologically in precisely adjusted flux in the glutaminolysis pathway, allowing the maintenance of critical levels of citric-acid-cycle intermediates and of a functionally appropriate resting phosphate potential, but avoiding a catabolic avalanche that would result in generation of inappropriately high levels of ATP or other coupling factors that might be generated by mitochondria. The actual rate of this basal flux in glutaminolysis remains to be determined. Hypersensitivity of the β-cell to pharmacological dosages of leucine as observed in hypoglycemia of otherwise normal individuals is interpreted as a manifestation of physiological deinhibition of the enzyme in fuel-depleted states, when glutamine may be an important substrate for subsistance metabolism of the cell.

Glutaminolysis in β-cells proceeds by several steps *(81,82)*. Glutamine enters the cell via Na^+-dependent and Na^+-independent transport across the cell membrane, enters the mitochondria by a carrier system, and is then deaminated by glutaminase to glutamate. Glutamate serves as substrate for several enzymes: aminotransferases for various α-ketoacids, glutamate decarboxylase, which produces γ-aminobutyrate, and GDH, which was discussed earlier. In view of the kinetic characteristics of the enzyme GDH *(77)*, the results with its nonmetabolized activator BCH *(69)* and based on the findings in the PHHI-GDH syndrome *(79,80)*, we suggest that GDH is the rate-controlling step for the glutaminolysis pathway in the pancreatic β-cell. It is further concluded that the activity of the enzyme is governed primarily by the energy status of the cell, dependent, most importantly, on the ambient glucose level and the activity of the glucose sensor glucokinase. It is concluded that it serves as an important anaplerotic step to maintain critical levels of citric-acid-cycle intermediates in the β-cell. This proposed role for GDH contrasts starkly with the situation in the liver where glutaminase is thought to be rate limiting *(83)*.

Metabolism of leucine, isoleucine, and valine was also studied intensively. Impetus for such studies came, in part, from the finding that the corresponding α-ketoacids are potent stimulators of insulin release even in the absence of glucose *(61,66,67,84,85)*. The interpretation of results obtained with these α-ketoacids is made difficult because transamination reactions may channel alanine (converted to pyruvate) or glutamate (converted to α-ketoglutarate) into the active metabolite pool. Furthermore, the branched-chain amino acids that are generated by transamination may stimulate GDH, as discussed earlier, and contribute indirectly to the generation of coupling factors from glutamate. The quantification of the relative contribution of these multiple auxiliary pathways has not been accomplished to date.

Even though leucine metabolism of β-cells is complex attempts have been made to identify critical enzymes that comprise and regulate relevant pathways *(86–88)*. The design of such studies was influenced by observations showing that prior exposure of islet tissue to high glucose desensitized β-cells to stimulation by leucine in the absence of glucose. This contrasts markedly with the effect that pretreatment of islets with high glucose has on a subsequent glucose stimulation, which is greatly potentiated. In an attempt to find a molecular explanation for the phenomenon, MacDonald's laboratory discovered that high glucose markedly depressed the expression of the E1α-subunit of the BCKDH, contrasting with the induction of pyruvate dehydrogenase and pyruvate carboxylase *(87)*. This led the investigators to the view that BCKDH determines leucine sensitivity of β-cells. The above studies are flawed by the omission of critical control experiments. For example, it was not determined whether insulin release as a result of KIC was impaired following high-glucose preincubation, as would be expected if reduced BCKDH is a critical event in the desensitization mechanism. Others found no evidence for reduced sensitivity to KIC in islets cultured for 6 d at the moderately high-glucose levels *(88)*. MacDonald and collaborators *(87)* discounted the potential regulatory role of GDH in the desensitization process, because the activity of the enzyme measured in islet cell extracts was not affected by prior glucose treatment. Such a conclusion does not consider the potential for short-term allosteric regulation of GDH by potential activators and inhibitors (e.g., ADP and GTP, respectively).

MITOCHONDRIA AS METABOLIC SIGNAL GENERATORS OF FUEL-STIMULATED β-CELLS

The importance of oxidative metabolism in the stimulus–secretion coupling of insulin release is illustrated by the finding that nutrient secretagogues increase islet respiration *(42,89)*, and that agents that interfere with mitochondrial electron transport or oxidative phosphorylation are potent inhibitors of insulin release *(90)*. However, pyruvate, the end product of aerobic glycolysis, fails to stimulate insulin secretion *(91,92)*. Studies with an inhibitor of pyruvate transport into mitochondria or an inhibitor of the TCA cycle suggest that metabolism of glucose-derived pyruvate in mitochondria or in the TCA cycle is not well correlated with glucose-induced insulin secretion *(93)*. Therefore, it was argued that NADH generated by the glycolytic enzyme glyceraldehydes 3-phosphate dehydrogenase (GAPDH) and then transferred into mitochondria for oxidative metabolism and ATP production through various NADH shuttles (e.g., the glycerol phosphate shuttle and the malate–aspartate shuttle) might be sufficient to initiate insulin release when glucose is elevated *(94,95)*. There seemed to be no critical role for pyruvate oxidation in metabolic coupling when glucose is the stimulus. However, this scenario must be reconciled with the fact that certain fuels that are exclusive mitochondrial substratets (e.g., glutamine plus branched-chain amino acids or their nonmetabolized analog BCH) cause insulin release in the total absence of glucose. Thus, mitochondrially generated metabolic coupling factors are sufficient to initiate insulin release and are as effective as glucose under defined conditions. A plausible minimal model for fuel-stimulated insulin release, including that resulting from glucose, must incorporate the mitochondrial component of signal generation as essential. However, the distinction can be made that in the case of glucose stimulation of the β-cell, the major mitochondrial contribution comes from H^+ shuttles rather than from oxidation of glucose-derived pyruvate. It is also important to note that mitochondrial activation may generate unidentified mitochondrial factors, distinct from ATP, that directly trigger insulin exocytosis, as discussed by Wollheim and colleagues in recent publications *(96–98)*. This group screened molecules derived from mitochondrial metabolism for their secretagogue activity in permeabilized β-cells and suggested glutamate as a candidate for the putative messenger, a proposal requiring much additional scrutiny. These authors also address a critical role of Ca^{2+} for activating mitochondrial dehydrogenases *(96,97)*. The calcium indicator, aequorin, was introduced into β-cell mitochondria by a targeted expression system and was used to monitor the intramitochondrial Ca^{2+} levels in intact islet cells exposed to glucose or methylpyruvate but also to succinate or α-glycero-P following permeabilization of the cell membrane. The data suggested that energizing the mitochondria by various fuels enhances Ca^{2+} uptake, which could then lead to activation of mitochondrial dehydrogenases, an event that may be essential for the generation of metabolic coupling factors. The intramitochondrial enzymes pyruvate dehydrogenase (PDH), 2-oxoglutarate (2-OG) dehydrogenase, and NAD-linked isocitrate dehydrogenase are all Ca^{2+} sensitive *(24)*. PDH is converted from its inactive phosphorylated form into its active dephosphorylated form when islets are stimulated with glucose or high extracellular Ca^{2+} *(99)*, in keeping with the Ca^{2+} sensitivity of PDH-P phosphatase *(100)*. Furthermore, islets mitochondria contain a high activity of the flavin-linked α-glycerophosphate (α-GP) dehydrogenase, which is also activated by Ca^{2+} *(101)*. Therefore, it has been suggested that the increased respiration seen in glucose-stimulated islets is a consequence of stimulation of these dehydrogenases by the elevated Ca^{2+}, a mechanism designed to cover the rising energy demand of secretion *(99,100)*. However, it is a striking observation made by many that glucose and other fuel secretagogues stimulate respiration of islet tissue and that this stimulation of respiration is independent of extracellular Ca^{2+} *(102)*. Lack of extracellular Ca^{2+} does, however, reduce the oxidation of glucose to CO_2 and H_2O *(102)*. This result is consistent with the view that the enhancement of respiration by high glucose is the result of a mass action effect, in part explained by highly efficient hydrogen shuttles, but that precise regulation of intermediary metabolism and generation of metabolic coupling factors from glucose is subject to fine control by mitochondrial Ca^{2+} levels *(3)*.

Eto et al. *(103)* have shown that inhibition of both shuttles (the glycerol phosphate shuttle and the malate–aspartate shuttle) was associated with the suppression of glucose-induced increases in NAD(P)H autofluorescence, mitochondrial membrane potential, and mitochondrial ATP content to 25–30% of the normal state, and insulin secretion was abolished. Abolition of the NADH shuttle system resulted in ~50% reduction of the TCA cycle activity, so contribution of the TCA cycle and NADH shuttle system to mitochondrial ATP production may be approximately equal in the physiological state. Based on these data, the authors propose a plausible model for glucose-induced insulin secretion: Glucose stimulation of β-cells can both produce NADH in the cytosol and provide pyruvate for the TCA cycle. Cytosolic NADH can be transferred into mitochondria through the NADH shuttles, and, concomitantly, it leads to an increase in $[Ca^{2+}]_m$ because of an altered mitochondrial membrane potential, thereby activating pyruvate oxidation in the TCA cycle. The NADH shuttles thus would contribute to critical quantities of ATP generation to trigger insulin secretion. When NADH shuttles are halted, the activity of the TCA cycle is also decreased by approx 50%, at least in part because of concurrent inhibition of Ca^{2+} entry into mitochondria. The resultant severe decrease in mitochondrial ATP synthesis to approx 25% of the normal state no longer maintains glucose-induced insulin secretion. Thus, defects in the generation of mitochondrial metabolic signals through the NADH shuttles might contribute to the impairment of glucose-induced insulin secretion of NIDDM.

The importance of the mitochondrial contribution in fuel-stimulated insulin release is highlighted by recent reports about diabetes syndromes that develop as a result of mitochondrial lesions. Mutations of the mitochondrial genome may become manifest as impaired β-cells function both in man *(104,105)* and in a rat model of diabetes mellitus *(106,107)*.

The forgoing discussion demonstrates that mitochondrial involvement in fuel-stimulated insulin release remains a critical and fruitful area of future research.

NEURAL AND ENDOCRINE REGULATION OF INSULIN RELEASE

Neural and endocrine factors have been shown to greatly affect fuel-induced insulin release *(6)*. Acetylcholine, the neurotransmitter of the vagus, strongly potentiates glucose-stimulated insulin release, but it is not effective in the absence of glucose. In contrast, the catecholamines, adrenaline and noradrenaline, block stimulated insulin release. Muscarinic and α-adrenergic receptors mediate these effects of the parasympathetic and sympathetic nervous systems. The secretory response of β-cells to fuel stimulation is also markedly enhanced by the gut hormone GLP-1 *(108)*, a member of the glucagon family, which is released into the portal circulation when a meal is digested. The physiological importance of GLP-1 is strikingly demonstrated by comparing the stimulatory efficacies of equivalent glucose loads given orally (which induce GLP-1) or intravenously (which do not). Ingested glucose is significantly more effective. Several investigators have suggested that priming by enteric hormones (GLP-1) and/or neural stimulation (vagal acetylcholine) are absolutely necessary for fuels, particularly glucose, to be effective stimuli, suggesting that β-cells are not intrinsically competent as fuel-sensor cells *(108)*.

At least two sets of observations contradict this concept, however. First, a significant fraction of isolated single β-cells studied electrophysiologicaly, optically, and by other approaches show characteristic electrical, ionic, and secretory responses when stimulated with glucose in the absence of neuroendocrine factors, clearly demonstrating their competency *(109,110)*. Second, various cultured β-cell lines respond to fuels, including glucose, amino acids and fatty acids, without prior priming by neurotransmitters and hormones. Therefore, it remains reasonable to take the position that β-cells are able to respond to glucose directly, that it is glucose that enables β-cells to respond to other fuels, and that the role of transmitters of the autonomic nervous system and enteric hormones is to potentiate or curb the action of fuel molecules, depending on the momentary need of the organism. Much effort is currently devoted to assess the therapeutic potential of GLP-1 and related compounds for the long-term treatment of type 2 diabetes *(111)*.

OUTLOOK

Substrate control of insulin secretion defines the pancreatic β-cell as unique, contrasting it with most other secretory cells that are primarily controlled by neuroendocrine factors. Much progress has been made in the last three decades to characterize the metabolic pathways that are involved. Information on glucose metabolism is most extensive and most advanced. Clearly defined pathological syndromes have recently been discovered in man that are caused by genetic defects in critical pathways of β-cell fuel metabolism, including permanent neonatal diabetes mellitus (PNDM-GK), MODY-2, and PHHI-GK (permanent hyperinsulinemic hypoglycemia in infancy), all caused by mutations of the glucokinase gene. PHHI-GDH (caused by mutations of GDH) and sulfonylurea receptor (SUR-1)/KIR-6.2-related hyperinsulinemic hypoglycemia (caused by mutations of the sulfonylurea receptor or the inward rectifying K-channel complex of β-cells) are equally instructive about the metabolic basis of insulin release. Molecular genetic approaches have been successfully applied to critically test prevailing hypotheses in this area (e.g., the role of glucose transporters, the glucokinase glucose sensor hypothesis, the role of glutamate dehydrogenase as pacemaker of glutaminolysis, the critical role of adenine nucleotides as modifiers of ion channels, and the significance of lipid-related molecules as metabolic coupling factors). A wide range of biophysical and physiological chemical approaches are being applied with increasing success to the question of substrate controlled insulin release (e.g., Ca^{2+} imaging, or ^{31}P- and ^{13}C-NMR in dynamic studies exploring matrix embedded cultured β-cells, as illustrated by selected samples [Figs. 2–6]). Vigorous attempts are being made to develop pharmacological agents that might modify critical metabolic pathways of β-cells and thus influence insulin secretion. Glucokinase is a striking example: A class of very potent GK-activator drugs has been discovered *(112–114)*. Those compounds increase the affinity of glucose for GK and increase the catalytic rate of enzyme. This enhances glucose stimulation of insulin release in the β-cell and glucose disposal in the liver. The drugs are very effective orally in the animal model of type 2 diabetes and have considerable promise for application in man. Molecular bioengineering approaches take advantage of the wealth of fundamental knowledge about substrate-controlled insulin release in attempts to develop implantable cell-based devices that may aid or replace impaired β-cells in diabetes *(115)*. It is safe to predict much progress in this area of pre-eminent medical relevance in the years to come.

REFERENCES

1. Epple A, Brinn JE. The Comparative Physiology of the Pancreatic Islets. Springer-Verlag, Berlin, 1987.
2. Matschinsky FM, Collins HW. Essential biochemical design features of the fuel-sensing system in pancreatic β-cells. Chem Biol 1997;4:249–257.
3. Matschinsky FM. Banting Lecture 1995. A lesson in metabolic regulation inspired by the glucokinase glucose sensor paradigm. Diabetes 1996;45:223–241.

4. Newgard CB, Matschinsky FM. Substrate control of insulin release. In: Jefferson L, Cherrington A, eds. Handbook of Physiology. Oxford University Press, Oxford 2001, Vol. 2, pp. 125–151.
5. Matschinsky FM, Sweet IR. Annotated questions and answers about glucose metabolism and insulin secretion of β-cells. Diabetes Rev 1996;4:130–144.
6. Liang Y, Matschinsky FM. Mechanism of action on non glucose insulin secretagogues. Am Rev Nutr 1994;14:59–81.
7. Bell GI, Kayano T, Buse JB, Burant CF, Takeda J, Lin D, et al. Molecular biology of mammalian glucose transporters. Diabetes Care 1990;13:198–208.
8. Thorens B, Sarkar HK, Kaback HR, Lodish HF. Cloning and functional expression in bacteria of a novel glucose transporter in liver, intestine, kidney and beta-pancreatic islet cells. Cell 1988;55:281–290.
9. Johnson JH, Newgard CB, Milburn JL, Lodish HF, Thorens B. The high K_m glucose transporter of islets of Langerhans is functionally similar to the low affinity transporter of liver and has an identical primary sequence. J Biol Chem 1990;265:6548–6551.
10. DeVos A, Heimberg H, Quartier E, Huypens P, Bouwens L, Pipeleers D, et al. Human and rat beta cells differ in glucose transporter but not in glucokinase gene expression. J Clin Invest 1995;96:2489–2495.
11. Ferrer J, Benito C, Gomis R. Pancreatic islet GLUT-2 glucose transporter mRNA and protein expression in humans with and without NIDDM. Diabetes 1995;44:1369–1374.
12. Meglasson MD, Matschinsky FM. Pancreatic islet glucose metabolism and regulation of insulin secretion. Diabetes Metab Rev 1986;2:163–214.
13. Wilson JE. Regulation of mammalian hexokinase activity. In: Beitner R, ed. Regulation of Carbohydrate Metabolism. CRC, Boca Raton, FL, 1984, pp. 45–85.
14. Johnson JH, Ogawa A, Chen L, Orci L, Newgard CB, Alam T, et al. Underexpression of β-cell high Km glucose transport in noninsulin-dependent diabetes. Science 1990;250:546–549.
15. Froguel PH, Zouali H, Vionnet N, Velho G, Vaxillaire M, Sun F, et al. Familial hyperglycemia due to mutations in glucokinase:definition of a subtype of diabetes mellitus. N Engl J Med 1993;328:697–702.
16. Perales MA, Sener A, Malaisse WJ. Hexose metabolism in pancreatic islets: the glucose-6-phosphate riddle. Mol Cell Biochem 1991;101:67–71.
17. Khan AV, Chaudramouli V, Gotenson CG, Ahren B, Schumann WC, Low H, et al. Evidence for presence of glucose cycling in pancreatic islets of the ob/ob mouse. J Biol Chem 1989;264:9732–9733.
18. Sekine N, Cirulli V, Regazzi R, Brown LJ, Gine E, Tamarit-Rodriguez J, et al. Low lactate dehydrogenase and high mitochondrial glycerol phosphate dehydrogenase in pancreatic β-cells. J Biol Chem 1994;269:4895–4902.
19. Voet D, Voet JG. Electron transporter and oxidative phosphorylation. In: Voet D, Voet JG, eds. Biochemistry. Wiley, New York, 1990, pp. 528–557.
20. Nelson DL, Cox MM. Oxidative phosphorylation and photophosphorylation. In: Nelson DL, Cox MM, eds. Lehninger Principles of Biochemistry. Worth Publishers, New York, 2000, pp. 659–715.
21. Darley-Usmar V, Ragan I, Smith P, Wilson M. The proteins of the mitochondrial inner membrane and their role in mitochondria. In: Darley-Usmar V, Schapira AH, eds. DNA, Proteins and Disease. Portland, Chapel Hill, NC, 1994, pp. 1–25.
22. Liang Y, Bai G, Doliba N, Buettger C, Wang L, Berner DK, et al. Glucose metabolism and insulin release in mouse βHC9 cells as model for wildtype pancreatic β-cells. Am J Physiol 1996;270:E846–E857.
23. Berman HK, Newgard CB. Fundamental metabolic differences between hepatoyctes and islet β-cells revealed by glucokinase overexpression. Biochemistry 1998;37:4543–4552.
24. Prentki M, Matschinsky FM. Ca^{2+}, cAMP and phospholipid-derived messengers in coupling mechanism of insulin secretion. Physiol Rev 1987;67:1185–1248.
25. McGarry JD. What if Minkowski had been ageusic? An alternative angle on diabetes. Science 1992;258:766–770.
26. Prentki M, Corkey BE. Are the β-cell signaling molecules malonyl CoA and cytosolic long chain-CoA implicated in multiple tissue defects of obesity and NIDDM? Diabetes 1996;45:273–283.
27. Newgard CB, McGarry JD. Metabolic coupling factors in pancreatic beta-cell signal transduction. Annu Rev Biochem 1995;64:689–719.
28. Corkey BE, Glennon MC, Chen KS, Deeney JT, Matschinsky FM, Prentki M. A role for malonyl-CoA in glucose-stimulated insulin secretion from clonal pancreatic β-cells. J Biol Chem 1989;264:21,608–21,612.

29. Prentki M, Vischer S, Glennon MC, Regazzi R, Deeney JT, Corkey BE. Malonyl-CoA and long chain acyl-CoA esters as metabolic coupling factors in nutrient-induced insulin secretion. J Biol Chem 1992;267:5802–5810.
30. McGarry JD, Woeltje KF, Kuwajima M, Foster DW. Regulation of ketogenesis and the renaissance of carnitine palmitoyltransferase. Diabetes Metab Rev 1989;5:271–284.
31. Chen S, Ogawa A, Ohneda M, Unger RH, Foster DW, McGarry JD. More direct evidence for a malonyl-CoA–carnitine palmitoyltransferase I interaction as a key event in pancreatic β-cell signalling. Diabetes 1994;43:878–883.
32. Cook DL, Hales N. Intracellular ATP directly blocks K^+-channels in pancreatic β-cells. Nature 1984;311:269–271.
33. Ashcroft FM, Harrison DE, Aschroft SHJ. Glucose induces closure of single potassium channels in isolated rat pancreatic β-cells. Nature 1984;312:446–448.
34. Misler S, Falke LC, Gillis K, McDaniel ML. A metabolite-regulated potassium channel in rat pancreatic B cells. Proc Natl Acad Sci USA 1986;83:7119–7123.
35. Atwater I, Mears D, Rojas E. Electrophysiology of the pancreatic β-cell, In: Leroith D, Taylor SI, Olefsky JM, eds. Diabetes Mellitus (A Fundamental and Clinical Text). Lippincott–Raven, New York, 1996, pp. 78–102.
36. Misler S, Pressel DM, Barnett DW. Stimulus transduction in metabolic sensor cells. In: Speralakis N, ed. Cell Physiology Source Book. Academic, San Diego, CA, 1998, pp. 652–667.
37. Gembal M, Detimary P, Gilon P, Gao Z-Y, Henquin JC. Mechanisms by which glucose can control insulin release independently from its action on adenosine triphosphate-sensitive K channels in mouse β-cells. J Clin Invest 1993;91:871–880.
38. Ganesan S, Calle R, Zawalich K, Greenawalt K, Zawalich W, Rasmussen H. Immunocytochemical location of α-protein kinase C in rat pancreatic β-cells during glucose-induced insulin secretion. J Cell Biol 1992;119:313–324.
39. Calle R, Ganesan S, Smallwood JI, Rasmussen H. Glucose-induced phosphorylation of myristolated alanine-rich C kinase substrate (MARCKS) in isolated rat pancreatic islets. J Biol Chem 1992;267:18,723–18,727.
40. Prentki M, Glennon MC, Geschwind J-F, Matschinsky FM, Corkey BE. Cyclic AMP raises cytosolic Ca^{2+} and promotes Ca^{2+} influx in a clonal pancreatic β-cell line (HIT T-15). FEBS Lett 1987;220(1):103–107.
41. Albano JDM, Barnes GD. Factors affecting the saturation assay of cyclic AMP in biological systems. Anal Biochem 1974;60:130–141.
42. Hutton JC, Malaisse WJ. Dynamics of O_2 consumption in rat pancreatic islets. Diabetologia 1980;18:395–405.
43. Hopkins WF, Fatherazi S, Peter-Riesch B, Corkey BE, Cook DL. Two sites for adenine-nucleotide regulation of ATP-sensitive potassium channels in mouse pancreatic beta-cells and HIT cells. J Membr Biol 1992;129:287–295.
44. Balasse EO, Ooms HA. Role of plasma free acids in the control of insulin secretion in man. Diabetologia 1973;9:145–151.
45. Liang Y, Matschinsky FM. Content of CoA-esters in perifused rat islets stimulated by glucose and other fuels. Diabetes 1991;40:327–333.
46. Vara E, Tamarit-Rodriguez J. Effects of L-leucine on palmitate metabolism and insulin release by isolated islets of fed and starved rats. Endocrinology 1986;119:404–407.
47. Vara E, Tamarit-Rodriguez J. Glucose stimulation of insulin secretion in islets of fed and starved rats and its dependence on lipid metabolism. Metabolism 1986;35:266–271.
48. Tamarit-Rodriguez J, Vara E, Tamarit J. Starvation-induced secretory changes of insulin, somatostatin, and glucagon and their modification by 2-bromostearate. Horm Metab Res 1984;16:115–119.
49. Tamarit-Rodriguez J, Vara E, Tamarit J. Starvation-induced changes of palmitate metabolism and insulin secretion in isolated rat islets stimulated by glucose. Biochem J 1984;221:317–324.
50. Bedoya FJ, Ramirez R, Arilla E, Goberna R. Effect of 2-bromostearate on glucose-phosphorylating activities and the dynamics of insulin secretion in islets of Langerhans during fasting. Diabetes 1984;33:858–863.
51. Stein DT, Esser V, Stevenson BE, Lane KE, Whiteside JH, Daniels MB, et al. Essentiality of circulating fatty acids for glucose-stimulated insulin secretion in the fasted rat. J Clin Invest 1996;97:2728–2735.
52. Stein DT, Stevenson BE, Chester MW, Basit M, Daniels MB, Turley SD, et al. The insulinotropic potency of fatty acids is influenced profoundly by their chain length and degree of saturation. J Clin Invest 1997;100:398–403.

53. Unger RH. Lipotoxicity in the pathogenesis of obesity-dependent NIDDM: genetic and clinical implications. Diabetes 1995;44:863–870.
54. Katahira H, Nagamatsu S, Ozawa S, Nakamichi Y, Yamaquchi S, Furukawa H, et al. Acute inhibition of proinsulin biosynthesis at the translational level by palmitic acid. Biochem Biophys Res Commun 2001;282(2):507–510.
55. Chan CB, De Leo D, Joseph JW, McQuaid TS, Ha XF, Xu F, et al. Increased uncoupling protein-2 levels in beta-cells are associated with impaired glucose-stimulated insulin secretion: mechanism of action. Diabetes 2001;50(6):1302–1310.
56. Antinozzi P, Prentki M, Segall L, McGarry JD, Newgard CB. Molecular or pharmacologic perturbation of the link between glucose and lipid metabolism is without effect on glucose-stimulated insulin secretion: a re-evaluation of the long-chain acyl CoA hypothesis. J Biol Chem 1998;273(26):16,146–16,154.
57. Chen G, Koyama K, Ynan X, Lee Y, Zhou YT, O'Doherty R, et al. Disappearance of body fat in normal rats induced by adenovirus-mediated leptin gene therapy. Proc Natl Acad Sci USA 1996;93:14,795–14,799.
58. Dobbins RL, Chester MW, Daniels MB, McGarry JD, Stein DT. Circulating fatty acids are essential for efficient glucose-stimulated insulin secretion after prolonged fasting in humans. Diabetes 1998;47(10):1613–1618.
59. Sugden MC, Bulmer K, Holness MJ. Fuel-sensing mechanisms integrating lipid and carbohydrate utilization. Biochem Soc Trans 2001;29:272–278.
60. Wahren J, Felig P. Effect of protein ingestion on splanchnic and leg metabolism in normal man and in patients with diabetes mellitus. J Clin Invest 1976;57:987–999.
61. Fajans S, Floyd JL, Knopf RF, Conn JW. Effects of amino acids and proteins on insulin secretion in man. Recent Prog Horm Res 1967;23:617–656.
62. Felig Ph. Amino acid metabolism in man. Annu Rev Biochem 1975;44:933–955.
63. DeFronzo RA, Felig Ph. Amino acids in uremia: insight gained from normal and diabetic man. Am J Clin Nutr 1980;33:1378–1386.
64. Pagliara AS, Stillings SN, Hover BA, Martin DM, Matschinsky FM. Glucose modulation of amino acid induced glucagon and insulin release in the isolated perfused rat pancreas. J Clin Invest 1974;54:819–832.
65. Braunstein AE, Bychkov SM. A cell-free enzymic model of 1-amino-acid dehydrogenase (1′ deaminase). Nature 1939;144:751–752.
66. Matschinsky FM, Fertel R, Kotler-Brajtburg J, Stillings S, Ellerman J, Raybaud F, et al. Factors governing the action of small calorigenic molecules on the islets of Langerhans. In: Mussacchia XJ, Breitenbach RP, eds. 8th Midwest Conference on Endocrinology and Metabolism. University of Missouri–Columbia Press, Columbia, 1973, pp. 63–87.
67. Matschinsky FM, Ellerman J, Stillings S, Raybaud F, Pace C, Zawalich W. Hexoses and insulin secretion. In: Hasselblatt A, Bruchhausen FV, eds. Handbook of Experimental Pharmacology, New Series. Springer-Verlag, Berlin, 1975, pp. 79–114.
68. Sener A, Malaisse WJ. The stimulus secretion coupling of amino acids induced insulin release: insulinotropic action of branched-chained amino acids at physiological concentrations of glucose and glutamine. Eur J Clin Invest 1981;11:455–460.
69. Sener A, Malaisse-Lagae F, Malaisse WJ. Stimulation of pancreatic ilset metabolism and insulin release by a non metabolizable amino acid. Proc Natl Acad Sci USA 1981;78:5460–5464.
70. Panten U, Zielmann S, Langer J, Zunkler BJ, Lenzen S. Regulation of insulin secretion by energy metabolism in pancreatic β-cell mitochondria. Studies with a non-metabolizable leucine analogue. Biochem J 1984;219:189–196.
71. Malaisse-Lagae F, Sener A, Garcia-Morales P, Valverde I, Malaisse WJ. The stimulus-secretion coupling of amino acid-induced insulin release. Influence of a nonmetabolized analog of leucine on the metabolism of glutamine in pancreatic islets. J Biol Chem 1982;257:3754–3758.
72. Malaisse WJ, Carpinelli AR, Lebrun P, Herchulz A, Sener A. The stimulus–secretion coupling of amino acid-induced insulin release. IV. Ionic response to L-leucine and L-glutamine. Pflugers Arch 1981;391:112–118.
73. Malaisse WJ, Hutton JC, Carpinelli AR, Herchuelz A, Sener A. The stimulus–secretion coupling of amino acid-induced insulin release: metabolism and cationic effects of leucine. Diabetes 1980;29:431–437.
74. Malaisse WJ, Sener A, Malaisse-Lagae F, Welsh M, Matthews DE, Bier DM, et al. The stimulus–secretion coupling of amino acid-induced insulin release. Metabolic response of pancreatic islets of L-glutamine and L-leucine. J Biol Chem 1982;257:8731–8737.

75. Sener A, Malaisse-Lagae F, Malaisse WJ. The stimulus–secretion coupling amino acid-induced insulin release. XII. Contrasting effects of L-leucine and a nonmetabolized analog upon islet metabolism and insulin secretion. Horm Metab Res 1982;14:459–463.
76. Gao Z, Li G, Najafi H, Wolf BA, Matschinsky FM. Glucose regulation of glutaminolysis and its role in insulin secretion. Diabetes 1999;47:1535–1542.
77. Hudson RC, Daniel RM. Glutamate dehydrogenase: distribution, properties, and mechanism. Exp Biochem Physiol 1993;106B:767–792.
78. Bryla J, Michalek M, Nelson J, Erecinska M. Regulation of glutamate dehydrogenase activity in rat islets of Langerhans and its consequences on insulin release. Metabolism 1994;43:1187–1195.
79. Weinzimer SA, Stanley CA, Berry GT, Yudkoff M, Tuchman M, Thornton PS. A syndrome of congenital hyperinsulinism and hyperammonemia. J Pediatr 1997;130:661–664.
80. Stanley CA, Lien KY, Hsu BYL, Burlina AB, Greenberg CR, Hopwood NJ, et al. Hyperinsulinism and hyperammonemia in infants with regulatory mutation of glutamate dehydrogenase. N Engl J Med 1998;338(19):1352–1357.
81. Michalik M, Nelson J, Erecinska M. Glutamate production in islets of Langerhans: properties of phosphate-activated glutaminase. Metabolism 1992;41:1319–1326.
82. Curthoys NP. Regulation of glutaminase activity and glutamine metabolism. Annu Rev Nutr 1995;15:133–159.
83. Low SY, Salter M, Knowles RG, Pogson CI, Rennie MJ. A quantitative analysis of the control of glutamine catabolism in rat liver cells. Use of selective inhibitors. Biochem J 1993;295:617–624.
84. Lenzen S, Schmidt W, Rustenbeck I, Panten U. 2-Ketoglutarate generation in pancreatic β-cell mitochondria regulates insulin secretory action of amino acids and 2-ketoacids. Biosci Rep 1986;6:163–169.
85. Knopf RF, Fajans SS, Floyd JG Jr, Conn JW. Comparison of experimentally induced and naturally occurring sensitivity to leucine hypoglycemia. J Clin Endocrinol Metab 1963;23:579.
86. MacDonald MJ, Fahien LA, McKenzie DI, Moran SM. Novel effects of insulin secretagogues on capacitation of insulin release and survival of cultured pancreatic islets. Am J Physiol (Endocr Metab 22) 1990;259:E548–E554.
87. MacDonald MJ, McKenzie DI, Kaysen JH, Walker TM, Moran SM, Fahien LA, et al. Glucose regulates leucine-induced insulin release and the expression of the branched chain ketoacid dehydrogenase E1 alpha subunit gene in pancreatic islets. J Biol Chem 1991;266:1335–1340.
88. Siegel EG, Wollheim CB, Janjic D, Ribes G, Sharp GW. Involvement of Ca^{2+} in the impaired glucose-induced insulin release from islets cultured at low glucose. Diabetes 1983;32:993–1000.
89. Hellerstrom C. Effects of carbohydrates on oxygen consumption of isolated pancreatic islets of mice. Endocrinology 1967;81:105–112.
90. Aleyassine H. Energy requirements for insulin release from rat pancreas in vivo. Endocrinology 1970;87:84–89.
91. Lenzen S. Effects of α-ketocarboxylic acids and 4-pentenoic acid on insulin secretion from the perfused rat pancreas. Biochem Pharmacol 1979;27:1321–1324.
92. Sener A, Kawazu S, Hutton JC, Boschero AC, Devis G, Somers G, et al. The stimulus secretion coupling of glucose-induced insulin release. Biochem J 1978;176:217–232.
93. Dukes ID, McIntyre MS, Mertz RJ, Philipson LH, Roe MW, Spencer B, et al. Dependence on NADH produced during glycolysis for beta-cell glucose signaling. 3rd. J Biol Chem 1994;269(15): 10,979–10,982.
94. MacDonald MJ. High content of mitochondrial glycerol-3-phosphate dehydrogenase in pancreatic islets and its inhibition by diazoxide. J Biol Chem 1981;256(16):8287–8290.
95. MacDonald MJ. Evidence for the malate aspartate shuttle in pancreatic islets. Arch Biochem Biophys 1982;213(2):643–649.
96. Maechler P, Kennedy ED, Pozzan T, Wollheim CB. Mitochondrial activation directly triggers the exocytosis of insulin in permeabilized pancreatic β-cells. EMBO J 1997;16:3833–3841.
97. Kennedy ED, Rizzalo R, Theler JM, Pralong WF, Bastianutto C, Pozzan T, et al. Glucose stimulated insulin secretion correlates with changes in mitochondrial and cytosolic Ca^{2+} in aequorin-expressing INS-1 cells. J Clin Invest 1996;98:2524–2538.
98. Maechler P, Wollheim CB. Mitochondrial glutamate acts as a messenger in glucose-induced insulin exocytosis. Nature 1999;402:685–689.
99. McCormack JG, Longo EA, Corkey BE. Glucose-induced activation of pyruvate dehydrogenase in isolated rat pancreatic islets. Biochem J 1990;267:527–530.
100. McCormack JG, Halestrap AP, Denton RM. Role of calcium ions in regulation of mammalian intramitochondrial metabolism. Physiol Rev 1990;70(2):391–425.

101. Rasschaert J, Malaisse WJ. Hexose metabolism in pancreatic islets. Glucose-induced and Ca^{2+}-dependent activation of FAD-glycerophosphate dehydrogenase. Biochem J 1991;278:335–340.
102. Erecinska M, Bryla J, Michalik M, Meglasson MD, Nelson D. Energy metabolism in islets of Langerhans. Biochem Biophys Acta 1992;1101:273–295.
103. Eto K, Tsubamoto Y, Terauchi Y, Sugiyama T, Kishimoto T, Takahashi N, et al. Role of NADH shuttle system in glucose-induced activation of mitochondrial metabolism and insulin secretion. Science 1999;283:981–985.
104. Gerbitz KD, Gempel K, Brediczka D. Mitochondria and diabetes. Genetic, biochemical and clinical implications of the cellular energy circuit. Diabetes 1996;45:113–126.
105. Kadowaki T. Maternally inherited diabetes and deafness: new subtype of diabetes mellitus. In: LeRoith D, Taylor SI, Olefsky JM, eds. Diabetes Mellitus, A Fundamental and Clinical Text. Lippincott–Raven, New York, 1996, pp. 591–595.
106. Mathews CE, McGraw RH, Berdanier CD. A point mutation in the mitochondrial DNA of diabetes prone BHE cdb rats. FASEB J 1995;9:1638–1642.
107. Liang Y, Bonner-Weir S, Wu YJ, Berdanier CD, Berner DK, Efrat S, et al. In situ glucose uptake and glucokinase activity of pancreatic islets in diabetic and obese rodents. J Clin Invest 1994;93:2473–2481.
108. Holz GG, Habener JF. Signal transduction cross talk in the endocrine system: pancreatic β-cells and the glucose competency concept. Trends Biochem Sci 1992;17:388–393.
109. Pralong WF, Bartley C, Wollheim CB. Single islet β-cell stimulation by nutrients: relationship between pyridine nucleotides, cytosolic Ca^{2+} and secretion. EMBO J 1990;9:53–60.
110. Meda P. Molecular biology of gap junction proteins. In: Draznin B, LeRoith D, eds. Molecular Biology of Diabetes, Part 1. Humana, Totowa, NJ, 1994, pp. 333–356.
111. Juhl CB, Schmitz O, Pincus S, Holst JJ, Veldhuis J, Porksen N. Short-term treatment with GLP-1 increases pulsatile insulin secretion in type II diabetes with no effect on orderliness. Diabetologia 2000;43(5):583–588.
112. Doliba N, Vatamaniuk M, Najafi H, Boettger C, Collins H, Grippo J, et al. Novel pharmacological glucokinase activators enhance glucose metabolism, respiration and insulin release in isolated pancreatic islets demonstrating a unique therapeutic potential. Diabetes 2001;50:359A (abstract).
113. Grimsky J, Sarabu R, Bizzarro F, Coffey J, Chu C, Corbett W, et al. Allosteric activation of islet and hepatic glucokinase: a potential new approach to diabetes therapy. Diabetes 2001;50:115A (abstract).
114. Cuesta-Munoz A, Boettger C, Davis E, Shiota C, Magnuson M, Grippo J, et al. Novel pharmacological glucokinase activators enhance glucose metabolism, respiration and insulin release in isolated pancreatic islets demonstrating a unique therapeutic potential. Diabetes 2001;50:109A (abstract).
115. Newgard CB, Clark S, BeltrandelRio H, Hohmeier HE, Quaade C, Normington K. Engineered cell lines for insulin replacement in diabetes: current status and future prospects. Diabetologia 1997;40:S42–S47.

7 Prevention and Correction of Hypoglycemia

Relevance to Type 1 Diabetes

Philip E. Cryer, MD

CONTENTS

INTRODUCTION

Hypoglycemia is the limiting factor in the glycemic management of diabetes because it generally precludes maintenance of euglycemia. Improving glycemic control while minimizing hypoglycemia in type 1 diabetes mellitus (T1DM) and advanced type 2 diabetes (T2DM) involves both application of the principles of aggressive therapy—patient education and empowerment, frequent self-monitoring of blood glucose, flexible insulin regimens, individualized glycemic goals, and ongoing professional guidance and support—and implementation of hypoglycemia risk reduction. Iatrogenic hypoglycemia is the result of the interplay of therapeutic insulin excess and compromised physiological and behavioral defenses against falling plasma glucose concentrations in T1DM and advanced T2DM. Relative or absolute insulin excess occurs when insulin doses are excessive, ill-timed, or of the wrong type, when exogenous glucose delivery, endogenous glucose production, or insulin clearance are decreased or when insulin-independent glucose utilization or sensitivity to insulin are increased. However, these conventional risk factors explain only a minority of episodes of severe hypoglycemia. More potent risk factors include absolute insulin deficiency, a history of severe hypoglycemia, and aggressive therapy *per se* as evidenced by lower glycemic goals, lower hemoglobin A1C levels, or both. These are clinical surrogates of compromised glucose counterregulation, the clini-

From: *Contemporary Endocrinology: Type 1 Diabetes: Etiology and Treatment*
Edited by: M. A. Sperling © Humana Press Inc., Totowa, NJ

cal syndromes of defective glucose counterregulation (the result of absent decrements in insulin and absent increments in glucagon with attenuated increments in epinephrine), and hypoglycemia unawareness (the result of reduced autonomic [sympathochromaffin] activation causing reduced warning symptoms of developing hypoglycemia). The unifying concept of hypoglycemia-associated autonomic failure in T1DM posits that (1) periods of relative or absolute therapeutic insulin excess in the setting of absent glucagon responses lead to episodes of hypoglycemia, (2) these episodes, in turn, cause reduced autonomic (including adrenomedullary) responses to falling glucose concentrations on subsequent occasions, and (3) these reduced autonomic responses result in both reduced symptoms of developing hypoglycemia (i.e., hypoglycemia unawareness) and—because epinephrine responses are reduced in the setting of absent glucagon responses—impaired physiological defenses against developing hypoglycemia (i.e., defective glucose counterregulation). Thus, a vicious cycle of recurrent hypoglycemia is created and perpetuated. Hypoglycemia risk reduction includes, first, addressing the issue of hypoglycemia—the patient's awareness of and concerns about it, and its frequency, severity, timing and clinical settings—in every patient contact. Then, it requires application of the principles of aggressive therapy, consideration of both the conventional risk factors and those indicative of compromised glucose counterregulation, and appropriate regimen adjustments, including a 2- to 3-wk period of scrupulous avoidance of hypoglycemia in patients with hypoglycemia-associated autonomic failure. With this approach, the goals of improving glycemic control and minimizing hypoglycemia are not incompatible.

HYPOGLYCEMIA IN DIABETES: THE CLINICAL CONTEXT

Glycemic control is a fundamentally important component of the comprehensive management of diabetes mellitus because it prevents or delays the long-term specific complications of diabetes (retinopathy, nephropathy, and neuropathy) and may reduce its atherosclerotic complications *(1–3)*. However, iatrogenic hypoglycemia is the limiting factor *(4,5)* in the glycemic management of both T1DM *(1,2,6–8)* and T2DM *(3,9)* both conceptually and in practice. Were it not for the potentially devastating effects of hypoglycemia, particularly on the brain, glycemic control would be rather easy to achieve. Administration of enough insulin (or any effective medication) to lower plasma glucose concentrations to or below the nondiabetic range would eliminate the symptoms of hyperglycemia, prevent diabetic ketoacidosis and the nonketotic hyperosmolar syndrome, almost assuredly prevent retinopathy, nephropathy, and neuropathy, and likely reduce atherosclerotic risk. However, the devastating effects of hypoglycemia are real and the glycemic management of diabetes is therefore complex.

Because of the barrier of iatrogenic hypoglycemia, euglycemia, even near euglycemia, cannot be achieved and maintained safely in most patients with T1DM *(1,2)* and many with T2DM *(3)*. As a result, retinopathy, nephropathy, and neuropathy develop or progress in some patients with T1DM *(1,2)* or T2DM *(3)* despite aggressive attempts to achieve glycemic control. Indeed, the inability to maintain euglycemia consistently over time may well explain the limited impact of aggressive glycemic therapy on the atherosclerotic complications of diabetes *(1–3)*.

In T1DM, aggressive attempts to achieve glycemic control increase the risk of severe, at least temporarily disabling, iatrogenic hypoglycemia (i.e., that requiring the assistance of another individual) more than threefold. That was documented in both of the controlled clinical trials with sample sizes large enough to demonstrate beneficial effects of intensive therapy on the long-term complications of diabetes, the Diabetes Control and Complications Trial (DCCT) *(1,6,7)*, and the Stockholm Diabetes Intervention Study *(2,8)*. It was confirmed in a meta-analysis that also included 12 smaller controlled clinical trials of intensive therapy *(10)*. However, it is possible to reduce the risk of hypoglycemia during aggressive therapy of T1DM. For example, the sixfold increased risk of severe hypoglycemia during intensive therapy in the feasibility phase of the DCCT *(6)* was reduced by half in the full-scale trial *(1,7)*.

The impact of iatrogenic hypoglycemia on the lives of people with diabetes should not be underestimated. Because of the interplay of therapeutic insulin excess and compromised physiological and behavioral defenses against falling plasma glucose concentrations, as discussed later in this chapter, people with T1DM are at ongoing risk for episodes of hypoglycemia *(3)*. Those attempting to achieve glycemic control suffer untold numbers of episodes of asymptomatic hypoglycemia—plasma glucose levels may be lower than 50 mg/dL (2.8 mmol/L) as much as 10% of the time—and an average of two episodes of symptomatic hypoglycemia per week. They suffer an episode of severe, at least temporarily disabling, hypoglycemia, often with seizure or coma, every year or two on average. Although seemingly complete recovery from even severe hypoglycemia is the rule, permanent neurological deficits can result. It has been estimated that 2–4% of deaths of people with T1DM are caused by hypoglycemia *(3,11)*. In addition, hypoglycemia can cause recurrent or even persistent psychosocial morbidity. The reality of hypoglycemia, the rational fear of hypoglycemia, or both, can be a barrier to glycemic control. Iatrogenic hypoglycemia is generally less frequent in T2DM *(3)*. However, it occurs during treatment with sulfonylureas or other insulin secretagogues (and has been reported in patients treated with metformin) or with insulin. The frequency of hypoglycemia approaches that in T1DM in those who reach the insulin-deficient end of the spectrum of T2DM *(9)*. Indeed, in one series, the frequency of severe hypoglycemia was similar in patients with T2DM and T1DM matched for duration of insulin therapy *(12)*. It is notable that the United Kingdom Prospective Diabetes Study investigators concluded that, over time, hypoglycemia becomes limiting in the treatment of T2DM, just as it is in the treatment of T1DM *(9)*.

Given the now well-established long-term benefits of glycemic control and the short-term potentially devastating effects of iatrogenic hypoglycemia, it is clear that the goals of both reducing mean glycemia and minimizing hypoglycemia are important for people with diabetes. Minimizing the risk of hypoglycemia in T1DM involves both application of the principles of aggressive therapy—patient education and empowerment, frequent self-monitoring of blood glucose, flexible insulin regimens, individualized glycemic goals, and ongoing professional guidance and support—and implementation of hypoglycemia risk reduction. As discussed later in this chapter, hypoglycemia risk reduction requires consideration of the roles of both therapeutic insulin excess and compromised physiological and behavioral defenses against developing hypoglycemia. This clinical approach will be developed in the context of the physiology of glucose counterregulation—the mechanisms that normally prevent or rapidly correct hypoglycemia—and its pathophysiology in T1DM as it relates to a comprehensive view of the clinical risk factors for iatrogenic hypoglycemia.

PHYSIOLOGICAL PREVENTION OR CORRECTION OF HYPOGLYCEMIA

Systemic Glucose Balance

Glucose is an obligate metabolic fuel for the brain under physiological conditions *(4)*. (The brain can utilize other circulating substrates, including ketones such as β-hydroxybutyrate, but the blood levels of these seldom rise high enough for them to enter the brain in quantity and thus partially replace glucose, except during prolonged fasting.) Because of its unique dependence on glucose oxidation as an energy source and because it cannot synthesize glucose or store more than a few minute's supply as glycogen, the brain requires a continuous supply of glucose from the circulation. At normal plasma glucose concentrations the rate of glucose transporter (GLUT-1) mediated blood-to-brain glucose transport down a concentration gradient exceeds that of brain glucose metabolism. However, when arterial glucose concentrations fall below the physiological range blood-to-brain glucose transport falls and ultimately becomes limiting to brain glucose metabolism and thus its functions and even its survival. Given the immediate survival value of maintenance of the plasma glucose concentration, it is not surprising that physiological mechanisms that very effectively prevent or rapidly correct hypoglycemia have evolved.

Rates of endogenous glucose influx into and of glucose efflux out of the circulation are normally coordinately regulated—largely by the plasma glucose-lowering (regulatory) hormone insulin and the plasma glucose-raising (counterregulatory) hormones glucagon and epinephrine—such that systemic glucose balance is maintained, hypoglycemia (as well as hyperglycemia) is prevented, and a continuous supply of glucose to the brain is assured *(4)*. This is accomplished despite wide variations in the influx of exogenous glucose (feeding vs fasting) and in the efflux of endogenous glucose (e.g., exercise vs rest). Hypoglycemia develops when rates of glucose appearance in the circulation [the sum of exogenous glucose delivery from ingested carbohydrates and regulated endogenous glucose production from the liver—via both glycogenolysis and gluconeogenesis—and to a lesser extent from the kidneys—via gluconeogenesis *(13)*] fail to keep pace with rates of glucose disappearance from the circulation (the sum of ongoing brain glucose metabolism and regulated glucose utilization by tissues such as muscle and fat as well as the liver and kidneys, among others).

Physiology of Glucose Counterregulation

The physiological postabsorptive arterial plasma glucose concentration in healthy humans is approx 70–110 mg/dL (3.9–6.1 mmol/L). Falling plasma glucose concentrations normally elicit a characteristic series of responses *(14–16)* (*see* Fig. 1). Insulin secretion decreases (favoring increased hepatic [and renal] glucose production and decreased glucose utilization by tissues other than the brain) as plasma glucose concentrations decline within the physiological range. The arterialized venous glycemic threshold for decreased insulin secretion is approx 80–85 mg/dL (approx 4.4–4.7 mmol/L). Decreased insulin secretion is the first defense against hypoglycemia *(3)*. The secretion of glucose counterregulatory (plasma glucose raising) hormones—glucagon and epinephrine as well as cortisol and growth hormone—increases as plasma glucose concentrations fall just below the physiological range. The arterialized venous glycemic thresholds for their secretion are approx 65–70 mg/dL (approx

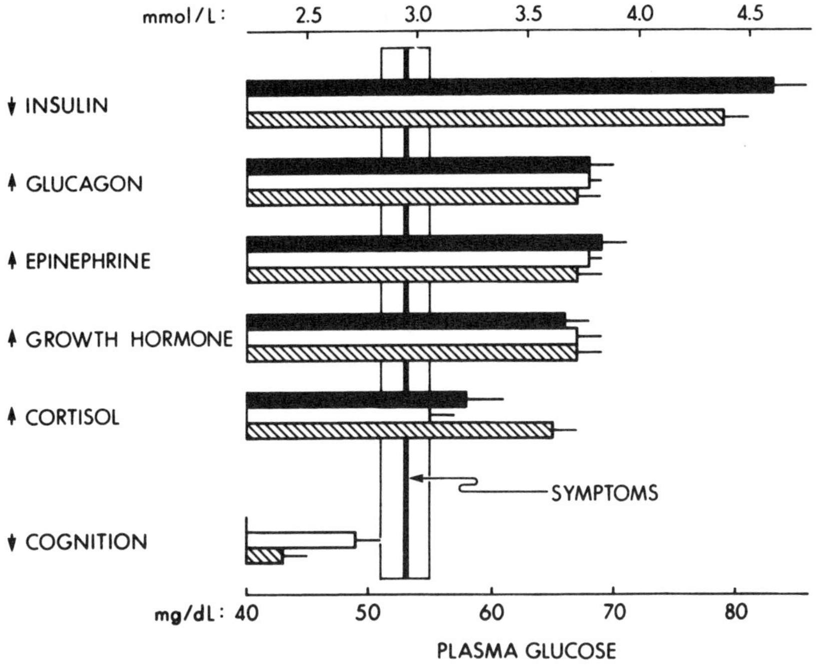

Fig. 1. Arterialized venous glycemic thresholds for responses to falling plasma glucose concentrations. Drawn from data in refs. *14* (solid columns), *15* (open columns), and *16* (crosshatched columns). (Modified from ref. *75*, reproduced with permission of the American Diabetes Association.)

3.6–3.9 mmol/L). Glucagon stimulates glucose production largely by increasing hepatic glycogenolysis. Increased glucagon secretion is the second defense against hypoglycemia *(4)*. Epinephrine stimulates hepatic (and renal) glucose production largely by mobilizing gluconeogenic substrates from peripheral tissues such as skeletal muscle and fat. It also limits glucose utilization by these insulin-sensitive tissues. Albeit demonstrably involved, epinephrine is not normally critical to the prevention or correction of hypoglycemia. However, epinephrine, the third defense against hypoglycemia, becomes critical when glucagon is deficient *(4)*. Thus, decrements in insulin and increments in glucagon and epinephrine stand high in the hierarchy of redundant glucose counterregulatory factors. Hypoglycemia develops or progresses when glucagon and epinephrine are deficient and insulin is present *(4)*.

Cortisol and growth hormone, which support glucose production and limit glucose utilization after a lag of several hours, are involved in the defense against prolonged hypoglycemia but are not critical to the correction of even prolonged hypoglycemia or to the prevention of hypoglycemia after an overnight fast *(17)*. To the extent to which they are involved, glucose autoregulation, sympathetic neural activation, and effects of substrates other than glucose (and fatty acids that may mediate part of the glucose-raising actions of catecholamines) play quantitatively minor roles *(4)*.

The physiology of glucose counterregulation, just summarized, is illustrated in Fig. 2.

Age and gender affect the glucose counterregulatory responses to falling plasma glucose concentrations. Children have greater epinephrine and neurogenic symptom responses to hypoglycemia and to falling glucose levels late after glucose ingestion

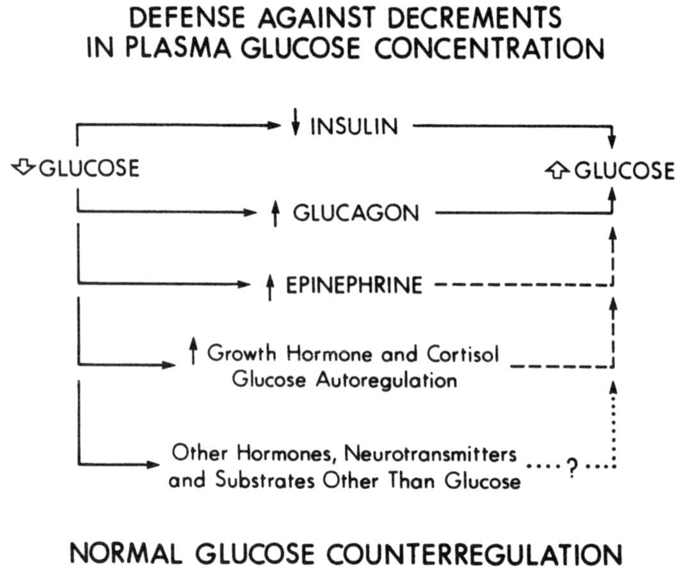

Fig. 2. Summary of the physiology of glucose counterregulation, the mechanisms that normally prevent or rapidly correct hypoglycemia.

than adults *(18–20)*. This appears to be the result of glycemic thresholds for the epinephrine responses at higher plasma glucose concentrations in children *(19,20)*. The glucagon, growth hormone, and cortisol responses to hypoglycemia are similar in children and adults *(18,19)*. In general, men have greater neuroendocrine and metabolic responses to hypoglycemia than women *(21–24)*. This appears to be the result of greater sensitivity to a given level of hypoglycemia in men because the glycemic thresholds are similar in men and women *(23,24)*. The mechanism(s) of these age and gender differences is not known.

Clinical Manifestations of Hypoglycemia

Glucose concentrations lower than those that activate the glucose counterregulatory defenses, just summarized, cause symptoms of hypoglycemia and, ultimately, brain dysfunction *(14–16)*. The arterialized venous glycemic thresholds for symptoms are approx 50–55 mg/dL (approx 2.8–3.1 mmol/L); those for cognitive impairment are ≤ 50 mg/dL (≤ 2.8 mmol/L).

Neuroglycopenic symptoms *(25)* such as behavioral changes, confusion, fatigue, seizure, and loss of consciousness are the direct result of widespread central nervous system (CNS) neuronal glucose deprivation. If hypoglycemia is prolonged and severe, this mechanism can cause permanent brain damage and even death. Neurogenic (autonomic) symptoms *(25)* are the result of the perception of physiological changes caused by the CNS-mediated autonomic (sympathochromaffin) discharge triggered by glucose deprivation from glucose-sensitive neurons in the brain (and perhaps in other sites, including the portal vein). They include both adrenergic (adrenomedullary epinephrine-mediated and sympathetic neural or adrenomedullary norepinephrine-mediated) symptoms such as palpitations, tremor and anxiety, and cholinergic (sympathetic neural acetylcholine-mediated) symptoms such as sweating, hunger, and paresthesias.

Dynamic Glycemic Thresholds

In healthy subjects, the glycemic thresholds for responses to falling arterial glucose concentrations—decreased insulin secretion, increased counterregulatory hormone secretion, symptoms, and cognitive dysfunction—are remarkably reproducible from laboratory to laboratory *(14–16)*. Nonetheless, these thresholds are dynamic, not static. They shift to higher plasma glucose concentrations in people with poorly-controlled diabetes *(26,27)*, who often have symptoms of hypoglycemia at higher than normal glucose levels, and to lower plasma glucose concentrations in people who suffer recurrent hypoglycemia such as those with well-controlled diabetes *(27)* or with an insulinoma *(28)*, who often tolerate subnormal glucose levels without symptoms.

CLINICAL RISK FACTORS FOR HYPOGLYCEMIA AND THE PATHOPHYSIOLOGY OF GLUCOSE COUNTERREGULATION IN DIABETES

Conventional Risk Factors: Insulin Excess

The conventional risk factors for iatrogenic hypoglycemia in T1DM *(4)* are based on the premise that relative or absolute therapeutic insulin excess, which must occur from time to time because of the gross pharmacokinetic imperfections of all current insulin replacement regimens, is the sole determinant of risk.

Relative or absolute therapeutic insulin excess occurs when (1) insulin doses are excessive, ill-timed, or of the wrong type, (2) the influx of exogenous glucose is decreased (such as during the overnight fast or following missed meals or snacks), (3) insulin-independent glucose utilization is increased (such as during exercise), (4) endogenous glucose production is decreased (such as following alcohol ingestion or administration of other drugs and with loss of renal parenchyma), (5) sensitivity to insulin is increased (such as following exercise, in the middle of the night, with glycemic control, with increased fitness, weight loss, or both, or with administration of certain drugs), and (6) insulin clearance is decreased (such as in renal failure).

These are the issues that people with diabetes and their health care providers deal with routinely as they attempt to minimize iatrogenic hypoglycemia. However, it became clear early in the DCCT that these conventional risk factors explain only a minority of episodes of severe iatrogenic hypoglycemia *(6)*. Indeed, in a multivariate model, none was found to be significant statistically. Clearly, we must look beyond these risk factors if we are to understand the majority of episodes of severe hypoglycemia in T1DM.

Comprehensive Risk Factors: Interplay of Insulin Excess and Compromised Glucose Counterregulation

Iatrogenic hypoglycemia in T1DM is more appropriately viewed as the result of the interplay of relative or absolute therapeutic insulin excess (the conventional risk factors) and compromised glucose counterregulation. Three clinically well-documented risk factors for iatrogenic hypoglycemia in T1DM are (1) absolute insulin deficiency (i.e., C-peptide negativity) *(7,29,30)*, (2) a history of severe hypoglycemia *(7,30)*, and (3) aggressive glycemic therapy *per se*, as evidenced by lower glycemic goals or lower hemoglobin A1C levels *(7,30)*. [Obviously, iatrogenic hypoglycemia occurs in people with diabetes who are not C-peptide negative, have no history of severe hypoglycemia, and are not practicing aggressive glycemic therapy. Nonetheless, these are associated with a substantially increased risk of hypoglycemia *(7,29,30).*] These three risk factors are clinical surrogates of compromised physiological and behavioral defenses against falling plasma glucose concentrations—the clinical syndromes of defective glucose counterregulation and of hypoglycemia unawareness and the pathophysiological concept of hypoglycemia-associated autonomic failure.

Pathophysiology

As the person with T1DM becomes absolutely insulin deficient over the first few months or years of clinical T1DM, circulating insulin levels—then simply the passive result of absorption of exogenous insulin—do not fall as plasma glucose levels decline. The first defense against hypoglycemia is lost.

Over the same time frame, the glucagon response to hypoglycemia is lost in T1DM *(31,32).* This is a selective defect; the glucagon responses to other stimuli are largely, if not entirely, intact. Its mechanism is unknown, but it is tightly linked to, and potentially attributable to, absolute insulin deficiency *(29).* Thus, the clinical hypoglycemia risk factor of C-peptide negativity *(7,29,30)* indicates that the first defense against hypoglycemia—decreased insulin secretion—is lost and predicts accurately that the second defense against hypoglycemia—increased glucagon secretion—is lost. Therefore, patients with established (i.e., C-peptide negative) T1DM are largely dependent on the third defense against hypoglycemia—increased epinephrine secretion.

The epinephrine response to hypoglycemia is attenuated in many patients with T1DM *(32–35),* particularly those with the other clinical risk factors for hypoglycemia such as a history of severe hypoglycemia or aggressive glycemic therapy *per se,* as evidenced by lower glycemic goals, lower hemoglobin A1C levels, or both. The former indicates and the latter implies recurrent episodes of prior hypoglycemia. In contrast to the absent glucagon response, the attenuated epinephrine response represents a threshold shift; an epinephrine response can be elicited, but lower plasma glucose concentrations are required *(27,35).* This threshold shift to lower plasma glucose concentrations is largely the result of recent antecedent iatrogenic hypoglycemia. Recent antecedent hypoglycemia reduces autonomic (including adrenomedullary epinephrine) and symptomatic, among other, responses to a given level of subsequent hypoglycemia in nondiabetic individuals *(36–40)* and in patients with T1DM *(35,41,42).* It shifts the glycemic thresholds for the responses to lower plasma glucose concentrations. As a result, it also impairs glycemic defense against hyperinsulinemia and developing hypoglycemia in T1DM *(35).* In addition to this functional threshold shift, there may well be an anatomical component (i.e., loss of adrenomedullary chromaffin cells) to the reduced epinephrine response in patients with classical diabetic autonomic neuropathy *(43,44).*

Defective Glucose Counterregulation

The development of an attenuated epinephrine response to falling glucose levels—loss of the third defense against hypoglycemia—is a critical pathophysiological event. Patients with T1DM who have combined deficiencies of their glucagon and epinephrine responses have been shown in prospective studies to suffer severe hypoglycemia at rates 25-fold *(45)* or more *(46)* higher than those with absent glucagon but intact epinephrine responses during aggressive glycemic therapy. They have the clinical syndrome of *defective glucose counterregulation.*

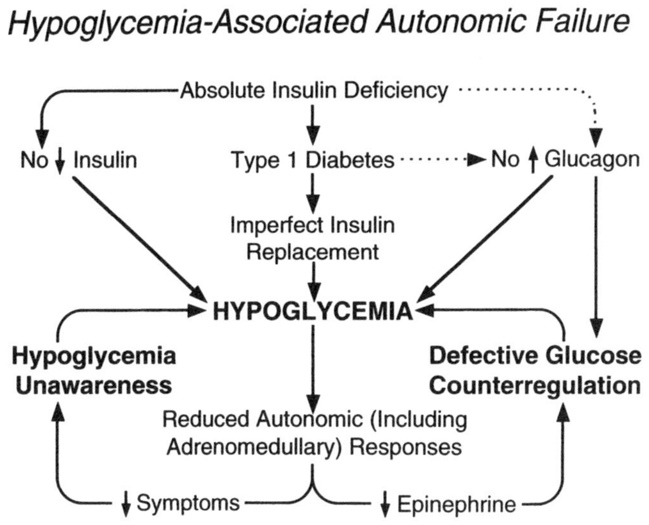

Fig. 3. The concept of hypoglycemia-associated autonomic failure in type 1 diabetes. (Reproduced with permission of the American Diabetes Association from ref. *48.*)

Hypoglycemia Unawareness

By reducing the autonomic, specifically the sympathochromaffin, responses to subsequent hypoglycemia, recent antecedent iatrogenic hypoglycemia also causes loss of the warning, largely if not exclusively neurogenic, symptoms of developing hypoglycemia *(35,41,42)* that previously allowed the patient to recognize that glucose levels were falling and prompted the appropriate behavioral response (e.g., ingestion of food) to abort the episode. Thus, the first manifestation of a hypoglycemic episode is neuroglycopenia, and it is often too late for the patient to recognize and self-treat the episode. This is the clinical syndrome of *hypoglycemia unawareness.* It, too, has been shown in a prospective study to be associated with a high frequency of severe iatrogenic hypoglycemia *(47).*

Hypoglycemia-Associated Autonomic Failure

The concept of hypoglycemia-associated autonomic failure in T1DM, a functional disorder distinct from the fixed autonomic failure of classical diabetic autonomic neuropathy, was formulated *(48)* and then verified experimentally *(35,49–52)* to unify the pathogenesis of the clinical syndromes of defective glucose counterregulation and hypoglycemia unawareness.

The concept of *hypoglycemia-associated autonomic failure* in T1DM (*see* Fig. 3) posits that (1) periods of relative or absolute therapeutic insulin excess in the setting of absent glucagon responses lead to episodes of hypoglycemia, (2) these episodes, in turn, cause reduced autonomic (including adrenomedullary epinephrine) responses to falling glucose concentrations on subsequent occasions, and (3) these reduced autonomic responses result in both reduced symptoms of, and therefore the behavioral response to, developing hypoglycemia (i.e., hypoglycemia unawareness) and—because epinephrine responses are reduced in the setting of absent glucagon responses—

impaired physiological defenses against developing hypoglycemia (i.e., defective glucose counterregulation). Thus, a vicious cycle of recurrent hypoglycemia is created and perpetuated.

Perhaps the most compelling support for the concept of hypoglycemia-associated autonomic failure in T1DM is the finding, in three independent laboratories *(52–54)*, that hypoglycemia unawareness and, at least in part, the reduced epinephrine component of defective glucose counterregulation are reversible after as little as 2 wk of scrupulous avoidance of iatrogenic hypoglycemia. This involves a shift of glycemic thresholds for autonomic and symptomatic responses back toward higher plasma glucose concentrations.

The basic mechanism(s) of hypoglycemia-associated autonomic failure remains to be determined. There is evidence that it is mediated by the cortisol response to previous hypoglycemia *(55,56)*. Evidence, obtained with the Kety–Schmidt technique, that it involves increased brain glucose uptake during hypoglycemia, has been reported *(57,58)*. However, evidence that recent antecedent hypoglycemia does not increase blood-to-brain glucose transport or cerebral glucose metabolism, measured with [1-^{11}C]glucose and positron-emission tomography, has been presented *(59)*. The latter data do not exclude regional increments in blood-to-brain glucose transport. Alternatively, the alteration may lie beyond the blood-brain barrier.

Consistent with the concept of hypoglycemia-associated autonomic failure in T1DM, recent antecedent hypoglycemia also shifts glycemic thresholds for hypoglycemic cognitive dysfunction to lower plasma glucose concentrations *(49–51)* and impairs detection of hypoglycemia in the clinical setting *(50)* in patients with T1DM. In addition to shifting the thresholds for adrenomedullary (plasma epinephrine) and parasympathetic (plasma pancreatic polypeptide) responses to lower plasma glucose concentrations, recent antecedent hypoglycemia has been reported to reduce the sympathetic neural response to subsequent hypoglycemia *(35,40,56)* although the latter has been questioned *(60)*.

There is also evidence that reduced sensitivity to catecholamines, measured as a reduced heart rate response to the β-adrenergic agonist isoproterenol, contributes to the pathogenesis of hypoglycemia unawareness in T1DM *(61–64)*. Hypoglycemia has been reported to reduce β-adrenergic sensitivity, tested about 10 h later, in T1DM (but not in nondiabetic individuals) *(63)*. Thus, it is conceivable that both reduced activation of the sympathochromaffin system and reduced sensitivity to released catecholamines might play a role in the pathogenesis of hypoglycemia unawareness and defective glucose counterregulation induced by recent antecedent iatrogenic hypoglycemia. Fritsche et al. *(64)* reported a patient with a 55-yr history of T1DM whose hypoglycemia unawareness was reversed following a period of scrupulous avoidance of hypoglycemia. That reversal was associated with increased sensitivity of the cardiac chronotropic response to isoproterenol. Although the epinephrine response to hypoglycemia was surprisingly robust, albeit subnormal, prior to reversal, the epinephrine response following reversal was not reported. Thus, the extent to which reversal of hypoglycemia unawareness was the result of enhanced sympathochromaffin secretory responses, enhanced sensitivity to those responses, or both is unknown.

The extent to which these pathophysiological concepts, developed in T1DM, apply to patients with T2DM remains to be assessed in detail. However, they may well apply to those approaching the insulin-deficient end of the spectrum of T2DM because

Table 1
Comprehensive Risk Factors for Hypoglycemia in Diabetes

Premise: Iatrogenic hypoglycemia in type 1 diabetes is the result of the interplay of therapeutic insulin excess and compromised glucose counterregulation.

1. Absolute or relative therapeutic insulin excess (the conventional risk factors)
   - Insulin doses excessive, ill-timed, wrong type
   - Decreased food intake
   - Increased glucose utilization (e.g., exercise)
   - Decreased glucose production (e.g., alcohol)
   - Increased sensitivity to insulin (e.g., after exercise, during the night, glycemic control, weight loss)
   - Decreased insulin clearance (e.g., renal failure)
2. Compromised glucose counterregulation
   - Absolute insulin deficiency (C-peptide negativity)

     β-cell destruction: No ↓ in insulin in response to ↓ glucose

     Unknown: No ↑ in glucagon in response to ↓ glucose
   - History of severe hypoglycemia or aggressive therapy *per se* (lower glucose goals, lower HbA1C)

     Episodes of hypoglycemia: Attenuated autonomic (including ↑ epinephrine) activation and symptoms in response to ↓ glucose (defective glucose counterregulation and hypoglycemia unawareness)

hypoglycemia becomes limiting to glycemic control in such patients *(9)*. Indeed, in one series, the frequency of severe hypoglycemia was found to be similar in patients with T2DM and T1DM matched for duration of insulin therapy *(12)*. This issue is complicated by the fact that some patients with apparent T2DM may actually have late-onset T1DM *(65)*. Nonetheless, patients with advanced T2DM have recently been reported to have reduced glucagon responses to hypoglycemia *(66)*, a key feature of defective glucose counterregulation in T1DM. Such patients also have reduced epinephrine and neurogenic symptom responses following recent antecedent hypoglycemia *(66)*, key features of hypoglycemia unawareness, and defective glucose counterregulation in T1DM.

The concept of hypoglycemia-associated autonomic failure in T1DM is illustrated in Fig. 3 and the comprehensive risk factors for iatrogenic hypoglycemia in T1DM, viewed in the context of the interplay of therapeutic insulin excess and compromised glucose counterregulation, are outlined in Table 1.

HYPOGLYCEMIA RISK REDUCTION IN DIABETES

Current Approaches

Clearly, every effort must be made to minimize the risk of iatrogenic hypoglycemia and eliminate the risk of severe hypoglycemia while pursuing the greatest degree of glycemic control that can be achieved safely in an individual person with diabetes. Hypoglycemia risk reduction involves (1) addressing the issue of hypoglycemia in every patient contact, (2) applying the principles of aggressive glycemic therapy, and (3) considering each of the comprehensive risk factors for hypoglycemia.

In addition to questioning the patient about episodes of symptomatic and biochemical hypoglycemia and looking for low values in the self-monitoring of blood glucose (SMBG) log, it is important to assess the patient's awareness of hypoglycemia. A history of hypoglycemia unawareness identifies that clinical syndrome (and also implies defective glucose counterregulation). It is also important to determine the extent to which the patient is concerned about the reality or the possibility of hypoglycemia. Fear of hypoglycemia can be a barrier to glycemic control. If episodes of hypoglycemia are identified, their frequency, severity, timing, and clinical contexts need to be determined.

Once the problem of iatrogenic hypoglycemia is recognized, it is appropriate to review the treatment plan with respect to the principles of aggressive glycemic therapy. These include (1) patient education and empowerment, (2) frequent SMBG, (3) flexible insulin (or other drug) regimens, (4) rational, individualized glycemic goals, and (5) ongoing professional guidance and support. Particularly in T1DM, but also in advanced T2DM, glycemic control is achieved safely by a well-informed, thoughtful person with diabetes who must make judgments about the management of his or her diabetes several times each day. The patient must be given the resources to make those judgments.

In the context of these therapeutic principles, hypoglycemia risk reduction requires consideration of both the conventional risk factors that lead to episodes of absolute or relative insulin excess—insulin (or other drug) dose, timing, and type, patterns of food ingestion and of exercise, interactions with alcohol or other drugs, and altered sensitivity to or clearance of insulin—and the risk factors for compromised glucose counterregulation that impair physiological and behavioral defenses against developing hypoglycemia (*see* Table 1). The underlying principle is that iatrogenic hypoglycemia is the result of the interplay of insulin excess and compromised glucose counterregulation rather than insulin excess alone.

As discussed earlier in this chapter, the clinical surrogates of risk attributable to compromised glucose counterregulation, include absolute deficiency—which may be apparent from a history of ketosis-prone diabetes requiring insulin therapy from diagnosis, although it is now recognized that absolute insulin deficiency can sometimes develop more gradually in late onset T1DM *(65)* or advanced T2DM *(66)*—and a history of recurrent hypoglycemia or, absent that, aggressive glycemic therapy *per se* as evidenced by lower glycemic goals, lower hemoglobin A1C levels, or both. It is possible to test for defective glucose counterregulation, with an insulin infusion test *(45,46)*, but that is generally neither practical nor useful given the now recognized dynamic nature of hypoglycemia unawareness and the reduced epinephrine component of defective glucose counterregulation discussed earlier in this chapter. On the other hand, a diagnosis of partial or complete hypoglycemia unawareness can be made from the history. Clinical hypoglycemia unawareness (which also suggests defective glucose counterregulation) implies recurrent antecedent iatrogenic hypoglycemia, whether that has or has not been documented. If such hypoglycemia is not apparent to the patient or to his or her family or in the SMBG log, it is probably occurring during the night. Indeed, hypoglycemia—including severe hypoglycemia—occurs most commonly during the night in people with T1DM *(1,6,7)*. That is typically the longest interdigestive period and time between SMBG and the time of maximal sensitivity to insulin *(67)*. In addition, sleep limits recognition of warning symptoms of developing hypoglycemia and thus the appropriate behavioral response and has been found to further reduce the epinephrine response to hypoglycemia *(68)* and, thus, to further compromise physiological defense against developing hypoglycemia.

In addition to regimen adjustments, approaches to the problem of nocturnal hypoglycemia include use of newer insulin analogs and bedtime treatments. Substitution of a preprandial rapid-acting insulin analog (e.g., lispro or aspart) for short-acting (regular) insulin during the day reduces the frequency of nocturnal hypoglycemia *(69)*. Substitution of a long-acting insulin analog (e.g., glargine) for neutral protamine Hagedorn (NPH) or ultralente insulin at bedtime may also reduce the frequency of nocturnal hypoglycemia *(70)*. Bedtime treatments intended to reduce nocturnal hypoglycemia include bedtime snacks, although the efficacy of these is largely limited to the first half of the night *(71)*. Experimental approaches include bedtime administration of uncooked cornstarch *(72,73)*, the glucagon-releasing amino acid alanine *(71)*, or the epinephrine-simulating β_2-adrenergic agonist terbutaline *(71)*.

Obviously, with a history of recurrent hypoglycemia, one should determine when it occurs and adjust the treatment regimen appropriately. With a basal-bolus insulin regimen, morning-fasting hypoglycemia implicates the long- or intermediate-acting basal insulin, daytime hypoglycemia implicates the rapid- or short-acting insulin, and night-time hypoglycemia may implicate either, all in the context of the other risk factors for insulin excess. A history of severe iatrogenic hypoglycemia—that requiring the assistance of another individual—is a clinical red flag. Unless it was the result of an easily remediable factor, such as a missed meal after insulin administration or vigorous exercise without the appropriate regimen adjustment, a substantive change in the regimen must be made. If it is not, the risk of recurrent severe hypoglycemia is unacceptably high *(7,30)*.

In a patient with hypoglycemia unawareness, a 2- to 3-wk period of scrupulous avoidance of iatrogenic hypoglycemia is advisable and can be assessed by the return of awareness of hypoglycemia. This has been accomplished without *(53–54)* or with minimal *(52)* compromise of glycemic control, but that required substantial involvement of health professionals. In practice, it can involve acceptance of somewhat higher glucose levels over the short term. However, with return of symptoms of developing hypoglycemia, empirical approaches to better glycemic control can be tried.

Bolli *(74)* has reviewed his views of practical approaches to achieving glycemic control while minimizing hypoglycemia in T1DM. That is also discussed later in this book (Chapters 10 and 18).

Future Approaches

Hypoglycemia is a fact of life for people with T1DM (and some with T2DM) who attempt to achieve near euglycemia *(1–4,6–10,30)*. Because of the pharmacokinetic imperfections of all current insulin replacement regimens, it is not practical to both maintain euglycemia and eliminate episodes of asymptomatic and even symptomatic hypoglycemia in T1DM. That awaits the ultimate goal of the prevention and cure of diabetes, or, in the shorter term, development of clinical strategies for perfect insulin replacement (e.g., transplantation of insulin-secreting cells or development of a closed-loop insulin replacement system), or for near-perfect insulin replacement coupled with measures that prevent, correct, or compensate for compromised glucose counterregulation *(5)*.

ACKNOWLEDGMENTS

The author gratefully acknowledges the contributions of his several colleagues who shaped the work that led to the views expressed in this chapter, the assistance of the staff of the Washington University General Clinical Research Center in the performance of our studies, and the assistance of Ms. Karen Muehlhauser in the preparation of the manuscript. The author's work cited was supported, in part, by U.S.P.H.S. grants R37 DK27085, M01 RR00036, P60 DK20579 and T32 DK01720 and by a grant and a fellowship award from the American Diabetes Association.

REFERENCES

1. The Diabetes Control and Complications Trial Research Group. The effect of intensive treatment of diabetes on the development and progression of long-term complications in insulin-dependent diabetes mellitus. N Engl J Med 1993;329:977–986.
2. Reichard P, Nilsson B-Y, Rosenqvist U. The effect of long-term intensified insulin treatment on the development of microvascular complications of diabetes mellitus. N Engl J Med 1993;329:304–309.
3. The United Kingdom Prospective Diabetes Study Group. Intensive blood-glucose control with sulfonylureas or insulin compared with conventional treatment and risk of complications in patients with type 2 diabetes. Lancet 1998;352:837–853.
4. Cryer PE. Hypoglycemia. Pathophysiology, Diagnosis and Treatment. Oxford University Press, New York, 1997.
5. Cryer PE. Hypoglycemia *is* the limiting factor in the management of diabetes. Diabetes/Metab Res Rev 1999;15:42–46.
6. The Diabetes Control and Complications Trial Research Group. Epidemiology of severe hypoglycemia in the Diabetes Control and Complications Trial. Am J Med 1991;90:450–459.
7. The Diabetes Control and Complications Trial Research Group. Hypoglycemia in the Diabetes Control and Complications Trial. Diabetes 1997;46:271–286
8. Reichard P, Berglund B, Britz A, Cars I, Nilsson BY, Rosenqvist U. Intensified conventional insulin treatment retards the microvascular complications of insulin-dependent diabetes mellitus: The Stockholm Diabetes Intervention Study after 5 years. J Intern Med 1990;230:101–108.
9. The United Kingdom Prospective Diabetes Study Group. A 6-year, randomized, controlled trial comparing sulfonylurea, insulin and metformin therapy in patients with newly diagnosed type 2 diabetes that could not be controlled with diet therapy. Ann Intern Med 1998;128:165–175.
10. Egger M, Davey Smith G, Stettler C, Diem P. Risk of adverse effects of intensified treatment in insulin-dependent diabetes mellitus: A meta-analysis. Diabet Med 1997;14:919–928.
11. Laing SP, Swerdlow AJ, Slater SD, Bothat JL, Burden AC, Waugh NR, et al. The British Diabetic Association Cohort Study. II. Cause-specific mortality in patients with insulin-treated diabetes mellitus. Diabet Med 1999;16:466–471.
12. Hepburn DA, MacLeod KM, Pell ACH, Scougal IJ, Frier BM. Frequency and symptoms of hypoglycemia experienced by patients with type 2 diabetes treated with insulin. Diabet Med 1993;10:231–237.
13. Stumvoll M, Meyer C, Mitrakou A, Nadkarni V, Gerich J. Renal glucose production and utilization: new aspects in humans. Diabetologia 1997;40:749–757.
14. Schwartz NS, Clutter WE, Shah SD, Cryer PE. Glycemic thresholds for activation of glucose counterregulatory systems are higher than the threshold for symptoms. J Clin Invest 1987;79:777–781.
15. Mitrakou A, Ryan C, Veneman T, Mokan M, Jensen T, Kiss I, et al. Hierarchy of glycemic thresholds for counterregulatory hormone secretion, symptoms and cerebral dysfunction. Am J Physiol 1991;260:E67–E74.
16. Fanelli C, Pampanelli S, Epifano L, Rambotti AM, Ciofetta M, Modarelli F, et al. Relative roles of insulin and hypoglycemia on induction of neuroendocrine responses to, symptoms of, and deterioration of cognitive function in hypoglycemia in male and female humans. Diabetologia 1994;37: 797–807.
17. Boyle PJ, Cryer PE. Growth hormone, cortisol, or both are involved in defense against, but are not critical to recovery from, prolonged hypoglycemia in humans. Am J Physiol 1991;260:E395–E402.
18. Amiel SA, Simonson DC, Sherwin RS, Lauritano AA, Tamborlane WV. Exaggerated epinephrine responses to hypoglycemia in normal and insulin-dependent diabetic children. J Pediatr 1987;110: 832–837.

19. Jones TW, Boulware SD, Kraemer DT, Caprio S, Sherwin RS, Tamborlane WV. Independent effects of youth and poor diabetes control on responses to hypoglycemia in children. Diabetes 1991;40:358–363.
20. Jones TW, Borg WP, Boulware SD, McCarthy G, Sherwin RS, Tamborlane WV. Enhanced adrenomedullary response and increased susceptibility to neuroglycopenia: mechanisms underlying the adverse effects of sugar ingestion in healthy children. J Pediatr 1995;126:171–177.
21. Amiel, SA, Maran A, Powrie, JK, Umpleby AM, Macdonald IA. Gender differences in counterregulation to hypoglycemia. Diabetologia 1993;36:460–464.
22. Davis SN, Cherrington AD, Goldstein RE, Jacobs J, Price L. Effects of insulin on counterregulatory response to equivalent hypoglycemia in normal females. Am J Physiol 1993;265:E680–E689.
23. Fanelli C, Pampanelli S. Epifano L, Rambotti AM, Ciofetta M, Modarelli F, et al. Relative roles of insulin and hypoglycaemia on induction of neuroendocrine responses to, symptoms of, and deterioration of cognitive function in hypoglycaemia in male and female humans. Diabetologia 1994;37:797–807.
24. Davis S, Shavers C, Costa F. Differential gender related neuroendocrine responses to hypoglycemia are due to alterations in CNS drive and not glycemic thresholds. Diabetes 1997;46:17A (abstract).
25. Towler DA, Havlin CE, Craft S, Cryer P. Mechanisms of awareness of hypoglycemia: Perception of neurogenic (predominantly cholinergic) rather than neuroglycopenic symptoms. Diabetes 1993;42:1791–1798.
26. Boyle PJ, Schwartz NS, Shah SD, Clutter WE, Cryer PE. Plasma glucose concentrations at the onset of hypoglycemic symptoms in patients with poorly controlled diabetes and in nondiabetics. N Engl J Med 1988;318:1487–1492.
27. Amiel SA, Sherwin RS, Simonson DC, Tamborlane WV. Effect of intensive insulin therapy on glycemic thresholds for counterregulatory hormone release. Diabetes 1988;37:901–907.
28. Mitrakou A, Fanelli C, Veneman T, Perriello G, Platanisoto D, Rambotti A, et al. Reversibility of hypoglycemia unawareness in patients with an insulinoma. N Engl J Med 1993;329:834–839.
29. Fukuda M, Tanaka A, Tahara Y, Ikegami H, Yamamoto Y, Kumahara Y, et al. Correlation between minimal secretory capacity of pancreatic β-cells and stability of diabetic control. Diabetes 1988;37:81–88.
30. Mühlhauser I, Overmann H, Bender R, Bott U, Berger M. Risk factors for severe hypoglycaemia in adult patients with type 1 diabetes—a prospective population based study. Diabetologia 1997;41:1274–1282.
31. Gerich JE, Langlois M, Noacco C, Karam JH, Forsham PH. Lack of glucagon response to hypoglycemia in diabetes: evidence for an intrinsic pancreatic alpha cell defect. Science 1973;182:171–173.
32. Bolli G, De Feo P, Compagnucci P, Cartechini MG, Angeletti G, Santeusanio F, et al. Abnormal glucose counterregulation after subcutaneous insulin in insulin dependent diabetes mellitus: interaction of anti-insulin antibodies and impaired glucagon and epinephrine secretion. Diabetes 1983;32:134–141.
33. Boden G, Reichard GA Jr, Hoeldtke RD, Rezvani I, Owen OE. Severe insulin-induced hypoglycemia associated with deficiencies in the release of counterregulatory hormones. N Engl J Med 1981;305:1200–1205.
34. Hirsch BR, Shamoon H. Defective epinephrine and growth hormone responses in type 1 diabetes are stimulus specific. Diabetes 1987;36:20–26.
35. Dagogo-Jack SE, Craft S, Cryer PE. Hypoglycemia-associated autonomic failure in insulin dependent diabetes mellitus. J Clin Invest 1993;91:819–828.
36. Heller SR, Cryer PE. Reduced neuroendocrine and symptomatic responses to subsequent hypoglycemia after one episode of hypoglycemia in nondiabetic humans. Diabetes 1991;40:223–226.
37. Davis MR, Shamoon H. Counterregulatory adaptation to recurrent hypoglycemia in normal humans. J Clin Endocrinol Metab 1991;73:995–1001.
38. Widom B, Simonson DC. Intermittent hypoglycemia impairs glucose counterregulation. Diabetes 1992;41:1597–1602.
39. Veneman T, Mitrakou A, Mokan M, Cryer P, Gerich J. Induction of hypoglycemia unawareness by asymptomatic nocturnal hypoglycemia. Diabetes 1993;42:1233–1237.
40. Davis SN, Shavers C, Mosqueda-Garcia R, Costa F. Effects of differing antecedent hypoglycemia on subsequent counterregulation in normal humans. Diabetes 1997;46:1328–1335.
41. Davis MR, Mellman M, Shamoon H. Further defects in counterregulatory responses induced by recurrent hypoglycemia in IDDM. Diabetes 1992;41:1335–1340.
42. Lingenfelser T, Renn W, Sommerwerck U, Jung ME, Buettner UW, Zaiser-Kaschel H, et al. Compromised hormonal counterregulation, symptom awareness, and neurophysiological function after recurrent short-term episodes of insulin-induced hypoglycemia in IDDM patients. Diabetes 1993;42:610–618.
43. Bottini P, Boschetti E, Pampanelli S, Ciofetta M, Del Sindaco P, Scionti L, et al. Contribution of autonomic neuropathy to reduced plasma adrenaline responses to hypoglycemia in IDDM: evidence for a nonselective defect. Diabetes 1997;46:814–823.

44. Meyer C, Grobmann R, Mitrakou A, Mahler R, Veneman T, Gerich J, et al. Effects of autonomic neuropathy on counterregulation and awareness of hypoglycemia in type 1 diabetic patients. Diabetes Care 1998;21:1960–1966.
45. White NH, Skor D, Cryer PE, Bier DM, Levandoski L, Santiago JV. Identification of type 1 diabetic patients at increased risk for hypoglycemia during intensive therapy. N Engl J Med 1983;308:485–491.
46. Bolli GG, De Feo P, De Cosmo S, Perriello G, Ventura MM, Masssi-Benedetti M, et al. A reliable and reproducible test for adequate glucose counterregulation in type 1 diabetes. Diabetes 1984;33:732–737.
47. Gold AE, MacLeod KM, Frier BM. Frequency of severe hypoglycemia in patients with type 1 diabetes with impaired awareness of hypoglycemia. Diabetes Care 1994;17:697–703.
48. Cryer PE. Iatrogenic hypoglycemia as a cause of hypoglycemia-associated autonomic failure in IDDM: a vicious cycle. Diabetes 1992;41:255–260.
49. Hvidberg A, Fanelli CG, Hershey TG, Terkamp C, Craft S, Cryer PE. Impact of recent antecedent hypoglycemia on hypoglycemic cognitive dysfunction in nondiabetic humans. Diabetes 1996;45: 1030–1036.
50. Ovalle F, Fanelli CG, Paramore DS, Hershey T, Craft S, Cryer PE. Brief twice weekly episodes of hypoglycemia reduce detection of clinical hypoglycemia in type 1 diabetes mellitus. Diabetes 1998;47:1472–1479.
51. Fanelli CG, Paramore DS, Hershey T, Terkamp C, Ovalle F, Craft S, et al. Impact of nocturnal hypoglycemia on hypoglycemic cognitive dysfunction in type 1 diabetes mellitus. Diabetes 1998;47: 1920–1927.
52. Dagogo-Jack S, Rattarasarn C, Cryer PE. Reversal of hypoglycemia unawareness, but not defective glucose counterregulation, in IDDM. Diabetes 1994;43:1426–1434.
53. Fanelli CG, Pampanelli S, Epifano L, Rambotti AM, Vincenzo AD, Modarelli F, et al. Long-term recovery from unawareness, deficient counterregulation and lack of cognitive dysfunction during hypoglycemia following institution of rational intensive therapy in IDDM. Diabetologia 1994;37:1265–1276.
54. Cranston I, Lomas J, Maran A, Macdonald I, Amiel S. Restoration of hypoglycemia unawareness in patients with long duration insulin-dependent diabetes mellitus. Lancet 1994;344:283–287.
55. Davis SN, Shavers C, Costa F, Mosqueda-Garcia R: Role of cortisol in the pathogenesis of deficient counterregulation after antecedent hypoglycemia in normal humans. J Clin Invest 1996;98:680–691.
56. Davis SN, Shavers C, Davis B, Costa F. Prevention of an increase in plasma cortisol during hypoglycemia preserves subsequent counterregulatory responses. J Clin Invest 1997;100:429–438.
57. Boyle PJ, Nagy RJ, O'Connor AM, Kempers SF, Yeo RA, Qualls C. Adaptation in brain glucose uptake following recurrent hypoglycemia. Proc Natl Acad Sci USA 1994;91:9352–9356.
58. Boyle PJ, Kempers SF, O'Connor AM, Nagy RJ. Brain glucose uptake and unawareness of hypoglycemia in patients with insulin dependent diabetes mellitus. N Engl J Med 1995;333:1726–1731.
59. Segel S, Fanelli C, Dence C, Markham J, Videen T, Paramore D, et al. Blood-to-brain glucose transport is not increased following hypoglycemia. Diabetes 2001;50:1911–1917.
60. Paramore DS, Fanelli CG, Shah SD, Cryer PE. Hypoglycemia *per se* stimulates sympathetic neural as well as adrenomedullary activity but, unlike the adrenomedullary response, the forearm sympathetic neural responses is not reduced following recent hypoglycemia. Diabetes 1999;48:1429–1436.
61. Berlin I, Grimaldi A, Payan C, Sachon C, Bosquet F, Thervet F, et al. Hypoglycemic symptoms and decreased β-adrenergic sensitivity in insulin dependent diabetic patients. Diabetes Care 1987;10:742–747.
62. Korytkowski M, Mokan M, Veneman T, Mitrakou A, Cryer P, Gerich JE. Reduced β-adrenergic sensitivity in insulin dependent diabetic patients. Diabetes Care 1998;21:1939–1943.
63. Fritsche A, Stumvoll M, Grüb M, Sieslack S, Renn W, Schmülling R-M, et al. Effect of hypoglycemia on β-adrenergic sensitivity in normal and type 1 diabetic subjects. Diabetes Care 1998;21:1505–1510.
64. Fritsche A, Stumvoll M, Häring H-U, Gerich JE. Reversal of hypoglycemia unawareness in a long-term type 1 diabetic patient by improvement of β-adrenergic sensitivity after prevention of hypoglycemia. J Clin Endocrinol Metab 2000;85:523–525.
65. Turner R, Stratton I, Horton V, Manley S, Zimmet P, Mackay IR, et al., for the UKPDS Group. Autoantibodies to islet cell cytoplasm and glutamic acid decarboxylase for prediction of insulin requirement in type 2 diabetes. Lancet 1997;350:1288–1293.
66. Segel SA, Paramore DS, Cryer PE. Defective glucose counterregulation in type 2 diabetes. Diabetes 2000;49:A131 (abstract).
67. Perriello G, De Feo P, Torlone E, Fanelli C, Santeusanio F, Brunetti P, et al. The dawn phenomenon in type 1 (insulin dependent) diabetes mellitus: magnitude, frequency, variability, and dependence on glucose counterregulation and insulin sensitivity. Diabetes 1991;34:21–28.

68. Jones TW, Porter P, Sherwin RS, Davis EA, O'Leary P, Frazer F, et al. Decreased epinephrine responses to hypoglycemia during sleep. N Engl J Med 1998;338:1657–1662.
69. Heller SR, Amiel SA, Mansell P, the U.K. Lispro Study Group. Effect of the fast acting insulin analog lispro on the risk of nocturnal hypoglycemia during intensified insulin therapy. Diabetes Care 1999;22:1607–1611.
70. Ratner RE, Hirsch IB, Neifing JL, Garg SK, Mecca TE, Wilson CA, for the U.S. Study Group of Insulin Glargine in Type 1 Diabetes. Less hypoglycemia with insulin glargine in intensive insulin therapy for type 1 diabetes. Diabetes Care 2000;23:639–643.
71. Saleh TY, Cryer PE. Alanine and terbutaline in the prevention of nocturnal hypoglycemia in IDDM. Diabetes Care 1997;20:1231–1236.
72. Ververs MTC, Rouwé C, Smit GPA. Complex carbohydrates in the prevention of nocturnal hypoglycaemia in diabetic children. Eur J Clin Nutr 1993;47:268–273.
73. Kaufman FR, Devgan S. Use of uncooked cornstarch to avert nocturnal hypoglycemia in children and adolescents with type 1 diabetes. J Diabetes Complications 1996;10:84–87.
74. Bolli GB. How to ameliorate the problem of hypoglycemia in intensive as well as nonintensive treatment of type 1 diabetes. Diabetes Care 1999;22(Suppl 2):B43–B52.
75. Cryer PE. Hypoglycemia: the limiting factor in the management of IDDM: Diabetes 1994;43:1378–1379.

8 Nonautoimmune Forms of Diabetes

Neonatal Diabetes, DIDMOAD–Wolfram Syndrome, and Related Syndromes

Timothy G. Barrett, PhD, MB

Contents

INTRODUCTION

Diabetes mellitus is the name given to a heterogeneous group of disorders characterized by intolerance to glucose. The most common form of childhood onset diabetes (type 1) has an autoimmune basis, but there are many syndromes in which diabetes mellitus is a component (*see* Table 1). Although individually rare, collectively they make up about 5% of children seen in diabetes clinics. Some, like Wolfram syndrome, are associated with insulin deficiency; others, like Rabson–Mendenhall syndrome, are associated with insulin resistance. The importance of these syndromes for children lies in the recognition of treatable complications, and for their parents, the possibility of genetic testing in future pregnancies. The scientific importance is enormous, as they demonstrate a wide variety of different mechanisms by which glucose metabolism can be disrupted and may contribute to the genetic heterogeneity of the more common type 1 and type 2 diabetes. This is because some of the clinic population, who are not troubled

From: *Contemporary Endocrinology: Type 1 Diabetes: Etiology and Treatment*
Edited by: M. A. Sperling © Humana Press Inc., Totowa, NJ

Table 1
Inherited Diabetic Syndromes

Maturity Onset Diabetes of the Young (MODY)
MODY 1,2,3,4,5
"Mitochondrial" diabetes
Diabetes and deafness resulting from "3243" mutation
Kearn–Sayre syndrome
Pearson's syndrome
Neonatal diabetes
Transient neonatal diabetes
Permanent neonatal diabetes
Insulin-deficient syndromes
Wolcott–Rallison
Wolfram–DIDMOAD
Thiamine-responsive diabetes (TRMA)
Syndromes of insulin resistance
Rabson–Mendenhall
Leprechaunism
Syndromes of uncertain insulin status
Bardet–Biedl (probable insulin resistance)
Alstrom (probable insulin resistance)
Prader–Willi

DIDMOAD, diabetes insipidus, diabetes mellitus, optic atrophy, and deafness; TRMA, thiamin-responsive megaloblastic anemia.

by the other features of these disorders, may be heterozygotes for various recessive syndromes. This review will discuss several diabetic syndromes for which there have been significant recent advances in our understanding. Many of these disorders are inherited, so the review inevitably has a genetic bias.

MATURITY-ONSET DIABETES OF THE YOUNG

Maturity-onset diabetes of the young (MODY) is an early-onset inherited form of diabetes, caused by defects in β-cell function. It was first described in a large family with autosomal dominant inheritance *(1),* and, subsequently, different genetically defined subgroups have been identified *(2).* Mildly elevated hyperglycemia may be asymptomatic and patients may be identified during intercurrent illness or on screening during pregnancy *(3).* The criteria for diagnosis *(2)* are as follows:

- Early-onset non-insulin-dependent diabetes. At least one family member diagnosed under 25 yr; non-insulin dependent if 5 yr after diagnosis the person is not on insulin or, if treated with insulin, has significant circulating C-peptide.
- Autosomal dominant inheritance. At least two and, ideally, three generations are affected with diabetes.

Maturity-onset diabetes of the young is thought to account for 1–2% of patients in adult type 2 diabetes clinics. The proportion in pediatric diabetes clinics is unknown, but it is probably much more common than the other single-gene defects described in this chapter. In a young person presenting with diabetes, the differential is usually

Table 2
Comparison of MODY, Type 1 Diabetes, and Type 2 Diabetes

MODY	*Type 1 diabetes*	*Type 2 diabetes*
β-cell dysfunction	β-cell failure	β-cell dysfunction and insulin resistance
Prevalence in children unknown	Prevalence 0.17% in US residents 0–19 yr	Prevalence 0.1–5.1% in US studies
	...ght	Up to 85% overweight at diagnosis
	... of	75–100% have family history in first- or second-degree relative
	... insulin	17–37% on insulin
		F>M
	...4 yr	Peak age of onset 12–14 yr
		ICA negative May be GAD positive HLA association unknown

...oxylase antibody; HLA, human leukocyte

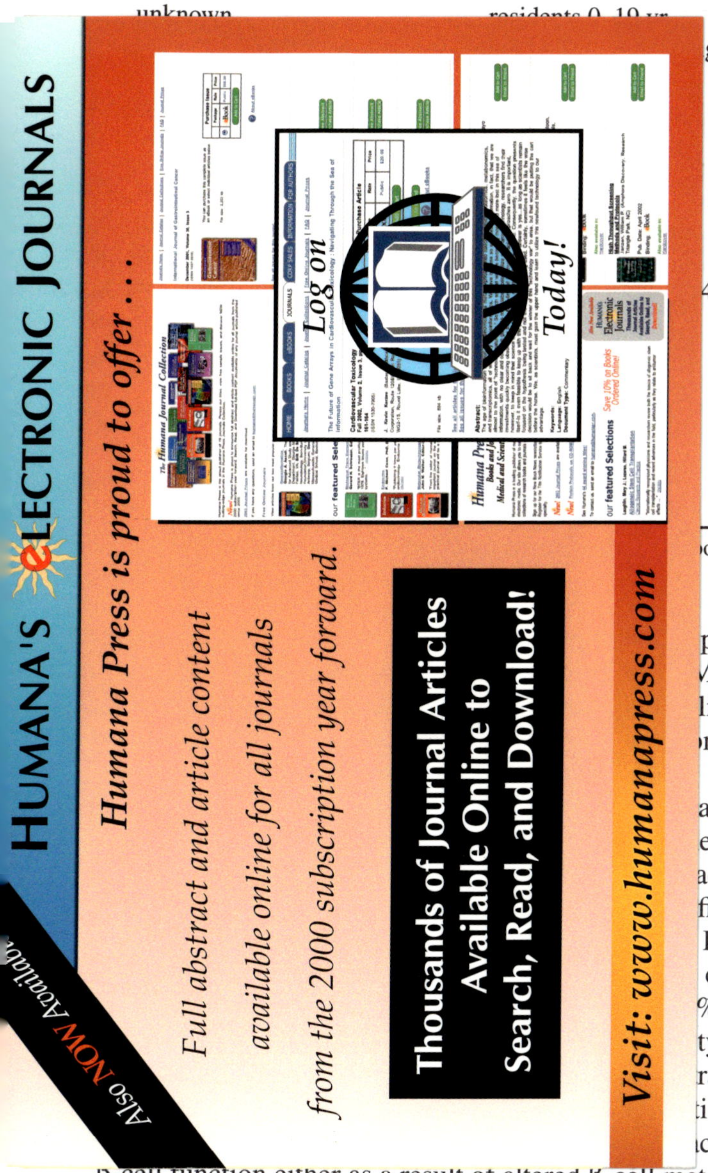

...pe 2 diabetes (*see* Table 2). In type ...MODY, one parent will be affected; ...likely to have type 2 diabetes or ...n with MODY may have an insulin

...as been unraveled, and at least five ...es described so far are glucokinase ...actors hepatocyte nuclear factor-1α ...fied in 1996 *(5,6)*, insulin promoter ... HNF-1β (MODY5) *(8)*. Defects in ... of patients with MODY, HNF-1α ...% of patients with MODY *(9)*.

...ty in MODY (MODY3) is a defec- ...ranscription factor that alters the ...tissues, including the liver, kidney, ...ctor result in a progressive loss of β-cell function either as a result of altered β-cell metabolism or abnormal β-cell development *(2)*. Patients with this form of MODY may have normal glucose tolerance in childhood, but develop symptomatic diabetes in adolescence or early adulthood. The mean age of diagnosis is 22 yr, but this may be many years after the development of diabetes. Initially, young patients with HNF-1α mutations may show normal or minimally elevated fasting blood glucose, but frank diabetes on the 2-h value of an oral glucose tolerance test. Significant retinopathy causing loss of sight or requiring laser

Table 3
Subgroups of MODY

MODY 1	*MODY 2*	*MODY 3*	*MODY 4*	*MODY 5*
HNF-4α	Glucokinase	HNF-1α	IPF-1	HNF-1β
Prevalence 5%	15%	70%	<1%	2%
Progressive glucose intolerance	Mild stable hyperglycemia	Progressive glucose intolerance	Progressive glucose intolerance	Progressive glucose intolerance
Onset 12–35 yr	Birth	12–28 yr	14–40 yr	12–28 yr
Microvascular complications	Complications rare	Microvascular complications	Microvascular complications	Microvascular complications; renal dysfunction, including renal cysts
Progressive requirement for treatment	Treatment in pregnancy	Progressive requirement for treatment	Progressive requirement for treatment	Progressive requirement for treatment

therapy is present in 14% of these patients *(2)*, and nephropathy is also reported. Young people with HNF-1α mutations are usually very sensitive to sulfonylureas and, indeed, may develop hypoglycemia on anything but the smallest doses. Treatment requirements are likely to increase as patients get older, because of the progressive deterioration in their glucose intolerance seen with HNF-1α mutations.

Mutations in the glucokinase gene are the second most common cause of MODY. The glucokinase gene encodes the enzyme glucokinase, which catalyzes the phosphorylation of glucose to glucose-6-phosphate. This is the rate-limiting step in β-cell metabolism leading to the secretion of insulin. Glucokinase has a low affinity for its substrate glucose and is not inhibited by its product glucose-6-phosphate. A glucokinase gene mutation reduces the enzyme's activity, causing an inappropriately low insulin secretion for a given glucose level and, hence, resulting in hyperglycemia. Over 80 mutations have been described in the glucokinase gene, clustering in exons 5, 6, 7, and 8, which code for the glucose-binding site of the enzyme *(10)*. This defect in β-cell sensing of glucose causes fasting glucose homeostasis to be reset about 2 mmol/L higher than normal. Despite this, β-cells do respond to a glucose load, so that ketoacidosis is rare. These patients have an elevated fasting blood glucose from birth (6–8 mmol/L). Mild deterioration in glucose tolerance occurs with age, but fasting glucose rarely exceeds 10 mmol/L. Children are rarely symptomatic and may only be diagnosed coincidentally while investigating intercurrent illness. Most young people do not need any treatment; the only exception to this is during pregnancy, when most women are treated with insulin. Microvascular complications are rare; it is not known whether patients are at risk from macrovascular complications, but they do have normal fasting lipids *(11)*.

About 5% of MODY patients have mutations in HNF-4α (MODY1). Mutations were found in a large family with MODY that was linked to chromosome 20q *(12)*. HNF-1α and HNF-4α interact to regulate the expression of many genes in widespread tissues, including the liver, kidney, and pancreas. Again, there is a defective insulin secretory response to an oral glucose load. This is a rare cause of MODY, and patients experience a progressive deterioration in glycemic control, with a risk of microvascular and macrovascular complications similar to MODY 3 and type 1 diabetes. Patients progress from normoglycemia to diabetes between 10 and 30 yr of age. As with HNF-1α mutations, some patients respond well to dietary measures and sulfonylureas.

An IPF-1 gene also known as PDX1 has been shown to be the cause of MODY in a single family (MODY4) *(7)*. IPF-1 is important in the regulation of insulin secretion and pancreas development. It has been implicated in a child with pancreatic agenesis associated with a homozygous frame-shift mutation *(13)*. The mean age of onset of diabetes of heterozygotes was 35 yr (range: 17–68) with only one of the eight diabetic members diagnosed under the age of 25 yr.

The transcription factors HNF-1α and HNF-4α are members of a complex transcriptional regulatory network that includes other homeodomain proteins. Another member of this transcription factor family, HNF-1β, was screened for mutations in MODY families, and a nonsense mutation was found in one family (MODY5) *(8)*. This is a relatively rare cause of MODY, with only six families published to date. These families are characterized by early-onset diabetes, which is similar to HNF-1α, and by renal abnormalities, which usually precede the diabetes, including renal cysts, proteinuria, and end-stage renal failure. Three different histologies have been described to date: oligomeganephronia, cystic renal dysplasia, and glomerulocystic disease.

MITOCHONDRIAL DIABETES

Patients with mitochondrial DNA (mtDNA) disease may have a clinical syndrome that involves mitochondrial dysfunction that is easy to identify. As an example, patients with mitochondrial encephalopathy with lactic acidosis and stroke-like episodes (MELAS) present in childhood with short stature and develop bilateral deafness in their teens, and then diabetes, seizures, stroke-like episodes, and an encephalopathy in their third or fourth decade *(14)*. Other patients have a constellation of clinical features that are highly suggestive of mitochondrial disease, but do not fall neatly into a specific syndrome category. An example is a history of migraine and diabetes. Finally, mitochondrial diseases may have a non-neurological presentation, such as diabetes alone. Between 0.5% and 1% of adult diabetic patients are thought to harbor a causative mtDNA mutation *(15)*.

Mitochondria are the intracellular organelles responsible for the generation of energy by the process of oxidative phosphorylation (OXPHOS). The human mtDNA is a 16,565-nucleotide double-stranded closed circular molecule that encodes 13 genes of OXPHOS, together with the structural ribosomal RNAs and transfer RNAs needed for their expression *(16)*. Mitochondrial diseases may result from either mutations of mtDNA or nuclear DNA, as genes from both genomes are needed to encode subunits of OXPHOS.

The most common cause of diabetes resulting from mitochondrial disorders is a point mutation at nucleotide pair 3243. The mutation has been described in families with a mild form of type 2 diabetes mellitus of adult onset and sensorineural deafness *(17–19)*. The diabetes associated with np3243 is usually diagnosed in the third to fifth decades of life, but it may present between the late teens and mid-eighties. Hyperglycemia is often mild and controlled by diet at diagnosis, but it tends to be progressive. The underlying pathogenesis is thought to be β-cell failure, with evidence of reduced insulin secretion in the presence of normal insulin sensitivity *(20)*. The same mitochondrial mutation may result in the less common, but severe, MELAS phenotype, as described earlier.

Deletions of mtDNA are generally clinically severe, of childhood onset, and, fortunately, less common. An example is Kearns–Sayre syndrome *(21)*. This is a sporadic multisystem disorder with progressive external ophthalmoplegia, retinal dystrophy, and at least one of the following: heart block, cerebellar ataxia, and raised cerebrospinal fluid (CSF) protein levels. Diabetes mellitus is a frequent finding, presenting in infancy and requiring treatment with insulin. The syndrome has been associated with the "common" mitochondrial deletion, of about 7 kb, but more recently, it has been shown that other rearrangements can cause this phenotype—in particular, duplications of mtDNA *(22)*. The same "common" mitochondrial deletion has been reported in another syndrome of sideroblastic anemia, exocrine pancreatic dysfunction, and lactic acidosis (Pearson syndrome) *(23)*. This is a rare disorder associated with onset of diabetes in early infancy; affected children do not usually survive beyond the first decade. One patient has been reported who progressed from Pearson syndrome in infancy to Kearns–Sayre syndrome in adulthood *(24)*.

The investigation of a child with suspected mitochondrial disease is complex; blood tests such as lactate are nonspecific. Magnetic resonance imaging (MRI) is helpful with neurological symptoms and may show cerebral and cerebellar atrophy. A muscle biopsy may reveal subsarcolemmal accumulations of mitochondria ("ragged red fibers"), and on histochemistry there may be cytochrome-*c* oxidase (COX, complex IV)-deficient fibers. Respiratory chain complex assays may also show a deficiency.

The underlying mechanism of diabetes in mitochondrial disorders is thought to be reduced insulin secretion (decreased first-phase insulin response, reduction in urinary C-peptide). Insulin secretion in response to postprandial glucose elevation depends on a sequence of metabolic events, including the uptake of glucose through the GLUT-2 transporter, phoshorylation of glucose by glucokinase, production of NADH and pyruvate by glycolysis, and stimulation of mitochondrial OXPHOS. As a result of OXPHOS stimulation, the ATP level rises, leading to closure of ATP-dependent potassium channels. The resulting depolarization of the membrane potential is followed by the opening of calcium channels, allowing an increased intracellular calcium level, which triggers insulin secretion. Thus, reduced ATP availability in the β-cells may compromise the whole pathway for insulin secretion in response to elevated glucose *(25)*.

NEONATAL DIABETES

Neonatal diabetes has been defined as hyperglycemia occurring within the first 6 wk of life in term infants *(26)*. A recent UK survey established an incidence of 1/400,000 live births, similar to a German study *(27)*. These infants present with intrauterine growth retardation, failure to gain weight adequately, and development of hyperglycemia, dehydration, and minimal ketosis. Endogenous insulin levels are usually low or undetectable, and exogenous insulin is usually required for a mean duration of 3 mo. Transient neonatal diabetes (TND) resolves by 18 mo of age, but type 2 diabetes may recur in early adulthood *(28,29)*. In the UK survey, 11 infants had TND, and the median age of resolution was 3 mo (range: 1–8 mo). There were two infants with permanent neonatal diabetes who were still diabetic at 4 and 6 yr of age, respectively. TND is distinct from classic type 1 diabetes, as patients do not have the common human leukocyte antigen (HLA) susceptibility haplotypes, and there is no evidence of autoimmunity. It is probable that transient and permanent neonatal diabetes have separate etiologies.

Two unrelated patients were initially described with TND and paternal isodisomy of chromosome 6 *(30)*. In uniparental disomy (UPD), both copies of genetic material are inherited from one parent. Isodisomy refers to the inheritance of two identical copies of a single parental chromosome. Uniparental isodisomy may be involved in disease pathogenesis in two ways. First, it can unmask a rare recessive disorder in the child of a carrier parent, the child, in effect, being functionally homozygous. Second, the inheritance of gene(s) from only one parent (UPD) can lead to disordered expression if that gene is imprinted. Imprinted genes are those in which expression depends on parental origin. Although UPD may not be the mechanism of all cases of TND, it is possible that an imprinted gene on chromosome 6 is central to the development and maturation of early fetal and neonatal pancreatic β-cell function and that overexpression of a gene(s) in the region of 6q21-23 may be responsible for TND. The gene has to be paternally expressed to cause TND, with no expression of the maternally inherited allele. Within the critical region of duplication on 6q, a differentially methylated CpG island was found that was methylated only on the maternally inherited chromosome 6 homolog *(31)*. All patients with paternal UPD of chromosome 6 showed a complete lack of methylation at this site.

Very recently, a cohort of 30 affected children have been reported who have been investigated for aberrations in chromosome 6 *(32)*. These patients could be divided into four groups. Group 1 had paternal UPD of chromosome 6 (11 children); group 2 had a duplication involving chromosome band 6q24, which was paternal in origin where tested (10 children); group 3 was 1 patient with a loss of methylation at a CpG island within the TND critical region; group 4 had no identifiable rearrangement of chromosome 6 (7 children). There were no significant clinical differences among the four groups. In group 2, two relatives of the TND patients who presented with type 2 diabetes and no early history of TND had inherited an identical duplication. It is not known whether imprinting abnormalities at 6q24 are involved in the more common type 1 and type 2 diabetes.

There has been no evidence of UPD in permanent neonatal diabetes. A number of disorders of pancreatic organogenesis have been implicated, including isolated absence of islet cells, pancreatic hypoplasia, and agenesis *(33,34)*, as well as Wolcott–Rallison syndrome. Recently, a child with pancreatic agenesis was described with a homozygous mutation of IPF-1 *(13)*. Heterozygosity for an IPF-1 mutation is recognized as a cause of MODY (MODY4).

WOLCOTT–RALLISON SYNDROME

Multiple epiphyseal dysplasia associated with permanent neonatal diabetes in three siblings was originally described in 1972 *(35)*. Children with this syndrome classically present with neonatal or early infancy onset, permanent insulin-requiring diabetes mellitus. There may or may not be an increased tendency to fractures of the long bones, and children walk with a waddling, lordotic gait, with genu valgum. Radiological investigations show epiphyseal dysplasia, with symmetrically small epiphyses, irregular in outline and poorly calcified. Other abnormalities include short stature, ectodermal dysplasia, and brown mottling of the teeth near the gums. Multisystemic manifestations include renal and hepatic dysfunction, mental retardation, and cardiac abnormalities. Of the 12 or so reported children in the literature, none survived beyond the teenage years; causes of death included renal and hepatic dysfunction. In one report of postmortem findings in a 4-yr-old *(36)*, there was severe pancreatic hypoplasia, with a reduction in pancreatic β-cells. In addition to Wolcott–Rallison syndrome, this child had a deletion of chromosome 15q11-12 in 65% of her cells. The disorder is inherited as an autosomal recessive trait. Recently, the translation initiation factor EIF2AK3 was found to be mutated in two unrelated families with this syndrome *(37)*. One family was of Tunisian origin and the other was from Pakistan; both were consanguineous, and in both, the mutations segregated with the disease. EIF2AK3 has a role in the regulation of protein translation and is highly expressed in pancreatic islet cells; presumably, it functions in maintaining the integrity of pancreatic β-cells. An EIF2AK3-related protein, PKR, has a role in the control of cell growth and apoptosis, raising the possibility that EIF2AK3 has a similar function that may be relevant to the characteristic pancreas β-cell destruction seen in these patients.

WOLFRAM SYNDROME

Wolfram syndrome is the inherited association of childhood-onset diabetes mellitus and optic atrophy *(38)*. As other complications were identified, the acronym DIDMOAD was coined (diabetes insipidus, diabetes mellitus optic atrophy, and deafness). This is a progressive, neurodegenerative disorder and many patients also develop urinary tract atony, ataxia, peripheral neuropathy, and psychiatric illness. We previously characterized the natural history of this condition in a UK nationwide series of 45 patients *(39)* (*see* Fig. 1). Diabetes mellitus presented at a median age of 6 yr, followed by optic atrophy at 11 yr. Optic atrophy is progressive, leading to vision of 6/60 or less in the better eye in a median of 8 yr *(40)*. Cranial diabetes insipidus occurred in 33 patients (73%), with sensorineural deafness (28, 62%) in the second decade; renal tract abnormalities (incontinence, neuropathic bladder [26, 58%]) presented in the third decade, followed by neurological complications (cerebellar ataxia, myoclonus [28, 62%]) in the fourth decade. There is a significant risk of psychiatric illness (incipient dementia, short- term memory loss, endogenous depression, mixed affective disorder) and suicide *(41)*. Other complications included gonadal atrophy and gastrointestinal dysmotility. The median age at death was 30 yr (range: 25–49), commonly caused by central respiratory failure with brainstem atrophy. The underlying pancreatic pathology is a selective loss of β-cells *(42)*.

In Wolfram patients with diabetes insipidus, there is loss of vasopressin neurons in the supraoptic nucleus, with a defect in vasopressin precursor processing *(43)*. We estimated the prevalence as 1/500,000 children in the United Kingdom, with a carrier frequency of 1 in 354. The prevalence has been estimated as 1/100,000 in a North American population, based on the 1/175 occurrence of optic atrophy in a juvenile diabetes clinic *(44)*.

The absence of affected parents and a high proportion of consanguinity suggested autosomal recessive inheritance, and genetic linkage studies linked Wolfram syndrome to the short arm of chromosome 4 *(45,46)*. A Wolfram syndrome gene has been positionally cloned (WFS1) *(47)* and identified by a candidate gene approach (Wolframin) *(48)*. It consists of 8 exons, encoding a polypeptide of 890 amino acids, predicted to have 9 transmembrane domains. The function is as yet unknown but is likely to be

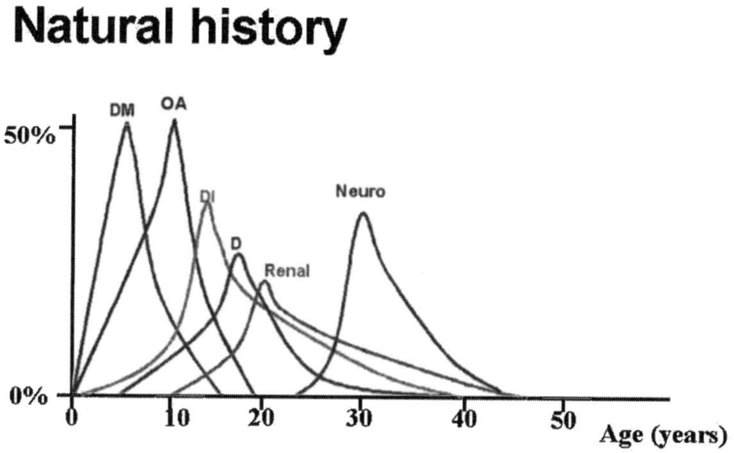

Fig. 1. Natural history of Wolfram syndrome. Abbreviations: DM, diabetes mellitus; OA, optic atrophy; DI, diabetes insipidus; D, deafness; Renal, neuropathic bladder; Neuro, ataxia, myoclonus, and so forth.

involved in pancreatic β-cell and neuronal cell survival. Northern analysis with human adult tissues shows WFS1 expression in the heart, brain, placenta, lung, liver, skeletal muscle, kidney, and pancreas *(47)*. High expression was found in pancreatic islets compared with the exocrine pancreas. In a mutation analysis of 30 patients from 19 British families, we identified 24 mutations in the WFS1 gene in 18 of the families *(49)*. Most patients were compound heterozygotes for two mutations, and there was no common founder mutation. There was no obvious correlation between observed mutations and disease severity. Most of the mutations produced truncation and subsequent loss of, or mutations in, the carboxy tail of the protein.

A high prevalence of diabetes has been noted in relatives of patients with Wolfram syndrome patients *(44)*, suggesting that heterozygote carriers may contribute to the genetic heterogeneity of diabetes in the general population. A genetic association study of 185 type 1 diabetes patients and 380 control subjects revealed the R456H missense mutation was significantly increased in the type 1 diabetes group compared to the control group ($p = 0.0005$) *(50)*. The patients with this missense mutation had an increased frequency of type 1 diabetes-resistant HLA-DRB1 alleles and reduced frequency of GAD antibodies, suggesting that WFS1 may have a role in the development of common type 1 diabetes on a nonautoimmune genetic basis.

A second locus has been mapped to chromosome 4q22-24 after linkage analysis of four consanguineous Jordanian families *(51)*. These patients had a different clinical picture, with the absence of diabetes insipidus and the presence of upper gastrointestinal ulceration and bleeding. There has been a report of "mitochondrial Wolfram syndrome" in a Spanish family, with all of the most common Wolfram complications resulting from deletions in the mitochondrial genome *(52)*. It is possible that mitochondrial function is disrupted because of mutations in a nuclear gene or that mutations in a nuclear gene deleteriously interact with the mitochondrial genome. However, an investigation of the UK cohort of 50 patients found no evidence supporting a role for mtDNA in Wolfram syndrome, no abnormal mitochondrial function, and no mtDNA mutations *(53)*.

The minimum ascertainment criteria for the diagnosis of Wolfram syndrome are the co-occurrence of childhood-onset (<15 yr) diabetes and progressive optic atrophy.

These criteria give a positive predictive value for Wolfram syndrome of 83% and a negative predictive value of 1%, based on the characterization of 45 patients *(39)*. The addition of further clinical features such as deafness does not increase the predictive value for Wolfram syndrome. Using these criteria, screening for Wolfram syndrome mutations will identify at least one mutation in WFS1 in 90% of patients and two mutations in 78% *(54)*. Exclusion of a WFS1 mutation in unaffected siblings may offer reassurance. However, the diagnosis of Wolfram syndrome remains essentially clinical, with mutation analysis used only to confirm the diagnosis.

THIAMIN-RESPONSIVE MEGALOBLASTIC ANEMIA SYNDROME

Thiamin-responsive megaloblastic anemia syndrome is also known as Roger's syndrome, after the first description in an 11-year-old girl *(55)*. The cardinal clinical manifestations of the syndrome are megaloblastic anemia, diabetes mellitus, and sensorineural deafness, all of which may respond in varying degrees to the administration of thiamin (vitamin B_1), 25 mg/d. The diabetes, which appears in childhood, is non-type-1 and nonautoimmune in nature; in some cases, the insulin requirement is reduced during thiamin therapy *(56,57)*. In addition to the cardinal findings for which the syndrome is named, some patients show cardiac arrythmias *(58–60)*, as well as abnormalities of the retina and the optic nerve, including optic atrophy *(59,61)*. The anemia may be variable and may present with a microcytic picture on blood film, evolving to a macrocytic film with increased iron stores and ringed sideroblasts on bone marrow aspirate.

The pathophysiology of this syndrome is unclear, but reduced activity of thiamin-dependent enzymes has been demonstrated in two patients, corrected in one by titrating with increasing concentrations of thiamin pyrophosphate *(62)*. Thiamin is thought to be taken up by cells via two mechanisms: an active process by a specific carrier and a passive diffusion process *(61)*. Once inside the cell, thiamin is phosphorylated to its metabolically active form, thiamin pyrophosphate (TPP). It then acts as a cofactor for several enzymes, including oxoglutarate dehydrogenase (OGDH) and pyruvate dehydrogenase (PDH). In thiamin-responsive diabetes, there may be defective TPP metabolism or a defect in TPP transport to its metabolically active sites.

The consanguinity of many of the families and the absence of affected parents suggested autosomal recessive inheritance. This was confirmed by a homozygosity mapping strategy where the gene was localized to chromosome 1p *(63)* and narrowed to a 4-cM region *(64)*. Recently, the vitamin transporter SLC19A2 has been identified as mutated in families with this syndrome *(65–67)*. The gene encodes a transmembrane protein (THTR-1), which functions as a high-affinity thiamine transporter *(66)*. The gene consists of six exons; exons 2 and 5 are highly conserved across species, and exon 2 contains a large extracellular loop, which may be responsible for recognition of thiamine. This is consistent with the fact that most mutations are found in exon 2 *(68)*. Exon 5 contains a G-protein receptor consensus sequence, which suggests that this intracellular region may interact with other proteins inside the cell. Because THTR-1 function is predicted to be absent in patients with this syndrome, presumably there must be a secondary transport process that acts to allow sufficient thiamin uptake to prevent the metabolic condition of severe thiamine deficiency. THTR-1 must have a critical role in glucose homeostasis.

SYNDROMES OF INSULIN RESISTANCE

Insulin resistance is an important feature of type 2 diabetes, and failure of insulin action in the peripheral insulin sensitive tissues, skeletal muscle, and adipose tissue is a major part of disease pathogenesis. Rare inherited syndromes of extreme insulin resistance have been vital in identifying genes involved in the insulin signaling pathway. One of these, Rabson–Mendenhall syndrome, consists of pineal hyperplasia, facial dysmorphism, phallic enlargement in males, short stature, acanthosis nigricans, and premature dentition. Diabetes mellitus presents between 3 and 7 yr of age, with death from ketoacidosis in the second decade. The diabetes is highly insulin resistant. Survivors develop later widespread microvascular disease *(69)*. The syndrome is caused by insulin-receptor mutations leading to defective binding capacity *(70)*. A model of treatment for this condition has been described, using monoclonal antibodies acting as a substitute for the normal ligand, thereby activating the defective receptor *(71)*. It is interesting that another inherited syndrome, leprechaunism (Donohue syndrome) is also associated with insulin-receptor mutations. This syndrome is characterized by intrauterine growth retardation and presentation in infancy with pachydermia, hypertrichosis, acanthosis nigricans, reduced subcutaneous fat stores, and coarse facies *(72)*. There is extreme hyperinsulinism, insulin resistance, and, paradoxically, often fasting hypoglycemia. Insulin binding to receptors is severely decreased. The diabetes is difficult to treat and may be complicated by renal disease similar to diabetic nephropathy *(73)*. Over 50 insulin-receptor mutations have been described, the vast majority in association with these extreme insulin-resistance syndromes. These mutations either abolish insulin receptor binding, disrupt the tyrosine kinase activity of the receptor, or interfere with the synthesis and expression of the receptor *(74)*. It is probable that leprechaunism, Rabson–Mendenhall syndrome, and type A insulin resistance (nonobese, nondysmorphic, severely insulin-resistant females with hirsutism, acanthosis nigricans, and menstrual disturbance) represent points on a continuum of increasingly severe receptor dysfunction, rather than completely distinct syndromes *(71)*. Mutations in the insulin receptor do not make a major contribution to the insulin resistance seen in more common disorders such as type 2 diabetes. Interest is now being focused on peroxisome proliferator-activated-receptor gamma (PPARγ), a nuclear receptor that is the target of thiazolidinedione drugs. Dominant negative mutations have been described in three individuals with diabetes mellitus as a result of severe insulin resistance and hypertension *(75)*.

BARDET–BIEDL SYNDROME

Bardet–Biedl syndrome (BBS) is an autosomal recessive condition characterized by rod-cone dystrophy (atypical retinitis pigmentosa), postaxial polydactyly, central obesity, mental retardation, hypogonadism, and renal dysfunction. Other features, not always present, include hepatic fibrosis, diabetes mellitus, reproductive abnormalities, endocrinological disturbances, short stature, developmental delay, and speech deficits. BBS is distinguished from the much rarer Laurence–Moon syndrome, in which retinal pigmentary degeneration, mental retardation, and hypogonadism occur in conjunction with progressive spastic paraparesis and distal muscle weakness, but without polydactyly *(76)*. BBS was first described in 1920 *(77)*, and the cardinal manifestations were described as retinal pigmentary dystrophy (retinitis pigmentosa), postaxial polydactyly, central obesity, mental retardation, and hypogenitalism *(78)*. The prevalence of BBS is about 1 in 125,000, and criteria for diagnosis have been published *(79)*. In this large survey of 109 BBS patients in the United Kingdom and their families, the average age at diagnosis was 9 yr, although parents first noticed abnormalities in their children at a mean age of 3 yr. Obesity only began to develop at around 2–3 yr, and retinal degeneration did not become apparent until a mean age of 8.5 yr. Only seven patients (6%) had non-insulin-dependent diabetes mellitus. However, only a minority of patients surveyed had undergone a fasting glucose measurement or glucose tolerance test, so the prevalence of diabetes may be much higher. Diabetes presented in adulthood and was thought to be the result of insulin resistance.

Recently, genetic heterogeneity has been confirmed with the finding of five gene loci, on chromosomes 11 (BBS1) *(80)*, 16 (BBS2) *(81)*, 3 (BBS3) *(82)* 15 (BBS4) *(83)*, and 2 (BBS5) *(84)*, each associated with a similar phenotype. Recently, Bardet–Biedl families from Newfoundland who had genetic linkage excluded from the known loci were found to be linked to markers on chromosome 2q31 (BBS6) *(85)*. Mutations were identified in a chaperonin-like gene, McKusick–Kaufman syndrome (MKKS). Most were frame-shift mutations that were likely to result in a severely truncated, nonfunctional protein. The MKKS protein shows similarity to type II chaperonins, which are responsible for folding a wide range of proteins. Spatial conformation is likely to be critical to this molecule and disruptions may reduce the efficiency or abolish the ability to fold target peptides. Presumably there are other BBS genes that encode proteins that interact with MKKS to form a multimeric chaperone unit. Molecules that require MKKS for correct folding may also be candidates for different aspects of the BBS phenotype.

ALSTROM SYNDROME

This syndrome was first described in 1959, when two of Alstrom's original patients died from renal failure *(86)*. The characteristic features of this syndrome appear to be pigmentary retinal degeneration, sensorineural hearing loss, childhood obesity, non-insulin-dependent diabetes mellitus, hyperlipidaemia, and chronic nephropathy. Features occasionally observed include acanthosis nigricans, hypogonadism, hypothyroidism, alopecia, short stature, and cardiomyopathy. A large kindred including eight affected patients has been described *(87)*. Hyperinsulinemia and hypertriglyceridemia with normal cholesterol levels were observed in most affected individuals tested. Non-insulin-dependent diabetes and growth retardation appeared to be age-related manifestations that occurred postadolescence. Younger affected children were not overtly hyperglycaemic and were normal or above average height for age.

A homozygosity mapping strategy has been used to link a disease-causing gene to chromosome 2p *(88)*. The same group has found a candidate mouse gene *(tub)* responsible for the phenotype tubby mouse *(89)*. These mice also suffer a strikingly similar phenotype to Alstrom patients. The authors postulate that the phenotypic features of tubby mice may be the result of cellular apoptosis triggered by expression of the mutated tub gene.

PRADER–WILLI SYNDROME

Prader–Willi syndrome (PWS) is a complex, multisystem disorder first described in 1956 *(90)*. It is diagnosed in about 1 in 10,000–15,000 people *(91)*, occurring in all sexes and races. Many of the manifestations are related to functional hypothalamic deficiency, and the clinical appearance in infancy differs markedly from that in childhood and adulthood *(92)*. The major features associated with PWS are decreased fetal activity, neonatal hypotonia and feeding difficulties, hyperphagia with obesity, and psychomotor and mental retardation. Characteristic features include narrow bifrontal diameter, almond-shaped palpebral fissures, narrow nasal bridge, and down-turned mouth with a thin upper lip. The children also have a characteristic body habitus, including sloping shoulders, heavy midsection, and genu valgum. Obesity is the major cause of morbidity and mortality in PWS. Diabetes may result from excessive obesity, as may cardiopulmonary compromise, hypertension, thrombophlebitis, chronic leg edema, and obstructive sleep apnea. Diabetes mellitus has been reported in as many as 7–20% of PWS patients, with age of onset usually in the teens. Consequently, the diagnosis has usually been made before diabetes develops. The diabetes was assumed to be the same as that occurring in obese individuals without PWS. However, in a case-control study, individuals with PWS did not show the predicted insulin resistance that is seen in obese children without the syndrome *(93)*. There was a suggestion that PWS children actually have normal or increased insulin sensitivity.

Prader–Willi syndrome is caused by the absence of normally active paternally inherited genes at chromosome 15(q11-q13); the maternally inherited genes are normally inactive owing to genetic imprinting. About 75% of patients have a 4-Mb deletion of the paternally contributed chromosome 15q. Most of the remaining patients have maternal uniparental disomy for chromosome 15. Presumably, there is an imprinting center within this deletion. Methylation is one mechanism by which genomic imprinting can occur, and methylation has been shown for several genes identified within the PWS region *(94)*.

SUMMARY

The main cause of diabetes in children is type 1 diabetes, which has an autoimmune basis and is insulin deficient. Type 2 diabetes is increasing in children, probably resulting from increasing obesity, and is associated with insulin resistance. Non-type-1, or non-type 2, diabetes account for up to 5% of children in pediatric diabetes clinics and are principally genetic, thus relatively stable in numbers over time. These children present difficult management problems and may have associated nonendocrine disorders. MODY is almost certainly the most common inherited diabetes disorder caused by a single-gene defect and is probably underdiagnosed. Other disorders such as Wolfram are multisystemic and have devastating consequences for the physical, educational, and emotional outlook of the child. These inherited diabetes syndromes are often misdiagnosed as type 1 diabetes initially, but present complex management problems. Collectively, they are important in revealing pathways of insulin metabolism, normal and abnormal. They are also candidate genes for contributing to the genetic heterogeneity of common type 1 and type 2 diabetes. As the causative genes are being identified, they are enabling us to offer genetic testing to siblings of affected children, mutational analysis to correlate the clinical pattern to the genotype, and novel therapeutic approaches that may have implications for the wider diabetic community.

ACKNOWLEDGMENTS

I am very grateful to Professor Andrew Hattersley who kindly revised the section on MODY. I am also grateful to Children Nationwide for supporting me. Research on

Wolfram syndrome reviewed in this article was supported by SPARKS (Sport Aiding Research in Kids), The Royal Society, The British Medical Association John William Clark Award, and The University of Birmingham Small Grants Scheme.

REFERENCES

1. Tattersall RB. Mild familial diabetes with dominant inheritance. Q J Med 1974;43:339–357.
2. Hattersley AT. Maturity-onset diabetes of the young: clinical heterogeneity explained by genetic heterogeneity. Diabet Med 1998;15:15–24.
3. Ellard S, Beards F, Allen L, et al. A high prevalence of glucokinase mutations in gestational diabetes subjects selected by clinical criteria. Diabetologia 2000;43:250–253.
4. Hattersley A, Turner R, Permutt M, et al. Linkage of type 2 diabetes to the glucokinase gene. Lancet 1992;339:1307–1310.
5. Yamagata K, Oda N, Kaisaki PJ, et al. Mutations in the hepatic nuclear factor 1 alpha gene in maturity-onset diabetes of the young (MODY3). Nature 1996;384:455–458.
6. Yamagata K, Furuta H, Oda N, et al. Mutations in the hepatocyte nuclear factor 4 alpha gene in maturity-onset diabetes of the young (MODY1). Nature 1996;384:458–460.
7. Stoffers D, Ferrer J, Clarke W, Habener J. Early-onset type-II diabetes mellitus (MODY4) linked to IPF1. Nat Genet 1997;17:138–139.
8. Horikawa Y, Iwasaki N, Hara M, et al. Mutation in hepatocyte nuclear factor-1β gene (TCF2) associated with MODY. Nat Genet 1997;17:384–385.
9. Hattersley AT. Heterogeneity in type 2 diabetes: lessons from maturity-onset diabetes of the young. Diabet Rev Int 1998;7(2):10–12.
10. Gidh-Jain M, Takeda J, Xu L, et al. Glucokinase mutations associated with non-insulin-dependent (type 2) diabetes mellitus have decreased enzymatic activity: implications for structure/function relationships. Proc Natl Acad Sci USA 1993;90:1932–1936.
11. Hattersley A. Maturity onset diabetes of the young. Bailliere's Clin Paediatr 1996;4:663–680.
12. Bell G, Xiang K, Newman M, et al. Gene for non-insulin-dependent diabetes mellitus (maturity-onset diabetes of the young subtype) is linked to DNA polymorphism on human chromosome 20q. Proc Natl Acad Sci USA 1991;88:1484–1488.
13. Stoffers D, Zinkin N, Stanojevic V, Clarke W, Habener J. Pancreatic agenesis attributable to a single nucleotide deletion in the human IPF1 gene coding sequence. Nat Genet 1997;15:106–110.
14. Hirano M, Ricci E, Koenigsberger M, et al. MELAS: an original case and clinical criteria for diagnosis. Neuromusc Disord 1992;2:125–135.
15. Maassen J, Kadowaki T. Maternally inherited diabetes and deafness: a new diabetes subtype. Diabetologia 1996;39:375–382.
16. Chinnery P, Howell N, Andrews R, Turnbull D. Clinical mitochondrial genetics. J Med Genet 1999;36:425–436.
17. Reardon W, Ross R, Sweeney M, et al. Diabetes mellitus associated with a pathogenic point mutation in mitochondrial DNA. Lancet 1992;340:1376–1379.
18. van den Ouweland J, Lemkes H, Ruitenbeek W, et al. Mutation in mitochondrial $tRNA^{Leu(uur)}$ gene in a large pedigree with maternally transmitted type II diabetes mellitus and deafness. Nat Genet 1992;1:368–371.
19. Ballinger S, Shoffner J, Hedaya E, et al. Maternally transmitted diabetes and deafness associated with a 10.4 kb mitochondrial DNA deletion. Nat Genet 1992;1:11–15.
20. Kadowaki T, Kadowaki H, Mori Y, et al. A subtype of diabetes mellitus associated with a mutation of mitochondrial DNA. N Engl J Med 1994;330:962–968.
21. Kearns T, Sayre G. Retinitis pigmentosa, external ophthalmoplegia, and complete heart block: unusual syndrome with histologic study in one of two cases. Arch Ophthalmol 1958;60:280–289.
22. Poulton J, Morten K, Weber K, Brown G, Bindoff L. Are duplications of mitochondrial DNA characteristic of Kearns–Sayre syndrome? Hum Mol Genet 1994;3:947–951.
23. Pearson H, Lobel J, Kocoshis S, et al. A new syndrome of refractory sideroblastic anemia with vacuolization of marrow precursors and exocrine pancreatic dysfunction. J Pediatr 1979;95:976–984.
24. Larsson N, Holme E, Kristiansson B, Oldfors A, Tulinius M. Progressive increase of the mutated mitochondrial DNA fraction in Kearns–Sayre syndrome. Pediatr Res 1990;28:131–136.
25. Gerbitz K, Gempel K, Brdiczka D. Mitochondria and diabetes. Diabetes 1996;45:113–126.
26. Shield J. Neonatal diabetes. In: Shield JPH, Baum JD, eds. Childhood Diabetes. Bailliere's Clin Paediatr, Elsevier, London, 1996;4:681–689.

27. von Muhlendahl K, Herkenhoff H. Long-term course of neonatal diabetes. N Engl J Med 1995;333:704–708.
28. Shield J, Baum J. Transient neonatal diabetes and later onset diabetes: a case of inherited insulin resistance. Arch Dis Child 1995;72:56–57.
29. Shield J, Gardner R, Wadsworth E, et al. Aetiopathology and genetic basis of neonatal diabetes. Arch Dis Child 1997;76:F39–F42.
30. Temple I, James R, Crolla J, et al. An imprinted gene(s) for diabetes? Nat Genet 1995;9:110–112.
31. Gardner R, Mackay D, Mungall A, Shield J, Temple I, Robinson D. An imprinted locus associated with transient neonatal diabetes mellitus. Hum Mol Genet 2000;9:589–596.
32. Temple I, Gardner R, Mackay D, Barber J, Robinson D, Shield J. Transient neonatal diabetes. Widening the understanding of the etiopathogenesis of diabetes. Diabetes 2000;49:1359–1366.
33. Dodge J, Lawrence K. Congenital absence of islets of Langerhans. Arch Dis Child 1977;52:411–419.
34. Lemons J, Ridenour R, Orsini E. Congenital absence of the pancreas and intra-uterine growth retardation. Pediatrics 1979;64:255–256.
35. Wolcott C, Rallison M. Infancy-onset diabetes mellitus and multiple epiphyseal dysplasia. J Pediatr 1972;80:292–297.
36. Thornton C, Carson D, Stewart F. Autopsy findings in the Wolcott–Rallison syndrome. Pediatr Pathol Lab Med 1997;17:487–496.
37. Delapine M, Nicolino M, Barrett T, Golamaully M, Lathrop M, Julier C. EIF2AK3, encoding translation initiation factor 2-α kinase 3, is mutated in patients with Wolcott–Rallison syndrome. Nat Genet 2000;25:406–409.
38. Wolfram DJ, Wagener HP. Diabetes mellitus and simple optic atrophy among siblings: report of four cases. Mayo Clin Proc 1938;13:715–718.
39. Barrett TG, Bundey SE, Macleod AF. Neurodegeneration and diabetes: UK nationwide study of Wolfram (DIDMOAD) syndrome. Lancet 1995;346:1458–1463.
40. Barrett T, Bundey S, Fielder A, Good P. Optic atrophy in Wolfram (DIDMOAD) syndrome. Eye 1997;11:882–888.
41. Swift R, Sadler D, Swift M. Psychiatric findings in Wolfram syndrome homozygotes. Lancet 1990;336:667–669.
42. Karasik A, O'Hara C, Srikanta S, et al. Genetically programmed selective islet β-cell loss in diabetic subjects with Wolfram's syndrome. Diabetes Care 1989;12:135–138.
43. Gabreels B, Swaab D, Kleijn D, et al. The vasopressin precursor is not processed in the hypothalamus of Wolfram syndrome patients with diabetes insipidus: evidence for the involvement of PC2 and 7B2. J Clin Endocrinol Metab 1998;83:4026–4033.
44. Fraser F, Gunn T. Diabetes mellitus, diabetes insipidus, and optic atrophy. An autosomal recessive syndrome? J Med Genet 1977;14:190–193.
45. Polymeropoulos MH, Swift RG, Swift M. Linkage of the gene for Wolfram syndrome to markers on the short arm of chromosome 4. Nat Genet 1994;8:95–97.
46. Collier D, Barrett T, Curtis D, et al. Linkage of Wolfram syndrome to chromosome 4p16.1 and evidence for heterogeneity. Am J Hum Genet 1996;59:855–863.
47. Inoue H, Tanizawa Y, Wasson J, et al. A gene encoding a transmembrane protein is mutated in patients with diabetes mellitus and optic atrophy (Wolfram syndrome). Nat Genet 1998;20:143–148.
48. Strom T, Hortnagel K, Hofmann S, et al. Diabetes insipidus, diabetes mellitus, optic atrophy and deafness (DIDMOAD) caused by mutations in a novel gene (wolframin) coding for a predicted transmembrane protein. Hum Mol Genet 1998;7:2021–2028.
49. Hardy C, Khanim F, Torres R, et al. Clinical and molecular genetic analysis of 19 Wolfram syndrome kindreds demonstrating a wide spectrum of mutations in WFS1. Am J Hum Genet 1999;65:1279–1290.
50. Awata T, Inoue K, Kurihara S, et al. Missense variations of the gene responsible for Wolfram syndrome (WFS1/wolframin) in Japanese: possible contribution of the Arg456His mutation to type 1 diabetes as a nonautoimmune genetic basis. Biochem Biophys Res Commun 2000;268:612–616.
51. El-Shanti H, Lidral AC, Jarrah N, Druhan L. Ajlouni K. Homozygosity mapping identifies an additional locus for Wolfram syndrome on chromosome 4q. Am J Hum Genet 2000;66:1229–1236.
52. Barrientos A, Casademont J, Saiz A, et al. Autosomal recessive Wolfram syndrome associated with an 8.5-kb mtDNA single deletion. Am J Hum Genet 1996;58:963–970.
53. Barrett T, Scott-Brown M, Seller A, Bednarz A, Poulton K, Poulton J. The mitochondrial genome in Wolfram syndrome. J Med Genet 2000;37:463–466.
54. Khanim F, Kirk J, Latif F, Barrett T. Mutation update: WFS1/Wolframin mutations in Wolfram syndrome. Hum Mutat 2001;17:357–367.

55. Rogers L, Porter F, Sidbury J. Thiamine-responsive megaloblastic anemia. J Pediatr 1969;74:494–504.
56. Borgna-Pignatti C, Marradi P, Pinelli L, Monetti N, Patrini C. Thiamine responsive anemia in DIDMOAD syndrome. J Pediatr 1989;114:405–410.
57. Mandel H, Berant M, Hazani A, Naveh Y. Thiamine-dependent beriberi in the thiamine-responsive anemia syndrome. N Engl J Med 1984;311:836–838.
58. Viana M, Carvalho R. Thiamine-responsive megaloblastic anemia, sensorineural deafness, and diabetes mellitus: a new syndrome? J Pediatr 1978;93:235–238.
59. Abboud M, Alexander D, Najjar S. Diabetes mellitus, thiamine-dependent megaloblastic anemia, and sensorineural deafness associated with deficient α-ketoglutarate dehydrogenase activity. J Pediatr 1985:107:537–541.
60. Poggi V, Rindi G, Patrini C, DeVizia B, Lorgo G, Andria H. Studies on thiamine metabolism in thiamine-responsive megaloblastic anemia. Eur J Pediatr 1989;148:307–311.
61. Rindi G, Patrini C, Laforenza U, et al. Further studies on erythrocyte thiamine transport and phosphorylation in seven patients with thiamine-responsive megaloblastic anemia. J Inherited Metab Dis 1994;17:667–677.
62. Barrett T, Poulton K, Baines M, McCowen C. Muscle biochemistry in thiamin-responsive anaemia. J Inherited Metab Dis 1997;20:404–406.
63. Neufeld E, Mandel H, Raz T, et al. Localization of the gene for thiamine-responsive megaloblastic anemia syndrome, on the long arm of chromosome 1, by homozygosity mapping. Am J Hum Genet 1997;61:1335–1341.
64. Raz T, Barrett T, Szargel R, et al. Refined mapping of the gene for thiamine-responsive megaloblastic anemia syndrome in a 4 cM region and evidence for genetic homogeneity. Hum Genet 1998;103:455–461.
65. Labay V, Raz T, Baron D, et al. Mutations in SLC19A2 cause thiamine-responsive megaloblastic anaemia associated with diabetes mellitus and deafness. Nat Genet 1999;22:300–304.
66. Fleming J, Tartaglini E, Steinkanp M, Schorderet D, Cohen N, Neufeld E. The gene mutated in thiamine-responsive anaemia with diabetes and deafness (TRMA) encodes a functional thiamine transporter. Nat Genet 1999;22:305–308.
67. Diaz G, Banikazemi M, Oishi K, Desnick R, Belb B. Mutations in a new gene encoding a thiamine transporter cause thiamine-responsive megaloblastic anaemia syndrome. Nat Genet 1999;22:309–312.
68. Raz T, Labay V, Baron D, et al. The spectrum of mutations, including 4 novel ones, in the thiamine-responsive megaloblastic anaemia gene SLC19A2 of eight families. Hum Mutat 2000;16:37–42.
69. O'Rahilly S, Moller D. Mutant insulin receptors in syndromes of insulin resistance. Clin Endocrinol (Oxford) 1992;36:121–132.
70. Krook A, Kumar S, Laing I, Boulton A, Wass J, O'Rahilly S. Molecular scanning of the insulin receptor gene in syndromes of insulin resistance. Diabetes 1994;43:357–368.
71. Krook A, Soos MA, Kumar S, Siddle K, O'Rahilly S. Functional activation of mutant human insulin receptor by monoclonal antibody. Lancet 1996;347:1586–1590.
72. Cantani A, Ziruolo M, Tacconi ML. A rare polydysmorphic syndrome: leprechaunism—review of 49 cases reported in the literature. Ann Genet 1987;30:221–227.
73. Ellis E, Kemp S, Frindik J, Elders M. Glomerulonephropathy in patient with Donohue syndrome (leprechaunism). Diabetes Care 1991;14:413–414.
74. Baynes K, Whitehead J, Krook A, O'Rahilly S. Molecular mechanisms of inherited insulin resistance. Q J Med 1997;90:557–562.
75. Barroso I, Gurnell M, Crowley V, et al. Dominant negative mutations in human PPARγ associated with severe insulin resistance, diabetes mellitus and hypertension. Nature 1999;402:880–883.
76. Laurence J, Moon R. Four cases of "retinitis pigmentosa" occurring in the same family, and accompanied by general imperfections of development. Ophthalmol Rev 1866;2:32–41.
77. Bardet G. Sur un syndrome d'obesite congenitale avec polydactylie et retinite pigmentaire (contribution a l'etude des formes clinique de l'obesite hypophysaire). Thesis, Paris, 1920.
78. Green J, Parfrey P, Harnett J, et al. The cardinal manifestations of Bardet–Biedl syndrome, a form of Lawrence–Moon–Biedl syndrome. N Engl J Med 1989;321:1002–1009.
79. Beales P, Elcioglu N, Woolf A, Parker D, Flinter F. New criteria for improved diagnosis of Bardet–Biedl syndrome: results of a population survey. J Med Genet 1999;36:437–446.
80. Leppert M, Baird L, Anderson K, Otterud D, Lupskin J, Lewis R. Bardet–Biedl syndrome is linked to DNA markers on chromosome 11q and is genetically heterogeneous. Nat Genet 1994;7:108–112.
81. Kwitek-Black A, Carmi R, Duyk G, et al. Linkage of Bardet–Biedl syndrome to chromosome 16q and evidence for non-allelic genetic heterogeneity. Nat Genet 1993;5:392–396.

82. Sheffield V, Carmi R, Kwitek-Black A, et al. Identification of a Bardet–Biedl syndrome locus on chromosome 3 and evaluation of an efficient approach to homozygosity mapping. Hum Mol Genet 1994;3:1331–1335.
83. Carmi R, Rokhlina T, Kwitek-Black A, et al. Use of a DNA pooling strategy to identify a human obesity locus on chromosome 15. Hum Mol Genet 1995;4:9–13.
84. Young T, Penny L, Woods M, et al. A fifth locus for Bardet–Biedl syndrome maps to 2q31. Am J Hum Genet 1999;64:900–904.
85. Katsanis N, Beales P, Woods M, et al. Mutations in MKKS cause obesity, retinal dystrophy and renal malformations associated with Bardet–Biedl syndrome. Nat Genet 2000;26:67–70.
86. Alstrom C, Hallgren B, Nilsson L, Asander H. Retinal degeneration combined with obesity, diabetes mellitus and neurogenous deafness: a specific syndrome (not hitherto described) distinct from the Laurence–Moon–Bardet–Biedl syndrome: a clinical, endocrinological and genetic examination based on. Acta Psychiatr Neuro Scand 1959;34:1–35.
87. Marshall J, Ludman M, Shea S, et al. Genealogy, natural history, and phenotype of Alstom syndrome in a large Acadian kindred and three additional families. Am J Med Genet 1997;73:150–161.
88. Collin G, Marshall J, Cardon L, Nishina P. Homozygosity mapping at Alstrom syndrome to chromosome 2p. Hum Mol Genet 1997;6:213–219.
89. Noben-Trauth K, Naggert J, North M, Nishina P. A candidate gene for the mouse mutation tubby. Nature 1996;380:534–538.
90. Prader A, Labhart A, Willi H. Ein Syndrom von Adipositas, Kleinwuchs, Kryptorchidismus und Oligophrenie nach myotoniergem Zustand im Neugeborenalter. Schweiz Med Wochenschr 1956;86:1260–1261.
91. Burd L, Vesely B, Martsolf J, Kerbeshian J. Prevalence study of Prader–Willi syndrome in North Dakota. Am J Med Genet 1989;37:97–99.
92. Cassidy S. Prader–Willi syndrome. J Med Genet 1997;34:917–923.
93. Zipf W. Glucose homeostasis in Prader–Willi syndrome and potential implications of growth hormone therapy. Acta Paediatr 1999;88(Suppl):115–117.
94. Mann M, Bartolomei M. Towards a molecular understanding of Prader–Willi and Angelman syndromes. Hum Mol Genet 1999;8:1867–1873.

II TREATMENT OF TYPE 1 DIABETES

9 Diabetic Ketoacidosis

Ram K. Menon, MD *and Mark A. Sperling,* MD

CONTENTS

INTRODUCTION

Diabetic ketoacidosis (DKA) is a potentially life-threatening medical emergency that reflects a state of metabolic decompensation in patients with insulin-dependent diabetes mellitus (IDDM) *(1–6)*. It should be distinguished from nonketotic hyperglycemic–hyperosmolar syndrome with which it shares some similarities in pathophysiology and treatment *(1)*. At least 25% of patients with new-onset diabetes mellitus type 1, especially children, will present in ketoacidosis *(2);* infections and silent or overt myocardial infarction may trigger decompensation to DKA *(1–6)*. However, the most common cause for DKA in patients with established diabetes is inadvertent or deliberate omission of insulin *(7)*. In this chapter, we provide an overview of the pathogenesis and management of DKA and describe in greater detail some of the unique features of DKA in children.

DEFINITION

Diabetic ketoacidosis is characterized by hyperglycemia, ketonemia with total ketones (β-hydroxybutyrate and acetoacetate) in serum exceeding 3 m*M,* and acidosis with blood pH lower than 7.3 or a serum bicarbonate lower than 15 meq/L *(1–7)*. A blood glucose concentration over 300 mg/dL is usually present in DKA. However, hyperglycemia is not a *sine qua non* for its diagnosis because DKA can occur with blood glucose less than 300 mg/dL and, rarely, even with normal blood glucose concentrations if, for example, vomiting with resulting reduced carbohydrate assimilation ensues while insulin administration is continued *(8)*. Ketonemia is usually diagnosed by demonstrating a positive sodium nitroprusside reaction (Acetest, Ketostix, Chemstrips UGK) with 1 : 2 dilution of serum or undiluted urine. Acidosis in DKA is predominantly the result of the accumulation of ketoacids and is thus characterized by an increased anion gap *(9)*. Other mechanisms contributing to acidosis include lactic aci-

From: *Contemporary Endocrinology: Type 1 Diabetes: Etiology and Treatment*
Edited by: M. A. Sperling © Humana Press Inc., Totowa, NJ

dosis from tissue hypoperfusion and hyperchloremic acidosis, particularly during therapy with intravenous fluids *(9–10)*. The spectrum of acidosis encountered in DKA usually extends from pure ketoacidosis to a mixture of keto, lactic, and hyperchloremic acidosis *(1–4,9,10)*. However, a patient may present with predominant hyperchloremic acidosis and, hence, normal anion gap *(9)*. Some suggest that patients with pure hyperchloremic acidosis may experience a slower recovery from their metabolic decompensation *(9)*. It should also be emphasized that the degree of acidosis bears no relation to the degree of hyperglycemia.

In addition to nonketotic hyperglycemic hyperosmolar coma, DKA should be distinguished from lactic acidosis, another metabolic condition that may be confused with DKA, which is characterized by blood lactate values (> 7 m*M*) rarely encountered in DKA *(9,10)*.

BIOCHEMICAL PATHOPHYSIOLOGY

Actions of Insulin and Glucagon

The cardinal hormonal alteration that triggers the metabolic decompensation of DKA is insulin deficiency accompanied by an excess of glucagon and the stress hormones epinephrine, norepinephrine, cortisol, and growth hormone *(2,3,6)*. Insulin stimulates anabolic processes in liver, muscle, and adipose tissues and thereby permits glucose utilization and storage of the energy as glycogen, protein, and fat (*see* Table 1). Concurrent with these anabolic actions, insulin inhibits catabolic processes such as glycogenolysis, gluconeogenesis, proteolysis, lipolysis, and ketogenesis. Insulin deficiency curtails glucose utilization by insulin-sensitive tissues, disinhibits lipolysis in adipose tissue, and enhances protein breakdown in muscle. Glucagon acting unopposed by insulin causes increased glycogenolysis, gluconeogenesis, and ketogenesis.

Although insulin and glucagon may be considered as the primary hormones responsible for the development of DKA, increased levels of the stress hormones epinephrine, norepinephrine, cortisol, and growth hormone play critical auxiliary roles. Epinephrine and norepinephrine activate glycogenolysis, gluconeogenesis, and lipolysis and inhibit insulin release by the pancreas. Cortisol elevates blood glucose concentration by decreasing glucose utilization in muscle and by stimulating gluconeogenesis. Growth hormone increases lipolysis and impairs insulin's action on muscle. The catabolic and metabolic effects of each of these counterregulatory hormones are accentuated during insulin deficiency *(2,3,6)*. Under experimental conditions, the hyperglycemic effect of all of these counterregulatory hormones infused together is greater than the sum of the effects of the individual hormones; that is, the effects are synergistic and not merely additive. Even in normal persons, high concentrations of these counterregulatory hormones can induce hyperglycemia and ketonemia, a phenomenon that may explain the rapid development of DKA during stress induced by infection, vomiting, trauma, and infarction (in patients with IDDM) *(1)*. Acute psychological stress induced by anger and rage may also precipitate DKA in some patients *(2,11)*. Indeed, there is consensus that although insulin deficiency *per se* is a prerequisite for the development of DKA, the complete features of metabolic decompensation characteristic of DKA are the result of the elevated levels and actions of the stress counterregulatory hormones *(1–7)*.

Table 1
Major Metabolic Events During the Fed and Fasted States

Tissue	*High-insulin (fed) state*	*Low-insulin (fasted) state*
Liver	Glucose uptake	Glucose production
	Glycogen synthesis	Glycogenolysis
	Lipogenesis	Absent lipogenesis
	Absent ketogenesis	Ketogenesis
	Absent gluconeogenesis	Gluconeogenesis
Muscle	Glucose uptake	Absent glucose uptake
	Glucose oxidation	Fatty acid α ketone oxidation
	Glycogen synthesis	Glycogenolysis
	Protein synthesis	Proteolysis and amino acid release
Adipose tissue	Glucose uptake	Absent glucose uptake
	Lipid synthesis	Lipolysis and fatty acid release
	Triglyceride uptake	Absent triglyceride uptake

Source: From ref. *2.*

Ketogenesis

The keto acids relevant to DKA are β-hydroxybutyric acid and acetoacetic acid *(2,3,6)*. The primary mode of keto acid generation is from free fatty acids (FFAs). Released from triglycerides in adipose tissue, FFAs are transported to the liver, where they are converted to acyl-CoA derivatives in the cytosol of hepatocytes. These acyl-CoA derivatives enter the mitochondria as carnitine esters via a process catalyzed by carnitine acyl transferase I (CAT I) (*see* Fig. 1). In the mitochondria, acyl-CoA is regenerated and subsequently oxidized to acetyl-CoA. Acetyl-CoA condenses with acetoacetyl-CoA to form β-hydroxy-β-methylglutaryl-CoA (HMGCoA), which then splits to form acetoacetate and acetyl-CoA. Acetoacetate is converted to β-hydroxybutyrate in the presence of NADH. The net metabolic effect of ketone formation is the accumulation of keto anions and the formation of three hydrogen ions for every triglyceride molecule metabolized to ketones *(3)*.

Low insulin and elevated glucagon concentrations facilitate the release of FFA from adipose stores; the opposite hormonal milieu of elevated insulin and low glucagon concentrations inhibits keto acid production. In the whole animal, keto acid generation is, to the greatest extent, regulated by the substrate, (i.e., FFA availability) *(3)*. The rate of accumulation of keto acids is dependent on the ability of the tricarboxylic acid (TCA) cycle to utilize acetyl-CoA and the rate at which acetyl-CoA is generated. Evidence indicates that overproduction of acetyl-CoA and not reduced TCA cycle activity is the major mechanism for the increase in keto acids in DKA *(3)*.

Acetone is a neutral compound with no effect on blood pH; it is formed by the nonenzymatic decarboxylation of acetoacetate. Acetone is metabolically of little importance, but it provides an important bedside clinical clue to the diagnosis of DKA because of its characteristic odor and excretion via expired air and urine. In the normal fasting state, the ratio of serum β-hydroxybutyrate to acetoacetate is of the order of 3 : 1. The rate of interconversion of acetoacetate and β-hydroxybutyrate depends on the cellular redox state (*see* Fig. 2). A reduced redox state, as encountered in DKA, favors the formation of β-hydroxybutyrate, whereas an increase in the redox state associated

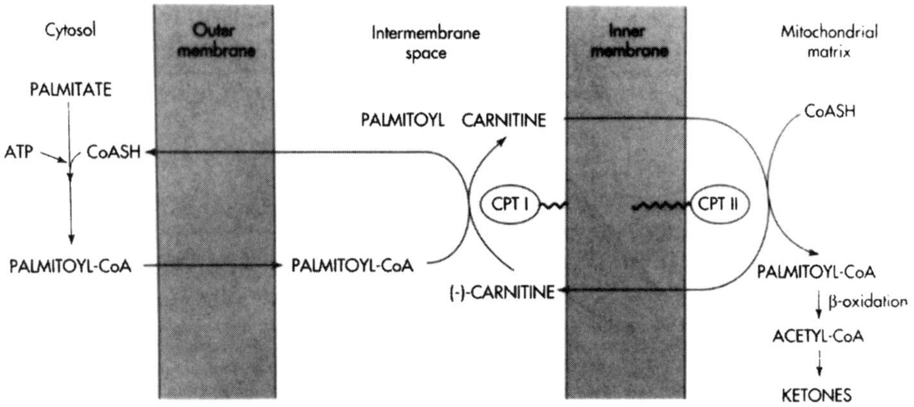

Fig. 1. Fatty acid oxidation system in the liver. The inner mitochondrial membrane is impermeable to long-chain fatty acyl-CoA but permeable to fatty acylcarnitine. Formation of the carnitine ester is catalyzed by carnitine palmitoyltransferase I (CPT I), the rate-limiting step in the sequence. This enzyme is inhibited by malony-CoA. The transesterification reaction is reversed inside mitochondria by CPT II. the majority of fatty acid molecules entering the mitochondria are converted to ketones, only a small amount of the acetyl-CoA generated being oxidized in the tricarboxylic acid cycle. (From Unger RH, Foster DW. Diabetes mellitus. In: Wilson JD, Foster DW, eds., Williams Textbook of Endocrinology, 7th ed. WB Saunders, Philadelphia, 1985.)

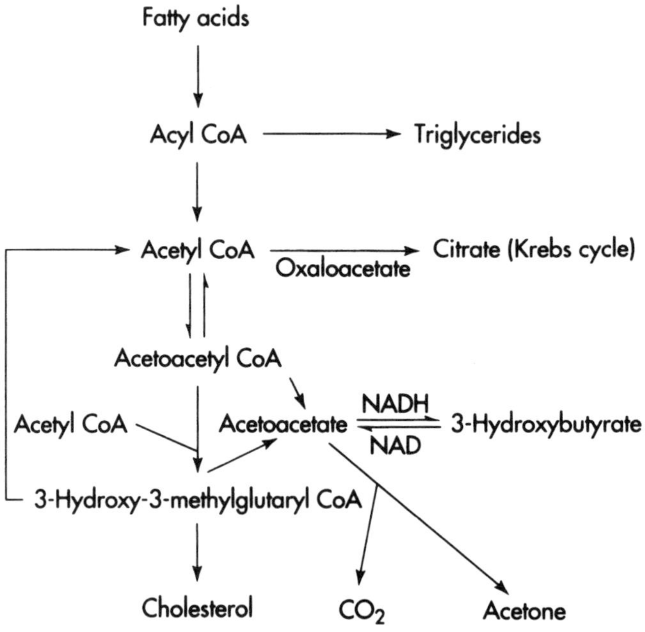

Fig. 2. Generation of ketone bodies. Simplified schema of the formation of the major ketone bodies: acetoacetate (AA). β-hydroxybutyrate (BHOB), and acetone. Note the preferential formation of BHOB from AA with acidosis and, conversely, the dissociation of BHOB to AA when acidosis resolves. The nitroprusside reaction commonly used to detect ketone bodies reacts strongly with AA, weakly with acetone, and not at all with BHOB. *See* text for significance.

with recovery from DKA favors the conversion of β-hydroxybutyric acid to acetoacetic acid. Thus, in severe DKA the ratio of β-hydroxybutyric acid to acetoacetic acid is usually about 7 : 1 and may even increase to 15 : 1 *(1–6)*. The nitroprusside reaction used in the semiquantitative and qualitative tests (Acetest, Ketostix, Chemstrips UGK) for ketonemia and ketonuria does not measure β-hydroxybutyric acid, reacts weakly with acetone, and predominantly measures acetoacetic acid. About 80% of the color reaction in the nitroprusside test is a result of acetoacetate, and acetoacetate comprises only one-third to one-fifteenth of the total ketone bodies in the circulation during DKA *(2)*. Thus, the usual bedside tests for ketones provide a gross underestimation of the total ketone body concentration. This laboratory artifact has important implications for the management of patients with DKA. First, the absence of a positive nitroprusside reaction does not necessarily imply the absence of ketoacidosis. Conversely, the persistence or even an increase in the color reaction of the nitroprusside test should not be assumed to be the result of a deteriorating metabolic response to treatment. This is because with improvement in the metabolic status of the patient, the concomitant increase in the cellular redox state results in the conversion of the "unmeasured" β-hydroxybutyric acid to "measured" acetoacetate and an apparent worsening of the ketonemic state. False-positive reactions for ketones with the nitroprusside reaction, although rare, can occur as a result of the presence of drugs such as captopril in the urine *(2,3)*.

Lactic Acidosis

Lactate is formed primarily as the end product of anaerobic metabolism of glucose *(10)*. Lactate can be synthesized by virtually every tissue in the body, although, under basal conditions, the daily lactate generation of 15–20 mmol/kg is predominantly derived from muscle, skin, erythrocytes, brain, and the gastrointestinal tract *(10)*. Under basal conditions, the daily rate of lactate production is balanced by a matching degree of utilization. Lactate can be converted back to glucose by the gluconeogenic enzymes pyruvate carboxykinase and phosphoenolpyruvate carboxykinase (*see* Fig. 3). Under basal conditions, the liver accounts for approximately two-thirds and the kidneys one-third of lactate consumption. Lactic acidosis caused by hypoxia results from an overproduction of lactate by skeletal muscle and the gastrointestinal tract, with a concomitant reduction in the capacity for lactate utilization by the liver and kidney. Although DKA *per se* does not result in an increase in blood lactic acid concentrations, severe DKA may be complicated by tissue hypoxia, which results in lactic acidosis.

Fluid and Electrolyte Losses

Fluid and electrolyte abnormalities are virtually universal in patients with DKA, and, if unrecognized or mismanaged, contribute significantly to the morbidity and mortality of DKA *(1–6)*. Fluid and electrolyte losses in DKA vary so that the extent of these losses is unpredictable in any given patient. However, estimates of losses that form the basis of the initial management of DKA have been formulated (*see* Table 2). It is emphasized that these recommendations are only guidelines, that each patient should be closely monitored, and that the response to the initial therapy dictates any subsequent changes.

Water and electrolyte losses from the extracellular compartment occur via osmotic diuresis brought about by hyperglycemia, via the respiratory tract because of hyperventilation as a result of metabolic acidosis and via the gastrointestinal tract because of vom-

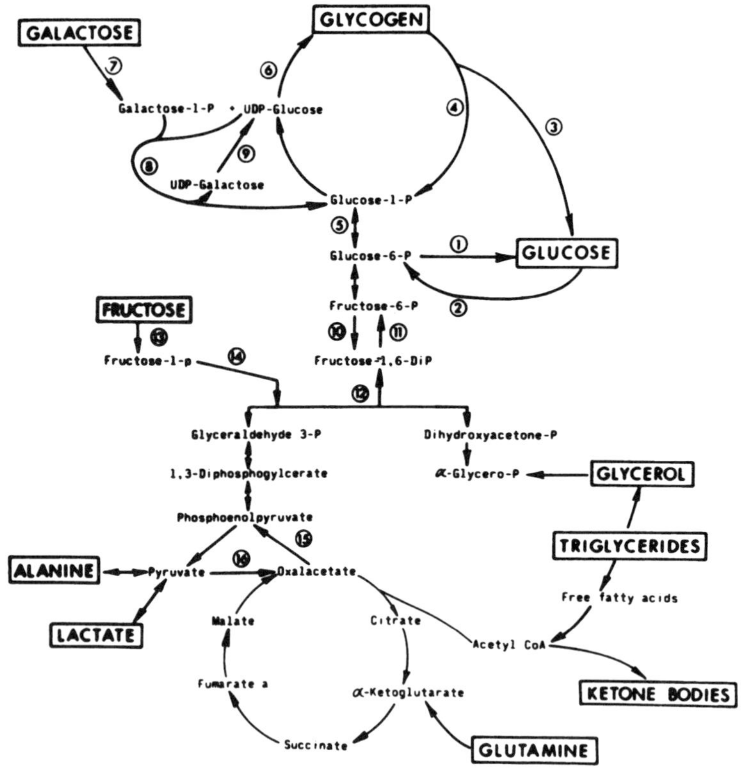

Fig. 3. Key metabolic pathways of intermediary metabolism. Disruption of the elements of these pathways may be pathogenetic in the development of hypoglycemia. Not shown is the hormonal control of these pathways: 1, glucose-6-phosphatase; 2, glucokinase; 3, amylo-1,6-glucosidase; 4, phosphorylase; 5, phosphoglucomutase; 6, glycogen synthetase; 7, galactokinase; 8, galactose-1-phosphate uridyl transferase; 9, uridine diphosphogalactose-4-epimerase; 10, phosphofructokinase; 11, fructose-1,6-diphosphatase; 12, fructose-1,6-diphosphate aldolase; 13, fructokinase; 14, fructose-1-phosphate aldolase; 15, phosphoenolypyruvate carboxykinase; 16, pyruvate carboxylase. [From Pagliara AS, et al. Hypoglycemia in infancy and childhood. J Pediatr 82:365 (Pt 1), 558, (Pt 2), 1973.]

iting. In DKA, there is an osmotically driven shift of water from the intracellular to the extracellular compartment. This phenomenon results in a clinical underestimation of the extent of dehydration and is responsible for the unusual laboratory finding of hyponatremia despite dehydration and hyperosmolarity. It is estimated that for every 3 m*M* increase in glucose, there will be a 1 m*M* fall in plasma sodium concentration. Spurious hyponatremia may also result from lipemic plasma because sodium is distributed only in water, but the volume of the sample taken into account for the calculation of sodium concentration includes the space occupied by lipids and other solids. This artifact can be avoided if special electrodes are used for the estimation of serum or plasma sodium concentration. Serum potassium levels in DKA are variable but tend to be at the upper limits of normal in the majority of patients at initial presentation. However, even when serum potassium is normal, there is almost always depletion of total-body potassium stores. Several factors contribute to these alterations of potassium balance. Serum potassium tends to be elevated because insulin deficiency *per se* will reduce the Na^+/K^+-ATPase activity with a decrease in sodium–potassium exchange across the cell membrane. In

Table 2
Fluid and Electrolyte Maintenance and Losses in Diabetic Ketoacidosis

Element	*Maintenance requirements*[a]	*Losses*[b]
Water	1500 mL/m^2	100 mg/kg (range: 60–100)
Sodium	45 meq/m^2	6 meq/kg (range: 5–13)
Potassium	35 meq/m^2	5 meq/kg (range: 4–6)
Chloride	30 meq/m^2	4 meq/kg (range: 3–9)
Phosphate	10 meq/m^2	3 meq/kg (range: 2–5)

[a] Maintenance is epxressed in surface area to permit uniformity because fluid requirements change as weight increases.

[b] Losses are expressed per unit of body weight because the losses remain relatively constant as a function of total body weight.

Source: From ref. *2.*

addition, acidosis will cause a movement of intracellular potassium to the extracellular–intravascular compartment in exchange for hydrogen ions moving into the cell along a concentration gradient. Hyperglycemia *per se* and impairment of renal function also tend to keep the serum potassium levels elevated. The potassium entering the intravascular compartment is then lost in part via osmotic diuresis and vomiting and in part via the actions of aldosterone, elevated in response to volume depletion.

Initiation of therapy may result in a rapid decrease in serum potassium levels with disastrous consequences if adequate potassium supplementation is not instituted, making hypokalemia one of the avoidable causes of fatality in DKA. Correction of acidosis, restoration of intravascular volume, administration of insulin, and improvement in renal function all tend to decrease extracellular concentration of potassium. In addition, if bicarbonate is provided, the hypokalemic effects of the above-mentioned factors are compounded *(12).* It is estimated that about one-quarter to one-half of the potassium administered during fluid replacement therapy is lost in the urine. Patients with urinary losses greatly exceeding these estimates (potassium sink) have been described; such patients are at a serious risk of hypokalemia. Hence, potassium supplements should be provided early in the course of therapy; contrary to the usual practice of avoiding potassium infusion in patients with renal failure, patients with DKA and compromised renal function may need careful potassium supplementation because insulin therapy will promote cellular uptake of extracellular potassium and favor the development of hypokalemia. These considerations about potassium balance in DKA emphasize the need for frequent and meticulous monitoring of serum potassium concentrations, with adjustments in the therapeutic regimen tailored to each individual patient's response rather than reliance on a "standard" protocol *(1–6,12,13).*

Disturbances in phosphorus homeostasis must also be considered during the management of patients with DKA. Because DKA is a catabolic state, it is accompanied by a shift of intracellular phosphate into the extracellular compartment, with subsequent loss via urine, leading to depletion of total-body phosphorus. As in the case of potassium, serum phosphate concentrations do not provide an accurate estimate of the total-body phosphate stores. Also, as with potassium, institution of insulin and fluid replacement therapy results in a shift of extracellular phosphate into the intracellular compartment and, therefore, frequently leads to a hypophosphatemic state *(1–4,13,14).*

Hypophosphatemia impairs insulin action and will result in a decrease in synthesis of ATP and other energy intermediates. Phosphate deficiency will also result in a depletion of 2,3-diphosphoglycerate (2,3-DPG). Depletion of 2,3-DPG leads to a shift in the oxygen–hemoglobin dissociation curve to the left; that is, it increases the affinity of hemoglobin for oxygen and hence decreases the amount of oxygen released to the tissues. Concurrent acidosis shifts the oxygen–hemoglobin dissociation curve to the right (Bohr effect) so that the effect of 2,3-DPG deficiency is offset by DKA. However, after institution of treatment, the amelioration of the acidotic state may unmask the deleterious effect of hypophosphatemia on tissue oxygen supply. Inclusion of phosphate in the therapeutic regimen is therefore recommended and has been shown to lead to the normalization of 2,3-DPG levels within 24 h, whereas without phosphate supplementation, this process may take 3–4 d *(13)*. Phosphate is recommended and usually provided as potassium phosphate. This form of replacement confers an additional advantage in that it facilitates a reduction in the amount of chloride administered as potassium chloride to replace potassium losses and thus helps to avoid the development of hyperchloremic acidosis. Despite these theoretical reasons for phosphate supplementation, clinical studies have, by and large, failed to substantiate an unequivocal advantage of phosphate therapy in terms of either decreased morbidity and mortality or shortened recovery time *(14)*. Hence, the decision to administer phosphate must be made on an individual basis and not as a routine measure, especially as there exists a danger of precipitating hyperphosphatemia and hypocalcemia *(14,15)*.

Precipitating Factors

The cardinal feature of DKA is a deficiency of insulin action brought about by an absolute or relative lack of insulin *(1,7,16)*. In newly diagnosed patients or when insulin therapy has been omitted, an absolute lack of insulin is responsible for the development of DKA *(7,16)*. In contrast, during acute illness, stress, most commonly the result of an infection, causes DKA to result from a relative deficiency of insulin, with insulin's action opposed by the surge in the counterregulatory hormones, glucagon, catecholamines, cortisol, and growth hormone *(1–4)*. Acute and severe emotional stress may be an important precipitating factor for DKA in children *(6,11)*. In most instances, emotional factors such as parental discord, peer pressure at school, and adolescent adjustment problems may serve to worsen an already disturbed metabolic state *(6,7)*. In rare instances, these factors may appear to be the sole precipitating cause for DKA. However, the most common precipitating change in patients with established diabetes is deliberate or inadvertent omission of insulin *(7)*. Deliberate omission of insulin resulting in recurrent episodes of ketoacidosis may be pathognomonic for an intolerable home environment and may signal the patient's plea to be removed from this situation. The use of steroids or other drugs that antagonize insulin action may also precipitate DKA in a patient taking insulin. Examples include "bursts" of steroids in patients with asthma, with cystic fibrosis-related diabetes, and after solid organ transplantation, where imminent rejection is treated by a combination of agents that inhibit insulin secretion such as cyclosporin or tacrolimus along with steroids that, together, can bring about diabetes and DKA *(2)*.

Clinical Features

Polyuria, polydipsia, and weight loss are nearly always present historically in a patient with DKA. Metabolic acidosis initiates hyperventilation to compensate for acidosis by respiratory alkalosis. This is the typical Kussmaul respiration: deep, sighing, and rapid. However, in severe acidemia, respiration may be depressed, with an absence of Kussmaul breathing. In very young children, especially those below the age of 1 yr, the rapidity of development of DKA may blur these symptoms, and the patient may present in coma without the parents noticing the classical triad of symptoms. The degree of cerebral obtundation is related to the degree of hyperosmolarity and may vary from drowsiness to deep coma *(3–6)*.

Vomiting is both a precipitating factor and a symptom of DKA. Acute abdominal pain is not uncommon in DKA and may simulate acute appendicitis or pancreatitis. Elevation in nonspecific serum amylase can occur in DKA, but without pancreatitis, serum lipase is normal *(17)*. In most cases, the abdominal pain, if not surgical in origin, resolves within a few hours of fluid and insulin treatment. Hence, it is recommended that a decision to intervene surgically be made only after an adequate trial of fluid and insulin therapy for DKA. However, appendicitis and other causes of a surgical abdomen must be carefully evaluated, including the possibility of bowel infarction from vascular obstruction in long-standing diabetes. Although, infection is the most common precipitating factor for DKA, the presence of an elevated white cell count with polymorphonuclear leukocytosis need not necessarily indicate acute infection; these findings may exist in DKA *per se* as part of an acute stress response. The presence of fever should be taken as an indicator of infection and excluded by clinical examination and appropriate laboratory tests.

The classical patient with DKA is characterized by dehydration, acidosis with hyperventilation, with varying degrees of cerebral obtundation, and peripheral circulatory compromise. Again, the most common precipitating factors following initial presentation are omission of insulin, infection, and, in adults, typical or atypical myocardial infarction *(1,7)*.

Laboratory Findings

Laboratory investigations in the management of DKA are required for three purposes: (1) diagnosis of DKA, to include blood glucose, blood acid–base status, and documentation of ketonemia; (2) identification of precipitating and complicating factors, to include complete blood count, serum electrolytes, renal function, chest X-ray, ECG, urine culture, and blood culture, if necessary; (3) monitoring the effect of the therapeutic regimen, to include serum electrolytes, glucose, phosphate, magnesium, calcium, ECG, acid–base status, and serum and urine ketones. Other investigations such as a cranial computed tomography (CT) scan or abdominal ultrasound may be indicated, depending on whether the evolution of cerebral edema or an acute surgical abdomen is being considered *(18)*.

Treatment

The goals of treatment are (1) correction of the metabolic disturbances, particularly hyperglycemia, ketonemia, and acidosis, (2) treatment of precipitating factors, (3) prevention and early identification of complications resulting from the therapy for DKA, and (4) prevention of recurrence.

Although there are broad guidelines and principles that should be adhered to in managing DKA, it cannot be overemphasized that the management must be individualized, depending on the patient's initial condition and response to therapy. Children younger than 2 yr of age or those with an arterial pH of less than 7.0, blood glucose greater than 1000 mg/dL, or altered mentation are best managed in an intensive care unit or an equivalent setting, where close monitoring of metabolic changes and meticulous supervision of therapy can be provided by experienced personnel. A flowsheet detailing the composition of intravenously administered fluid, oral fluid intake, fluid output, timing and dose of insulin administered, electrolyte and acid–base status, and clinical parameters (pulse, respiration, blood pressure, and conscious state) should be maintained; such a flowsheet is essential in monitoring the patient's progress. Bladder catheterization may be needed; urine bag collection or condom drainage usually provide an adequately accurate estimate of urine output in children. Repeated measurements of glucose, acid–base status, and serum electrolytes are obtained at 2-h intervals for the initial 8 h, at 4-h intervals for the next 16 h, and then every 6–12 h until acidosis is completely resolved and the patient is fully conscious and able to tolerate an adequate oral fluid intake without vomiting.

The varying requirements with age and the relatively small volumes involved in the computation of fluid and electrolyte requirements of a child with DKA dictate that these be more carefully calculated than those of a typical adult. The maintenance fluid requirement of a child changes as the child grows but is constant when expressed per unit of surface area; it is not constant when expressed per unit of body weight. In general, 1500 mL/m^2 is accepted as maintenance fluid requirement. By contrast, dehydration is expressed as a percentage of body weight; that is, 10% dehydration implies a loss of 10% of the body weight as water (*see* Table 3). Because different patients have different body weights, it is imperative to relate dehydration to an individual's weight. At presentation, clinical assessment usually underestimates the degree of dehydration. For practical purposes, it can generally be assumed that patients in DKA are initially at least 10% dehydrated. The total fluid to be administered is the sum of maintenance and estimated deficit plus ongoing losses. Table 4 outlines an example of a replacement procedure in a child of 30 kg and 1.0 m^2 in surface area. Clearly, this example can be modified to suit the weight and surface area of any individual patient in DKA but must take into consideration associated conditions such as cardiac or renal impairment. Replacement is extended over 36–48 h in order to reduce the likelihood of too rapid a drop in plasma osmolality, a factor implicated by some as predisposing to cerebral edema *(19–25)*. However, it is not proven that medical treatment can cause or prevent cerebral edema in children with DKA *(26–28)*. To reduce the potential for developing cerebral edema, the initial replacement fluid is generally recommended to consist of normal saline (0.9%) so that a gradual decrease in plasma osmolality is achieved. Potassium therapy is initiated in the second hour. Some of the potassium is given as the phosphate in order to provide phosphate repletion and to reduce the provision of excess chloride.

Fluid and electrolyte therapy alone often result in significant clinical and biochemical improvement *(13)*. Hydration alone benefits patients by restoring intravascular volume, decreasing blood concentrations of counterregulatory hormones, and improving insulin sensitivity of the tissues. It is recommended that insulin therapy be deferred until the second hour of fluid therapy, especially in established diabetics who may have received their dose of insulin within hours of presenting in ketoacidosis. However, insulin is absolutely essential to restore acid–base balance and resolve ketoacidosis *(2,3,7)*. The preferred method of insulin delivery is the continuous low-dose intravenous infusion, as outlined in Table 5. Glucose concentrations often reach levels of 200–300 mg/dL before acidosis is completely resolved. Therefore, it is important to continue insulin administration at

Table 3
Fluid and Electrolyte Losses Based on Assumed 10% Dehydration in a Child with Diabetic Ketoacidosis[a]

Fluid and electrolyte	*Approximate accumulated losses with 10% dehydration*	*Approximate requirements for maintenance (36 h)*	*Working total (36 h)*
Water (mL)	3000	2250	5500
Sodium (meq)	180	65	250
Potassium (meq)	150	50	200
Chloride (meq)	120	45	165
Phosphate (meq)	90	15	100

[a] Weight 30 kg; surface area, 1 m^2.
Source: From ref. *2*.

Table 4
Replacement Procedure for a Child (30 kg, 1 m^2) with Diabetic Ketoacidosis (10% Dehydration)

Approximate duration	*Fluid composition*	*Sodium*	*Potassium*	*Chloride*	*Phosphate (meq)*
Hour 1 (500 mL/h)	500 mL of 0.9% NaCI (normal saline)	75	—	75	—
Hour 2 (500 mL/h)	500 mL of 0.45% NaCI (0.5 normal saline) plus 20 meq of KCI	35	20	55	—
Hour 3–12 (200 mL/h for 10 h)	2000 mL of 0.45% saline with 30 meq/L of potassium phosphate	150	60	150	40
Subtotal (initial 12 h)	3000 mL	260	80	280	40
Next 24 h (100 mL/h)	0.2 Normal saline in 5% glucose with 40 meq/L of potassium as the phosphate	75	100	75	60
Total over 36 h	5400 mL	335	180	355	100

Bicarbonate therapy
For pH ≥ 7.10, no therapy necessary.
For pH between 7.00 and 7.10, 40 meq/m^2 of bicarbonate over 2 h, then re-evaluate.
For pH < 7.00, 80 meq/m^2 of bicarbonate over 2 h, then re-evaluate.
New diabetics < 2 yr of age with DKA and 10% dehydration or any diabetic with pH < 7.00 should be managed in an ICU or equivalent setting.

Note: All replacement values should be halved if dehydration is estimated to be 5%. Maintenance requirements remain the same.

the standard rate of 0.1 U/kg/h, (or occasionally 0.05 U/kg/h,) while adding 5% or even 10% glucose to the infusate in order to maintain glucose concentrations between 200 and 300 mg/dL until bicarbonate levels exceed 15 meq/L. Glucose contributes substantially to plasma osmolality, so the reason for maintaining glucose concentration in the range of 200–300 mg/dL is to prevent too rapid a fall in plasma osmolality, a factor implicated by some as predisposing to cerebral edema *(20–26)*.

Table 5
Continuous Low-Dose Intravenous Insulin Therapy for Diabetic Ketoacidosis

Priming dose: 0.1 U/kg regular insulin, intravenously.
Continuous intravenous infusion: 0.1 U/kg/h regular insulin beginning with second hour.
Directions for making insulin infusion: Add 50 U regular insulin (0.5 mL of U 100 insulin, i.e., 100 U/mL, therefore, 0.5 mL of U 100 = 50 U) to 49.5 mL of physiological saline solution (0.9% = normal saline).
Initially infuse at a rate of 0.1 U/kg/h (for 30-kg patient, infuse at a rate of 3.0 mL/h [i.e., 3 U/h]) using a separate infusion pump.
When the blood glucose concentration approaches 300 mg/dL and acidosis is resolved, discontinue the insulin infusion and start insulin therapy by subcutaneous injections of 0.2 to 0.4 U/kg at 6-h intervals; if acidosis persists, as glucose approaches 300 mg/dL, add glucose (D_5 or D_{10}) to insulin infusion.

The decision to switch from intravenous insulin therapy to subcutaneous administration of insulin is based on a stable cardiopulmonary status with normal peripheral perfusion and a blood glucose concentration near 300 mg/dL. Intravenous fluids and intravenous or subcutaneous insulin should be continued until the metabolic acidosis is corrected and the patient is able to tolerate food intake. Subcutaneous insulin therapy is initiated with regular (short acting) insulin given in a dose of 0.2–0.4 U/kg, with the subsequent dose being adjusted every 4–6 h, depending on the response as judged by the blood glucose levels and ketonuria.

Bicarbonate administration is not routinely recommended *(2,12)*. The role of bicarbonate therapy in the management of DKA remains unclear. Severe acidemia (pH < 7) is considered detrimental because of its negative inotropic effect, direct peripheral vasodilatory effect resulting in hypotension, depression of cerebral function, and antagonism of insulin's action. However, the provision of insulin and fluids generally corrects ketoacidosis and elevates the blood pH so that in most patients with DKA, a satisfactory outcome is achieved without the use of bicarbonate. We do not support the use of bicarbonate in patients with arterial pH greater than 7.0, because of the potential drawbacks to the use of bicarbonate for DKA *(2,6)*. Among these drawbacks is hypokalemia, an effect caused by alkolosis shifting potassium intracellularly so that potassium replacement should be carefully adjusted to meet this additional requirement. Other established side effects of bicarbonate therapy include impaired tissue oxygenation with leftward shift of the oxyhemoglobin dissociation curve, rebound alkalosis, sodium overload, and a paradoxical fall in cerebrospinal fluid pH while systemic acidosis is being corrected. This occurs because HCO_3 associates with H^+ to form H_2CO_3 and this dissociates to H_2O and CO_2; whereas CO_2 diffuses freely across the blood-brain barrier, HCO_3 diffuses poorly. Although there is no definite evidence for its efficacy even when the arterial pH is 7.0 or less, some authorities recommend that when the pH is 7.0 or below, 40–80 meq/m^2 (1–2 meq/kg of sodium bicarbonate) be infused over 2 h, followed by reassessment of the clinical status of the patient. Bicarbonate should never be given as a bolus except during cardiopulmonary resuscitation.

Complications

With appropriate therapy, complications of DKA itself are uncommon, but the overriding concern is the precipitating event itself. Precipitating or associated factors for DKA such as myocardial infarction, adult respiratory distress syndrome, mucormycosis, rhabdomyolysis, emphysematous cholecystitis, or malignant otitis externa should be considered in adults but are not usually a consideration in childhood *(1,29)*. Iatrogenic management complications include hypoglycemia, hypocalcemia from too vigorous a use of phosphate, and hypokalemia from inadequate potassium replacement *(1,4,6,15)*.

In children, the major complication of concern during treatment for DKA is cerebral edema and related intracerebral complications *(20–28,30–32)*. This complication of DKA remains a serious problem in children, who are at a disproportionately higher risk for developing clinical cerebral edema as compared to adults with DKA. Clinically relevant cerebral edema is estimated to occur in 0.7–1.0% of episodes of diabetic ketoacidosis in children *(26–28)*. The etiology of this potentially devastating sequence of events remains incompletely understood *(26–28)*. It is both practically and ethically difficult to conduct well-designed prospective studies because of the relatively small number of patients with this complication seen by any given physician or center. Thus, most of the data collated to date regarding this problem have been derived from retrospective studies amalgamating the experience of different physicians and treatment centers, the most recent of which identified approx 60 episodes of cerebral edema over 15 yr from a multicenter survey *(27)*.

Clinically, cerebral edema develops in patients, usually with new-onset diabetes, several hours after the institution of therapy when clinical and biochemical indices suggest improvement. Manifestations of cerebral edema include symptoms and signs of raised intracranial pressure such as headache, deterioration in consciousness, bradycardia, papilledema, development of fixed dilated pupils, and, occasionally, polyuria (secondary to diabetes insipidus), which may be misdiagnosed as osmotic diuresis resulting from hyperglycemia. CT scanning has revealed that subclinical cerebral edema is common in children being treated for DKA *(18)*.

Magnetic resonance imaging (MRI) and CT scanning have additionally indicated that at least some of these children have cerebral thrombosis and infarction in addition to cerebral edema *(26,31)*. In adults, monitoring by indwelling intrathecal catheters indicates that there is a rise in cerebrospinal fluid pressure in all patients during fluid and insulin therapy for DKA *(26)*. In children, subclinical cerebral edema may be present in the majority, as suggested by narrowing of the cerebral ventricles detected by CT scanning during treatment and restoration to normal ventricular size after recovery *(18)*. The cause of this syndrome is believed by some to be a rapid correction of osmotic disequilibrium between brain cells and extracellular fluid brought about by hypotonic fluids and by a precipitous lowering of the blood glucose concentration *(20–29)*. This hypothesis is based on the tenet that in response to the hyperosmolar state of hyperglycemia, brain cells generate "idiogenic osmoles," which increase the intracellular osmotic pressure, thereby maintaining the intracellular water content of these cells *(19)*. With institution of treatment, there is a decrease in the plasma osmolality as a result of hydration and lowering of the plasma glucose concentration. In this milieu, if idiogenic moles dissipate at a rate slower than the rate at which the plasma osmolality is being lowered, then cerebral edema may be precipitated because the brain cells are hyperosmolar with respect to the extracellular compartment *(20–28)*. Experiments in animals, such as the rat, have suggested taurine as one of the idiogenic osmoles that accumulates in DKA *(19,23)*. Other mechanisms and factors implicated in the pathogenesis of cerebral edema in DKA include a direct effect of insulin on the influx of Na^+, K^+, and water into brain cells, activation of the plasma membrane Na^+–H^+ exchanger because of acidosis with movement of Na^+ into the cells *(32)*, inappropriate secretion of antidiuretic hormone, administration of bicarbonate, and cerebral hypoxia resulting in toxic activation of the *N*-methyl-D-aspartate (NMDA) receptor *(28)*. Proof of a dominant role for any single one of these factors is tenuous because none of these mechanisms provides a satisfactory explanation for all of the salient epidemiological features of this complication. In the recent comprehensive survey of cerebral edema in children *(27,28)*, the factors that conferred increased risk were low partial pressure of arterial carbon dioxide and high serum urea nitrogen at presentation and treatment with bicarbonate *(27,33)*. All of these risk factors may reflect more severe metabolic decompensation and longer antecedent duration of metabolic disturbance before intervention. Thus, at the present time, there is no clear explanation for the unique susceptibility of infants and children and the relative lack of this complication in adults with DKA. Also, this complication is rare in the syndrome of nonketotic hyperosmolar coma where the initial hyperosmolarity is considerably greater than that usually encountered in DKA *(1)*. The observation that there is a preponderance of children with new-onset IDDM with this complication compared to children with established IDDM may, again, reflect severity and duration, because the diagnosis of diabetes mellitus has not been considered or recognized until DKA supervenes *(27,28)*. Thus, the only way to avoid cerebral edema is to avoid DKA. One reason why a majority have subclinical brain swelling, whereas only a few (approx 1%) manifest clinically apparent cerebral edema, may relate to the intracranial pressure-volume curve, which demonstrates a steep exponential rise in intracranial pressure beyond a critical volume of cerebral mass *(34)*. For these reasons, it is prudent to anticipate the possibility of clinical cerebral edema in all children treated for DKA and to avoid DKA by heightening awareness of diabetes as a potential diagnosis in unexplained weight loss or other vague symptoms *(2,27,28)*. Some authorities believe that the risks can be reduced by limiting the rate of fluid administration to 4.0 $L/m^2/d$ or less and avoiding the excessive use of bicarbonate *(20–25)*. It has also been suggested that fluid resuscitation in DKA should extend over 48 h and that crystalloid solutions with an average Na^+ concentration of 125 meq/L be utilized so that serum Na^+ levels increase as serum glucose levels decrease; hence, serum osmolality will remain relatively constant, and fluid shifts across the blood-brain barrier will be minimized *(25)*. We consider that in the absence of evidence to the contrary, it is advisable to moderate the rate of fluid administration and restrict the amount of free water provided during the initial phases of the rehydration protocol. As soon as intracranial hypertension is clinically suspected, measures should be taken to reduce brain swelling by the use of mannitol at 10–20 g/m^2/iv (0.25–1.0 g/kg iv) repeated at 2- to 4-h intervals if necessary, reducing the rate of fluid administration, and instituting hyperventilation therapy. Retrospective studies suggest that these measures, instituted promptly, are lifesaving and may avoid neurological sequelae *(30–31)*. Heroic measures such as cerebral decompression via craniotomy are usually desperate measures. Once clinically obvious, cerebral edema is associated with a mortality of about 70% and only 7–14% of these patients escape permanent impairment of neurological function *(31)*.

In summary, DKA is a medical emergency that dictates prompt and careful management, including close clinical and laboratory monitoring. Complications of DKA are uncommon in patients diagnosed promptly and managed appropriately. In adults, an underlying or precipitating event such as infection or infarction must be considered and managed. In children, prudent and prompt management usually results in excellent outcome and prognosis. Recurrent DKA reflects mostly deliberate omission of insulin, especially in adolescents and may be a plea for psychosocial intervention.

REFERENCES

1. Delaney MF, Zisman A, Kettyle WM. Diabetic ketoacidosis and hypergycemic hyperosmolar nonketotic syndrome. Endocrinol Metab Clin North Am 2000;29:683–705.
2. Sperling MA. Diabetes mellitus. In: Sperling MA, ed. Pediatric Endocrinology, 2nd ed. WB Saunders, Philadelphia 2002, pp.
3. Foster DW, McGarry JD. The metabolic derangements and treatment of diabetic ketoacidosis. N Engl J Med 1983;309:159–169.
4. Kitabchi AE, Wall BM. Diabetic ketoacidosis. Med Clin North Am 1995;79:9–37.
5. Lebovitz HE. Diabetic ketoacidosis. Lancet 1995;345:767–772.
6. Sperling MA. Diabetic ketoacidosis. Pediatr Clin North Am 1984;31:591–610.
7. Morris AD, Boyle DIR, McMahon AD, et al. Adherence to insulin treatment, glycaemic control, and ketoacidosis in insulin-dependent diabetes mellitus. Lancet 1997;350:1505–1510.
8. Munro JF, Campbell IW, McCuish AC, et al. Euglycaemic diabetic ketoacidosis. Br Med J 1973;2:578–580.
9. Adrogue HJ, Wilson H, Boyd AE, et al. Plasma acid–base patterns in diabetic ketoacidosis. N Engl J Med 1982;307:1603–1610.
10. Arieff AI. Pathogenesis of lactic acidosis. Diabetes Metab Rev 1989;5:637–649.
11. Winter RJ, Harris CJ, Phillips LS, et al. Diabetic ketoacidosis: induction of hypocalcemia and hypomagnesemia by phosphate therapy. Am J Med 1979;67:897–900.
12. Riley LJ, Cooper M, Narins RG. Alkali therapy of diabetic ketoacidosis: biochemical, physiologic, and clinical perspectives, Diabetes Metab Rev 1989;5:627–636.
13. Waldhausl W, Kleinberger G, Korn A, et al. Severe hyperglycemia: effects of rehydration on endocrine derangements and blood glucose concentrations, Diabetes 1979;28:577–584.
14. Fisher JN, Kitabchi AE. A randomized study of phosphate therapy in the treatment of diabetic ketoacidosis, J Clin Endocrinol Metab 1983;57:177–180.
15. Winter RJ, Harris CJ, Phillips LS, Green OC. Diabetic ketoacidosis. Induction of hypocalcemia and hypomagnesemia by phosphate therapy. Am J Med 1979;67:897–900.
16. Menon RK, Sperling MA. Childhood diabetes. Med Clin North Am 1988;72:1565–1576.
17. Moller-Petersen J, Andersen PT, Hjorne N, et al. Hyperamylasemia, specific pancreatic enzymes, and hypoxanthine during recovery from diabetic ketoacidosis, Clin Chem 1985;31(12):2001–2004.
18. Krane EJ, Rockoff, MA, Wallman JK, et al. Subclinical brain swelling in children during treatment of diabetic ketoacidosis, N Engl J Med 1985;312(18):1147–1151.
19. Arieff AI, Kleeman CR. Studies on mechanisms of cerebral edema in diabetic comas. Effects of hyperglycemia and rapid lowering of plasma glucose in normal rabbits. J Clin Invest 1973;52:571–583.
20. Duck SC, Weldon VV, Pagliara AS, et al. Cerebral edema complicating therapy for diabetic ketoacidosis. Diabetes 1976;25(2):111–115.
21. Duck SC, Wyatt DT. Factors associated with brain herniation in the treatment of diabetic ketoacidosis. J Pediatr 1988;113:10–14.
21. Harris GD, Fiordalisi I, Harris W, et al. Minimizing the risk of brain herniation during treatment of diabetic ketoacidemia: a retrospective and prospective study, J Pediatr 1990;117:22–31.
22. Hammond P, Wallis S. Cerebral oedema in diabetic ketoacidosis. Br Med J 1992;305:203–204.
23. Harris GD, Lohr JW, Fiordalisi I, Acara M. Brain osmoregulation during extreme and moderate dehydration in a rat model of severe DKA. Life Sci 1993;53:185–191.
24. Harris GD, Fiordalisi I, Finberg L, et al. Safe management of diabetic ketoacidemia. J Pediatr 1988;113(1):65–68.
25. Finberg L. Why do patients with diabetic ketoacidosis have cerebral swelling, and why does treatment sometimes make it worse? Arch Pediatr Adolesc Med 1996;150:785–786.
26. Muir A. Do doctors cause or prevent cerebral edema in children with diabetic ketoacidosis? Pediatr Diabetes 2000;1:209–216.
27. Glaser N, Barnett P, McCaslin I, et al. Risk factors for cerebral edema in children with diabetic ketoacidosis. N Engl J Med 2001;344:264–269.

28. Dunger DB, Edge JA. Predicting cerebral edema during diabetic ketoacidosis. N Engl J Med 2001;344:302–303.
29. Carroll P, Matz R. Adult respiratory distress syndrome complicating severely uncontrolled diabetes mellitus: report of nine cases and a review of the literature. Diabetes Care 1982;5:574–580.
30. Bello FA, Sotos JF. Cerebral oedema in diabetic ketoacidosis in children. Lancet 1990;336:64.
31. Rosenbloom AL. Intracerebral crisis during treatment of diabetic ketoacidosis. Diabetes Care 1990;13:22–33.
32. Van der Meulen JA, Klip A, Grinstein S. Possible mechanism for cerebral edema in diabetic edema in ketacidosis. Lancet 1987;2:306–308.
33. Assadi FK, John EG, Fornell MT, et al. Falsely elevated serum creatinine concentration in ketoacidosis. J Pediatr 1985;107:562–564.
34. Marmarou A, Shulman K, Rosende R. A nonlinear analysis of the cerebrospinal fluid system and intracranial pressure dynamic. J Neurosurg 1978;38:332–344.

10 Insulin Regimens for Type 1 Diabetes

Baiju R. Shah, MD, FRCPC and
Bernard Zinman, MDCM, FRCPC, FACP

Contents

PRINCIPLES OF INSULIN TREATMENT

Since insulin was first administered on January 11, 1922 *(1),* treatment of patients with type 1 diabetes has attempted to restore the metabolic abnormalities associated with autoimmune β-cell destruction and insulin deficiency. The ensuing decades have seen many advances in our understanding of insulin physiology, pharmacokinetics, and therapeutics, and the resultant development of purified insulin, recombinant human insulin, and insulin analogs. However, complete metabolic normalization with exogenous insulin therapy in such patients remains infrequent. The Diabetes Control and Complications Trial (DCCT) established conclusively that this inadequate metabolic control results in the long-term microvascular complications of diabetes *(2).* To minimize these complications, insulin-treatment regimens must mimic the complex secretion of insulin by the β-cells of the healthy pancreas. This task, however, remains a challenging goal *(3).*

Normal Insulin Physiology

The healthy pancreas secretes insulin into the portal system in response to daily variations in nutrient intake and energy expenditure. Polonsky et al. carefully characterized the normal 24-h insulin secretion of healthy subjects *(4).* They found that daily insulin secretion was pulsatile and could be divided into two components: a constant basal secretion rate and marked increases in insulin secretion following meals (Fig. 1). The basal component of insulin release, which comprises approximately 40% of the total 24-h insulin secretion, limits glucose release from the liver and free fatty acid

From: *Contemporary Endocrinology: Type 1 Diabetes: Etiology and Treatment*
Edited by: M. A. Sperling © Humana Press Inc., Totowa, NJ

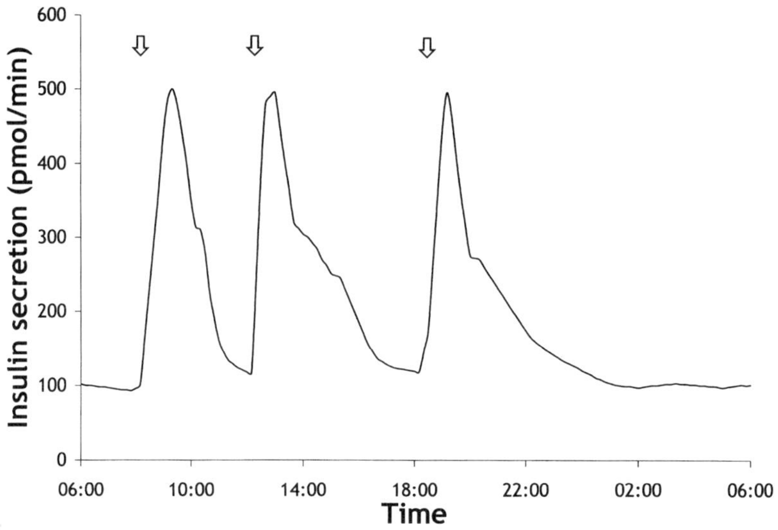

Fig. 1. Mean 24-h profiles of insulin secretion rates in normal subjects. Arrows indicate meals. Basal insulin comprises about 40% of total daily secretion, while abrupt pulses of insulin secretion up to five times basal levels follow ingestion of mixed meals. (Adapted from ref. *4*.)

release from adipose tissue. Following ingestion of a mixed meal, insulin secretion abruptly increases up to fivefold and then gradually falls back to the basal rate over the next 4 h before the subsequent meal. These insulin pulses, which limit postprandial excursions in plasma glucose concentration by inhibiting hepatic glucose production and increasing glucose uptake and storage, are triggered in response to various secretagogues from the diet, including glucose and amino acids.

Exercise and energy expenditure decrease insulin secretion. As glucose uptake and metabolism are increased with exercise, the β-cells maintain euglycemia by reducing the basal insulin secretion, thereby allowing increased glucose release from the liver *(5)*.

TYPES OF INJECTABLE INSULINS

A multitude of sources and types of insulin have been used clinically. The original insulin extracted by Banting, Best, Collip, and MacLeod was derived from a dog pancreas *(1)*. Insulins from cattle and swine of increasing purity soon became the principal source of injectable insulin. These have been replaced by recombinant human insulins developed in the 1980s. Furthermore, advances were made by changing the crystal structure and the media in which insulin was suspended, resulting in altered pharmacokinetics of insulin absorption from subcutaneous tissue *(6)*. More recently, molecular analogs to insulin with tailored pharmacokinetics have been developed (*see* Table 1).

Human Insulins

The first biosynthetic insulin became commercially available in the 1980s *(7)*. Regular recombinant human insulin is an identical polypeptide to endogenous insulin. However, in solution, regular insulin tends to form hexamers that must dissociate into dimers and then monomers before being absorbed from the subcutaneous tissue injection site into the systemic circulation *(8)*. This delay modifies the pharmacologic parameters of

Table 1
Pharmacokinetics of Human Insulins and Recently Developed Insulin Analog for Treatment of Type 1 Diabetes

	Action (h)		
Insulin	*Onset*	*Peak*	*Duration*
Meal insulins			
Regular	0.5	2–5	6–8
Lispro	0.25	0.25	2–4
Aspart	0.25	0.75	2–5
Basal insulins			
NPH	2–3	5–7	13–16
Lente	2–3	7–12	Up to 18
Ultralente	3–4	8–10	Up to 20
Glargine	2	–	24

regular insulin: The onset of biological action is about 30 min after injection, the peak effect is after 2–5 h, and the duration of action up to 8 h.

The duration of insulin activity can be lengthened by changing its suspension, creating the basal insulins. Neutral protamine Hagedorn (NPH) insulin is formed by complexing the insulin with protamine, whereas the lente series is formed by crystallizing insulin with zinc and acetate. These insulins are poorly absorbed from subcutaneous tissue, prolonging their onset, peak, and duration of action. However, as indicated in Table 1, these insulins show significant interpatient and intrapatient variability in their pharmacokinetics.

Premixed insulins, made up of defined proportions of meal and basal insulins, are valuable in the treatment of type 2 diabetes, but are generally not appropriate for use in type 1 diabetes.

Since its introduction, insulin has been life sustaining for patients with type 1 diabetes, and thus is often available without prescription. Although it is relativly inexpensive in the developed world, in many developing countries with limited health care resources, it is not routinely available *(9)*. Indeed, children with type 1 diabetes in sub-Saharan Africa often do not live longer than 1 yr *(10)*.

Animal Insulins

Beef and pork insulins, extracts from the pancreases of cows and pigs, were the only preparations commercially available for most of the history of insulin therapy. They differ from endogenous human insulin by one and three amino acids, respectively. Although they are well absorbed after subcutaneous injection, the amino acid changes slow their absorption slightly compared with recombinant human insulins *(11)*. Additionally, nonhuman insulins are more likely to result in anti-insulin antibody formation *(12)*. These antibodies affect the activity and absorption characteristics of insulin, making its pharmacologic effects more unpredictable. Furthermore, production of animal insulins is dependent on a supply of bovine and porcine pancreases, whereas human insulins are produced synthetically. Because recombinant human insulin is produced more economically than animal insulin and has captured the larger share of the insulin market, some pharmaceutical companies have stopped making animal insulins altogether.

Insulin Analogs

Regular insulin is not truly "rapid acting," as its slow dissociation from hexamers to monomers when injected subcutaneously results in nonphysiologic plasma profiles, even if administered 0.5 h before a meal, as recommended. The delayed absorption results in early postprandial hyperglycemia, with an increased risk of subsequent hypoglycemia several hours after the meal. To address this problem, meal insulin analogs have been developed with amino acid substitutions that change the structure of the molecule and accelerate its absorption after subcutaneous injection *(13)*.

The protein structure of human insulinlike growth factor 1 (IGF-1) is similar to that of human insulin. One of the differences between these two molecules is that the 28th and 29th amino acids in the B-chain of insulin, proline and lysine, are reversed in IGF-1. The observation that IGF-1 has reduced multimer formation led to the development of insulin lispro, with an amino acid sequence identical to insulin except for reversal of these two amino acids: lysine–proline *(14)*. The resulting conformational change reduces dimer formation of lispro by a factor of 300 compared to regular human insulin while maintaining identical biological activity at the insulin receptor. The pharmacokinetics of lispro exhibit a more rapid onset of action, rapid time to peak activity, higher peak of activity, and shorter duration of action. Patients may, therefore, inject lispro insulin immediately before eating. It became the first commercially available synthetic insulin analog, released in 1996.

Numerous studies have documented the effectiveness of lispro in controlling early and late postprandial hyperglycemia *(15)*. It reduces the risk of severe and nocturnal hypoglycemia compared with regular human insulin *(16,17)*. Additionally, the pharmacokinetics of lispro remain constant despite escalating doses, whereas the peak and duration of activity of regular insulin are prolonged with larger doses *(18)*. However, improvement in glycosylated hemoglobin values with lispro treatment has not been consistently documented.

Another rapidly acting insulin analog in clinical practice is insulin aspart. Aspartic acid replaces proline at the B28 position of the molecule. Its negative charge causes repulsion from other aspart molecules, so they remain as monomers and dimers in solution *(19)*. The pharmacokinetic profile of aspart reveals more rapid onset, peak, and duration of activity compared with subcutaneously injected regular insulin *(20)*. Randomized double-blinded trials have demonstrated that aspart provides better postprandial glucose control *(21,22)* and fewer episodes of hypoglycemia *(16,23)* than regular human insulin.

Insulin analogs are also used to provide more physiologic basal insulin action than the traditional basal insulins. For example, lispro complexed with protamine, neutral protamine lispro, has been formulated as a basal insulin. Its pharmacokinetics are similar to NPH insulin and the clinical responses in controlling overnight glycemia are the same *(24)*. Glargine is an insulin analog with prolonged peakless activity and has several molecular modifications compared with regular human insulin. Two arginine molecules are added to the C-terminus of the B-chain, making the molecule soluble at a more acidic pH, and an acid-sensitive asparagine molecule in the A-chain is replaced with a more stable glycine molecule *(25)*. These changes cause glargine to form a microprecipitate in the neutral pH of the subcutaneous tissue, resulting in long-lasting and smooth insulin absorption. Unlike NPH, it does not have a peak action; rather, after increasing for 4 h after injection, its activity remains at a plateau for many hours *(26)*.

In clinical trials, glargine has been demonstrated to give better fasting glucose control *(27,28)* and less nocturnal hypoglycemia than NPH *(29)*.

The development of a series of insulin analogs with improved pharmacokinetic profiles can be expected in the next few years, improving our ability to replace insulin more physiologically.

INSULIN REGIMENS

The purpose of insulin treatment in a patient with newly diagnosed type 1 diabetes is to reverse and correct the symptoms of hyperglycemia and ketosis caused by insulin deficiency. In addition, insulin resistance can be caused by hyperglycemia itself and restoring euglycemia pharmacologically may improve insulin sensitivity sufficiently to allow the residual insulin secretion from the remaining β-cells to prevent ketosis. This early period of pancreatic functional recovery is termed the "honeymoon phase." However, even these β-cells will eventually fail, and long-term insulin replacement therapy will be required. Other short-term goals of therapy include restoration of lost lean body mass, and improvement of exercise capacity and the patient's sense of well-being.

The long-term treatment of choice for type 1 diabetes is an intensive management program, which requires four components:

- *Regular self-monitoring of blood glucose* throughout the day to evaluate the efficacy of the treatment program.
- *An intensive insulin regimen* that reproduces normal pancreatic insulin secretion as closely as possible. It must provide basal insulin replacement, along with boluses of insulin in response to meals.
- *A motivated and skilled patient* who must be willing to monitor glucose control and learn how to respond to and adjust the insulin regimen and the other components of the intensive therapy.
- *A dedicated interdisciplinary team* to support the patient and his or her family.

The goal of such an intensive program is to keep blood glucose concentrations as close to the normal range as possible without excessive hypoglycemia. The DCCT established in 1993 that the complications of diabetes are reduced with intensive treatment. For example, the intensive-treatment group of the study had a relative risk reduction of 76% for developing retinopathy and of 54% for progression of retinopathy compared to conventional therapy *(2)*. The relative risk of proteinuria was reduced by 54% and of neuropathy by 60% *(2)*. Macrovascular disease may have also been diminished with improved glucose control, although these findings were not conclusive. The relative risk reduction for macrovascular events of 41% was not statistically significant *(30)*.

Insulin therapy is initiated on an inpatient basis if the presenting feature of diabetes is ketoacidosis. Indeed, intravenous insulin administration is often required initially. Likewise, initiation of therapy in children may require inpatient management.

As previously stated, daily physiologic insulin secretion by the healthy pancreas is divided equally into basal secretion and episodic pulse secretion in response to meals. Unfortunately, our ability to reproduce this physiologic pattern of insulin release with subcutaneously injected insulin remains imperfect, despite increasing understanding of insulin action and dose adjustment *(3)*.

Intensive Insulin Regimens

The insulin regimens that best accomplish the goals of an intensive management program are multiple daily injections (MDI) of insulin and continuous subcutaneous insulin infusion (CSII).

Four injections of insulin per day are required in MDI regimens. Meal insulins are given in three boluses per day to emulate physiologic insulin pulses with meals, controlling postprandial hyperglycemia. Rapidly acting insulin analogs are the meal insulin of choice because of their superior pharmacokinetic characteristics.

In the healthy pancreas, basal insulin secretion controls hepatic glucose release and provides insulin replacement interprandially. This action is particularly important in dietary practices with a long time between meals. Basal insulin replacement is accomplished with a fourth insulin injection of NPH, lente, ultralente, or glargine at bedtime. However, this single bedtime dose may not be adequate to cover daytime basal requirements, particularly for patients using very rapidly acting analogs as their meal insulin. Indeed, up to one-quarter of such patients receiving a single injection of NPH or ultralente at bedtime will have unacceptable glucose control before dinner *(31)*; these patients require extra basal insulin to be given before their breakfast, too.

The CSII regimens most closely mimic physiologic insulin secretion and were shown to improve glucose control more effectively than MDI *(32)*. A small pump attached to or kept under clothing delivers insulin continuously via a cannula into the subcutaneous tissue. Patients program the pump to deliver a basal rate of insulin. Then, prior to eating, patients can administer a bolus of insulin to counter postprandial hyperglycemia. Lispro used in CSII provides improved control and lower rates of hypoglycemia compared to regular insulin *(33,34)*. Aspart has been shown to be as efficacious as lispro in CSII *(35)*.

CSII therapy gives patients maximum flexibility over the timing of meals. Because the basal insulin infusion continues at all times, a meal can be delayed or even skipped without consequence; in MDI regimens, bolus injections must be given every few hours as the insulin activity from the previous dose ends. However, CSII also has some limitations. Undetected pump malfunction may result in interruption in the delivery of insulin, placing the patient at risk for hyperglycemia and ketoacidosis. In some patients, cellulitis or a subcutaneous abscess may develop at the insertion site of the cannula; this risk can be reduced by changing the cannula location every 2 d. Finally, the pump and the supplies required for its operation are expensive, limiting the widespread use of CSII therapy.

Starting Insulin Doses for Intensive Regimens

The typical starting daily dose of insulin is 0.5 U/kg of body weight, although most patients with type 1 diabetes eventually need about 0.6–0.7 U/kg. However, the total daily dose may be substantially changed in certain circumstances. In pregnancy, doses decrease in the first trimester, but then may increase substantially during the second and third trimesters. This effect is further described in Chapter 19. During adolescence, circulating growth hormone counteracts insulin activity, and daily doses up to 1.5 U/kg body wt may be needed. In contrast, young children may be treated with smaller amounts of insulin to reduce the risk of hypoglycemic reactions.

Of the total daily insulin dose, approx 40% is delivered as basal insulin. In MDI regimens, this is administered as a dose of one of the basal insulins at bedtime, whereas in CSII treatment, it is administered continuously divided over 24 h. Usual basal rates for CSII vary

Step 1: Determine total daily dose

Sum of current insulin doses *or* 0.5 units × body weight (kg)

For example, a patient weighing 72 kg: 0.5 × 72 = 36 units per day

Step 2: Determine basal requirements

40% of total daily dose

MDI: Give as basal insulin subcutaneously at bedtime

NPH 14 units subcutaneously at bedtime

CSII: Give as a continuous infusion divided over 24 hours

Lispro 0.6 units/hour

Step 3: Determine meal requirements

35% of remaining insulin before breakfast, 30% before lunch, 35% before dinner

MDI: Give as meal insulin subcutaneously before each meal

Lispro 8 units subcutaneously before breakfast
Lispro 6 units subcutaneously before lunch
Lispro 8 units subcutaneously before dinner

CSII: Give as infusion boluses before each meal

Lispro 8 units bolus before breakfast
Lispro 6 units bolus before lunch
Lispro 8 units bolus before dinner

Fig. 2. Suggested algorithm to determine starting doses at initiation of intensive insulin therapy.

between 0.6 and 1.2 U/h. The remaining insulin is divided as insulin boluses before each meal; usually, less insulin is required before lunch than before breakfast or dinner (Fig. 2). To further improve glucose control, patients may also administer small doses of a rapidly acting insulin before snacks at any time of day. Because of its delayed onset of action, if regular insulin is used as the meal insulin in MDI, it must be given about 30 min prior to eating, whereas lispro and aspart can be given immediately before or even after eating. Rapidly acting analogs are the preferred meal insulin for intensive regimens.

Dose Adjustment

Although these calculated doses are good estimates of the amount of insulin needed before each meal, the actual amount given should be adjusted based on three variables:

- *Preprandial glucose.* Patients must self-monitor their blood glucose level before each meal. If the preprandial glucose concentration is higher than a predetermined target, a higher dose of insulin is required. In practice, the insulin dose given is adjusted, based on a variable insulin dose schedule (Fig. 3). Trends or patterns recognized in the self-monitored glucose results over time are analyzed to determine if changes in the basic dose schedule are required. Care must be taken to ensure that adjustments in response to habitually abnormal glucose determinations are made to the appropriate insulin. For example, if predinner blood glucose concentrations are consistently elevated, the dose schedule for meal insulin given before lunch needs to be increased. If fasting glucose levels are regularly low, the overnight basal insulin dose should be decreased.
- *Anticipated carbohydrate intake.* Patients are taught "carbohydrate counting," in which the carbohydrate content of a meal can be estimated by measuring the quantity of food or evaluating portion size and dividing it into its various groups, including starches, fruits, and milk products. Once they determine their individual insulin requirements per gram of carbohydrate intake for a given meal, patients may further modify the dose of insulin given in anticipation of a change in carbohydrate intake, just as a functioning pancreas secretes more insulin in response to a high-carbohydrate meal than a low-carbohydrate meal. Most individuals require an additional 1 U of insulin per extra 10 g of carbohydrate with meals.

Blood glucose (mg/dL)	Units of meal insulin (lispro or regular)				Bedtime basal insulin
	Breakfast	Lunch	Dinner	Snack	
< 69	3	2	3	0	10
70–109	6	4	6	0	
110–149	6	4	8	0	
150–189	8	5	10	2	
190–209	8	6	12	2	
210–289	10	7	14	4	
290–360	12	8	16	4	
≥ 360	14	10	18	5	

Fig. 3. Variable insulin dose scale. Rather than using fixed insulin doses for each meal, patients can adjust their dose based on the results of blood glucose monitoring. Higher insulin doses are given when preprandial glucose levels are higher than desired. (Example for illustrative purposes only.) (Adapted from the Leadership Sinai Centre for Diabetes, Mount Sinai Hospital, Toronto, ON, Canada.)

- *Physical activity.* Patients must also modify their insulin doses in anticipation of moderate to intense exercise. When using MDI treatment, the bolus insulin dose given before the meal prior to the exercise may have to be reduced by 50%. This varies with individuals, and patients are encouraged to use self-monitoring of blood glucose to determine their individual responses to a given exercise. Those using CSII regimens can also adjust their basal insulin infusion rate in response to exercise. Patients must also be alert for the delayed hypoglycemic effects of exercise, which may occur up to 24 h after completion of the activity. Adjustment in basal insulin requirements as well as other meal boluses may be required.

A further adjustment available with CSII therapy occurs for some patients in whom the release of the counterregulatory hormone growth hormone in the early waking hours (0500–0800) can lead to early morning hyperglycemia, the "dawn phenomenon." Insulin infusion pumps can be preprogrammed to increase the basal insulin infusion rate during these hours to counteract this problem.

"Split–Mixed" Insulin Therapy

Studies such as the DCCT have shown that intensive insulin therapy reduces a patient's risk of developing the long-term complications of type 1 diabetes. Unfortunately, many patients are unable or unwilling to comply with the dosing regimens and frequent monitoring required for intensive therapy. For such patients, a treatment regimen using "split–mixed" insulin doses may be required. These regimens require two daily injections of a mixture of meal insulin with basal insulin.

For many patients, the basal insulin injected as part of the dose before dinner peaks in the night, causing nocturnal hypoglycemia and compensatory early morning hyperglycemia. A solution for such patients is to divide the predinner insulin dose, giving the meal component before dinner and the basal component at bedtime. The three-times-daily insulin injection regimen is a hybrid between "split–mixed" therapy and MDI therapy and is also attractive for patients for whom insulin administration before lunch may be inconvenient.

Starting Doses

As with intensive subcutaneous insulin therapy, the starting total daily dose of insulin should be 0.5 U/kg body wt, although most patients ultimately require 0.6–0.7 U/kg.

Step 1: Determine total daily dose
Sum of current insulin doses *or* 0.5 units × body weight (kg)
For example, a patient weighing 72 kg: 0.5 × 72 = 36 units per day

Step 2: Determine each dose
$^2/_3$ of daily total before breakfast, $^1/_3$ before dinner
24 units before breakfast, 12 units before dinner

Step 3: Determine components of each dose
$^2/_3$ of each dose as basal insulin, $^1/_3$ as meal insulin
NPH 16 units + regular 8 units subcutaneously before breakfast
NPH 8 units + regular 4 units subcutaneously before dinner

Fig. 4. Suggested algorithm to determine starting doses at initiation of "split–mixed" insulin therapy.

The dose given before breakfast replaces the physiologic insulin pulses after breakfast and lunch and the basal insulin secretion during the day. Similarly, the dose before dinner replaces the dinner bolus and the overnight basal rate. A starting algorithm for each component of the "split–mixed" regimen is detailed in Fig. 4. This therapy is clearly inferior to MDI and CSII and does not approximate physiologic insulin secretion. Specific deficiencies of the regimen are the absence of an insulin bolus for lunch, the potential for the basal insulin injected before dinner to peak in the middle of the night and the risk of nocturnal hypoglycemia, and the reduction of versatility to modify therapy from day to day. "Split–mixed" therapy provides suboptimal insulin replacement and should be used as a last resort.

Dose Adjustment

In addition to generating a nonphysiologic insulin profile, "split–mixed" therapy also affords the patient less flexibility in dose adjustment in response to the quantity and timing of meals and exercise. Changes to insulin dosing may need to be anticipated hours in advance of the event, as only two injections per day are given. Large changes in the basal component of each dose risk provoking hypoglycemia or hyperglycemia; for example, increasing the prebreakfast NPH in anticipation of a high-carbohydrate breakfast may result in hypoglycemia before lunch. An alternate solution is to keep the timing and carbohydrate content of meals constant from day to day so that dose adjustment is not required.

Risks of Insulin Therapy

Insulin is a life-sustaining medication for patients with type 1 diabetes. However, it does have important risks of which patients must be informed. Many of these risks increase as glycemic targets approach physiologic levels and the hemoglobin A1c is near normal.

The most feared complication of insulin treatment is hypoglycemia, because it can be potentially life threatening. Hypoglycemia results when too much insulin is given relative to the baseline glucose level, the carbohydrate intake, and the patient's level of activity. The DCCT established that the risk of hypoglycemia was directly proportional to the intensity of glucose control *(2)*. Patients in the intensively treated arm of the study experienced a threefold frequency of severe hypoglycemia compared to the conventionally treated arm *(36)*. However, increased hypoglycemia with intensive therapy is not due to the regimen *per se,* but rather to the glycemic target selected for these patients. Excessive hypoglycemia is best managed by raising the premeal and bedtime glycemic targets. Hypoglycemia is discussed in further detail in Chapter 18.

The other major risk of insulin therapy is weight gain. Insulin promotes fat storage in adipocytes and protein synthesis in muscles. It participates in many other growth and anabolic pathways. In addition, patients who experience improved control with intensive therapy eliminate glucosuria, go into positive caloric balance, and provoke further weight gain. In the DCCT, patients treated with intensive insulin therapy had a substantially higher incidence of obesity than those given conventional therapy *(36)*.

PRACTICAL ASPECTS OF INSULIN ADMINISTRATION

Regardless of the specific treatment regimen, insulin is currently primarily administered by subcutaneous injection. The most commonly used sites are the abdomen, anterior thigh, dorsal arm and buttock—using other areas with less subcutaneous fat may result in intramuscular injection of insulin, which is more painful and results in more rapid systemic absorption *(37)*. Abdominal injections are preferred, using the entire abdominal surface. It has a larger area than other sites, and absorption is rapid and the most consistent. For example, insulin injected into a limb that is subsequently exercised is more rapidly absorbed compared to absorption from the same site without exercise, primarily because of increased blood flow *(38)*. Rotating injection sites within the same anatomic area reduces the risk of lipohypertrophy at the injection sites while maintaining stable absorption patterns from day to day. Other factors that affect absorption are temperature, focal massage, and injection depth *(39)*.

Syringes

Insulin is most commonly injected using disposable plastic syringes. It is supplied in multiple-use vials with a concentration of 100 U/mL. Suspended insulins, such as NPH or lente, must be mixed before being drawn up, to ensure uniformity of the injected material. Air roughly equivalent in volume to the insulin to be removed is injected into the vial, and then the insulin is drawn up into the syringe. If basal and meal insulins are being mixed in the same syringe, the meal insulin is drawn before the suspended basal insulin. The insulin is then injected into the subcutaneous fat.

Pens and Cartridges

An alternative to syringes is the pen-and-cartridge system of insulin administration. The insulin is supplied in small 1.5- or 3-mL cartridges that are placed into a delivery device, or pen. The patient dials up the amount of insulin to be administered, attaches a needle to the pen, and inserts it into the subcutaneous fat. A plunger is depressed and the insulin dose is delivered. Disposable pens, with the insulin already loaded, are also available.

Insulin pens allow more accurate dosing *(40)* and make insulin administration easier *(41)*, particularly in public places. They are ideal for patients with visual or motor impairments for whom drawing up insulin is difficult. However, pens do not allow mixing of insulins, so patients taking different types of insulin simultaneously must inject themselves separately for each. Pens are particularly valuable for MDI regimens and are quickly becoming the method of choice for delivering insulin.

Novel Routes of Insulin Delivery

Research is ongoing to find alternative routes of insulin delivery *(42)*. Although oral administration of insulin would be convenient and improve patient compliance, most formulations have been limited by enzymatic destruction of insulin in the digestive system. More recent work has encapsulated insulin into synthetic microscopic beads, which allow slow insulin release once they are absorbed systemically *(43)*. The bioavailability of intranasal insulin is rendered unpredictable by even minor changes in the nasal mucosa from infections or irritation *(42)*. However, absorption across the alveoli appears more consistent, and large-scale clinical trials of inhaled insulin are underway *(44)*.

Pancreas transplantation is offered in many centers, usually following or simultaneously with renal transplantation. Islet cell transplantation has been evaluated as a less morbid alternative, but, as yet, only one center reports long-term success *(45)*. These procedures are discussed in detail in Chapters 29 and 30.

MONITORING GLUCOSE CONTROL

A fundamental component of any insulin treatment regimen for type 1 diabetes is monitoring of glucose control. Rapid home measurement of glucose levels allows immediate assessment of control. Glycosylated hemoglobin levels reflect intermediate-term glucose control over several months. Long-term glucose control is reflected by the development of the microvascular and macrovascular complications of diabetes.

Self-Monitoring of Blood Glucose

The most powerful monitoring tool is capillary blood glucose monitoring *(46)*. A small lancet pricks a patient's fingertip to obtain a small drop of blood that is placed on a testing strip. With electrochemical methods, the glucose concentration of this drop can be determined in 5 to 30 s.

Patients with type 1 diabetes are encouraged to monitor blood glucose frequently. By determining glucose levels before a meal, patients can decide whether their insulin dose needs adjustment to counteract an already high glucose level. In addition, by recording each value in a "log book," patients can quickly develop a profile of their overall glucose control at various times of day and so can make informed changes to their insulin regimen. Many meters have memory features or accompanying computer software to chart values and identify glucose control trends.

For patients using intensive therapy, monitoring is recommended before each meal and at bedtime. In addition, glucose monitoring in the postprandial period, usually 2 h after eating, can often guide adjustments to meal insulin doses and improve overall control. This is particularly valuable for patients with on-target premeal glucose levels but inappropriately elevated hemoglobin A1c. Measurements taken in the early hours of the morning can help detect nocturnal hypoglycemia resulting from inappropriately high evening basal insulin doses. Some patients are unable or unwilling to monitor so frequently; these patients should be encouraged either to perform frequent monitoring for short intervals, or to monitor episodically at varying times of day, thereby creating a profile of glucose control over several days.

Newer methods of glucose monitoring being investigated include monitors that measure subcutaneous glucose concentrations every 5 min as a reflection of blood glucose concentrations *(47)*. These devices have the potential to provide a continuous profile of glucose levels throughout the day, which will presumably allow for much finer adjustment of intensive insulin therapies.

Glycosylated Hemoglobin

The impaired glucose metabolism of patients with diabetes results in higher than normal concentrations of glucose in the circulation. Glucose is a reactive carbohydrate that becomes nonenzymatically irreversibly bound to other proteins in the blood, including hemoglobin A. These glycosylated electrophoretically fast hemoglobins are named hemoglobin A1a, A1b, and A1c; however, most clinical laboratories only measure A1c. The proportion of hemoglobin molecules that are hemoglobin A1c reflects the overall glucose control over the preceding 3–4 mo and can, therefore, be used to evaluate a patient's treatment regimen if measured regularly *(48)*. However, only capillary blood glucose monitoring can determine exactly when, during the day, glucose control is poor and which insulin doses have to be modified.

Falsely low hemoglobin A1c may be seen in patients with hemoglobinopathies, which limit the ability of hemoglobin to be glycosylated. In pregnancy, increased red blood cell turnover results in a low hemoglobin A1c that may not reflect glucose control. Hemoglobin A1c measurements may be falsely elevated in patients with hemoglobin F or with carbamylated or acetaldehyde-bound hemoglobins. Finally, if hemoglobin A1c levels are higher than expected based on the glucose control recorded in a capillary monitoring "log book," meter error or log book falsification must be suspected.

In addition to accurately reflecting intermediate-term glucose control, hemoglobin A1c levels are known to be highly correlated with the long-term development of microvascular disease. The DCCT showed that for every 10% reduction of hemoglobin A1c, the risk of developing each of retinopathy, proteinuria or neuropathy was reduced by 30–45% *(2,49)*. Therefore, patients with type 1 diabetes should strive for hemoglobin A1c levels as near normal as possible (Table 2).

ADJUSTING TREATMENT DURING ILLNESS OR SURGERY

Only half of the total daily secretion of insulin by the healthy pancreas controls the glycemic response to meals; the other half is the 24-h basal requirement. Therefore, patients with type 1 diabetes who stop eating must continue to administer insulin to meet basal requirements. Without it, free fatty acid release from adipose tissue will be unsuppressed, leading to hepatic ketone production and diabetic ketoacidosis. Indeed, the physiologic stress associated with the illness or surgery that caused the patient to stop eating also stimulates the release of counterregulatory hormones that antagonize insulin action and may cause hyperglycemia despite decreased caloric intake.

When not eating, patients are instructed to monitor their blood glucose concentration every 4 h. If blood glucose levels are high, extra insulin is given to counteract them; if they are low, insulin doses are reduced by around 50%, but never stopped altogether. Patients are encouraged to drink sugar-rich fluids to maintain their carbohydrate intake, but if unable to tolerate even this diet, intravenous dextrose may be required.

Patients should also be wary of the development of ketoacidosis when ill. Excess counterregulatory hormones released in response to an illness can promote ketogenesis,

Table 2
Targets of Glucose Control

	Normal	*Goal*	*Additional action suggested*
Average preprandial plasma glucose, mg/dL (mmol/L)	< 110 (< 6.1)	90–130 (5.0–7.2)	< 90/> 150 (< 5.0/> 8.3)
Average bedtime plasma glucose, mg/dL (mmol/L)	< 120 (< 6.7)	110–150 (6.1–8.3)	< 110/> 180 (< 6.1/> 10.0)
Hemoglobin A1c, %	< 6	< 7	> 8

Source: ref. *50*.

even when exogenous insulin is continued. Traditionally, patients check for the development of ketoacidosis using "dipsticks" that change color when placed in urine containing ketones. However, a newly developed capillary blood monitor that also measures concentrations of β-hydroxybutyrate may aid in preventing and managing ketoacidosis *(51)*.

A similar approach may be used for patients who are having minor surgical procedures. Although usual insulin doses can accompany the usual diet on the day before surgery, patients will usually not be eating for several hours preoperatively. On the morning of surgery, half the patient's usual basal insulin dose is given without bolus insulin to control ketosis. Intravenous dextrose maintains the blood sugar level. Postoperatively, patients may resume usual insulin dosing based on the anticipated carbohydrate content of the meal they will eat.

If patients are going to be without oral intake for a prolonged time, such as during and after major surgery, insulin should be delivered intravenously to control glucose levels and ketone formation. Regular insulin is administered along with a dextrose solution to ensure some ongoing carbohydrate source. Because patients are not eating and therefore do not require the bolus component of their usual therapy and because systemic absorption of insulin from subcutaneous tissue is not complete, the amount of insulin infused intravenously over 24 h is approximately half the total daily dose of all subcutaneous insulins. Monitoring of blood glucose must be performed regularly to ensure that the glucose concentration is maintained at a safe level, and the infusion rate is modified accordingly. Urine or blood ketones should be checked regularly if the glucose level is high. Because the half-life of intravenous insulin is only a few minutes, patients will become acutely insulin deficient and risk developing ketoacidosis if the intravenous infusion is interrupted for any reason. Similarly, once the patient begins eating, the infusion must be continued for at least 1 h after the first subcutaneous insulin dose is given, to ensure that the action of the subcutaneous dose has started before the infusion is stopped.

REFERENCES

1. Banting FG, Best CH, Collip JB, Campbell WR, Fletcher AA. Pancreatic extracts in the treatment of diabetes mellitus. Can Med Assoc J 1922;12:141–146.
2. Diabetes Control and Complications Trial Research Group. The effect of intensive treatment of diabetes on the development and progression of long-term complications in insulin-dependent diabetes mellitus. N Engl J Med 1993;329:977–986.
3. Zinman B. The physiologic replacement of insulin: an elusive goal. N Engl J Med 1989;321:363–370.

4. Polonsky KS, Given BD, Van Cauter E. Twenty-four-hour profiles and pulsatile patterns on insulin secretion in normal and obese subjects. J Clin Invest 1988;81:442–448.
5. Levitt NS, Hirsch L, Rubenstein AH, Polonsky KS. Quantitative evaluation of the effect of low-intensity exercise on insulin secretion in man. Metabolism 1993;42:829–833.
6. Burge MR, Schade DS. Insulins. Endocrinol Metabol Clin North Am 1997;26:575–598.
7. Chance RE, Kroeff EP, Hoffmann JA, Frank BH. Chemical, physical, and biologic properties of biosynthetic human insulin. Diabetes Care 1981;4:147–154.
8. Kang S, Brange J, Burch A, Volund A, Owens DR. Subcutaneous insulin absorption explained by insulin's physicochemical properties. Evidence from absorption studies of soluble human insulin and insulin analogues in humans. Diabetes Care 1991;14:942–948.
9. Yudkin JS. Insulin for the world's poorest countries. Lancet 2000;355:919–921.
10. Makame M for the Diabetes Epidemiology Research International Study Group. Childhood diabetes, insulin, and Africa. Diabet Med 1992;9:571–573.
11. Gulan M, Gottesman IS, Zinman B. Biosynthetic human insulin improves postprandial glucose excursions in type 1 diabetes. Ann Intern Med 1987;107:506–509.
12. Fineberg SE, Galloway JA, Fineberg SN, Goldman J. Effects of species of origin, purification levels and formulation on insulin immunogenicity. Diabetes 1983;32:592–599.
13. Lee WL, Zinman B. From insulin to insulin analogues: progress in the treatment of type 1 diabetes mellitus. Diabet Rev 1998;6:73–88.
14. Holleman F, Hoekstra JBL. Insulin lispro. N Engl J Med 1997;337:176–183.
15. Heinemann L, Heise T, Wahl LC, et al. Prandial glycaemia after a carbohydrate-rich meal in type I diabetic patients: using the rapid acting insulin analogue [Lys(B28), Pro(B29)] human insulin. Diabet Med 1996;13:625–629.
16. Brunelle RL, Llewelyn J, Anderson JH, Gale EAM, Koivisto VA. Meta-analysis of the effect of insulin lispro on severe hypoglycemia in patients with type 1 diabetes. Diabetes Care 1998;21:1726–1731.
17. Heller SR, Amiel SA, Mansell P. Effect of the fast-acting insulin analog lispro on the risk of nocturnal hypoglycemia during intensified insulin therapy. Diabetes Care 1999;22:1607–1611.
18. Woodworth J, Howey D, Bowsher R, Lutz S, Santa P, Brady P. [Lys(B28), Pro(B29)] human insulin: dose-ranging vs. Humulin R. Diabetes 1993;42(Suppl 1):54A.
19. Kang S, Creagh FM, Peters JR, Brange J, Vølund A, Owens DR. Comparison of subcutaneous soluble human insulin and insulin analogues (Asp^{B9}, Glu^{B27}; Asp^{B10}; Asp^{B28}) on meal-related plasma glucose excursions in type I diabetic subjects. Diabetes Care 1991;14:571–577.
20. Heinemann L, Kapitza C, Starke AAR, Heise T. Time-action profile of the insulin analogue B28Asp. Diabet Med 1996;13:683–684.
21. Lindholm A, McEwen J, Riis AP. Improved postprandial glycemic control with insulin aspart. Diabetes Care 1999;22:801–805.
22. Raskin P, Guthrie RA, Leiter L, Riis A, Jovanovic L. Use of insulin apart, a fast-acting insulin analog, as the mealtime insulin in the management of patients with type 1 diabetes. Diabetes Care 2000;23:583–588.
23. Home PD, Lindholm A, Hylleberg B, Round P. Improved glycemic control with insulin aspart. Diabetes Care 1998;21:1904–1909.
24. Janssen MM, Casteleijn S, Deville W, Popp-Snijders C, Roach P, Heine RJ. Nighttime insulin kinetics and glycemic control in type 1 diabetes patients following administration of an intermediate-acting lispro preparation. Diabetes Care 1997;20:1870–1873.
25. Bolli GB, Owens DR. Insulin glargine. Lancet 2000;356:443–445.
26. Heinemann L, Linkeschova R, Rave K, Hompsech B, Sedlak M, Heise T. Time-action profile of the long-acting insulin analog insulin glargine (HOE901) in comparison with those of NPH insulin and placebo. Diabetes Care 2000;23:644–649.
27. Pieber TR, Eugène-Jolchine I, Derobert E. Efficacy and safety of HOE 901 versus NPH insulin in patients with type 1 diabetes. Diabetes Care 2000;23:157–162.
28. Rosenstock J, Park G, Zimmerman J, the U.S. Insulin Glargine (HOE 901) Type 1 Diabetes Investigator Group. Basal insulin glargine (HOE 901) versus NPH in patients with type 1 diabetes on multiple daily insulin regimens. Diabetes Care 2000;23:1137–1142.
29. Ratner RE, Hirsch IB, Neifing JL, et al. Less hypoglycemia with insulin glargine in intensive insulin therapy for type 1 diabetes. Diabetes Care 2000;23:639–643.
30. Lawson ML, Gerstein HC, Tsui E, Zinman B. Effect of intensive therapy on early macrovascular disease in young individuals with type 1 diabetes. Diabetes Care 1999;22:B35–B39.

31. Zinman B, Ross C, Campos RV, Strack T. The Canadian Lispro Study Group. Effectiveness of human ultralente versus NPH insulin in providing basal insulin replacement for an insulin lispro multiple daily injection regimen. Diabetes Care 1999;22:603–608.
32. Hanaire-Broutin H, Melki V, Bessières-Lacombe S, Tauber J-P, the Study Group for the Development of Pump Therapy in Diabetes. Comparison of continuous subcutaneous insulin infusion and multiple daily injection regimens using insulin lispro in type 1 diabetic patients on intensified treatment. Diabetes Care 2000;23:1232–1235.
33. Zinman B, Tildesley H, Chiasson JL, Tsui E, Strack T. Insulin lispro in CSII: results of a double-blind crossover study. Diabetes 1997;46:440–443.
34. Renner R, Pfutzner A, Trautmann M, Harzer O, Sauter K, Landgraf R. Use of insulin lispro in continuous subcutaneous insulin infusion treatment: results of a multicenter trial. Diabetes Care 1999;22:784–788.
35. Bode B, Weinstein R, Bell D, et al. Comparison of insulin aspart with buffered regular insulin and insulin lispro in continuous subcutaneous insulin infusion: a randomized study in type 1 diabetes. Diabetes Care 2002;25:439–444.
36. The Diabetes Control and Complications Research Group. Adverse events and their association with treatment regimens in the Diabetes Control and Complications Trial. Diabetes Care 1995;18: 1415–1427.
37. Vaag A, Handberg A, Lauritzen M, Henriksen JE, Pedersen KD, Beck-Nielsen H. Variation in absorption of NPH insulin due to intramuscular injection. Diabetes Care 1990;13:74–76.
38. Koivisto VA, Felig P. Effects of leg exercise on insulin absorption in diabetic patients. N Engl J Med 1978;298:79–83.
39. Skyler JS. Insulin pharmacology. Med Clin North Am 1988;72:1337–1354.
40. Lteif AN, Schwenk WF. Accuracy of pen injectors versus insulin syringes in children with type 1 diabetes. Diabetes Care 1999;22:137–140.
41. Graff MR, McClanahan MA. Assessment by patients with diabetes mellitus of two insulin pen delivery systems versus a vial and syringe. Clin Ther 1998;20:486–496.
42. Saudek CD. Novel forms of insulin delivery. Endocrinol Metabol Clin North Am 1997;26:599–610.
43. Musabayane CT, Munjeri O, Bwititi P, Osim EE. Orally administered, insulin-loaded amidated pectin hydrogel beads sustain plasma concentrations of insulin in streptozotocin-diabetic rats. J Endocrinol 2000;164:1–6.
44. Laube BL, Benedict GW, Dobs AS. The lung as an alternative route of delivery for insulin in controlling postprandial glucose levels in patients with diabetes. Chest 1998;114:1734–1739.
45. Shapiro AMJ, Lakey JRT, Ryan EA, et al. Islet transplantation in seven patients with type 1 diabetes mellitus using a glucocorticoid-free immunosuppressive regimen. N Engl J Med 2000;343:230–238.
46. Terent A, Hagfall O, Cederholm U. The effect of education and self-monitoring of blood glucose on glycosylated hemoglobin in type I diabetes: a controlled 18-month trial in a representative population. Acta Med Scand 1985;217:47–53.
47. Maran A, Crepaldi C, Tiengo A, et al. Continuous subcutaneous glucose monitoring in diabetic patients. Diabetes Care 2002;25:347–352
48. Nathan DM, Singer DE, Hurxthal K, Goodson JD. The clinical information value of the glycosylated hemoglobin assay. N Engl J Med 1984;310:341–346.
49. Diabetes Control and Complications Trial Research Group. The relationship of glycemic exposure (HbA1c) to the risk of development and progression of retinopathy in the Diabetes Control and Complications Trial. Diabetes 1995;44:968–983.
50. American Diabetes Association. Standards of medical care for patients with diabetes mellitus. Diabetes Care 2002;25(Suppl 1):S33–S49.
51. Byrne HA, Tieszen KL, Hollis S, Dornan TL, New JP. Evaluation of an electrochemical sensor for measuring blood ketones. Diabetes Care 2000;23:500–503.

11 Relationship Between Metabolic Control and Complications in Diabetes

Therapeutic Implications of the Diabetes Control and Complications Trial

Saul Genuth, MD

CONTENTS

INTRODUCTION

The Diabetes Control and Complications Trial (DCCT) was organized in 1982 in order to address definitively the question of whether the long-term complications of type 1 diabetes were directly related to hyperglycemia and whether the risks of these complications could be significantly reduced by lowering blood glucose levels to near normal. The question was of great scientific and public health importance. It was also a question of special clinical poignancy: First because a peak in the incidence of type 1 diabetes occurs peripubertally around ages 11–13 yr *(1),* a period heralding profound physical and emotional change; catastrophic late complications often followed after 15–25 yr of established disease *(2,3),* and life expectancy was previously shortened to an average age of death of 49 *(4),* and second, because attempts to maintain normal glycemia require highly disciplined regimens which limit flexible lifestyles for children and adolescents as well as adults and can be intrusive into family life.

A retrospective and prospective body of observational cohort studies and fragmentary evidence from several small randomized clinical trials conducted in the 1970s *(5)*

From: *Contemporary Endocrinology: Type 1 Diabetes: Etiology and Treatment*
Edited by: M. A. Sperling

provided preliminary evidence to adherents of "tight metabolic control" because of their *belief* that this form of treatment would prevent the dire long-term consequences of type 1 (and type 2) diabetes. This belief was buttressed by key animal experiments *(6)* and, increasingly, by new descriptions of mechanisms that could link hyperglycemia to diabetic retinopathy, nephropathy, and neuropathy *(7–11)*. On the other hand, the lack of clear proof that tight metabolic control did have long-term benefits persuaded some clinicians to favor looser metabolic control with less rigid blood glucose goals that were thought more readily achievable and, therefore, less likely to detract so much from the quality of life of children and adolescents.

The initiation of the DCCT was also stimulated by the development of self blood glucose monitoring, the resurrection of multiple daily insulin injection (MDI) programs with each dose of regular insulin guided by premeal blood glucose values, the introduction of external continuous subcutaneous insulin infusion (CSII) therapy, and the development of glycated hemoglobin tests [referred to generically in this chapter as HbA1c with a nondiabetic range of 4.05–6.05 *(12)*], which permitted accurate assessments of the average level of blood glucose over the preceding 4- to 12-wk periods of time. In addition, quantitative methods for measuring retinopathy, early nephropathy, and neuropathy had been developed *(13)*. Thus, all of the necessary components were in place to launch the DCCT.

In the planning phase of the DCCT, there was considerable discussion whether to include children or even adolescents in the trial. The safety of regimens aimed at normal glycemia was unproven in these patients. Their ability to complete a complex set of measurements repeatedly and their long-term adherence to a research protocol were questioned. Most importantly, their ability to maintain or even achieve near-normal average levels of blood glucose was subject to considerable doubt. Fortunately, as it turned out, the importance of testing the glucose hypothesis in nonadults won out over the concerns, and a cohort of adolescent subjects aged 13–15 yr was recruited. This permitted the conclusions of the DCCT regarding the efficacy and safety of "tight metabolic control" with intensive treatment to be applied with confidence to this critically important group of patients.

SUMMARY OF THE OVERALL DCCT RESULTS

The DCCT ended the controversy as to whether the degree of metabolic control of type 1 diabetes influences the development of long-term complications *(14)*. The DCCT was a prospective randomized trial that compared the effects of intensive treatment (IT) with those of conventional treatment (CT) on retinopathy, nephropathy, and neuropathy in subjects with type 1 diabetes. IT was aimed at producing normoglycemia (preprandial blood glucose levels of 70–120 mg/dL, HbA1c < 6.0%) and consisted of MDI (three to four daily daily injections) or CSII, frequent self blood glucose monitoring, monthly clinic visits, and frequent telephone contact with the treatment team. CT was aimed at producing clinical well-being, defined as freedom from symptoms of hyperglycemia and from inordinate hypoglycemia and consisted of no more than two insulin injections per day, urine or blood glucose monitoring, and routine quarterly visits to the clinic. A total of 1441 subjects aged 13–39 yr were studied; 726 were in a primary prevention cohort with diabetes duration 1–5 yr, no retinopathy by 7 field stereo fundus photographs, and urinary albumin excretion rate (AER) < 40 mg/24 h; 715 comprised a secondary intervention cohort with diabetes duration 1–15 yr, minimal to mild nonproliferative retinopathy, and AER < 200 mg/24 h. The mean baseline HbA1c was 8.8% in the primary cohort and 9.0% in the secondary cohort. Each cohort was separately randomized to IT and CT, and adolescents were included in all four of the treatment groups thus formed.

The trial was ended by the Data Safety and Quality Committee after a mean follow-up time of 6.5 yr *(14)*. The results showed that intensive treatment of type 1 diabetes reduces the risk of retinopathy *(15,16)*, nephropathy *(17)*, and neuropathy *(18,19)* by 39–63% when compared with conventional treatment. These risk reductions were evident in both the primary prevention cohort and the secondary intervention cohort of patients. The benefits of IT relative to CT did not become evident until approx 3 yr had elapsed *(14)*, but the risk reductions became progressively greater as the earliest randomized patients were followed for up to 9 yr of treatment. The lower rates of complications in IT patients were associated with median HbA1c levels of 7.2% (1.20 times upper limit of normal [ULN]) as opposed to 8.9% (1.48 times ULN) in the CT patients *(14)*. The difference of 1.7% in median HbA1c corresponded to a difference in mean daytime blood glucose levels of 76 mg/dL (231–155 mg/dL) *(14)*. These lower, but still above normal, levels of glycemia in the IT group were accompanied by a threefold greater risk of severe hypoglycemic episodes and by an increase in weight gain *(14,20)*.

This chapter will discuss the pertinence of the DCCT results to the present management of type 1 diabetes in adults and especially in children and adolescents. The younger age group will be emphasized when the available data allow, because their specific results have received less broad dissemination and application of these results to younger patients may be more controversial and difficult. However, some caveats are in order first. The DCCT subjects were not a random population based sample of type 1 diabetes, and few minority patients (i.e., of African or other racial/ethnic backgrounds) were studied. Treatment teams in each DCCT clinic were professionally diverse, consisting of physicians, nurses, dietitians, mental health professionals, and social workers with ample support *(21)*. All diabetes care and supplies were free to the patients with the generous support of the National Institute of Diabetes, Digestive and Kidney Diseases (NIDDK) and with supplementary assistance from industry. A constantly reinforced research goal, frequent telephone and clinic contacts, and numerous varied adherence activities all led to strong bonding between the DCCT personnel and the research patients. This accounted for remarkable compliance with assigned treatment in both treatment groups and a 99% participation in final follow-up measurements *(14)*.

BENEFITS OF INTENSIVE TREATMENT IN ADOLESCENTS

The DCCT *a priori* analytical plan included a stratified analysis of the main outcomes by adolescent status at baseline and these results have been published separately *(22)*. One hundred ninety-five (13.5%) of the 1441 DCCT subjects were classified as adolescent; 125 were in the primary prevention cohort and 70 were in the secondary intervention cohort. They were 13–17 yr of age and at least Tanner stage 2 on entry (41% were age 13–14, 47% were age 15–16, and 12% were age 17). Of primary cohort adolescents with diabetes duration 1–5 yr, 37% had sustecal stimulated C-peptide levels > 0.2 mmol/L but < 0.5 mmol/mL, whereas none of the adolescents with duration > 5 yr had levels > 0.2. In the primary cohort, duration of diabetes was 38 mo (of which, 32 mo were considered postpubertal). In the secondary cohort, these durations were 93 mo and 48 mo, respectively. Insulin doses averaged 0.90 U/kg in the primary

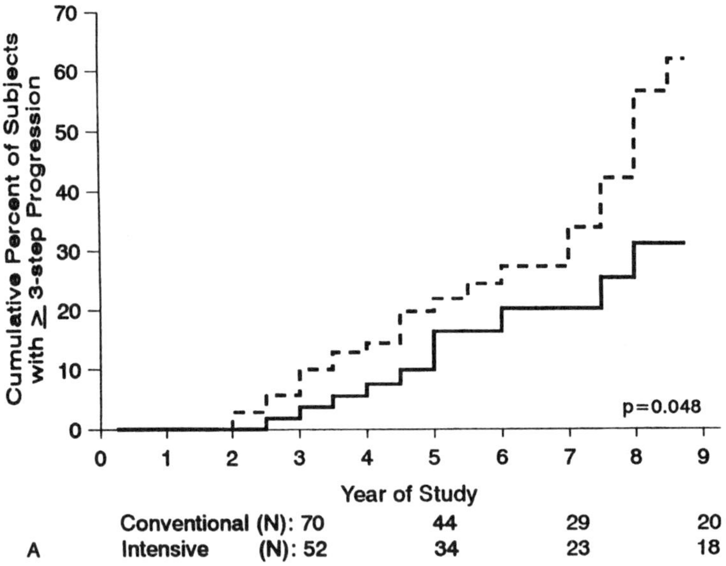

Fig. 1. Cumulative incidence of adolescent DCCT primary prevention subjects whose retinopathy progressed from none at baseline three or more steps on the Early Treatment Diabetic Retinopathy Study (ETDRS) scale and was sustained on a second photograph taken 6 mo later. Solid line: intensive treatment; dashed line: conventional treatment. (From ref. *22*.)

cohort and 1.04 U/Kg in the secondary cohort. Mean baseline HbA1c was 9.2% in the primary cohort and 10.0% in the secondary cohort. Seventy-four percent of the secondary cohort had only microaneurysms on their baseline fundus photographs and their mean AER was 28 mg/24 h.

Over an average DCCT follow-up time of 7.4 yr in the adolescents, the mean HbA1c in the intensive group was 8.1%, compared to 9.8% in the conventional group *(22)*. These values were each 0.8% higher than those maintained in the respective DCCT adult groups *(22)*. Every 3 mo, a seven-sample capillary blood glucose profile (3 premeal and $1^1/_2$ h postmeal and bedtime) was obtained. The mean values of all these blood glucoses were 177 mg/dL in the intensive group and 260 mg/dL in the conventional group. These values were each about 25 mg/dL higher than those recorded in the whole DCCT cohort. Of note, the total daily insulin dose required for IT did not differ significantly from that required for CT during the first year of treatment (1.03 vs 0.97 U/kg) when the HbA1c nadir of 7.6% was reached with IT; nor did these doses differ from the pre-DCCT doses. Thus, the key to maintaining a lower-level HbA1c with IT was more physiological distribution and better coordination of insulin with caloric intake and exercise throughout the day.

Figures 1 and 2 show the cumulative incidence of progression of retinopathy, defined conservatively as a sustained three-step worsening on the retinopathy scale, in the adolescent primary and secondary cohorts. IT reduced the progression significantly in each cohort (53%, $p < 0.048$, 70%, $p < 0.01$, respectively. Figure 3 demonstrates that intensive treatment also reduced the cumulative incidence of microalbuminuria in the secondary cohort (55%, $p < 0.042$). Table 1 presents the absolute rates of retinopathy and nephropathy as events per 100 patient-years and the risk reductions produced by IT *(22)*. There

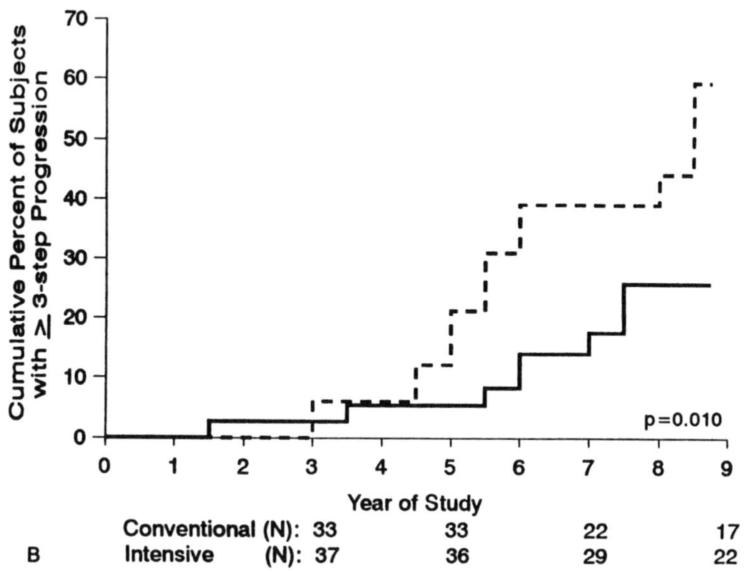

Fig. 2. Cumulative incidence of adolescent DCCT secondary intervention subjects whose retinopathy progressed from its baseline level three or more steps on the ETDRS scale and was sustained on a second photograph taken 6 mo later. Solid line: intensive treatment; dashed line: conventional treatment. (From ref. *22.*)

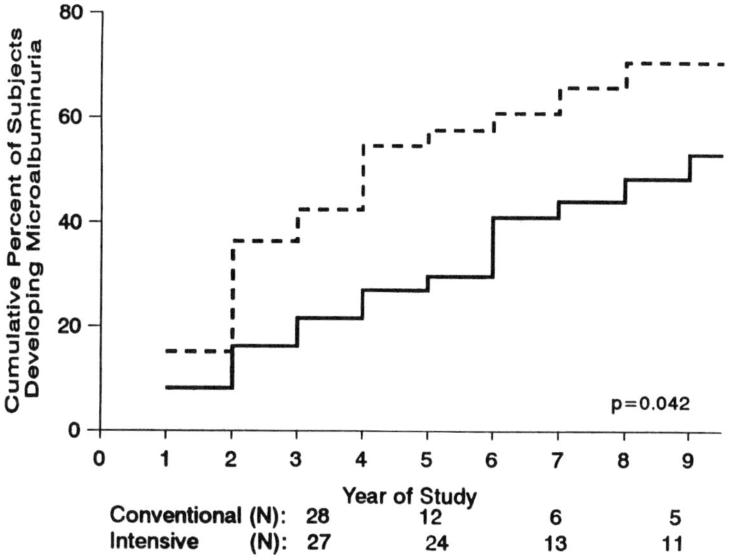

Fig. 3. Cumulative incidence of microalbuminuria in adolescent secondary intervention DCCT subjects who had none at baseline. Solid line: intensive treatment; dashed line: conventional treatment. (From ref. *22.*)

was a 61% reduction in retinopathy risk in the combined cohort ($p < 0.02$) and a 55% reduction in risk of developing microalbuminuria in the secondary cohort ($p < 0.05$). Seven adolescents developed confirmed clinical neuropathy during conventional treatment vs three during intensive treatment (numbers too small to yield statistical significance). However, median and peroneal motor and sensory peripheral nerve

Table 1
Rates of Retinopathy and Nephropathy (Events/100 Patient-Years) and Risk Reductions Produced by IT and CT

	Primary prevention cohort			*Secondary intervention cohort*		
Complications	*CT*	*IT*	*Risk reduction, (%)*	*CT*	*IT*	*Risk reduction, (%)*
Retinopathy[a]						
Any	23	18	30	—	—	—
≥ 3-Step progression	6.2	3.2	53[b]	7.4	2.9	70[b]
Nephropathy						
Urinary albumin > 40 mg/24 h	7.1	5.8	10	12.7	6.6	55[b]

[a] Sustained on at least two fundus photographs 6 mo apart.
[b] $p < 0.05$.

conduction velocities all decreased during CT, whereas they remained the same or increased during IT ($p < 0.04$ to < 0.001) *(22)*. In summary, IT of adolescents consistently reduced the risks of retinopathy, nephropathy, and neuropathy compared to CT, just as it did in the DCCT adults *(14,22)*.

These benefits were associated with an absolute reduction in HbA1c of about 2% and a reduction in mean blood glucose of 83 mg/dL. Thus, a straightforward conclusion from these data is that adolescents, like adults, should be encouraged to adopt and practice IT of their diabetes, aimed at normal glycemia.

ADVERSE EFFECTS OF IT IN ADOLESCENTS

The benefits of IT, however, need to be balanced against the major observed adverse effects: hypoglycemia and weight gain. Hypoglycemia is of special concern because the plasma glucose level at which adrenergic warning signs appear tends to fall with IT *(23,24)*. In addition, the brain requires glucose as an oxidative substrate during each hypoglycemic episode *(25)*. For these reasons, lapses into impaired judgment, confusion, coma, and convulsions become more frequent *(23)*. A predilection for events to occur during sleep poses an additional danger *(26,27)*.

The event rate for severe hypoglycemia (defined as *requiring* treatment by another person) was 86 per 100 patient-years in the adolescents treated intensively compared to 57 per 100 patient-years in the adults so treated *(22)*. For hypoglycemic events resulting in coma or seizure, these respective rates were 27 and 14 per 100 patient-years, respectively *(22)*. The relative risks of severe hypoglycemic events with IT vs CT were 2.9 in adolescents and 3.3 in adults. Eighty-two percent of intensively treated vs 45% of conventionally treated adolescents had at least one severe hypoglycemic event during the course of the DCCT. The comparable percentages for hypoglycemic coma/seizure were 63% and 25%, respectively. Some adolescents suffered multiple events. The overall risk of severe hypoglycemia increases as HbA1c falls *(14)*, an important point in selecting HbA1c targets for children and adolescents with type 1 diabetes. However, this inverse relationship does not entirely explain the increase in hypoglycemia associated with IT *(28)*.

Despite these high frequencies of severe hypoglycemia, there was no measurable difference of quality of life or in neuropsychological function test scores between the two treatment groups in the whole DCCT cohort, nor between subjects who did or did not suffer hypoglycemia, nor between those who had multiple events and those who did not *(29)*. Although these results and other reports *(30)* provide some reassurance of safety, long-term delayed central nervous system consequences of severe hypoglycemia cannot be ruled out until extended follow-up studies of the cohort are completed.

With regard to weight gain also, the adolescent cohort mirrored results in the whole DCCT cohort. Within the first 5 yr, the intensively treated adolescent females and males gained 4.0 kg and 3.2 kg, respectively—more weight than their conventionally treated counterparts *(22)*. Because growth in height was the same in the two treatment groups, the body mass index (BMI) increased approx 2 more units with intensive than with conventional treatment in both genders. In the whole DCCT cohort, the risk of becoming overweight was almost twofold greater with IT *(31)*. In the first year of IT, weight gain was positively correlated with the entry HbA1c level and with the subsequent decrease in HbA1c, suggesting that much of the early weight gain could be accounted for by improved glycemic control *(31)*. Intensively treated adolescents who experienced severe hypoglycemia also gained more weight than those subjects who did not have such events *(22)*.

There may be important health implications for those DCCT patients who gained the most weight on IT. When the weight gain was stratified by quartiles, those patients in the highest quartile of weight gain had higher BMI and waist–hip ratios, higher triglycerides, low-density lipoprotein (LDL) cholesterol and apolipoprotein B levels with increases in the dense LDL fractions, lower high-density lipoprotein (HDL) cholesterol and lipoprotein A1 levels, and higher blood pressure than those in the lowest quartile of weight gain *(32)*. Another study has shown that this atherogenic dyslipidemic tendency was also more likely seen in DCCT subjects with elevated urinary AER *(33)*, another risk factor for cardiovascular disease. Moreover, IT, although it reduced total and LDL cholesterol levels and triglycerides levels, did not significantly decrease cardiovascular event rates in the whole DCCT cohort *(34)*. Placed together, these observations have been interpreted to indicate that IT may be unveiling an inherent but latent insulin resistance syndrome, with its attendant risk of cardiovascular complications *(32)*, independent from the patients' type 1 diabetes. Although this suggestion is speculative at present, extended follow-up studies and appropriate future genotyping of the DCCT subjects who gained the most weight on intensive treatment (including those who were adolescent at entry into the DCCT) should confirm or deny this hypothesis.

In adolescents, the rigors of IT did not interfere with education (a mean of 14 yr at DCCT closeout in both treatment groups) or marrying (19 vs 22 marriages) *(35)*, both important developmental achievements. The comparable figures for the adults on IT and adults on CT were 15 and 15 yr of education and 195 and 197 marriages *(35)*. One adolescent in the IT group died of a motor vehicle accident unrelated to hypoglycemia, and one adolescent in the CT group committed suicide *(35)*. By comparison, there were six deaths of adults on IT and three adults died while on CT, with one fatal motor vehicle accident in each group possibly caused by hypoglycemia *(14)*.

FACTORS INFLUENCING THE RISK OF COMPLICATIONS

Although the most important accomplishment of the DCCT was the clear-cut demonstration that IT was superior to CT by reducing the risks of microvascular and neuropathic complications, the wealth of collected data permitted further analyses leading to a better understanding of the factors influencing these risks. Despite the fact that these analyses were performed with data from the whole DCCT cohort, there is no reason to believe that they do not apply to the adolescents, who were too few in number to analyze similarly as a separate group.

The most immediate question raised by the DCCT results was whether IT worked by lowering blood glucose. To explore this issue, the risk of retinopathy progression (sustained three-step worsening on the Early Treatment of Diabetic Retinopathy Study scale) was analyzed as a function of the mean HbA1c prior to the event or nonevent *(36)*. Figure 4 shows the result of this modeling and demonstrates clearly an exponential relationship within each treatment group. For each 10% *decrease* in HbA1c (i.e., 10.0 → 9.0, 9.0 → 8.1, 8.0 → 7.2, 7.0 → 6.3), the risk of retinopathy progression was *reduced* 45% in the CT group and 43% in the IT group. These nearly identical risk relationships in the two groups support the premise that the difference in outcomes between the two groups was related to the difference in mean levels of glycemia between them. Similar results were obtained when development of microaneurysms in the primary cohort, microalbuminuria, and neuropathy were modeled against HbA1c in like manner *(36)*.

Others have reported that there is a glycemic threshold around 8.0% HbA1c, below which no further risk of microalbuminuria *(37)* or retinopathy *(38)* is demonstrable. Because of the therapeutic importance such a threshold would have, the DCCT research group reanalyzed their data with models explicitly designed to reveal a threshold, if one existed *(39)*. No threshold could be demonstrated with this largest prospectively collected set of complications data. Thus, to completely prevent retinopathy, nephropathy, and neuropathy, complete normalization of blood glucose will almost certainly be required.

However, it must also be appreciated that because of the exponential nature of the relationship, the absolute risk of retinopathy decreases less for any proportional decrement in HbA1c as one approaches the nondiabetic HbA1c range *(36)*. For example, a decrease in HbA1c from 11.0% to 9.9%, a 10% decrease, reduces the absolute risk of retinopathy progression by 7.23 events per 100 patient-years (12.69 to 4.46); by contrast, a decrease in HbA1c from 7.0% to 6.3% (also a 10% decrease) reduces the absolute risk of retinopathy by 0.67 events per 100 patient years (1.17 to 0.50). Given the huge numbers of patients with type 1 diabetes worldwide (to say nothing of those with type 2 diabetes), this even smaller decrease in total numbers of retinopathy events is not inconsequential to society and to public health. Nonetheless, how much benefit the preadolescent, adolescent, or adult patient gains in striving for normal glycemia must be balanced against how much extra risk that individual patient incurs, especially for severe hypoglycemia.

Time of exposure also increases the risk of retinopathy associated with any level of hyperglycemia *(36)*. This is shown in Fig. 5 using data from the conventional treatment group. Exposure to a mean HbA1c of 11% for less than 3 yr yields the same rate of retinopathy as exposure to a HbA1c of 8% for 9 yr. The message is clear: The less time we allow a patient to be exposed to high levels of blood glucose, the better; the sooner we can safely start each patient on IT, the better. The latter point is illustrated by still other data from the whole DCCT cohort. The reduction in risk of retinopathy with IT versus CT was related to the duration of type 1 diabetes prior to entering the study *(16)*. For durations of 1, 5, 10, and 15 yr, the respective reductions in risk, using intensive

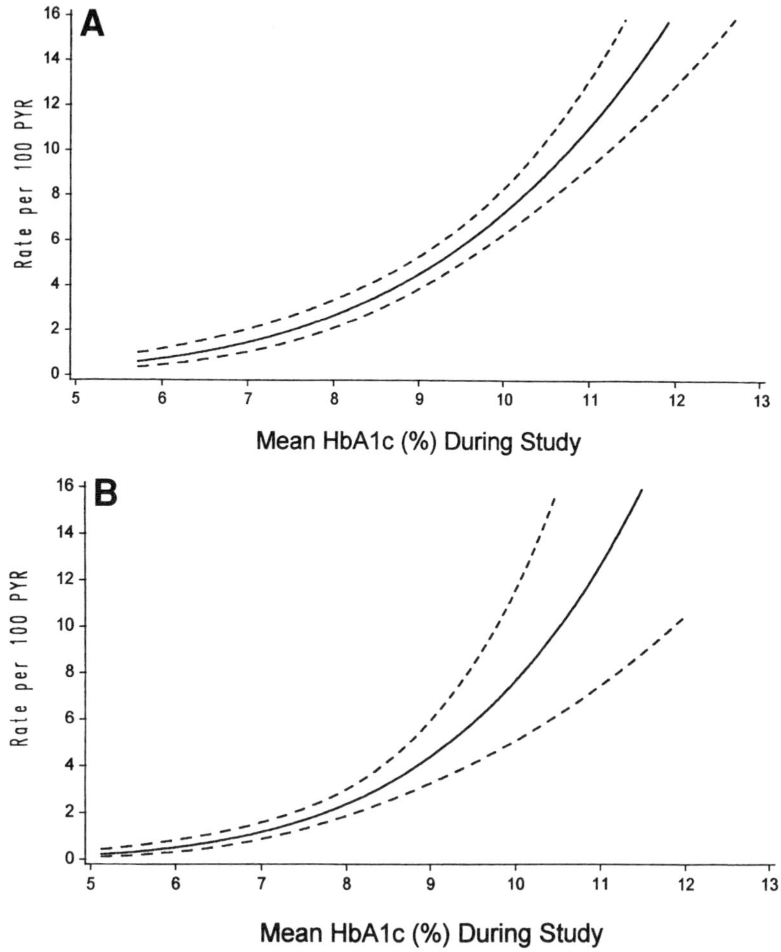

Fig. 4. Absolute risk of sustained retinopathy progression as a function of the mean HbA1c up to the time of the event in conventional group **(A)** and intensive group **(B)** of the entire DCCT cohort using a Poisson regression model. The risk gradients are not significantly different between the two treatment groups. (From ref. *36* © 1995 American Diabetes Association.)

treatment, were 92%, 77%, 64%, and 53%. Starting IT after 1 yr of type 1 diabetes was therefore almost twice as effective as starting it after 15 yr duration.

A related benefit of beginning IT is the preservation of C-peptide (i.e., insulin) secretion. Over half (855) of the DCCT cohort had type 1 diabetes duration of 1–5 yr at entry to the trial *(40)*. Of these, 303 (35%) were C-peptide responders as defined earlier. One hundred thirty-eight (45%) of these C-peptide responders were assigned to IT and 165 (55%) to CT. Those responders randomly assigned to CT rapidly lost their responsiveness (on average after 2–3 yr) *(40)*. By contrast, those responders randomly assigned to IT had extended responsiveness and higher mean C-peptide levels for 5 yr. The risk of completely losing β-cell function over the course of the DCCT was reduced 57% by IT compared to CT *(40)*.

Substantial benefits accrued to those IT patients who retained significant β-cell function. HbA1c was significantly lower at DCCT baseline (8.3% vs 9.4%) *(41)* and

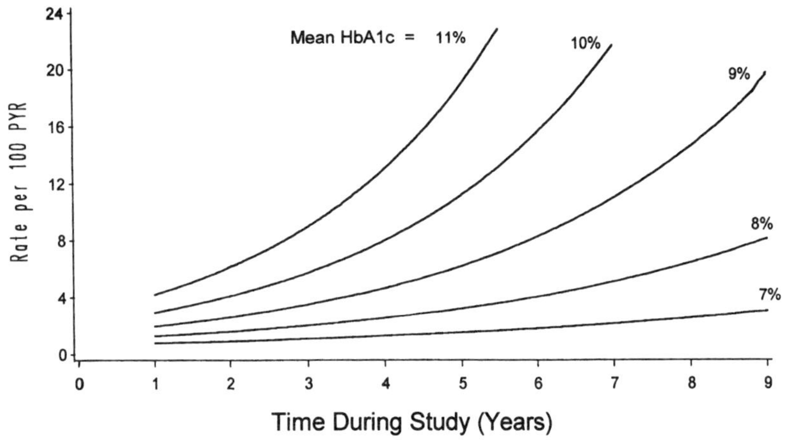

Fig. 5. Absolute risk of sustained retinopathy progression as a function of follow-up time and HbA1c. Note that the rate of retinopathy at any particular time-point is greater at higher HbA1c levels. Conversely, at lower HbA1c levels, it takes a longer time to reach any given rate of retinopathy. Both factors combine to increase the total glycemic exposure and thereby increase the rate of development of retinopathy. (From ref. *36* © 1995 American Diabetes Association.)

remained so for the first 4 yr of the DCCT *(40)*. The average difference was 0.4% lower in C-peptide responders. This benefit was lost after 2 yr of CT. The adjusted relative risks for progression of retinopathy and for development of microalbuminuria over the entire course of the DCCT for IT C-peptide responders vs nonresponders were 0.50 (95% confidence interval [CI]: 0.28–0.88) and 0.73 (95% CI: 0.36–1.46), respectively *(40)*. Moreover, the relative risk of suffering hypoglycemic coma or seizure was 0.38 (95% CI: 0.25–0.59). None of these benefits accrued to the CT C-peptide responders who lost their β-cell function more quickly. All of these observations emphasize and support the importance of beginning IT as early as safely possible in the course of type 1 diabetes.

The adverse hyperglycemic effects on the eyes and kidneys exhibit a carryover effect manifested by a kind of "metabolic memory" displayed by these target organs. The entry level of HbA1c was itself a significant, positive risk factor for subsequent progression of retinopathy, particularly in the CT group *(36)*. This was explained only partly by the fact that the entry-level HbA1c predicted the mean HbA1c during the trial. The prior duration of type 1 diabetes was also a significant positive risk factor for progression of retinopathy. These effects of prior glycemic exposure (HbA1c × time) were vividly illustrated by the time-course of response to intensive treatment. Not until 3–4 yr of DCCT treatment did the reduced risk of retinopathy with IT become evident in the whole DCCT cohort *(14)* or in the adolescent group specifically (Figs. 1 and 2). Again, this observation speaks for early initiation of intensive therapy.

Of the DCCT cohort, 95% are participating in an extended follow-up study called Epidemiology of Diabetes Interventions and Complications (EDIC). The effects of prior DCCT IT vs CT have been analyzed 4 yr after the closeout of the DCCT *(42)*. Within 1 yr, HbA1c in the former IT group rose about 1%, whereas HbA1c in the former CT group fell about 1%. During the entire 4 yr of EDIC, median HbA1c levels in the whole cohort of former intensively treated and conventionally treated subjects were 7.9% and 8.2%, respectively *(42)*. Despite this virtual equalization of glycemic control

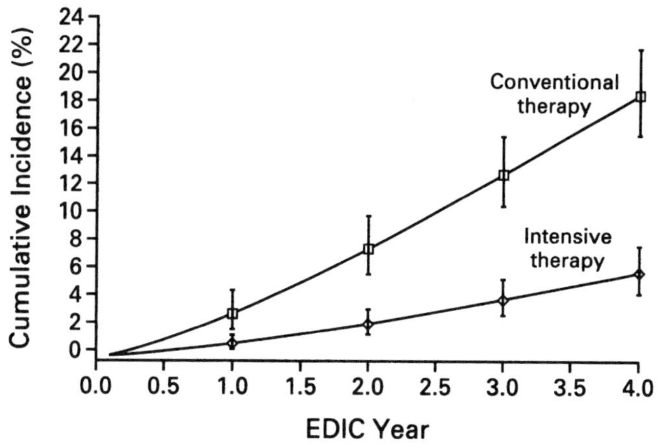

Fig. 6. Cumulative incidence of further progression of retinopathy from the end of the DCCT throughout the initial 4 post-DCCT (EDIC) years. Note the continued reduction in risk of retinopathy in the *former* intensive treatment group compared to the *former* conventional treatment group even after the DCCT had ended. (From ref. *42* © 2000 Massachusetts Medical Society. All rights reserved.)

for the ensuing 4 yr, the previous intensively treated patients continued to exhibit the advantages of their former therapy. The risk of a sustained three-step progression of retinopathy, from DCCT baseline, was reduced 75% after 4 yr of EDIC compared to 76% at DCCT closeout *(42)*. Even more important, the risks of clinically significant macular edema (CSME) and of requiring retinal photocoagulation for either CSME or proliferative retinopathy were reduced 46–56% in IT patients compared to former CT patients at DCCT closeout and still 52–58% after 4 yr of EDIC *(42)*. When the progression of retinopathy from the retinopathy status at DCCT closeout over the subsequent 4 yr of EDIC was specifically analyzed (Fig. 6), this risk was reduced 60–83% for various outcomes *(42)*. Parallel results were observed when development of microalbuminuria or progression to macroalbuminuria (AER > 300 mg/d) was analyzed *(42)*. All of these continued differences in later outcomes resulted from an average of 6.5 yr of prior IT versus CT and were strongly statistically significant.

The same trends were seen when the former DCCT adolescents on IT and CT were analyzed as a separate group *(43)*. However, the statistical significance of the continuing differences in various outcomes was weaker or marginal because of the much smaller numbers of subjects and events. Most of the DCCT adolescents—now young adults in EDIC—stated that they were still practicing IT. The mean HbA1c levels in the former IT and CT subjects were 8.4% and 8.5%, respectively. The risks of a three-step progression from DCCT baseline and of new proliferative diabetic retinopathy were further reduced 67% ($p = 0.03$), and 85% ($p = 0.06$), respectively. None of the former IT patients, compared to 5.6% of the former CT patients, have, thus far, required photocoagulation therapy during the 4 yr of EDIC. It was found that 9.9% of the former CT group vs 1.3% of the former IT group progressed to AER > 300 mg/d ($p = 0.08$). Thus, any significant period of intensive treatment, such as 6.5 yr, casts a beneficial glow for at least 4 yr thereafter, even if the HbA1c rises modestly. This is analogous to the adverse shadow cast by the first 3–4 yr of CT at the beginning of the DCCT (Fig. 1) *(14,22)*. Naturally, this observation is not to be taken as an argument for using IT for limited periods of time. The sum total of all these DCCT–EDIC observations of glycemic exposure supports the biological view that there is a momentum factor in retinopathy and nephropathy contributed to by the combination of glycemic level and time. The process of tissue damage builds up slowly, but in an accelerated fashion at higher HbA1c levels (Fig. 5), it decelerates slowly at lower HbA1c levels (Fig. 2), but also resumes its progression slowly after a period of time at lower HbA1c levels (Fig. 6). The clinical lesson of the DCCT is that intensive treatment with the preservation of β cell function should begin early and be sustained for as long as possible.

Genetic and Tissue Factors Affecting Complications

Late in its course, the DCCT also conducted a family study looking for familial clustering of retinopathy or nephropathy *(44)*. Two hundred forty-one first-degree relatives of 217 DCCT probands were studied, measuring their HbA1c level, determining their duration of diabetes, and assessing retinopathy and nephropathy status. First-degree relatives of DCCT probands with severe nonproliferative diabetic retinopathy, clinically significant macular edema, or having undergone photocoagulation were more likely to exhibit these signs of severe retinopathy than were first-degree relatives of DCCT probands without such severe retinopathy *(44)*. The risk ratio was 3.1 ($p < .05$). Moreover, first-degree relatives of DCCT probands with microalbuminuria were more likely to have microalbuminuria, macroalbuminuria, or end-stage renal disease than first-degree relatives of DCCT probands who did not have microalbuminuria. The risk ratio was 5.6 ($p < .001$). These observations suggest that involvement of genetic factors is increasing the risk of complications. These risk ratios persisted even when adjusted for HbA1c levels *(44)*.

In an ancillary study, 216 DCCT subjects volunteered to have a skin biopsy performed near the end of the trial *(45)*. The collagen was extracted from the skin and the levels of glycated collagen (furosine) and of the advanced glycation end products, pentosidine and carboxymethyllysine, were measured. In addition, the acid and pepsin solubility of the collagen was determined, as indicators of its elasticity. When all of these parameters were combined into a single panel reflecting collagen abnormalities that result from hyperglycemia, the degree of retinopathy, nephropathy, and neuropathy of the patients was correlated with their panels of collagen abnormalities. These collagen abnormalities explained as much as 51% of the variance in the complications, a contribution similar to or greater than that of the HbA1c level itself in some cases. The association of the complications with the collagen abnormalities was also independent of HbA1c levels *(45)*.

Taken together, the above observations suggest the existence of genetic factors that could increase or decrease the susceptibility of tissue to hyperglycemic damage. When it becomes possible to easily and accurately determine each individual patient's vulnerability to diabetic complications, it will also be possible to determine each individual's relative need for intensive treatment of hyperglycemia. This, in turn, will enable us to focus our resources on those patients who absolutely require intensive treatment of type 1 diabetes and spare those patients, who may not require equally rigorous treatment in order to avoid long-term complications, from its burdens and hazards. Nonetheless, normoglycemia should be a goal for all patients, if it can be achieved without the hazards of hypoglycemia, the health and social burdens of obesity, and serious disruption of lifestyle.

APPLICATION OF DCCT RESULTS IN THE COMMUNITY

How well can the DCCT results be extended to typical type 1 patients in typical diabetes care settings? Following the conclusion of the DCCT, both treatment groups were informed of the results of the trial and of the benefits and risks of intensive treatment. The intensive-treatment group was encouraged to continue that regimen, whereas the conventional-treatment group was strongly advised to adopt intensive treatment by learning to implement it before the DCCT clinics ceased managing their diabetes.

During the first two post-DCCT years, 95% of the former intensive-treatment group and 70% of the former conventional-treatment group reported practicing intensive treatment *(46)*. During these 2 yr, the median HbA1c of the former intensive group rose to 7.9% and that of the former conventional group fell to 8.1% *(46)*. Only 46% of intensive-treatment subjects and 36% of conventional-treatment subjects reported monitoring blood glucose four or more times per day *(47)*.

The best overall results with intensive treatment has been reported by an Italian group. One hundred twenty-four patients were started on intensive treatment at the time of diagnosis of type 1 during the period from 1981 to 1994; 112 patients remained on intensive treatment during those years *(24)*. The mean HbA1c was 7.2% (1.31 × ULN, with a range of 0.82–2.27). The patients, followed as outpatients every 2–3 mo, were recently offered free consultation 24 h/d by cellular telephone. This degree of commitment to achieving superior metabolic results might be very difficult for most practitioners to offer to more than a few patients.

More "real-life" results are seen in a cross-sectional analysis of over 3000 type 1 diabetic patients selected randomly at 31 diabetes centers in 16 European countries *(48)*. The mean HbA1c in approximate DCCT equivalents was 8.4%, varying among the centers from a low of 7.2% to a high of 11.8%. These results were reported after a HbA1c<7.0% had already been a consensus goal of treatment for several years in Europe *(49)*.

Given the reductions in retinopathy, nephropathy, and neuropathy in the DCCT adolescents randomized to intensive treatment, how well is such treatment being implemented in children and adolescents? A review of the published experience indicates the results are mixed. In a population-based sample of over 600 children and adolescents in western Australia, the mean HbA1c was 9.1% (1.47 × ULN); the mean HbA1c was 8.9% in children < 6 yr of age compared to 9.3% in those age 12–18 *(50)*. Except for a few of the older patients, the majority was injecting insulin only twice a day.

In a Belgian public university hospital, one pediatric diabetologist and nurse reported a mean HbA1c of 6.6% (1.20 × ULN) in a consecutive unselected group of 144 type 1 diabetic children and adolescents. Of these patients, 90% administered only two daily injections of insulin, but they performed self blood glucose monitoring an average of three to four times a day *(51)*. This unusually good compliance with monitoring and the excellent HbA1c results may be partly explained by the fact that the families of these children paid for very little of this care.

In a 1992 report from France, 205 adolescent type 1 diabetic patients were randomly assigned to remain on 2 injections or be switched to 3 injections of insulin per day *(52)*. The group taking three injections decreased HbA1c from 9.8% (1.46 × ULN) to 9.3%, whereas the group taking two injections increased HbA1c from 9.5% to 9.8%. The small difference in final outcome of 0.5% was statistically significant. A larger difference of 1.4% was observed in patients whose HbA1c was > 11.2% at entry. Neither group experienced a change in the rate of hypoglycemia and the three-injection regimen was as acceptable to the patients and the families as the two-injection regimen.

In 1995, a cross-sectional nationwide study was conducted in 2579 children with type 1 diabetes receiving care in 206 treatment centers in France *(53)*. Most of the children were still injecting insulin twice daily but reporting an average of almost three self blood glucose measurements daily. The mean HbA1c of the entire cohort was 9.0% (1.48 × ULN). Of these children, one-third had a HbA1c < 8.0%, a value similar to the median HbA1c in the DCCT intensively treated adolescents; however, almost one-sixth still had a HbA1c > 11.0%, much higher than the median HbA1c of the conventionally treated adolescents in the DCCT. Despite the less than optimal degree of glycemic control, the rate of severe hypoglycemia was 45 per 100 person-years.

Two years after the appearance of the DCCT results, a survey conducted in 1995 in 22 pediatric diabetic centers (15 in Europe, 4 in the United Kingdom, and 1 each in Japan, the United States, and Canada) reported HbA1c levels in 2873 children and adolescents *(54,55)*. In approximate DCCT equivalence, mean HbA1c was 8.3% (8.0% in those < 11 yr of age and 8.6% in those age 12–18). The HbA1c level in the teenagers was closer to that of the adolescents on IT in the DCCT (8.1%) than to the HbA1c of the DCCT adolescents on CT (9.8%). There was much disparity in the results; the mean HbA1c ranged from 7.3% to 9.9% among the centers, with an upward skew in the distribution. About one-third of the pediatric patients was injecting insulin three or more times daily and about one-third of this group had HbA1c levels below 7.7%. There was no correlation between the daily number of injections and HbA1c level. A lower HbA1c level was seen in patients whose daily dose contained a higher fraction of short-acting insulin. The event rate of severe hypoglycemia was 22 per 100 patient-years *(54)*, about that of the DCCT conventionally treated adolescents.

In one of the DCCT sites with a reference HbA1c laboratory, the mean HbA1c in the pediatric diabetic clinic has been tracked yearly from 1983 to 1999 (Fig. 7) *(56)*. Patients over 18 yr of age and with < 1 yr diabetes duration were excluded. The mean age and duration remained steady over the years as patients entered and exited the clinic, although the overall number of patients increased. Prior to the DCCT results, HbA1c was stable at 8.6% from 1983 to 1990, decreased slightly to 8.4% from 1990 to 1993, and then dropped more sharply to 7.9% in the post-DCCT 1993–1999 interval.

Another DCCT site has reported a research cohort study comparing 25 adolescents who chose CSII to 50 who chose MDI for intensive therapy in 1995–1998 *(57)*. After 6 mo, the mean HbA1c fell from 8.8% to 8.1% (nondiabetic range: 4.3–6.3%) in the MDI group and from 8.4% to 7.7% in the CSII group; the decrements in HbA1c were equal at 0.7%. However, by 12 mo, the mean HbA1c has risen slightly to 8.3% in the MDI group, whereas it declined further to 7.5% in the CSII group. The latter value was quite similar to that achieved by the DCCT adolescent intensively treated subjects at 12 mo. The CSII group used less total insulin dose than the MDI group (1.05 vs 1.49 U/kg/d) and had a lower incidence of severe hypoglycemia (76 vs 134 events per 100 patient-years) and manifestations of coma or seizure (24 vs 46 events/per 100 patient-years). Both groups reported improvement in a variety of psychosocial outcomes measured, including quality of life, depression, and diabetes self-efficacy. CSII users found coping with diabetes less difficult than did MDI users. Although these early results are encouraging, the CSII group was self-selected. It also remains to be seen how long beyond 12

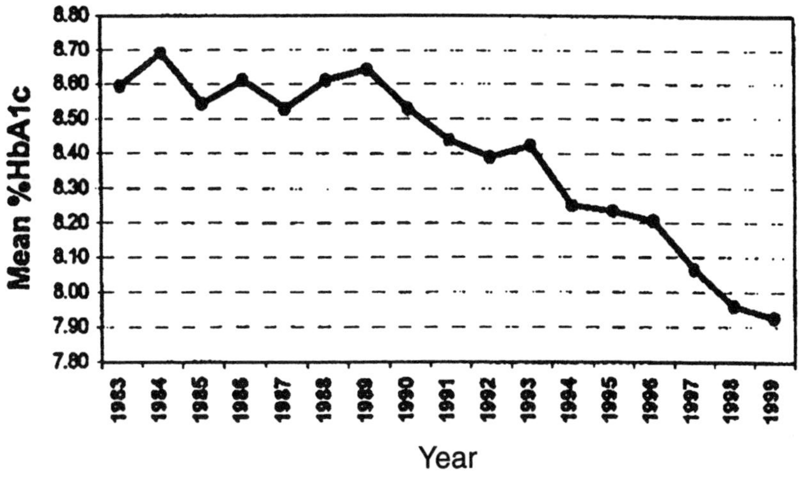

Fig. 7. The secular trend in HbA1c in the diabetes clinic of an academic institution that participated in the DCCT. Note the decline beginning in 1989–1990 but increasing further after announcement of the DCCT results in 1993. (From ref. *56* © 2000 American Diabetes Association.)

mo that the HbA1c can be kept down and whether similar results can be achieved outside of research centers and without the availability of research-grade resources.

SUMMARY

The DCCT has shown incontrovertibly that intensive treatment of type 1 diabetes significantly reduces the long-term incidence of retinopathy, nephropathy, and neuropathy in type 1 diabetic patients, including adolescents 13 yr of age and older. Intensive treatment is more effective when begun early, at a time when it may help maintain some residual endogenous insulin secretion. The efficacy and safety of intensive treatment in children less than 13 yr of age remains unproven.

Moreover, there is still debate as to whether control of diabetes during the prepubertal years affects the risk of complications *(58–61)* and there remains concern about the long-range effects of hypoglycemia suffered by children *(62–64)*. The ability to translate the now proven benefits of intensive treatment into daily adult and pediatric practice remains limited. Recent reports suggest that glycemic control in adolescents can be improved to near DCCT intensive treatment adolescent levels with relative safety when adequate resources are utilized in specialty centers. The development of point of care HbA1c instruments *(65)* and synthetic insulin analogs that better mimic basal insulin secretion *(66,67)* or mealtime bursts of insulin release *(68,69)* portend more efficacious and possibly safer intensive treatment. Ultimately, the promise of the DCCT that diabetic complications can be prevented in all type 1 diabetic patients most likely will be fulfilled by islet transplantation *(70)*.

REFERENCES

1. LaPorte RE, Matsushima M, Chang YF. Prevalence and incidence of insulin-dependent diabetes. Diabetes in America, 2nd ed. National Institutes of Health, Washington, DC, 1995.
2. Deckert T, Pulsen JE, Larsen M. Prognosis of diabetics with onset before the age of thirty-one. I. Causes of death and complications. Diabetologia 1978;14:363–370.

3. Nathan DM. Long-term complications of diabetes mellitus. N Engl J Med 1993;328:1676–1685.
4. Deckert T, Pulsen JE, Larsen M. Prognosis of diabetics with onset before the age of thirty-one. II. Factors influencing the prognosis. Diabetologia 1978;14:371–377.
5. Genuth SM. The case for blood glucose control. Adv Int Med. 1995;40:573–623.
6. Engerman R, Bloodworth JMB Jr, Nelson S. Relationship of micro-vascular disease in diabetes to metabolic control. Diabetes 1977;26:760–769.
7. Vlassara H, Bucala R, Striker L. Pathogenic effects of advanced glycosylation: biochemical, biologic, and clinical implications for diabetes and aging. Lab Invest 1994;70:138–148.
8. Brownlee M. Negative consequences of glycation. Metabolism 2000;49:9–13.
9. Baynes JW, Thorpe SR. Role of oxidative stress in diabetic complications: a new perspective on an old paradigm. Diabetes 1999;48:1–9.
10. Carrington AL, Litchfield JE. The aldose reductase pathway and nonenzymatic glycation in the pathogenesis of diabetic neuropathy: a critical review for the end of the 20th century. Diabetes Rev 1999;7:275–299.
11. Ishii H, Daisuke K, King GL. Protein kinase C activation and its role in the development of vascular complications in diabetes mellitus. J Mol Med 1998;76:21–31.
12. The DCCT Research Group. Feasibility of centralized measurements of glycated hemoglobin in the Diabetes Control and Complications Trial: A multicenter study. Clin Chem 1987;33:2267–2271.
13. The DCCT Research Group. The Diabetes Control and Complications Trial (DCCT) design and methodologic considerations for the feasibility phase. Diabetes 1986;35:530–545.
14. The DCCT Research Group. The effect of intensive treatment of diabetes on the development and progression of long-term complications in insulin-dependent diabetes mellitus. N Engl J Med 1993;329:977–986.
15. The DCCT Research Group. The effect of intensive diabetes treatment on the progression of diabetic retinopathy in insulin-dependent diabetes mellitus. Arch Opthalmol 1995;113:36–51.
16. The DCCT Research Group. Progression of retinopathy with intensive versus conventional treatment in the diabetes control and complications trial. Ophthalmology 1995;102:647–661.
17. The DCCT Research Group. Effect of intensive therapy on the development and progression of diabetic nephropathy in the Diabetes Control and Complications Trial. Kidney Int 1995;47:1703–1720.
18. The DCCT Research Group. The effect of intensive diabetes therapy on the development and progression of neuropathy. Ann Intern Med 1995;122:561–568.
19. The DCCT Research Group. Effect of intensive diabetes treatment on nerve conduction in the diabetes control and complications trial. Ann Neurol 1995;38:869–880.
20. The DCCT Research Group. Adverse events and their association with treatment regimens in the diabetes control and complications trial. Diabetes Care 1995;18:1415–1427.
21. The DCCT Research Group. Implementation of treatment protocols in the Diabetes Control and Complications Trial. Diabetes Care 1995;18:361–376.
22. The DCCT Research Group. Effect of intensive diabetes treatment on the development and progression of long-term complications in adolescents with insulin-dependent diabetes mellitus: Diabetes Control and Complications Trial. J Pediatr 1994;125:177–188.
23. Cryer PE. Hypoglycemia: the limiting factor in the management of IDDM. Diabetes 1994;43:1378–1389.
24. Pampanelli S, Fanelli C, Lalli C, et al. Long-term intensive insulin therapy in IDDM: effects on HbA1c, risk for severe and mild hypoglycaemia, status of counterregulation and awareness of hypoglycaemia. Diabetologia 1996;39:677–686.
25. Wahren J, Ekberg K, Fernqvist-Forbes E, et al. Brain substrate utilisation during acute hyperglycaemia. Diabetologia 1999;42:812–818.
26. Gale EAM, Tattersal RB. Unrecognized nocturnal hypoglycemia in insulin-treated diabetes. Lancet 1979;1:1049–1052.
27. The DCCT Research Group. Epidemiology of severe hypoglycemia in the Diabetes Control and Complications Trial. Am J Med 1991;90:450–459.
28. The DCCT Research Group. Hypoglycemia in the Diabetes Control and Complications Trial. Diabetes 1997;46:271–286.
29. The DCCT Research Group. Effects of intensive diabetes therapy on neuropsychological function in adults in the Diabetes Control and Complications Trial. Ann Intern Med 1996;124:379–388.
30. Kramer L, Fasching P, Madl C, et al. Previous episodes of hypoglycemic coma are not associated with permanent cognitive brain dysfunction in IDDM patients on intensive insulin treatment. Diabetes 1998;47:1909–1914.
31. The DCCT Research Group. Weight gain associated with intensive therapy in the Diabetes Control and Complications Trial. Diabetes Care 1988;11:567–573.

32. Purnell JQ, Hokanson JE, Marcovina SM, et al. Effect of excessive weight gain with intensive therapy of type 1 diabetes on lipid levels and blood pressure. Results from the DCCT. JAMA 1998;280: 140–146.
33. Sibley SD, Hokanson JE, Steffes MW, et al. Increased small dense LDL and intermediate-density lipoprotein with albuminuria in type 1 diabetes. Diabetes Care 1999;22:1165–1170.
34. The DCCT Research Group. Effect of intensive diabetes management on macrovascular events and risk factors in the Diabetes Control and Complications Trial. Am J Cardiol 1995;75:894–903.
35. The DCCT Research Group. Influence of intensive diabetes treatment on quality-of-life outcomes in the Diabetes Control and Complications Trial. Diabetes Care 1996;19:195–203.
36. The DCCT Research Group. The relationship of glycemic exposure (HbA_{1c}) to the risk of development and progression of retinopathy in the Diabetes Control and Complications Trial. Diabetes 1995;44:968–983.
37. Krolewski AS, Laffel LMB, Krolewski M, et al. Glycosylated hemoglobin and the risk of microalbuminuria in patients with insulin-dependent diabetes mellitus. N Engl J Med 1995;332:1251–1255.
38. Warram JH, Manson JE, Krolewski As. Glycosylated hemoglobin and the risk of retinopathy in insulin-dependent diabetes mellitus. N Engl J Med 1995;332:1035–1036.
39. The DCCT Research Group. The absence of a glycemic threshold for the development of long-term complications: the perspective of the Diabetes Control and Complications Trial. Diabetes 1996;45: 1289–1298.
40. The DCCT Research Group. Effect of intensive therapy on residual B-cell function in patients with type 1 diabetes in the Diabetes Control and Complications Trial. A randomized, controlled trial. Ann Intern Med 1998;128:517–523.
41. The DCCT Research Group. Effects of age, duration and treatment on insulin-dependent diabetes mellitus on residual B-cell function: observations during eligibility testing for the Diabetes Control and Complications Trial (DCCT). J Clin Endocrinol Metab 1987;65:30–36.
42. The DCCT/EDIC Research Group. Retinopathy and nephropathy in patients with type 1 diabetes four years after a trial of intensive therapy. N Engl J Med 2000;342:381–389.
43. White NH, Cleary PA, Dahms W, et al. Prolonged effects of DCCT intensive therapy (INT) in adolescents on diabetes complications after four years of follow-up in Epidemiology of Diabetes Interventions and Complications (EDIC). Diabetes 2000;49(Suppl 1):A47–A48.
44. The DCCT Research Group. Clustering of long-term complications in families with diabetes in the Diabetes Control and Complications Trial. Diabetes 1997;46:1829–1839.
45. Monnier VM, Bautista O, Kenny D, et al. Skin collagen glycation, glycoxidation, and crosslinking are lower in subjects with long-term intensive versus conventional therapy of type 1 diabetes. Relevance of glycated collagen products versus HbA_{1c} as markers of diabetic complications. Diabetes 1999;48:870–880.
46. EDIC Study Group. Epidemiology of Diabetes Interventions and Complications (EDIC): design, implementation, and preliminary results of a long-term follow-up of the Diabetes Control and Complications Trial cohort. Diabetes Care 1999;22:99–111.
47. Kolterman O, Lorenzi G. Self-care practices and outcomes in the DCCT cohort two years post-completion: EDIC follow-up study. Diabetes 1996;45:124A.
48. The EURODIAB IDDM Complications Study Group. Microvascular and acute complications in IDDM patients: the EURODIAB IDDM complications study. Diabetologia 1994;37:278–285.
49. European IDDM Policy Group. Consensus guidelines for the management of insulin-dependent (type 1) diabetes. Diabet Med 1993;10:990.
50. Davis EA, Keating B, Byrne GC, et al. Hypoglycemia: incidence and clinical predictors in a large population-based sample of children and adolescents with IDDM. Diabetes Care 1997;20:22–25.
51. Dorchy H, Roggemans M-P, Willems D. Glycated hemoglobin and related factors in diabetic children and adolescents under 18 years of age: a Belgian experience. Diabetes Care 1997;20:2–6.
52. Bourgnères PF, Landais P, Mairesse AM, et al. Improvement of diabetic control and acceptability of a three-injection insulin regimen in diabetic adolescents. Diabetes Care 1993;16:94–102.
53. Rosilio M, Cotton J-B, Wieliczko M-C, et al. Factors associated with glycemic control: a cross-sectional nationwide study in 2,579 French children with type 1 diabetes. Diabetes Care 1998;21:1146–1153.
54. Mortensen HB, Hougaard P. Comparison of metabolic control in a cross-sectional study of 2,873 children and adolescents with IDDM from 18 countries. Diabetes Care 1997;20:714–720.
55. Mortensen HB, Robertson KJ, Aanstoot H-J, et al. Insulin management and metabolic control of type 1 diabetes mellitus in childhood and adolescence in 18 countries. Diabet Med 1998;15:752–759.

56. Rohlfing CL, Little RR, Wiedmeyer H-M, et al. Improved glycemic control in childhood diabetes: a 16-year study. Diabetes 2000;49:A93–A94.
57. Boland EA, Grey M, Oesterle A, et al. Continuous subcutaneous insulin infusion: a new way to lower risk of severe hypoglycemia, improve metabolic control, and enhance coping in adolescents with type 1 diabetes. Diabetes Care 1999;22:1779–1784.
58. Kostraba JN, Dorman JS, Orchard TJ. Contribution of diabetes-duration before puberty to development of microvascular complications in IDDM subjects. Diabetes Care 1989;12:686–693.
59. Donaghue KC, Fung ATW, Hing S, et al. The effect of prepubertal diabetes duration on diabetes: microvascular complications in early and late adolescence. Diabetes Care 1997;20:77–80.
60. Danne T, Kordonouri O, Hövener G, et al. Diabetic angiopathy in children. Diabet Med 1997;14:1012–1025.
61. Lobefalo L, Verrotti A, Della Loggia G, et al. Diabetic retinopathy in childhood and adolescence: effect of puberty. Diabet Nutr Metab 1997;10:193–197.
62. Ryan CM, Atchison J, Puczynski S. Mild hypoglycemia associated with deterioration of mental efficiency in children with insulin dependent diabetes mellitus. J Pediatr 1990;117:32–38.
63. Ryan C, Vega A, Drash A. Cognitive deficits in adolescents who developed diabetes early in life. Pediatrics 1985;75:921–927.
64. Northam EA, Anderson PJ, Werther GA, et al. Neuropsychological complications of IDDM in children 2 years after disease onset. Diabetes Care 1998;21:379–384.
65. Cagliero E, Levina EV, Nathan DM. Immediate feedback of HbA_{1c} levels improves glycemic control in type 1 and insulin-treated type 2 diabetic patients. Diabetes Care 1999;22:1785–1789.
66. Lepore M, Pampanelli S, Fanelli CG, et al. Pharmacokinetics and dynamics of s.c. injection of insulin glargine, NPH and ultralente in T1DM: comparison with CSII. Diabetes 2000;49(Suppl 1):A9.
67. Pieber TR, Eugene-Jolchine I, Derobert E, et al. Efficacy and safety of HOE 901 versus NPH insulin in patients with type 1 diabetes. Diabetes Care 2000;23:157–162.
68. Chase HP, Peery BN, Shepherd ME, et al. The impact of the DCCT and of humalog treatment on glycohemoglobin (HbA1c) and hypoglycemia in type 1 diabetes. Diabetes 1999;48:A100.
69. Mudaliar SR, Lindberg FA, Joyce M, et al. Insulin aspart (B28 Asp-insulin): a fast-acting analog of human insulin: absorption kinetics and action profile compared with regular human insulin in healthy nondiabetic subjects. Diabetes Care 1999;22:1501–1506.
70. Shapiro J, Lakey JRT, Ryan EA, et al. Islet transplantation in seven patients with type 1 diabetes mellitus using a glucocorticoid-free immunosuppressive regimen. N Engl J Med 2000;343:230–238.

12 Open- and Closed-Loop Insulin Delivery Systems and Glucose Sensors

John C. Pickup, *MA, BM, BCh, DPhil, FRCPath*

CONTENTS

INTRODUCTION

Insulin replacement in diabetes aims to mimic nondiabetic insulin delivery patterns: a constant basal level throughout the entire day, with boosts at mealtimes, and feedback control of blood glucose concentrations via the glucose sensor of the β-cell. With insulin injections, this is accomplished or attempted by the use of long-acting insulin formulations for the basal supply and short-acting insulin for meals, with capillary blood glucose self-monitoring for dose adjustment and feedback control. In the last 25 yr or so, there have been attempts to obtain near-normoglycemia in diabetes by an alternative strategy: simulating physiological insulin administration using various electromechanical infusion systems.

Insulin infusion is described as "open loop" when the delivery rate is preset, with prandial boosts activated by the patient or physician. The most widely used form of this in clinical practice is continuous subcutaneous insulin infusion (CSII), now commonly known as "insulin pump therapy." "Closed-loop" insulin delivery systems use a glucose sensor to measure blood or interstitial fluid glucose concentrations and automatically alter the insulin infusion rate to maintain euglycemia. This feedback-control technology is also known as an "artificial endocrine pancreas." Most open-loop pumps are worn externally on the body; implanted open-loop pumps are still largely experimental.

From: *Contemporary Endocrinology: Type 1 Diabetes: Etiology and Treatment*
Edited by: M. A. Sperling © Humana Press Inc., Totowa, NJ

OPEN-LOOP SYSTEMS

CSII

In the 1970s, several workers showed that strict blood glucose control can be achieved in type 1 and 2 diabetes using variable-rate continuous intravenous insulin infusion over a few days *(1–5)*. Although this can be extended to several months in selected ambulatory subjects *(6)*, the risks of septicemia and thrombosis exclude intravenous insulin infusion as a long-term therapeutic approach. At this time, we were exploring new ways of achieving prolonged near-normoglycemia in type 1 diabetes, specifically to test the links between diabetic control and microvascular complications, and CSII was proposed as a way of realizing this goal *(7)*. It was hoped that infusing the insulin subcutaneously, rather than intravenously, would be a safer, more practicable long-term treatment. It was immediately apparent that much improved blood glucose and intermediary metabolite control was obtainable in comparison with conventional injection regimens *(7–9)*, quickly confirmed by many groups *(10–13)*.

CSII uses a portable, battery-driven pump to infuse insulin at a variety of rates via a fine and flexible delivery cannula that terminates in an implanted needle. The usual infusion site is the abdomen. Pumps from the two main manufacturers at present (MiniMed-Medtronic and Disetronic) are syringe drivers, where a motor-driven leadscrew advances an actuator and depresses the plunger of a small syringe. Other technologies such as clockwork pumps and rotary peristaltic pumps have been abandoned. The basal and bolus rates are set electronically on modern pumps by keys or buttons, and basal rates can be preprogrammed to come into operation at set times in the day (e.g., an increased nocturnal rate in the hours before breakfast) (*see* the following subsection). Alarm systems usually include those for cannula blockage, low-battery state, and empty syringe.

STARTING PATIENTS ON CSII

Until recently, buffered short-acting (regular) insulin has been used for CSII, but the pump insulin of choice is probably now a monomeric insulin such as lispro (Humalog, Eli Lilly) *(14–17)*. Insulin aspart (NovoRapid, Novo Nordisk) seems to be an effective alternative monomeric insulin *(18)*, but there is less experience with it for CSII.

A typical initial infusion strategy (Fig. 1) is to administer, via the pump, 80% of the daily insulin dose on injections, half as the basal rate (average about 13 mU/kg/h or 0.9 U/h for adults) and half divided among the three main meals. Prandial boosts are given on average 30 min before the meal when using regular insulin and with the meal when using monomeric insulin. The basal rate is adjusted for the individual patient by using the fasting (prebreakfast) blood glucose concentration and the 0300 h value. The mealtime insulin dose is adjusted using blood glucose values after meals. The usual ratio of prandial : basal insulin is 45 : 55%.

In many patients receiving insulin injections, the blood glucose levels increase significantly between about 0300 and 0800 h; this is known as the "dawn phenomenon" *(19)* and is the result of a decrease in insulin sensitivity caused by nocturnal surges of growth hormone *(20,21)*, combined with a waning of insulin action as insulin levels decline from the previous evening's delayed-action insulin injection. This cause of poor control can be countered in CSII patients by an appropriate choice of nocturnal basal rate *(22)* or by setting the pump to automatically deliver an increased predawn

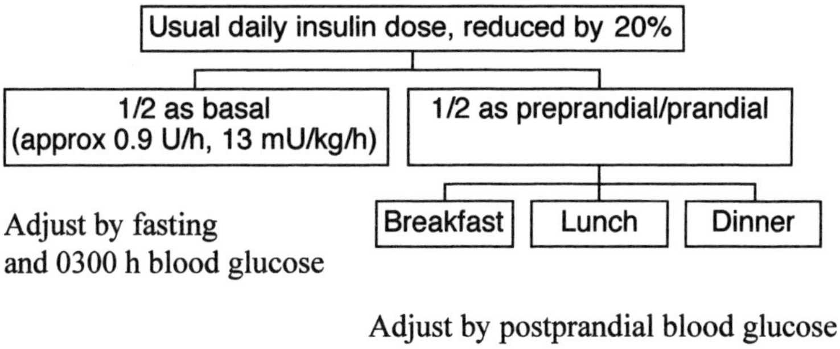

Fig. 1. An insulin infusion strategy for starting patients on continuous subcutaneous insulin infusion.

insulin rate *(23)*. Similarly, low glucose values at about 0300 h can be avoided by reducing the basal rate from midnight to 0300 h. Target blood glucose concentrations should be about 4–6 mmol/L (72–108 mg/dL) in the fasting state and <10 mmol/L (<180 mg/dL) after meals, and various algorithms have been published for adjusting insulin dosages on CSII according to blood glucose values *(24)*.

One of the most important aspects of starting pump therapy is a comprehensive education program. This should include explaining the principles of CSII and dosage adjustments, re-education about blood glucose self-monitoring, instructions for sport and exercise, action in case of hypoglycemia and hyperglycemia, intercurrent illness, ketonuria, pump malfunction, and infusion-site infection. Patients also should be supplied with insulin and syringes for emergency use. Moderate exercise, for example, can be performed without causing hypoglycemia by reducing the basal infusion rate by one-half for the duration of the exercise if this occurs more than 4 h after a meal or reducing the prandial insulin by one-half if exercise occurs shortly after a meal. Blood glucose monitoring after exercise is essential.

The Metabolic Effectiveness of CSII

There is no dispute that in most patients glycemic control is excellent on CSII. This was well shown in several randomized controlled studies testing the effect on diabetic microangiopathy of pump-induced strict control vs the glycemic control of conventional (nonoptimized) insulin injection therapy [e.g., early studies (in the 1980s) from the six-center Kroc Collaborative Group in the United States, Canada, and the United Kingdom *(25)*, the Steno Hospital Study in Copenhagen, Denmark *(26)*, and the Åker Hospital Study in Oslo, Norway *(27)*]. In the large Diabetes Control and Complications Trial (DCCT) in North America, which was reported in 1993 *(28)*, 34% of the intensively treated patients used CSII on a long-term basis (59% at some time). The glycated hemoglobin in the pump vs the nonoptimized injection-treated subjects was 6.8% vs 8.7–9.2%.

In the post-DCCT era, the main point of contention has been the performance of CSII compared to modern, optimized injection regimens or multiple-injection therapy (MIT). The advent of insulin pens, with their convenience and encouragement to use multiple injections, and vastly improved diabetes education of recent years might have enabled patients to match the strict control of CSII with ordinary injections. In 10 randomized, controlled trials of CSII vs MIT (often with relatively small numbers of subjects), glycated hemoglobin percentage was significantly lower in 6 *(29–34)* and similar in 4 of the studies *(27,35–37)*. A recent trial compared CSII using insulin lispro with optimized injection therapy using lispro and isophane *(34)* and concluded that pump therapy achieved the better control. Nonrandomized trials have generally involved larger numbers of patients and compared glycemic control on CSII to control in the same or other subjects on MIT. In several studies, control has been better on insulin pump therapy *(38–42)* and similar in others *(43,44)*. In the DCCT *(39)*, the 124 subjects who were randomly allocated to intensive therapy and chose CSII for more than 90% of the time had a glycated hemoglobin that was 0.2–0.4% lower (p <0.001) compared to those on MIT.

The use of monomeric insulin as the pump insulin now offers further opportunities to improve control with CSII. A number of randomized crossover trials of lispro vs regular human insulin *(14–17)* have shown lowered glycated hemoglobin and blood glucose levels, particularly after meals, with either no change in hypoglycemia or some reduction *(14)*.

It can be concluded that, in most patients, CSII is an effective form of intensive insulin therapy, in which the mean blood glucose level is similar to or slightly better than optimized injection therapy.

Potential Complications of CSII

The DCCT might have given the impression that insulin pump therapy increases the frequency of severe hypoglycemia, as the rate was found to be 2.8 times greater than during conventional injection treatment *(40)* (0.54 vs 0.19 episodes per patient-year, CSII vs injections). However, this is a much higher rate of hypoglycemia than many other studies that have demonstrated comparable degrees of glycemic control on the pump [e.g., 0.1 *(38)*, 0.22–0.39 *(44)*, 0.24 *(42)*, and 0.13 *(45)* episodes per patient-year]. Perhaps this reflected inexperience of pump and/or intensive therapy at some centers. In general, severe hypoglycemia is markedly less frequent on CSII, even when compared with nonoptimized injection regimens *(45)*, where the higher overall control would be expected to produce the lesser degrees of hypoglycemia.

Two recent studies emphasize the effectiveness of CSII in reducing hypoglycemia. Bode et al. *(44)* switched 55 type 1 diabetic subjects from MIT to CSII and found that although the glycated hemoglobin was similar on the two treatments (7.7% vs 7.4%, MIT vs CSII), the frequency of hypoglycemia was reduced by 84% in the first year and 81% in the second year of pump treatment (Fig. 2). Boland et al. *(42)* reported on 25 adolescents who chose CSII, as opposed to 50 who were treated by MIT. By 12 mo, pump patients were better controlled (glycated hemoglobin 8.3% vs 7.5%, p = 0.003, MIT vs CSII), and the rate of severe hypoglycemia was reduced nearly 50% in the pump group.

Some early reports showed that the frequency of diabetic ketoacidosis is increased on pump therapy compared to injections *(46–48)*. However, as doctors and patients gain experience with CSII, the frequency of CSII decreases *(46)*. There are many remediable factors that increase the likelihood of loss of control and ketoacidosis in pump patients, including poor knowledge of the correct techniques, use of unbuffered insulin, which can clog the delivery cannula *(49,50)*, and poor choice of patients (such as poorly motivated subjects, some ketoacidosis-prone brittle diabetic subjects, or patients who cannot or will not perform regular blood glucose monitoring). The first insulin pumps were also much less reliable than modern devices, lacked alarm features, and were subject to breakdown. Nevertheless, the CSII patient is at potential risk of ketoacidosis during illness or if the pump malfunctions because there is a much smaller depot of subcutaneous insulin at any

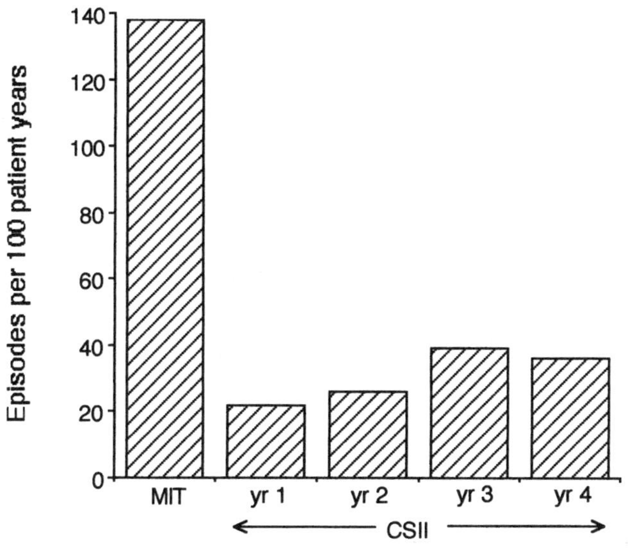

Fig. 2. Reduction in the frequency of severe hypoglycemia during CSII treatment. MIT, multiple insulin injections. (Adapted from ref. *44* with permission of the American Diabetes Association.)

one time than with injection therapy, and deliberate cessation of the pump shows that ketosis develops fairly quickly *(51)*. With meticulous education and training and proper choice of patients, the ketoacidosis rate is the same as on injections.

Infection at the site of infusion, sometimes with abscess, is more common than with injections; the organisms reported include *Staphylococcus aureus, S. epidermidis,* and *Mycobacterium fortuitum (52–54)*. It is possible that infection may be more common with certain insulin preservatives such as *m*-cresol *(53)*, but the risk can be substantially reduced by limiting the cannula use to 2 d, no reuse of cannulae, washing hands, cleaning the implantation site, and covering the implanted needle with a sterile dressing.

Special Groups: Pregnancy, Children, and Brittle Diabetes

Excellent control can be achieved with an insulin pump in most pregnant diabetic subjects *(55–58)*, but there is no evidence that the control is superior to MIT *(58)*. In the individual pregnant patient who fails to achieve strict control with MIT, a trial of CSII may be indicated.

Variable results have been reported for CSII in children. In highly motivated and well-supervised subjects, control can be comparable to that in adults *(59)*. On the other hand, some have reported less impressive control and high discontinuation rates *(60,61)*. In selecting children and young people for CSII, it is recommended that consideration be given to the patient's age, developmental and cognitive skills, and degree of supervision by adults *(62)*. The preschool child and those under about 8 yr are generally not capable of undertaking pump therapy; by age 10–12 yr, some type 1 diabetic children will be able to use CSII with some degree of independence. The mean age for starting pump therapy in one series of 83 pediatric patients was 13.6 yr *(62)*.

The type of "brittle" diabetes that most often occurs in adolescence or young adulthood and is characterized by frequent admissions to the hospital with ketoacidosis,

Table 1
Patient Prerequisites for Continuous Subcutaneous Insulin Infusion (CSII)

• Willing to use CSII
• Motivated to improve glycemic control
• History of compliance with conventional injection therapy
• Able to perform CSII procedures
• Able to perform frequent blood glucose self monitoring
• No significant psychological problems

apparent insulin resistance and severely disrupted lifestyle is, unfortunately, usually not helped by CSII *(63,64)*. Many of these subjects are suspected of deliberate interference with their treatment *(65)*, and the pump offers further opportunities for malefaction, such as inverting batteries, diluting pump insulin, and obstruction or dislodging the delivery cannula. There are some notable exceptions of ketoacidosis-prone patients who have improved on CSII *(66)*, but it is wise not to persist when an initial trial of an insulin pump is unsuccessful.

Clinical Indications for CSII

There is very variable use of CSII in different countries, with for example, an estimated 130,000 subjects on pump therapy in the United States, but only a few hundred in the United Kingdom. Countries where there is the largest takeup are generally those where CSII is recognized as an acceptable treatment mode for type 1 diabetes when prescribed and supervised by the physician and where there is reimbursement of pump costs by health insurance companies or national health schemes. For countries where there is only sporadic agreement by health authorities to fund pump therapy, it is helpful to recommend specific clinical indications, namely

- When a 2- to 3-mo trial of one or more intensive insulin injection regimens has failed to achieve good metabolic control because of frequent hypoglycemia or a marked dawn phenomenon, a trial of CSII is indicated.
- There may be a small number of individuals who have unacceptably poor control on MIT, short of hypoglycemia, who also would benefit from CSII. These might be pregnant diabetic subjects, for example, although pregnancy itself is not a general indication for CSII.
- Patients who simply prefer CSII as their form of intensive insulin therapy should probably be offered this treatment if funding is in place (private funds, agreement from insurance company, etc.), if there is supervision from a center knowledgeable about CSII, and if the patient meets the prerequisites for safe pump therapy (*see* Table 1).

Implantable Insulin Pumps

Insulin pumps that are totally implanted in the body and infuse insulin intravenously (iv) or intraperitoneally (ip) have been under development for some 20 yr *(67–69)*. However, unlike external pumps, they have yet to enter routine clinical practice, limited in large part by the relative invasiveness, cost, and occurrence of various complications. The advantages of implanted pumps include the pump being out of site and protected, the complete freedom from injection or insertion of a cannula needle, and easy insulin delivery to great veins or the peritoneal cavity. Intravenous infusion bypasses the vagaries of subcutaneous absorption while insulin is rapidly absorbed from the peritoneal cavity, much of it entering the portal bloodstream and being thus directed to the liver *(70)*. This may avoid peripheral hyperinsulinemia seen with most insulin regimens and the theoretical risk of accelerated atherosclerosis.

The three pumps that have undergone trial in recent years are the Infusaid, MiniMed and Siemens Promedos pumps, which have been used in several hundreds of diabetic subjects. There are no large-scale, long-term randomized trials of implanted pump therapy versus MIT in type 1 diabetes. However, one of the most informative studies randomly allocated 21 type 1 subjects to an implanted pump (iv or ip) or intensive subcutaneous insulin by CSII or MIT for 6 mo *(71)*. Overall control was similar (glycated hemoglobin 7.5% vs 7.8%, MIT/CSII vs implanted), but the standard deviation of blood glucose (a measure of glycemic fluctuations) was less during implanted pump therapy.

Large numbers of type 1 subjects have been treated by the EVADIAC (Evaluation dans le Diabete du Traitement par Implants Actifs) group of French centers *(72,73):* In 224 type 1 diabetic patients, glycated hemoglobin percentage was less during implanted pump therapy for 1–40 mo than during previous CSII/MIT (6.8% vs 7.4%, $p < 0.001$), as was the frequency of hypoglycemia (2.5 vs 15.2 episodes per 100 patient-years). Similar results were reported by the US/Italian Implantable Insulin Pump Trial Study Group *(74,75)*, in which control was slightly better on implanted pump compared to MIT/CSII (7.3% vs 7.9%, $p < 0.05$) and severe hypoglycemia was reduced from 33 to 4 episodes per 100 patient-years.

In a randomised controlled trial of 59 type 2 diabetic subjects treated by implantable pump and 62 by MIT, the glycated hemoglobin was similar (7.3% vs 7.5%, pump vs MIT), but, again, the standard deviation of blood glucose and (mild) hypoglycemia were less during pump therapy *(76)*.

At present, the high frequency of complications during implanted pump therapy *(77–79)* is a substantial hindrance to further clinical evaluation. A major problem is underdelivery caused by aggregation of insulin in the pump or catheter blockage caused by fibrin clots or omental encapsulation. Pump pocket problems include hematoma, skin erosion, local infection, abdominal pain, and pump migration. Electrical and mechanical pump failures occur occasionally.

A few cases of brittle diabetes characterized by extreme resistance to subcutaneous insulin, but usually more normal sensitivity to intravenous insulin, have been improved by implantable insulin pump therapy, although the reasons for this are not clear *(80,81)*. The success of direct infusion ip or iv hints at bypassing a subcutaneous barrier. However, as with many of the brittle diabetic patients of this type tried on CSII, deliberate malefaction is suspected and many think it possible that the inaccessible implanted pump simply offers less opportunity for tampering *(82)*.

GLUCOSE SENSORS

The most investigated glucose sensors are implanted needle-type amperometric (current measuring) enzyme electrodes *(83–90)*. In these devices, an enzyme—usually glucose oxidase—is immobilized at the tip of a charged platinum or carbon electrode. Either the hydrogen peroxide produced or oxygen consumed in the oxidation of glucose can be detected electrochemically:

$$\text{Glucose} + \text{oxygen} \xrightarrow{\text{glucose oxidase}} \text{hydrogen peroxide} + \text{gluconic acid},$$

$$H_2O_2 \xrightarrow{+700\text{ mV}} O_2 + 2H^+ + 2e^-,$$

$$O_2 + 4e^- + 4H^+ \xrightarrow{-700\text{ mV}} 2H_2O.$$

An alternative type of amperometric glucose sensor uses a small molecular-weight "mediator"—ferrocene is one example—to shuttle electrons between the enzyme and the underlying electrode, thereby bypassing oxygen as the final electron acceptor *(87,88)*. This technology was originally developed to be less sensitive to varying oxygen tension in the in vivo environment but is now used mostly for one-shot in vitro home blood glucose monitors (e.g., MediSense), rather than implanted sensors.

Enyzme electrodes were first described in the 1960s *(91)* and have been intensively investigated over the last 20 yr for continuous in vivo glucose sensing in diabetes. Many consider that the most appropriate implantation site is the subcutaneous tissue where there is good evidence that changes in interstitial fluid glucose levels measured by sensors follow closely glycemic changes *(83,87–90)*. Subcutaneous sensors have been implanted in animals and man for up to a week or so *(89)*. The main difficulties in translating this technology to routine patient management have been the unpredictable drift in in vivo responses and the apparently low glucose readings obtained from the subcutaneous tissue *(92)*, when independent methods suggest that plasma and tissue glucose are very similar *(93,94)*. This means that careful in vivo calibration of sensors is required. It is unclear why subcutaneous responses with the sensor are suppressed; possibly coating of the sensors with protein or electroactive substances are responsible.

The first implantable enzyme electrode to be commercialized (the Medtronic MiniMed's Continuous Glucose Monitoring System [CGMS]™) has received regulatory approval and has entered clinical practice. The sensor is worn for up to 3 d and readings are made every 10 s and averaged over 5 min. Data from the pager-sized monitor are downloaded to a computer to produce a graphical display and summary report of glucose trends *(95,96)*.

Because difficulties have been experienced over the last decade or so with the testing of implanted sensors, probably the result of bioincompatibility, alternative approaches have been devised to sample interstitial fluid. Microdialysis, for example, is based on the implantation into the subcutaneous tissue of a fine, hollow dialysis fiber that is perfused with isotonic fluid *(94,97,98)*. Glucose diffuses into the fiber and is transported to the outside of the body for measurement of glucose concentration by a sensor. The external sensor allows easy recalibration, if necessary, and there is generally a good correlation between perfusate-derived glucose readings and plasma glucose in many studies *(97,98)*.

Reverse iontophoresis is a further technique for extraction of interstitial glucose and has led to a recently approved commercial device (GlucoWatch® Biographer, Cygnus Inc) *(99–101)*. A small current is passed between two skin-surface electrodes and glucose is carried to the surface with the electro-osmotic flow of water. At the skin surface, the fluid is absorbed by a hydrogel patch containing glucose oxidase and the glucose concentration is measured with an electrochemical sensor (Fig. 3). The extraction and assay cycle takes 20 min, so three readings per hour can be taken. Sensors for temperature and sweating are incorporated, as these are confounding variables. The measurements need to be calibrated after a 3-h run-in period against a single blood glucose

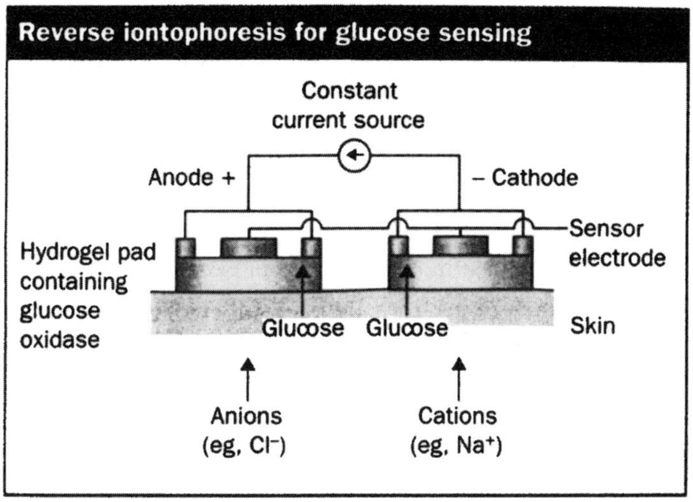

Fig. 3. The principle of reverse iontophoresis. With permission of The Lancet.

sample measured by conventional means such as finger-prick blood sample and reagent strip. There is generally good tracking of the blood glucose by the GlucoWatch®, although with an approx 18 min delay *(100,101)* (*see* Fig. 3).

The clinical use of both the Medtronic MiniMed and the Cygnus glucose sensing devices is, of course, yet to be explored in detail. We suspect that they will have advantages in detecting episodes of hypoglycemia and hyperglycemia that are not apparent from intermittent blood testing, thus allowing better adjustment of insulin dosages. With alarms for excursions outside preset limits, patients will have warning of actual or impending dangerous glycemic excursions, especially valuable for those without warning symptoms of hypoglycemia.

The ultimate patient-acceptable glucose sensor is thought by many to be a totally noninvasive technology either by exterior interrogation of a permanently implanted sensor or by analysis of radiation from the body. A number of groups are experimenting with glucose-sensitive molecules labeled with fluorescent probes that can be excited and emit light in the near-infrared region of the spectrum *(102,103)*. Because near-infrared light (about 600- to 1300-nm wavelength) passes through several centimeters of tissue, fluorescent sensors could be implanted or tattooed into the skin for exterior measurement.

Intrinsic glucose absorption peaks in the near-infrared spectroscopic region are small, but readings can be made by transmission or reflection through tissues such as the finger tip and oral mucosa *(104–106)*. With complex multivariate calibration, reasonably good correlation between spectroscopic and reference laboratory glucose concentrations can be shown *(104)*, but, at present, the precision is not good enough for clinical use *(107)*. It is likely that there are unpredictable spectral variations that are not the result of glucose changes, possibly alterations in temperature, light scattering, blood flow, tissue hydration, and other (nonglucose) metabolites that have absorption in a similar part of the near-infrared region.

Alternative, potentially noninvasive glucose sensing technologies include light scattering *(108)* and photoacoustic spectroscopy *(109)*, but these are at an early stage of development.

CLOSING THE LOOP

The first "artificial pancreas" was probably a device made by Kadish in the 1960s *(110)*, in which an autoanalyzer measured glucose levels in blood pumped from a peripheral vein and a simple servo-mechanism controlled insulin-, glucose-, or glucagon-containing syringe pumps. The first computer-controlled devices were reported by Albisser et al. *(111)* in Canada and Pfeiffer et al. *(112)* in Germany in 1974, again withdrawing blood from a vein and pumping it to an on-line glucose analyzer, with intravenous infusion of insulin according to preset algorithms. This type of artificial pancreas was a moderately large, bedside apparatus, commercialized as the Biostator. It was used for many short-term research studies such as investigating the effect of euglycemia on intermediary metabolite levels *(113)* and the potency and absorption kinetics of various insulin preparations *(114)*. Studies of the management of diabetes during childbirth *(115)*, ketoacidosis *(116)*, and surgery *(117)* were also reported, as was its use to determine subcutaneous insulin dosages in poorly controlled diabetic patients *(118)*.

However, the Biostator was perhaps too large and complex to sustain research or clinical interest. Closed-loop insulin delivery systems using needle-type glucose sensors were subsequently described in studies in animals and man *(119,120)* but have not yet been extensively exploited.

CONCLUSIONS

As we enter the 21st century, technology is advancing at an impressive pace. After many years of development, certain types of glucose sensors will soon be part of routine clinical practice; insulin pumps already are. Totally noninvasive glucose sensing is not yet a practical reality, but research in this field is extremely active. It seems unlikely that the stringent demands for safety will allow a completely automatic closed-loop insulin delivery system for routine use in the near future, but at least for many diabetic people this remains the eventual, most important goal of technology research in diabetes care.

REFERENCES

1. Slama G, Hautecouvature M, Assan R, Tchobroutsky G. One to five days of continuous insulin infusion on seven diabetic patients. Diabetes 1974;23:732–738.
2. Deckert T, Lørup B. Regulation of brittle diabetes by a preplanned infusion programme. Diabetologia 1976;12:573–579.
3. Hepp KD, Renner R, Funcke HJ, Mehnert H, Haerten R, Kresse H. Glucose homeostasis under continuous intravenous insulin therapy in diabetes. Horm Metab Res 1977;7(Suppl):72–76.
4. Service FJ. Normalisation of plasma glucose of unstable diabetes: studies under ambulatory fed conditions with pumped intravenous insulin. J Lab Clin Med 1978;91:480–489.
5. Genuth S, Martin P. Control of hyperglycemia in adult diabetics by pulsed insulin delivery. Diabetes 1977;26:571–581.
6. Irsigler K, Kritz H. Long-term continuous intravenous insulin therapy with a portable regulating apparatus. Diabetes 1979;28:196–203.
7. Pickup JC, Keen H, Parsons JA, Alberti KGMM. Continuous subcutaneous insulin infusion: an approach to achieving normoglycaemia. Br Med J 1978;i:204–207.
8. Pickup JC, Keen H, Parsons JA, Alberti KGMM, Rowe AS. Continuous subcutaneous insulin infusion: improved blood glucose and intermediary metabolite control in diabetes. Lancet 1979;i:1255–1258.

9. Pickup JC, White MC, Keen H, Kohner EM, Parsons JA, Alberti KGMM. Long-term continuous subcutaneous insulin infusion in diabetics at home. Lancet 1979;ii:870–873.
10. Tamborlane WV, Sherwin RS, Genel M, Felig P. Reduction to normal of plasma glucose in juvenile diabetes by subcutaneous administration of insulin with a portable infusion pump. N Engl J Med 1979;300:573–578.
11. Tamborlane WV, Sherwin RS, Genel M, Felig P. Restoration of normal lipid and amino acid metabolism in diabetic patients treated with a portable insulin-infusion pump. Lancet 1979;i:1258–1261.
12. Champion MC, Shepherd GAA, Rodger NW, Dupre J. Continuous subcutaneous insulin infusion in the management of diabetes mellitus. Diabetes 1980;29:206–212.
13. Mecklenburg RS, Benson JW, Becker NM, et al. Clinical use of the insulin infusion pump in 100 patients with type 1 diabetes. N Engl J Med 1982;307:513–518.
14. Melki V, Renard E, Lassman-Vague V, et al. Improvement of HbA1c and blood glucose stability in IDDM patients treated with lispro insulin analogue in external pumps. Diabetes Care 1998;21: 977–981.
15. Renner R, Pfützner A, Trautman M, Harzer O, Sauter K, Landgraf R. Use of insulin lispro in continuous subcutaneous insulin infusion treatment. Diabetes Care 1999;22:784–788.
16. Schmauss S, König A, Landgraf R. Human insulin analogue [LYS(B28), PRO(B29)]: the ideal pump insulin? Diabet Med 1998;15:247–249.
17. Zinman B, Tildesley H, Chiasson J-L, Tsui E, Strack T. Insulin lispro in CSII. Results of a double-blind crossover study. Diabetes 1997;46:440–443.
18. Bode B, McCulloch K, Strange P. Insulin aspart efficacy and safety compared to buffered regular insulin (Velosulin) for continuous subcutaneous insulin infusion. Diabetes 2000;49(Suppl 1):98A.
19. Schmidt MI, Hadji-Georgopoulos A, Rendell M, Margolis S, Kowarski A. The dawn phenomenon, an early morning glucose rise: implications for diabetic intraday blood glucose variation. Diabetes Care 1981;4:579–585.
20. Campbell PJ, Bolli G, Cryer PE, Gerich JE. Pathogenesis of the dawn phenomenon in patients with insulin-dependent diabetes mellitus. N Engl J Med 1985;312:1473–1479.
21. Perriello G, De Feo P, Fanelli C, Santeusanio F, Bolli G. Nocturnal spikes of growth hormone secretion cause the dawn phenomenon in type 1 (insulin-dependent) diabetes mellitus by decreasing hepatic (and extrahepatic) sensitivity to insulin in the absence of insulin waning. Diabetologia 1990;33:52–59.
22. Bending JJ, Pickup JC, Collins ACG, Keen H. Rarity of a marked "dawn phenomenon" in diabetic subjects treated by continuous subcutaneous insulin infusion. Diabetes Care 1985;8:28–33.
23. Koivisto VA, Yki-Järvinen H, Helve E, Sirkka-Liisa K, Pelkonen R. Pathogenesis and prevention of the dawn phenomenon in diabetic patients with CSII. Diabetes 1986;35:78–82.
24. Skyler JS, Seigler DE, Reeves ML. Optimising pumped insulin delivery. Diabetes Care 1982;5: 135–147.
25. Kroc Collaborative Study Group. Blood glucose control and the evolution of diabetic retinopathy and albuminuria. N Engl J Med 1984;311:365–372.
26. Lauritzen T, Frost-Larson K, Larsen HW, Deckert T. Effect of 1 year of near-normal blood glucose levels on retinopathy in insulin-dependent diabetes. Lancet 1983:i:200–204.
27. Dahl-Jørgensen K, Bringhman-Hansen O, Hanssen KF, et al. Effect of near-normoglycaemia for two years on progression of early diabetic retinopathy and neuropathy: the Oslo Study. Br Med J 1986;293:1195–1199.
28. The Diabetes Control and Complications Trial Research Group. The effect of intensive treatment of diabetes on the development and progression of long-term complications in insulin-dependent diabetes mellitus. N Engl J Med 1993;329:977–986.
29. Marshall SM, Home PD, Taylor R, Alberti KGMM. Continuous subcutaneous insulin infusion versus injection therapy: a randomised cross-over trial under usual diabetic clinic conditions. Diabet Med 1987;4:521–525.
30. Home PD, Capaldo B, Burrin JM, Worth R, Alberti KGMM. A crossover comparison of continuous subcutaneous insulin infusion (CSII) against multiple insulin injections in insulin-dependent diabetic subjects: improved control with CSII. Diabetes Care 1982;5:466–471.
31. Saurbrey N, Arnold-Larson S, Møller-Jensen B, Kühl C. Comparison of continuous subcutaneous insulin infusion with multiple insulin injections using the NovoPen. Diabet Med 1988;5:150–153.
32. Nathan DM, Lou P, Avruch J. Intensive conventional and insulin pump therapy in adult type 1 diabetes. A crossover study. Ann Intern Med 1982;97:31–36.

33. Helve E, Koivisto VA, Lehtonen A, Pelkonen R, Huttunen JK, Nikkilä EA. A crossover comparison of continuous insulin infusion and conventional injection treatment of type 1 diabetes. Acta Med Scand 1987;221:385–393.
34. Hanaire-Broutin H, Melki V, Bessierre-Lacombe S, Taube J. Comparison of continuous subcutaneous insulin infusion and multiple daily insulin injection regimens using insulin lispro in type 1 diabetic patients on intensified treatment. Diabetes Care 2000;23:1232–1235.
35. Schiffrin A, Belmonte MM. Comparison between continuous subcutaneous insulin infusion and multiple injections of insulin. Diabetes 1982;31:255–264.
36. Reeves ML, Seigler DE, Ryan EA, Skyler JS. Glycemic control in insulin-dependent diabetes mellitus. Comparison of outpatient intensified conventional therapy with continuous subcutaneous insulin infusion. Am J Med 1982;72:673–680.
37. Schmitz A, Sandahl-Christiansen J, Kjedahl Christiansen C, Hermansen K, Mogensen CE. Effect of pump versus pen treatment on glycaemic control and kidney function in long-term uncomplicated insulin-dependent diabetes mellitus (IDDM). Danish Med Bull 1989;36:176–178.
38. Chantelau E, Spraul M, Mühlhauser I, Gause R, Berger M. Long-term safety, efficacy and side effects of continuous subcutaneous insulin infusion treatment for type 1 (insulin-dependent) diabetes mellitus: a one centre experience. Diabetologia 1989;32:421–426.
39. Diabetes Control and Complications Trial Research Group. Implementation of treatment protocols in the Diabetes Control and Complications Trial. Diabetes Care 1995;18:361–376.
40. Haardt MJ, Berne C, Dorange C, Slama G, Selam J-L. Efficacy and indications of CSII revisited: the Hôtel Dieu cohort. Diabet Med 1997;14:407–408.
41. Bell D, Ovalle F. Better long term glycemic control with CSII than with multiple daily injections therapy. Diabetes 1998;47(Suppl 1):189A.
42. Boland EA, Grey M, Oesterle A, Fredrickson L, Tamborlane WV. Continuous subcutaneous insulin infusion. A new way to lower risk of severe hypoglycemia, improve metabolic control, and enhance coping in adolescents with type 1 diabetes. Diabetes Care 1999;22:1779–1784.
43. Knight G, Boulton AJM, Drury J, Ward JD. Long term glycaemic control by alternative regimens in a feasibility study of continuous subcutaneous insulin infusion. Diabetes Res 1986;3:355–358.
44. Bode BW, Steed RD, Davidson PC. Reduction in severe hypoglycemia with long-term continuous subcutaneous insulin infusion in type 1 diabetes. Diabetes Care 1996;19:324–327.
45. Bending JJ, Pickup JC, Keen H. Frequency of diabetic ketoacidosis and hypoglycemic coma during treatment with continuous subcutaneous insulin infusion. Am J Med 1985;79:685–691.
46. Peden NR, Bratten JT, McKendry JB. Diabetic ketoacidosis during long-term treatment with continuous subcutaneous insulin infusion. Diabetes Care 1984;7:1–5.
47. Mecklenburg RS, Benson EA, Benson JW, et al. Acute complications associated with insulin pump therapy. Report of experience with 161 patients. JAMA 1984;252:3265–3269.
48. Knight G, Jennings AM, Boulton AJM, Tomlinson S, Ward JD. Severe hyperglycaemia and ketoacidosis during routine treatment with an insulin pump. Br Med J 1985;91:371–372.
49. Mecklenburg RS, Guinn TS. Complications of insulin pump therapy: the effect of insulin preparation. Diabetes Care 1985;8:367–370.
50. Eichner HL, Selam J-L, Woertz LL, Cornblath M, Charles MA. Improved metabolic control of diabetes with reduction of occlusions during continuous subcutaneous insulin infusion. Diabet Nutr Metab 1988;1:283–287.
51. Pickup JC, Viberti GC, Bilous RW, et al. Safety of continuous subcutaneous insulin infusion: metabolic deterioration and glycaemic autoregulation after deliberate cessation of infusion. Diabetologia 1982;22:175–179.
52. Chantelau E, Lange G, Sonnenberg GE, Berger M. Acute cutaneous complications and catheter needle colonization during insulin-pump treatment. Diabetes Care 1987;10:478–482.
53. Van Faassen I, Razenberg PPA, Simoons-Smit AM, van der Veen EA. Carriage of *Staphylococcus aureus* and inflamed infusion sites with insulin pump therapy. Diabetes Care 1989;12:153–155.
54. Toth EL, Boychuk LR, Kirkland PA. Recurrent infection of continuous subcutaneous insulin infusion sites with Mycobacterium fortuitum. Diabetes Care 1995;18:1284–1285.
55. Rudolf M, Coustan D, Sherwin RS, Bates SE, Felig P, Genel M, et al. Efficacy of the insulin pump in the home treatment of pregnant diabetics. Diabetes 1981;30:891–895.
56. Potter JM, Reckless JPD Cullen DR. Effect of continuous insulin infusion and conventional regimes on 24-h variations of blood glucose and intermediary metabolites in the third trimester of diabetic pregnancy. Diabetologia 1981;21:534–540.

57. Kitzmiller JL, Younger AD, Hare JW, et al. Continuous subcutaneous insulin therapy during early pregnancy. Obstet Gynecol 1985;66:606–611.
58. Coustan DR, Reece A, Sherwin RS, et al. A randomised clinical trial of the insulin pump vs intensive conventional therapy in diabetic pregnancies. JAMA 1986;255:631–636.
59. Schiffrin AD, Desrosiers M, Aleyassine H, et al. Intensified insulin therapy in type 1 diabetic adolescents: a controlled trial. Diabetes Care 1984;7:107–119.
60. Greene SA, Smith MA, Baum JD. Clinical application of insulin pumps in the management of insulin dependent diabetes. Arch Dis Child 1983;58:578–581.
61. Brink SJ, Stewart C. Insulin pump treatment in insulin-dependent diabetes mellitis. Children, adolescents and young adults. JAMA 1986;255:617–621.
62. Kaufman FR, Halvorson M, Miller D, Mackenzie M, Fisher KF, Pitukcheewanont P. Insulin pump therapy in type 1 pediatric patients; now and into the year 2000. Diabet Metab Res Rev 1999;15:338–352.
63. Pickup JC, Home PD, Bilous RW, Keen H, Alberti KGMM. Management of severely brittle diabetes by continuous subcutaneous and intramuscular insulin infusions: evidence for a defect in subcutaneous insulin absorption. Br Med J 1981;282:347–350.
64. Pickup J, Williams G, Johns P, Keen H. Clinical features of brittle diabetic patients unresponsive to optimised subcutaneous insulin therapy (continuous subcutaneous insulin infusion). Diabetes Care 1983;6:279–284.
65. Schade DS, Drumm DA, Eaton RP, Sterling WA. Factitious brittle diabetes mellitus. Am J Med 1985;78:777–784.
66. Blackett PR. Insulin pump treatment for recurrent ketoacidosis in adolescence. Diabetes Care 1995;18:881–882.
67. Buchwald H, Barbosa J, Varco RL, et al. Treatment of a type II diabetic by a totally implantable insulin infusion device. Lancet 1981;i:1233–1235.
68. Irsigler K, Kritz H, Hagmuller G, et al. Long-term continuous intraperitoneal insulin infusion with an implantable remote controlled insulin infusion device. Diabetes 1981;30:1072–1075.
69. Schade DS, Eaton RP, Sterling WE, et al. A remotely programmable insulin delivery system: successful short-term implantation in man. JAMA 1982;247:1848–1853.
70. Schade DS, Eaton RP, Davis T, et al. The kinetics of peritoneal insulin absorption. Metabolism 1981;30:149–155.
71. Selam J-L, Raccah D, Jeandidier N, Lozano JL. Waxman K, Charles MA. Randomised comparison of metabolic control achieved by intraperitoneal insulin infusion with implantable pumps versus intensive subcutaneous insulin therapy in type 1 diabetic patients. Diabetes Care 1992;15:53–69.
72. Broussolle C, Jeandidier N, Hanaire-Broutin H. French experience of implantable insulin pumps. Lancet 1994;343:514–515.
73. Hanaire-Broutin H, Broussolle C, Jeandidier N, et al. Feasibility of intraperitoneal insulin therapy with programmable implantable pumps in IDDM. Diabetes Care 1995;18:388–392.
74. Selam J-L, Micossi P, Dunn FL, Nathan DM. Clinical trial of programmable implantable insulin pump for type 1 diabetes. Diabetes Care 1992;15:877–885.
75. Dunn FL, Nathan DM, Scavini M, Selam J-L, Wingrove TG. Long-term therapy of IDDM with an implantable insulin pump. Diabetes Care 1997;20:59–63.
76. Saudek CD, Duckworth WC, Giobbie-Huder A, et al. Implantable insulin pump vs multiple-dose insulin for non-insulin-dependent diabetes mellitus. A randomised clinical trial. JAMA 1996;276:1322–1327.
77. Renard E, Baldet P, Picot M-C, Jacques-Apostol D, Lauton D, Costalat G, et al. Catheter complications associated with implantable systems for peritoneal insulin delivery. Diabetes Care 1995;18:300–306.
78. Renard E, Bouteleau S, Jacques-Apostol D, Lauton D, Gibert-Boulet F, Bringer J, et al. Insulin underdelivery from implanted pumps using peritoneal route. Diabetes Care 1996;19:812–817.
79. Scavini M, Galli L, Reich S, Eaton RP, Charles MA, Dunne FL. Catheter survival during long-term insulin therapy with an implanted pump. Diabetes Care 1997;20:610–613.
80. Campbell IW, Irsigler K. Subcutaneous insulin resistance: treatment by implantable device. In: Pickup JC, ed. Brittle Diabetes. Blackwell Science, Oxford, 1985;pp. 289–300.
81. Wood DF, Goodchild K, Guillou P, Thomas DJ, Johnston DG. Management of "brittle diabetes" with a preprogrammable implanted insulin pump delivering intraperitoneal insulin. Br Med J 1990;301:1143–1144.

82. Tattersall RB. Brittle diabetes revisited: the third Arnold Bloom Lecture. Diabet Med 1997;14:99–110.
83. Shichiri M, Kawamori R, Yamasaki T, Hakui N, Abe H. Wearable-type artificial pancreas with needle-type glucose sensor. Lancet 1982;ii:1129–1131.
84. Abel P, Muller A, Fischer U. Experience with an implantable glucose sensor as a prerequesite of an artificial beta cell. Biomed Biochim Acta 1984;5:577–584.
85. Bindra DS, Zhang Y, Wilson GS, et al. Design and in vitro studies of a needle-type glucose sensor. Anal Chem 1991;63:1692–1696.
86. Armour JC, Lucisano JY, McKean BD, Gough DA. Application of chronic intravascular blood glucose sensor in dogs. Diabetes 1990;39:1519–1526.
87. Clarement DJ, Sambrook IE, Penton C, Pickup JC. Subcutaneous implantation of a ferrocene-mediated glucose sensor in pigs. Diabetologia 1986;29:817–821.
88. Pickup JC, Shaw GW, Claremont DJ. In vivo molecular sensing in diabetes mellitus: an implantable glucose sensor with direct electron transfer. Diabetologia 1989;32:213–217.
89. Moatti-Sirat D, Capron F, Poitout V, et al. Towards continuous glucose monitoring: in vivo evaluation of a miniaturised glucose sensor implanted for several days in rat subcutaneous tissue. Diabetologia 1992;35:224–230.
90. Rebrin K, Steil GM, Van Antwerp WP, Mastrototaro JJ. Subcutaneous glucose predicts plasma glucose independent of insulin: implications for continuous glucose monitoring. Am J Physiol 1999;40:E561–E571.
91. Updike SJ, Hicks GP. The enzyme electrode. Nature 1967;214:986–988.
92. Pickup J. In vivo glucose monitoring: Sense and sensorbility. Diabetes Care 1993;16:535–539.
93. Fischer U, Ertle R, Abel P, et al. Assessment of subcutaneous glucose concentration: validation of the wick technique as a reference for implanted electrochemical sensors. Diabetologia 1987;30:940–945.
94. Jansson P-A, Fowelin J, Smith U, Lönroth P. Characterization by microdialysis of intercellular glucose level in subcutaneous tissue of humans. Am J Physiol 1988;255:E218–E220.
95. Bode BW, Gross TM, Thornton KR, Mastrototaro JJ. Continuous glucose monitoring facilitates sustainable improvement in glycemic control. Diabetes 2000;49(Suppl 1):97A.
96. Gross TM, Ter Veer A, Spell J, Mastrototaro JJ. Continuous glucose monitoring in previously unstudied population subgroups. Diabetes 2000;49(Suppl 1):109A.
97. Meyerhof C, Bischof F, Sternberg F, Zier H, Pfeiffer EF. On line continuous monitoring of subcutaneous tissue glucose in men by combining portable glucosensor with microdialysis. Diabetologia 1992;35:1087–1092.
98. Hashiguchi Y, Sakakida M, Nishida K, Uemura T, Kajiwara K-I, Shichiri M. Development of a miniaturised glucose monitoring system with microdialysis sampling method. Diabetes Care 1994;17: 387–396.
99. Tamada JA, Bohannon NJV, Potts RO. Measurement of glucose in diabetic subjects using noninvasive glucose extraction. Nat Med 1995;1:1198–1201.
100. Garg SK, Potts RO, Ackerman NR, Fermi SJ, Tamada JA, Chase HP. Correlation of fingerstick blood glucose measurements with GlucoWatch Biographer glucose results in young subjects with type 1 diabetes. Diabetes Care 1999;22:1708–1714.
101. Tamada JA, Garg S, Jovanovic L, Pitzer KR, Fermi S, Potts RO. Noninvasive glucose monitoring. Comprehensive clinical results. JAMA 1999;282:1839–1844.
102. Rolinski OJ, Birch DJS, McCartney LJ, Pickup JC. A time-resolved near-infrared fluorescence assay for glucose: opportunities for trans-dermal sensing. J Photochem Photobiol B 2000;54:26–34.
103. Tolosa L, Szmacinski H, Rao G, Lakowicz JR. Lifetime-based sensing of glucose using energy transfer with a long lifetime donor. Anal Biochem 1997;250:102–108.
104. Robinson MR, Eaton RP, Haaland DM, Koepp GW, Thomas EV, Stallard BR, et al. Non-invasive glucose monitoring in diabetic patients: a preliminary evaluation. Clin Chem 1992:38:1618–1622.
105. Kajiwara K, Uemura T, Kishikawa H, Nishida K, Hashiguchi Y, Uehara M, et al. Non-invasive measuremnt of blood glucose concentrations by analysing Fourier transform infra-red absorbance spectra through oral mucosa. Med Biol Eng Comput 1993;31:S17–S22.
106. Marbach R, Koschinski T, Gries FA, Heise HM. Non-invasive blood glucose assay by near infrared diffuse reflectance spectroscopy of the human lip. Appl Spectrosc 1993;47:875–881.
107. Arnold MA. Non-invasive glucose monitoring. Curr Opin Biotechnol 1996;7:46–49.
108. Heinemann L, Schmelzeise Redeker G. Non-invasive continuous glucose monitoring in type 1 diabetic patients with optical glucose sensors. Diabetologia 1998;41:848–854.
109. MacKenzie HA, Ashton HS, Shen YC, Lindberg J, Rae P, Quan KM, et al. Blood glucose measurements by photoacoustics. Biomed Opt Spectrosc Diagn 1998;22:156–159.

110. Kadish AH. Automation control of blood sugar. A servomechanism for glucose monitoring and control. Trans Am Soc Artif Intern Organs 1963;19:363–367.
111. Albisser AM, Leibel BS, Ewart TG, Davidovac Z, Botz CK, Zingg W. An artificial endocrine pancreas. Diabetes 1974;23:389–396.
112. Pfeiffer EF, Thum CH, Clemens AH. The artificial beta-cell. A continuous control of blood sugar by external regulation of insulin infusion (glucose-controlled insulin infusion system). Horm Metab Res 1974;6:339–342.
113. Nosadini R, Noy GA, Nattrass M, et al. The metabolic and hormonal response to acute normoglycaemia in type 1 (insulin-dependent) diabetes: studies with a glucose controlled insulin infusion system (artificial endocrine pancreas). Diabetologia 1982;23:220–228.
114. Massi-Benedetti M, Burrin JM, Capaldo B, Alberti KGMM. A comparative study of the activity of biosynthetic human insulin and pork insulin using the glucose clamp technique in normal subjects. Diabetes Care 1981;4:163–167.
115. Nattrass M, Alberti KGMM, Dennis KJ, Gillibrand PN, Letchworth AT, Buckle AJL. A glucose controlled insulin infusion system for diabetic women during labour. Br Med J 1978;ii:599–601.
116. Pfeiffer EF, Kerner W. The artificial endocrine pancreas: its impact on the pathophysiology and treatment of diabetes mellitus. Diabetes Care 1981;4:11–26.
117. Schwarz SS, Horwitz DL, Zehfus B, et al. Use a glucose-controlled insulin infusion system (artificial beta cell) to control diabetes during surgery. Diabetologia 1979;16:157–164.
118. Lambert AE, Buysschaert M, Marchand E, Perard M, Wojcik S, Lambotte L. Determination of insulin requirements in brittle diabetic patients by the artificial pancreas. Diabetes 1978;27:825–833.
119. Shichiri M, Kawamori R, Hakui N, Asakawi N, Yamasaki Y, Abe H. The development of wearable-type artificial endocrine pancreas and its usefulness in glycaemic control of human diabetes mellitus. Biomed Biochem Acta 1984;43:561–568.
120. Rebrin K, Fischer U, Woedtke T, Abel P, Brunstein E. Automated feedback control of subcutaneous glucose concentration in diabetic dogs. Diabetologia 1989;32:573–576.

13 Living with Diabetes

Educating the Patient and Family with Type 1 Diabetes

Jean Betschart Roemer, MN, MSN, CPNP, CDE and Linda Siminerio, RN, PhD, CDE

CONTENTS

THE IMPACT OF DIABETES

It has long been recognized that treating and controlling diabetes is difficult. Diabetes is not an illness where a pill, an injection, or a particular diet is a cure. At best, there is hope to control it well. Optimal treatment demands dedication, motivation, energy, and knowledge. The best possible glycemic control can only be a result of diligence and commitment on the part of persons with diabetes, their family, and their health care providers. Diabetes and its treatment permeate daily living. A person with type 1 diabetes who is responsible in self-care must do the following:

- Consider food eaten and how it will affect blood glucose
- Exercise while balancing food and medication accordingly
- Take multiple daily injections of insulin or manage an insulin pump
- Perform multiple finger sticks to determine blood glucose and, hence, how much insulin to take
- Consider that there may be hypoglycemia or hyperglycemia whenever symptoms are felt
- Follow a reasonable schedule and plan of meals and exercise
- Maintain a log of records and events
- Visit a health care provider regularly
- Contemplate the possibility of developing serious complications

From: *Contemporary Endocrinology: Type 1 Diabetes: Etiology and Treatment*
Edited by: M. A. Sperling © Humana Press Inc., Totowa, NJ

Dealing with these issues on a daily basis can be a psychological burden for anyone. There are also enormous costs, especially for the uninsured or underinsured, compromising access to medical care and supplies, which are vital in supporting the rigors of care. Thus, it is common for those with diabetes and/or close members of their families to have guilt, sorrow, and depression *(1,2)*.

PSYCHOSOCIAL AND BEHAVIORAL CONSIDERATIONS

Persons with diabetes who cope well seem to find a balance as they fit diabetes into their daily living, rather than forcing life to revolve around diabetes. When the cares of diabetes take over and regulate the activities of daily living, an unhealthy imbalance has occurred. Although clinicians promote adherence to care, there can be a subtle expectation that a person with type 1 diabetes will not be able to adhere strictly to the diabetes regimen.

When those with diabetes have been unable to do the required tasks, their health care providers sometimes have labeled them as noncompliant or nonadherent. Diabetes literature has used the terms *compliance* and *noncompliance* to refer to patients' success in following their prescribed regimen. This is the historical model of the physician speaking and the patient doing as told, suggesting acquiescence or giving in to others. Experience teaches that education improves knowledge about diabetes and dietary concepts; yet, education does not necessarily improve adherence. Data from the Diabetes Control and Complications Trial (DCCT) indicate that few people will maintain regimens that do not fit their lifestyle, culture, and health care beliefs *(3)*.

Unfortunately, there has also been a tendency to treat adherence and metabolic control as interchangeable constructs. Health care providers have been known to assess patients' compliance and measure therapeutic success based solely on biological measures, such as HbA1c levels. The literature has not only failed to document a direct relationship between adherence and metabolic control *(4–6)*, but even when patients have followed their program reasonably, often there is far less than perfect control. Health care providers must take into consideration the numerous factors that influence or inhibit an individual's behaviors in maintaining good health. Also, measures of an individual's health should never be limited to metabolic ones. Psychosocial outcomes, such as quality of life, are equally, if not more, important in assessing a person's well-being.

It must also be recognized that adherence is not always consistent across all aspects of the diabetes regimen. Some people might always take their medication as prescribed, yet have more difficulty with dietary requirements. Others might follow their meal plan carefully but be slow to do monitoring. Still others might do the monitoring but fail to record insulin doses.

It has been reported that family support is associated with regimen adherence and that family conflict is associated with negative adherence *(7)*. When people function poorly, they usually have poor access to support and suffer a lack of resources, making it difficult for existing competencies to operate. One major and consistent discovery of social support research is that informal support from personal network members has powerful stress-buffering and health-promoting influences. When people know that others are interested and involved in their care, they are more likely to take care of themselves.

Thus, there has been recognition that many factors affect success in following a prescribed regimen. Diabetes impacts family life, work, and play. There can be relational, physical, and emotional changes. Vision, sexuality, energy, security, and a host of other aspects of everyday life are touched by the treatment regimen. Those with organized lives and structured schedules might do quite well in coping with their tasks. Others with more chaotic lifestyles or social and emotional barriers might become frustrated and unable to do what is required. At times, the relentless effort motivates the temptation to give up. Certainly, no mentally balanced person wants to be sick, experience complications, or face early mortality. Yet, many do not follow recommended management plans. Barriers primarily evolve from family dynamics, health beliefs, level of motivation, complexity of the requests, degree of support, coping skills, and current habits.

Although depression is not a complication of diabetes, it frequently is a consequence of the illness. The prevalence of depression in adults varies. Levels of diagnosable depression among those with diabetes are approximately three times the estimated prevalence in the population at large *(8)*. Depression also might be more severe in people with diabetes and has especially adverse effects. Difficulty evolves in treatment when clinical depression contributes to poor self-care, worsened glycemia, and deepened depression *(9)*.

Therefore, it is incumbent upon health care professionals to recognize the symptoms of clinical depression and treat it promptly. Although it remains unrecognized and untreated in a majority of cases, depression is responsive to psychotherapy *(10)*. It is important that health professionals do not attach to medical outcomes a patient's ability to adhere to the care plan. They must learn where the barriers to adherence exist and develop strategies to improve adherence by overcoming them.

THEORETICAL MODELS AND DIABETES EDUCATION

Theoretical models are used in diabetes education to provide structure in support of the concepts of education and research. The model is comprised of concepts that are integrated into a meaningful configuration *(11)*. There are a variety of theoretical models that consider broad concepts, as well as fine points of behavior.

Recently, the empowerment model has emerged, a model which has shifted the responsibility for diabetes care, putting the patient in the "driver's seat," with the health care team, family, and friends serving and acting as guides, supporters, and facilitators. Empowerment involves the discovery and development of patients' inherent capacity to be responsible for their own life. People are empowered when they have sufficient knowledge to make rational decisions, sufficient control and resources to implement those decisions, and sufficient experience to evaluate effectiveness *(12)*.

The Health Belief Model has become popular by helping us gain an understanding of a patient's health-related choices. It is hypothesized that adherence to medical advice depends on holding a particular set of beliefs. The beliefs that have been specified in the Health Belief Model include the following: a motive to comply; recognition that one has the disease and is susceptible to serious sequelae; that compliance would be beneficial in reducing problems; one has the ability to follow health recommendations; and the benefits of care outweigh the cost *(13)*.

The concept of self-efficacy has also served in identifying strategies to enhance diabetes self-care. The Self-Efficacy Model is used to learn more about patients' convictions and beliefs in their ability to carry out recommendations for care *(14)*. Patients might well believe in the recommended health plan but may not follow it, because it is perceived as being too difficult.

The Transtheoretical Model focuses on stages of behavioral change *(15)*. The central hypothesis is that not all individuals are prepared to take action to change their behavior at any given time. Stages included in this readiness model include precontemplation, contemplation, preparation, action, and maintenance. This model offers a new behavioral approach in helping diabetes educators identify where a patient is in the learning process and developing complementary interventions.

Although diabetes educators have been urged to use theoretical constructs as frameworks for developing educational plans, behavioral research related to diabetes has had little conceptual rigor. Educators and behavioral scientists need to embrace and study the considerable complexity that surrounds diabetes self-management education. With the demands of evidenced-based research in the development of treatment strategies, guidelines, and, ultimately, reimbursement, rigorous evaluation is critical.

Diabetes Self-Management Education

The process whereby people with chronic diseases, such as diabetes, learn to take care of their disorders has traditionally been termed "patient education." However, this designation has changed and is currently termed "self-management training," "self-management education," or "patient education" *(16)*. Diabetes self-management education (DSME) is the cornerstone of treatment for all people with diabetes.

The goal of self-management education is to provide patients with the knowledge, skills, and motivation to manage their diabetes successfully on a daily basis. To meet this goal, diabetes education must include the following:

- Teaching patients and their families new information
- Training them in various skills and treatment procedures
- Assisting them in devising methods to incorporate diabetes into their lifestyle
- Helping them reconcile their quality of life so they can be motivated to manage the disease

Currently, DSME is acknowledged as the most fully developed of all of the fields of patient education *(17)*. In order to recognize the importance of quality diabetes education services and to promote diabetes education, the International Diabetes Federation (IDF), the Canadian Diabetes Association (CDA), and the American Diabetes Association (ADA) have adopted standards for diabetes education *(18–20)*.

Because diabetes education is provided by a diverse group of health and lay professionals around the world with varying degrees of training and education, development of uniform standards that can apply to all corners of the world becomes difficult. In response to this problem, the IDF standards include two stages: basic and optimal. Basic and optimal standards according to the Consultative Section on Education of the IDF are defined in Table 1. This staged format allows for quality improvement but does not set a task that cannot be achieved in areas with limited resources.

Both the ADA and the IDF have also adopted processes for recognizing quality diabetes education programs based on their standards. In the United States, the recognition efforts based on the standards (listed in Table 2) are resulting in an increase in reimbursement practices by both federal and state laws.

Diabetes nutrition education has also gained acceptance and recognition. Medical nutrition therapy (MNT) defined in the ADA Nutritional Recommendations for Persons with Diabetes underscores the importance of individualized nutrition education *(21)*.

Table 1
Stages of Diabetes Education

Basic (technical level)	
The basic standards of education describe the minimum level of education service required to meet the needs of the people with diabetes. Basic education is technical in nature. Its practitioners work under supervision and use appropriate resources and consultation to meet client needs. Practitioners may be either lay people or health professionals. "Basic" standards may represent the most desirable level of education available in the local context of resources, staffing, or culture. In other localities, "basic" standards may define a first step in the evolution of diabetes education services toward the professional level.	
Optimal (professional level)	
The enhanced standards of diabetes education define a standard of excellence to which the professional educator should adhere. Professional educators are capable of independent practice, conducted without supervision and in collaboration with the other members of the multidisciplinary team. In addition to minimal transfer of knowledge and skill, as defined by the basic standards, practice at the enhanced level includes decision-making and problem-solving, both as an activity of the provider and as skills passed on to the client.	

Source: ref. *19.*

The four-step model used for both DSME and MNT is based on the teaching–learning process. In providing either DSME and/or MNT, the educational process should always include the following:

- A thorough patient assessment
- Development of an individualized plan that includes goal setting
- An intervention that includes provision of appropriate educational tools and strategies for implementing the plan
- Continuous follow-up, monitoring, and evaluation of patient progress with regard to cognitive, medical, and behavioral outcomes

The Diabetes Educator

The DCCT substantiated the commitment to education, the value of a multidisciplinary team, and the expanded role of nurses and dietitians. Since the DCCT report in 1993 *(22),* the roles and responsibilities of diabetes educators have changed greatly. The study validated the need for dietitians and nurses to increase their involvement in patient management in order to achieve optimal glucose control *(23,24).* Investigators in the study realized that intensive management was far more than increased frequency of monitoring or additional injections of insulin. It required careful follow-up to monitor progress toward individualized goals and support to reinforce management skills. Such complexities extend beyond the scope of sole practitioners whose training may be limited to medical management. In order to achieve metabolic outcomes with intensive therapy, health care professionals skilled in the teaching–learning process and behavioral strategies were needed. Inclusion of these individuals and adoption of this model is relatively new to diabetes, and as it evolves, it will require shifts in how diabetes providers view their roles and relationships both with patients and each other *(25).*

Diabetes educators have been recognized as essential providers of diabetes care in the United States and are gaining recognition throughout the world. A diabetes educator

Table 2
National Standards for Diabetes Self-Management Education (DSME)

Standard 1. The DSME entity will have documentation of its organizational structure, mission statement, and goals and will recognize and support quality DSME as an integral component of diabetes care.

Standard 2. The DSME entity will determine its target population, assess educational needs, and identify the resources necessary to meet the self-management educational needs of the target population(s).

Standard 3. An established system (committee, governing board, advisory body) involving professional staff and other stakeholders will participate annually in a planning and review process that includes data analysis and outcome measurements and addresses community concerns.

Standard 4. The DSME entity will designate a coordinator with academic and/or experiential preparation in program management and the care of individuals with chronic disease. The coordinator will oversee the planning, implementation, and evaluation of the DSME entity.

Standard 5. DSME will involve the interaction of the individual with diabetes with a multifaceted education instructional team, which may include a behaviorist, exercise physiologist, ophthalmologist, optometrist, pharmacist, physician, podiatrist, registered dietitian, registered nurse, other health care professionals, and paraprofessionals. DSME instructors are collectively qualified to teach the content areas. The instructional team must consist of at least a registered dietitian and a registered nurse. Instructional staff must be Certified Diabetes Educators (CDEs) or have recent didactic and experiential preparation in education and diabetes management.

Standard 6. The DSME instructors will obtain regular continuing education in the areas of diabetes management, behavioral interventions, teaching and learning skills, and counseling skills.

Standard 7. A written curriculum, with criteria for successful learning outcomes, shall be available. Assessed needs of the individual will determine which content areas listed below are delivered.

Standard 8. An individualized assessment, development of an educational plan, and periodic reassessment between participant and instructor(s) will direct the selection of appropriate educational materials and interventions.

Standard 9. There shall be documentation of the individual's assessment, education plan, intervention, evaluation, and follow-up in the permanent confidential education record. Documentation also will provide evidence of collaboration among instructional staff, providers, and referral sources.

Standard 10. The DSME entity will utilize a continuous quality improvement process to evaluate the effectiveness of the education experience provided and determine opportunities for improvement.

Source: ref. *16.*

is a health care professional who has mastered a core of knowledge and skill in the biological and social sciences, communication, counseling, and education and who has experience in the care of patients with diabetes. The role of the diabetes educator can be assumed by various health care professionals, including, but not limited to, nurses, physicians, dietitians, social workers, podiatrists, exercise physiologists, and pharmacists. In order to assure high professional standards and to identify for the patient competencies and quality education, the American Association of Diabetes Educators (AADE) *(26)* and the Australian Diabetes Educator Association have established

Table 3
Standards of Practice for Diabetes Educators

Standard I. Assessment. The diabetes educator should conduct a thorough, individualized needs assessment.
Standard II. Use of resources. The diabetes educator should strive to create an educational setting conducive to learning with adequate resources to facilitate the learning process.
Standard III. Planning. The written educational plan should be developed from information obtained on the needs assessment and based on the components of the educational process. The plan is coordinated with other members of the team.
Standard IV. Implementation. The diabetes educator should provide individualized education based on a progression from basic survival skills to advanced information for self-management.
Standard V. Documentation. The diabetes educator should completely and accurately document the educational experience.
Standard VI. Evaluation and outcome. The diabetes educator should participate in an annual review of the quality and outcome of the education process.
Standard VII. Multidisciplinary collaboration. The diabetes educator should collaborate with the multidisciplinary team of health care professionals and integrate their knowledge and skills to provide a comprehensive educational experience.
Standard VIII. Professional development. The diabetes educator should assume responsibility for professional development and pursue continuing education to acquire current knowledge and skills.
Standard IX. Professional accountability. The diabetes educator should accept responsibility for self-assessment of performance and peer review to assure the delivery of high-quality diabetes education.
Standard X. Ethics. The diabetes educator should respect and uphold the basic human rights of all persons.

Source: The 1999 Scope of Practice for Diabetes Educators and the Standards of Practice for Diabetes Educators. American Association of Diabetes Educators. Diabetes Educ 2000;26:53–59.

standards and scopes of practice for diabetes educators *(27)*. The AADE Standards of Practice for Diabetes Educators are presented in Table 3.

The Scope of Practice provides definitions of diabetes education while providing statements of beliefs regarding the educational process. The primary focus for the diabetes educator is the patients and their families. The content of the educational experience should include the following topics:

- Pathophysiology of diabetes
- Nutrition
- Pharmacologic interventions
- Exercise
- Self-monitoring
- Prevention and management of the acute and chronic complications
- Psychosocial adjustment
- Problem-solving skills
- Stress management
- Use of the health care delivery system

The Scope of Practice and Standards of Practice provide a framework for health care professionals who teach people with diabetes. In recent years, the scope of practice for diabetes has expanded to involve advanced practice roles that may have been previously considered to be medical management. In order to meet the needs of all individuals who require diabetes education in the prevention and treatment of the disease, diabetes educators will need to be recognized and accepted by a variety of disciplines. In order to assure that the educational process is effective, those providing this service must be trained in the proper steps of delivery, as well as the use of behavioral strategies.

BEHAVIORAL STRATEGIES

All of these efforts are an attempt to raise the quality of standard care for people with diabetes. Since 1990 there has been a large focused effort to employ both diabetes education and behavioral strategy in order to improve outcomes. Increased follow-up care and comprehensive curricula are part of the trend. A meta-analysis by Roter *(28)* revealed that a combined educational/behavioral focus is more effective than a single-focus intervention and that larger programs produced weaker effects. The behavioral strategies include skill building, practice activities, behavioral modeling, contracting, rewards, and mail/phone reminders. The goal of diabetes education is to transfer knowledge and produce behavioral change, which includes initiating new behaviors and modifying old ones *(29)*. Patient education necessarily promotes the avoidance of rigidity and poor self-care by fostering sound judgments and wise decisions in diabetes management.

Since the discovery of insulin in the early 1920s, it has been widely recognized that education is a cornerstone in the treatment of diabetes *(30)*. Knowledge alone, however, is insufficient *(31)*. The basic premise of a behavioral approach is that behavior is controlled by antecedents. The operative conditioning of stimulus response of the Skinner rats is basic to behavioral interventions. Building on this theory are four principles of behavioral intervention, better known as behavior modification techniques:

- Behavior is monitored at regular intervals.
- Goals are set for behavior change.
- Physical and social environment are altered.
- Behavior change is reinforced.

These techniques have potential for incorporation into the therapeutic alliance if the person is motivated to change habits. Behavior modification includes extended and frequent intervention and follow-up.

Few educators use one approach to the exclusion of others *(32)*. Educators base their approaches on their own values and understanding of the purposes and methods of patient education, as well as the needs of the patient. The patient will have varying needs and tolerance for autonomous decision-making in their diabetes self-care. Therefore, educational strategies must of necessity be flexible.

In this era of measuring outcomes, educators must also be vigilant in evaluating strategies and patient outcomes with the understanding that knowledge improvement is relevant only to the degree that it leads to other kinds of changes, such as improvement in self-care behavior, glycemic control, and quality of life. Therefore, imparting and assessing knowledge serve only as a fundamental and necessary first step in promoting positive medical, behavioral, and psychosocial outcomes *(33)*. Biological factors are important only to the extent that they predict (or are associated with) an impact on key patient behaviors and long-term outcomes such as physical and social functioning,

Table 4
Childhood and Adolescent Diabetes Mellitus Educational Checklist

At diagnosis: survival education
- How to administer and store insulin
- How to monitor blood glucose and urine ketones
- Recognizing and treating hypoglycemia
- Who and when to call
- Beginning meal planning

Within 1–2 mo of diagnosis: in-depth assessment and review
- The cause of diabetes
- Properties of insulin and how to make adjustments
- Use of blood glucose monitoring data
- Meal planning
- Adjusting for exercise
- Sick day guidelines
- Diabetic ketoacidosis (DKA) prevention/treatment
- Hypoglycemia identification, recognition, prevention, and treatment

Yearly: in-depth assessment and re-education
- Age appropriate education, including all of the above should include peer pressure, alcohol, sexual education, smoking prevention, eating disorders, including bulimia/anorexia and obesity, family adjustment, travel, diabetes-associated complications assessment, and ongoing barriers to control.

Source: Adapted from Brink SJ, New England Diabetes and Endocrinology Center (NEDEC) and Brink S, Moltz K. The message of the DCCT for children and adolescents. Diabetes Spectrum 1997;10:259–267.

hospitalization, and mortality. Behavior, not physiology, should be the primary outcome for health education and should be evaluated on a continuum *(34)*.

DIABETES EDUCATION FOR CHILDREN AND ADOLESCENTS

The burdens of diabetes management present medical, cognitive, behavioral and psychosocial challenges for the child and family. Diabetes care requires families to learn and carry out complex treatment regimens. Children with diabetes and their parents must acquire a cognitive understanding of diabetes and learn self-management skills that include monitoring blood glucose levels, recognizing and treating hypoglycemia and hyperglycemia, and food and exercise regulation, along with insulin administration. In the case of a child, education for diabetes management is necessary for both the child and the parent(s) and/or caregiver(s) and special considerations are necessary.

An individualized assessment of the child's maturity level, developmental stage, family and social supports, eating habits, and school and sports schedules is critical. The assessment should also be sensitive to cultural, cognitive, socioeconomic, and environmental determinants in developing a realistic, comprehensive, individualized teaching plan. After a careful assessment, the educator may find that some children and families will be able to master complicated management routines, whereas others may only be able to handle basic skills. The components of basic and advanced levels of education are listed in Table 4.

It is important to provide education for the child on a continuum with age-appropriate teaching methods and tools. Creative, innovative methods are necessary in order to engage the child in the educational process. For example, use of role-play, stories, diabetes camping programs, computer programs, and support groups have been shown to be effective methods for diabetes education interventions. Setting behavioral goals that are realistic, age appropriate, shared among the child, family and health care provider, and planned to achieve success are important when implementing the educational process. Whenever possible, the diabetes educational process should include mechanisms to measure the success of the goals and outcomes.

BEHAVIORAL AND PSYCHOSOCIAL CONSIDERATIONS IN CHILDREN WITH DIABETES

Illness in childhood has physical, psychological, and emotional implications for both the child and the family. The burdens of diabetes management present medical, cognitive, behavioral, and psychosocial challenges. Diabetes care requires families to learn and carry out complicated treatment regimens. Adhering to these regimens is also very difficult *(35)*. Along with learning these skills, parents must encourage adherence and even do the tasks when necessary. The way in which a family deals with these responsibilities of care can determine the effectiveness with which diabetes is managed at home *(36)*. It has been reported that the two most important psychosocial issues concerning families of youngsters with diabetes are how the responsibilities of diabetes management are defined and supported within the family and when responsibilities are transferred from parent to child.

Recently, recommendations about appropriate ages at which responsibilities should be transferred to children with diabetes have shifted significantly as a result of pertinent studies. Transference of responsibilities is no longer based on chronological age but on cognitive maturity *(37)*. Rather than encouraging total independence, health care providers are recommending a sharing of responsibilities between the child and the parent, even through adolescence *(38–40)*.

Parents, often perceiving the ill child as vulnerable, become overprotective, complicating roles in providing diabetes care. The demands of care affect the lifestyle of the child and the family. When integration of these regimens into pre-existing family routines is necessary, family functioning can be challenged. Along with burdensome treatment tasks, children often experience emotional distress. There is a sense of loss of health, wholeness and perfection, belief of a harmony in life, and complete freedom of choice. The safety and predictability of normal life are replaced with a sense of vulnerability, need for control, and blame of self, parents, and others *(40)*.

Emotional stress for the parents is related to the loss of a child's health, guilt, and the uncertainty of short-term problems and long-term complications associated with the disease. These components can be seen both in the child's and parents' perception of their quality of life. Emotionally stressed families must develop positive coping skills to become successful in managing the disease and, therefore, need access to support from health care providers, other family members, and community resources *(41)*.

The diagnosis and long-term management of diabetes presents a formidable challenge to the child and family. Treatment of chronic illness must include collaboration with the child's family to minimize adverse psychological effects while ensuring psychosocial management *(42)*. Therefore, when providing diabetes education to children and their families, cognitive, behavioral, and psychosocial aspects need to be considered when developing and implementing the educational plan.

SUMMARY

The importance of social and emotional impacts upon those with diabetes and their families is critical. This is every bit as much a part of treatment as medication itself. The challenges of daily life with diabetes can be devastating. Health care professionals must assist persons with diabetes and their families in learning diabetes management skills, as well as helping them translate knowledge into daily practices based on sound judgment and understanding of the issues involved. Although children and adolescents with diabetes have special needs, the task of translating knowledge into behavior is similar.

Theoretical models provide a framework for assisting the learning and translation process. They promote patient learning and self-management skills in an optimal way. Standardization of educational programs and national and international standards for diabetes educators are efforts to elevate the quality of care. Still, an individualized approach that addresses personal barriers to adherence and provides motivation to overcome obstacles results is the most successful intervention.

REFERENCES

1. Betschart J. Parents' understanding of and guilt over their children's blood glucose control. Diabetes Educ 1987;13:4;398–401.
2. Peyrot M, Rubin RR. Levels and risks of depression and anxiety symptomatology among diabetic adults. Diabetes Care 1997;20:585–590.
3. The DCCT Research Group. Influence of intensive therapy on quality of life outcomes in the Diabetes Control and Complications Trial. Diabetes Care 1996;19:195–203.
4. Glasgow R, McCaul KD, Schaefer LC. Self-care behaviors and glycemic control in type 1 diabetes. J Chronic Dis 1987;40:399–412.
5. Glasgow R, Toobert DJ, Riddle M, Donnelly J, Mitchell DJ, Calder, D. Diabetes-specific social learning variables and self-care behaviors among persons with type II diabetes. Health Psychol 1989;8,285–303.
6. Johnson SB, Freund A, Silverstein J, Hanson CA, Malone J. Adherence—health status relationships in childhood diabetes. Health Psychol 1990;8:606–631.
7. Hauser S, Jacobson A, Lavori P, et al. Adherence among children and adolescents with insulin-dependent diabetes mellitus over a four-year longitudinal follow-up: II, immediate and long-term linkages with family milieu. J Pediatr Psychol 1990;15:527–542.
8. Lustman PJ, Clouse RE, Alrakawi A, et al. Treatment of major depression in adults with diabetes: a primary care perspective. Clin Diabetes 1997;15:122–126.
9. Rubin R. Psychosocial disorders. In: Funnell M, ed. A Core Curriculum for Diabetes Education, 3rd ed. American Association of Diabetes Educators, Washington, DC, 1998, pp. 144–146.
10. Lustman PJ, Griffith LS, Clouse RE. Recognizing and managing depression in patients with diabetes. In: Anderson BJ, Rubin RR, eds. Practical Psychology for Diabetes Clinicians: How to Deal with the Key Behavioral Issues Faced by Patients and Health-Care Teams. American Diabetes Association, Washington, DC, 1996, pp. 143–154.
11. Fain JA, Nettles A, Funnell MM, Charron-Prochownik D. Diabetes patient education research: an integrative literature review. Diabetes Educ 1999;25(Suppl):7–15.
12. Anderson RM, Funnell MM, Barr PA, et al. Learning to empower patients: results of a professional education program for diabetes educators. Diabetes Care 1991;14(2):584–590.
13. Becker MH. The Health Belief Model and Personal Health Behavior. Health Educ Monogr 1974;2:324–473.
14. Bandura A. Self-efficacy: toward a unifying theory of behavior change. Psychol Rev 1970;84:191–215.
15. Ruggerio L, Prochaska JO. Readiness for change: application of the transtheoretical model to diabetes. Diabetes Spectrum 1993;6:22–60.
16. National Standards for Diabetes Self-Management Education Programs and American Diabetes Association. Diabetes Care 2000;23:682–689.
17. Redman B. The Practice of Patient Education, 8th ed. Mosby, St. Louis, MO, 1997, p. 264.
18. Funnell M, Haas LB. National Standards for Diabetes Self-Management Education. Diabetes Care 1995;18:100–116.

19. International Diabetes Federation Consultative Section on Education. International Consensus Standards of Practice for Diabetes Education, Bakersville Press, Bakersville, UK, 1997.
20. Canadian Diabetes Association, Diabetes Educator Section. Standards for Diabetes Education in Canada (2000) Education in Canada 1995.
21. American Diabetes Association. Nutrition recommendations and principles for people with diabetes mellitus. Diabetes Care 1994;17:519–524.
22. Diabetes Control and Complications Research Group. The effect of intensive treatment of diabetes on the development and progression of long-term complications in insulin-dependent diabetes mellitus. N Engl J Med 1993;329:977–986.
23. The DCCT Research Group. Expanded role of the dietitian in the Diabetes Control and Complications Trial: implications for clinical practice. J Am Diet Assoc 1993;93:758–767.
24. The DCCT Research Group. The Diabetes Control and Complications Trial: the trial coordinator perspective. Diabetes Educ 1993;13:236–241.
25. Siminerio L. Defining the role of the health education specialist in the United States. Diabetes Spectrum 1999;12:152–157.
26. The American Association of Diabetes Educators. The 1999 scope of practice for diabetes educators and the standards of practice for diabetes educators. AADE 2000 Resource Guide.
27. Australian Diabetes Educators Association. National Standards of Practice for Diabetes Educators. ACT, Canberra, 1989.
28. Roter DL, Hall JA, Merisca R, et al. Effectiveness of interventions to improve patient compliance: a meta-analysis. Med Care 1998;36:1138–1161.
29. Peyrot M. Behavior Change in Diabetes Education. Executive Summary of the Diabetes Educational and Behavioral Research Summit. American Association of Diabetes Educators, Washington, DC, 1999.
30. Assal J, Muhlhauser I, Pernet A, et al. Patient education as the basis for diabetes care in clinical practice and research. 1985.
31. Brown SA. Diabetes Education Interventions: State of the Science. Executive Summary of the Diabetes Educational and Behavioral Research Summit. Association of Diabetes Educators, Washington, DC, 1999.
32. Anderson RM. Educational Principles and Strategies. In: Funnell, M. ed. A Core Curriculum for Diabetes Education, 3rd ed. American Association of Diabetes Educators, Washington, DC, 1998, p. 6.
33. Peyrot M. Evaluation of patient education programs: how to do it and how to use it. Diabetes Spectrum 1996;9;2:86–93.
34. Kaplan RM. Behavior as the central outcome in health care. Am Psychol 1990;14:1211–1220.
35. Arslanian S, Becker D, Drash A. Diabetes in the child and adolescent. In: Kappy MS, Blizzard RM, Migeon, CJ, eds. Wilkins—The Diagnosis and Treatment of Endocrine Disorders in Childhood and Adolescence, 4th ed. Charles C Thomas, Springfield, IL, 1994, pp. 961–1027.
36. Hauser S, Solomon ML. Coping with diabetes: views from the family. In: Ahmed R, Ahmed N, eds. Coping with Juvenile Diabetes, Charles C Thomas, Springfield, IL, 1985, pp. 234–266.
37. Follansbee, DM. Assuming responsibility for diabetes care: what age, what price? Diabetes Educ 1989 15:347–352.
38. Kohler E, Hurwitz LS, Milan D. A developmentally staged curriculum for teaching self-care to the child with insulin-dependent diabetes mellitus. Diabetes Care 1982;5:30–35.
39. Ingersoll G, Orr D, Herrold AJ, Golden M. Cognitive maturity and self-management among adolescents with insulin-dependent diabetes mellitus. J Pediatr 1986;108:620–623.
40. Anderson BJ, Auslander WF, Jung KC, Miller JP, Santiago JV. Assessing family sharing of diabetes responsibilities. J Pediatr 1990;4:477–492.
41. Citrin W, Tapp J, Wine H. Diabetes counseling issues: the patient and family. In Pediatric and Adolescent Diabetes Medicine, Year Book Publishing, Chicago, IL, 1987, pp. 369–390.
42. Sargent, AJ. The sick child and the family. J Pediatr 1983:102,982–987.

14 Nutritional Management in Type 1 Diabetes

Christine A. Beebe, MS, RD, LD, CDE

CONTENTS

INTRODUCTION

The goal of medical nutrition therapy (MNT) for individuals with type 1 diabetes is to modify food intake to prevent diabetes-related acute and chronic complications while achieving and maintaining an optimal quality of life. The goal of MNT for health care professionals is to facilitate the person with type 1 diabetes and their families in doing so, while considering each person as an individual with cultural and personal food and lifestyle preferences. Nutrient intake should be modified to attain metabolic outcomes that have been defined by the American Diabetes Association (ADA) *(1)*:

- Near-normal blood glucose levels
- Optimal serum lipid parameters
- Optimal blood pressure levels

Additional goals of MNT in persons with type 1 diabetes include *(2)* the following:

- Promoting overall health and well-being
- Modifying nutrient intake and lifestyle to prevent and treat complications such as nephropathy, neuropathy, obesity, and cardiovascular disease (CVD) risk
- Providing for adequate growth and development in youth
- Providing for successful pregnancy outcomes

The challenge of MNT in diabetes is that the person with diabetes is responsible for 99% of the day-to-day management of the disease. As health care professionals, we provide the knowledge and skill to make the necessary nutrition modifications; how-

From: *Contemporary Endocrinology: Type 1 Diabetes: Etiology and Treatment*
Edited by: M. A. Sperling © Humana Press Inc., Totowa, NJ

ever, we must recognize that the person with diabetes ultimately makes the choice of what to eat, how much to eat, and when. Because type 1 diabetes spans the life cycle from infancy to old age, dietary and behavior modification principles and strategies are unique to each stage.

NUTRITIONAL FACTORS AFFECTING BLOOD GLUCOSE CONTROL

Blood glucose control, as measured by HbA1c, reflects the combined effect of fasting blood glucose levels, postprandial blood glucose excursions, and mean blood glucose values throughout the day. Nutrition interventions affect both fasting and postprandial values. Fasting blood glucose is determined by hepatic glucose production through the night and influenced by degree of insulin resistance and available insulin. Because individuals with type 1 diabetes produce little or no insulin, the amount and type of insulin provided during nighttime hours will determine fasting glucose levels. Previous days physical activity enhances insulin sensitivity, increases muscle glucose uptake, and, subsequently, may result in nighttime hypoglycemia. In turn, bedtime food intake in excess of insulin coverage can increase nighttime blood glucose levels.

In contrast, the postprandial blood glucose period, defined as up to 6 h after a meal, is predominantly the result of food intake, particularly carbohydrate absorption and the availability of insulin to cover the carbohydrate load *(3)*. Glucagon secretion and its interaction with available insulin will influence postprandial response through effects on liver and peripheral glucose metabolism. Carbohydrate and protein consumption influence both glucagon and insulin secretion.

Amount of Carbohydrate

Individuals with normal glucose tolerance experience a dose-related rise in postprandial blood glucose up to 60–75 g of carbohydrate consumed *(4)*. Consuming more carbohydrate does not increase blood glucose beyond 140 mg/dL primarily because insulin secretion keeps up with entry of glucose into the blood. In type 1 diabetes, in which insulin secretion is absent or very low, the larger the dose of carbohydrate, the greater the blood glucose response. Studies in individuals with type 1 diabetes show a strong relationship between the premeal short- or rapid-acting insulin dose and the postprandial blood glucose response based on total carbohydrate content of the meal *(5,6)*. Thus, for individuals with type 1 diabetes, learning to calculate and adjust insulin dose to total carbohydrate intake is the primary nutritional strategy used to optimize glycemic control. The optimal amount of carbohydrate to consume in the diet differs with each individual and should be based on preference. Carbohydrate foods such as fruits, vegetables, whole grains, and cereals provide necessary vitamins, minerals, fiber, and phytonutrients such as lycopene and anthoxanthines—all considered essential to a healthy diet. As a result, the ADA recommends 60–70% of total caloric intake be derived from a combination of carbohydrate and monounsaturated fat (*see* Table 1); in other words, approx 50% of the diet should come from carbohydrates *(2)*. Decreasing the carbohydrate intake to a level less than 40% in an effort to attenuate postprandial blood glucose levels results in a diet that can be too high in fat and protein.

Type of Carbohydrate

Despite the strong relationship between total carbohydrate intake and insulin requirement, postprandial blood glucose response to a mixed meal is not always predictable. In

Table 1
Individualizing Nutrition Interventions in Type 1 Diabetes

Guidelines in stepwise priority	*Daily implementation*
1. USDA Food Guide Pyramid for overall health	• 2–3 Servings fruit • 3–4 Servings vegetables • Whole grains • Sugar in context of healthy diet • Salt in moderation; < 2400 mg/d if hypertensive • Limit alcohol 1 Drink/d for women 2 Drinks/d for men
2. Carbohydrate counting to reduce glucose excursions	• Total carbohydrate goals/meal and snacks • Design insulin: carbohydrate regimen • Evaluate individual food glycemic response • Alternative sweeteners
3. Fat modification to reduce CVD risk	• Restrict SFA to ≤ 10% total calories ≤ 7% if LDL > 100 mg/dL • Restrict PUFA to ≤ 10% calories; fish at least twice a week • Preferred fat is MUFA • Total fat ≤ 25% of calories for weight loss
4. Vitamin/mineral supplementation	Women Folic acid: 400 μg if child-bearing age Calcium: to intake of 1000–1200 mg/d

Abbreviations: LDL, low-density lipoprotein; SFA, saturated fatty acid; PUFA, polyunsaturated fatty acid; MUFA, monounsaturated fatty acid; CVD, cardiovascular disease; USDA, United States Department of Agriculture.

a classic study illustrating this point, subjects with type 1 diabetes experienced a larger and longer postprandial blood glucose response when consuming a pizza meal despite equivalent amounts of carbohydrate, protein, and fat, as a standard meal *(7)*. It is now well accepted that the magnitude and nature of the postprandial blood glucose rise is proportional to the rate of digestion and absorption of carbohydrate in the meal. Several factors can influence the rate of digestion and absorption to a carbohydrate challenge, including premeal blood glucose values. Hyperglycemia before eating slows gastric emptying and results in a more prolonged glycemic response *(8)*, whereas hypoglycemia speeds emptying and results in a faster, higher, and earlier peak response *(9)*. The presence of some organic acids in foods, such as in sourdough bread or tannic acid in tea and wine, appears to slow gastric emptying and flatten the blood glucose response *(10)*.

The optimal type of carbohydrate is considered to be one that will yield a relatively flat postprandial blood glucose response. The Glycemic Index (GI) of foods is a classification of carbohydrate-rich foods based on their postprandial blood glucose and insulin response *(11)*. It is expressed as the percentage of blood glucose rise over 2–3 h from 50 g of carbohydrate from a particular food compared with the blood glucose response to 50 g of glucose. Foods are ranked from a GI of 20 to over 100 (pure glucose).

Research in this area has done much to dispel the myth that sugar or sucrose raises blood glucose more than starch *(12)* and provided evidence that carbohydrate foods can yield variable blood glucose and insulin responses both between and within food groups such as fruits, vegetables, and cereal grains *(13)*. Because blood glucose response of a carbohydrate food is directly related to the rate of glucose digestion and absorption from the gastrointestinal tract and is not a function of simple or complex carbohydrate, these terms (i.e., simple and complex) have been discouraged by the World Health Organization (WHO) *(14)*.

Digestible Starch

The molecular nature of a starch is one factor that alters the rate of digestion. Amylose, comprised of straight chains of glucose molecules, is a form of starch that is slowly digested and absorbed compared to amylopectin, made up of branched chains. Both amylose and amylopectin are present in various amounts in all starch-containing foods. Wheat starch, containing a greater percentage of amylopectin, yields a greater glucose response than oat starch, which is higher in amylose and viscous fibers. The ratio of amylopectin to amylose is about 70 : 30 in most starches and accounts for the rapid blood glucose effect of most starches *(15)*.

Cooking, as with potatoes, and processing, as in grinding apples for applesauce, soften the starch granule and expose it for easier enzymatic breakdown, raising blood glucose levels higher and faster *(16)*. This concept supports the principle that starches should be used in their whole-grain unprocessed form such as whole wheat breads and whole grain cereals whenever possible.

Nondigestible Starch

Some foods such as raw cornstarch contain naturally existing resistant starches that are higher in amylose, producing a flatter glycemic response *(17)*. This attribute has spurred the development of designer foods such as snack bars that contain a combination of sucrose and raw cornstarch that can be used with the intent to prevent hypoglycemia *(18)*. There is no evidence at present that the use of resistant starch has long-term benefit in type 1 diabetes; however, the clinical value in individuals at high risk for nighttime hypoglycemia may prove beneficial. Fiber such as that found in grains, beans, nuts, seeds, fruits, and vegetables is a form of carbohydrate that is indigestible and therefore does not contribute to the postprandial blood glucose rise. Furthermore, viscous soluble fibers found in oats and pectin limit enzyme access to other digestible carbohydrates in the gut, limiting postprandial glucose levels *(19)*. Early studies demonstrated a beneficial effect of fiber on glycemic control in type 1 diabetes, but they were complicated by the poor glycemic control of individuals and the small number of subjects *(20)*. More recent studies illustrate that large amounts of fiber may be required to effect long-term glycemic control and the effects are not consistent and modest at best. A diet containing 50 g of fiber with a GI of 70% resulted in a 24% drop in mean daily blood glucose concentrations and an HbA1c improvement of 0.5%, after 6 mo in persons with type 1 diabetes, compared to a diet containing 15 g of fiber with a GI of 90% *(21)*. In contrast, 56 g of fiber did not have an effect in another study in type 1 diabetes *(22)*.

Compliance with such high-fiber diets has been good in studies dispelling concerns that a high-fiber intake cannot be consumed through natural foods *(21,22)*. Because the average American consumes about 13 g of dietary fiber per day, progression to a high-fiber intake needs to be gradual and requires a good deal of motivation.

Persons with type 1 diabetes who adjust their insulin to carbohydrate intake may need to take into account if a food contains 5 g of fiber or more per serving and subtract the 5 g or more from the total grams of carbohydrate per serving. Benefits of fiber in diabetes also include optimal overall gastrointestinal function and the low-density lipoprotein (LDL) cholesterol lowering effect validated in nondiabetic individuals and recommended in the National Cholesterol Education Program Guidelines *(23)*.

Sugars and Sugar Alternatives

Sugar or sucrose (glucose + fructose) does not elevate blood glucose to a greater extent than starch *(24)*. Glucose is rapidly and easily absorbed but represents only one-half of the sucrose molecule. As fructose passes through the liver after absorption, it is metabolized and does not immediately or directly contribute to blood glucose elevation. As much as 10–17% of total calories as sugar, consistent with typical US intake, has shown no detrimental effect on blood glucose control in type 1 diabetes *(2,25)*. Consumption of sugar-rich foods is recommended in moderation and in the context of a healthy diet (potentially one serving daily) while counting gram for gram as a carbohydrate.

Treating hypoglycemia correctly is crucial to effectively managing diabetes. Although any form of carbohydrate will raise blood glucose, sugar in the form of glucose tablets, candy, soda, juice, or milk is traditionally used. Pure glucose or sucrose in tablets or a solution elevate blood glucose equally as well when treating hypoglycemia, providing a response within 10 min and alleviating symptoms within 15 min *(26)*. Approximately 15- to 20-g portions of these carbohydrates will elevate blood glucose levels approx 50 mg/dL when hypoglycemia is in the range of 50–70 mg/dL *(27)*. Levels less than this may require 30 g to bring the blood glucose levels back to normal within 15–30 min. Traditional treatments such as orange juice and milk can require over 40-g portions of carbohydrate to be as effective *(28)*.

Alternative sweeteners are available for the purpose of reducing calories and carbohydrate intake. Fructose is used as an alternative sweetener and is particularly abundant in soft drinks and fruit beverages, which accounts for two-thirds of fructose intake in the United States. Although blood glucose response is slightly flatter, concern has been raised that in large quantities, fructose (20% of calories) elevates serum cholesterol levels *(29)*. Sugar alcohols, such as sorbitol and mannitol, provide fewer calories (2–3 cal/g) than sucrose, glucose, or fructose and raise blood glucose to a lesser extent *(30)*. Yet, there are no published studies illustrating a long-term benefit in glycemic control or body weight to their regular use. Because sugar alcohols have a laxative effect when consumed in more than 20-g portions or 50 g daily, they should be used with caution in small children to prevent diarrhea *(31)*.

Non-nutritive sweeteners currently approved as safe by the Food and Drug Administration are aspartame, saccharine, acesulfame K, and sucralose. Because of their intense sweetening capacity, they do not contribute calories or carbohydrates to the meal plan and can be used freely in the diet *(2)*. However, rarely are alternative sweeteners used alone in a food except in diet drinks and some candies or gelatins. Other sources of carbohydrates may be present in combination with non-nutritive sweeteners in foods such as ice creams or desserts, requiring that total carbohydrate content per serving be calculated.

Although research has provided valuable explanations for varying blood glucose responses to individual foods and mixed meals, the clinical significance of the GI remains controversial. Indeed, clinical intervention trials in type 1 diabetes have yielded inconclusive results in that while post-meal blood glucose levels may be lower *(32,33)*, overall blood glucose control as measured by HbA1c is not improved *(22,34)*. Adding the GI requirement to total carbohydrate counting adds another level of complexity to an

Table 2
Recommended Daily Energy Intake

	Average energy allowance (kcal)		
Category	*Age (yr)*	*Per kg*	*Per day*
Infants	0.0–0.5	108	650
	0.5–1.0	98	850
Children	1–3	102	1300
	4–6	90	1800
	7–10	70	2000
Males	11–14	55	2500
	15–18	45	3000
	19–24	40	2900
	25–50	37	2900
	51+	30	2300
Females	11–14	47	2200
	15–18	40	2200
	19–24	38	2200
	25–50	36	2200
	51+	30	1900
Pregnant	1st trimester		+0
	2nd trimester		+300
	3rd trimester		+300
Lactating			+500

Source: From Food and Nutrition Board, National Research Council. Recommended Dietary Allowances, 10th ed. National Academy Press, Washington, DC, 1989.

already regimented diet. A study in children found that choosing carbohydrate portions from a list of low-glycemic index foods reduced the HbA1c by 0.3% and improved quality of life after 12 mo when compared to a carbohydrate-counting exchange-type regimen *(35)*. With the advent of rapid-acting insulin analogs, postprandial elevations with meals can be covered with insulin injections such that the greatest benefit to using low-GI foods may be between meals and as snacks when insulin concentration is waning. Nonetheless, consuming whole-grain, high-fiber, unprocessed foods with the potential for producing a flatter blood glucose response and enhancing general health is recommended as the first step in nutrition therapy for diabetes (*see* Table 1).

Carbohydrate Counting

Carbohydrate counting is a technique commonly used to quantify the total amount of carbohydrate consumed at a meal or snack *(36)*. Two basic techniques can be employed: One counts grams of carbohydrate using food labels and written sources to provide information on the grams of carbohydrate per serving in a food and the second uses a modified exchange system where carbohydrate-containing foods are classified in 15-g servings. One "carb" is equivalent to 15 g of carbohydrate. An individual's usual carbohydrate intake at meals and snacks can be assessed and used to establish carbohydrate goals for each meal and snack (*see* Table 2). The availability of rapid-acting insulin provides a means to establish an insulin-to-carbohydrate ratio for each meal.

The ratio is determined by body weight and trial and error (e.g., 1 U insulin : 15 g of carbohydrate is a good place to start in the average adult). On the other hand, the ratio for a 7-yr-old child may be 1 : 30. The insulin : carbohydrate ratio can then be adjusted until postprandial blood glucose goals are achieved.

In the Diabetes Control and Complications Trial (DCCT), reduction in HbA1c was related to self-reported adherence to the diet regimen *(37)*. Individual dietary components identified were adjusting insulin dose to food intake and blood glucose fluctuations and not deviating from the snack schedule. If an individual chooses to maintain a fixed dose of insulin at meals from day to day, then the carbohydrate intake must be consistent or fixed, as well. Deviations of more than 5–10 g could produce deviations in postprandial blood glucose levels. Most individuals, however, should and generally prefer to learn to adjust their insulin dose to total carbohydrate intake. Adjusting insulin dose to carbohydrate intake allows for more flexibility in the timing and quantity of food eaten at meals. If more or less carbohydrates are desired at a meal, the insulin dose can be adjusted accordingly. Rapid-acting insulin, because of its quick absorption time (5–15 min) is equally effective whether taken immediately before or immediately after a meal *(38)*. This attribute allows for tremendous flexibility in eating and a subsequent improved quality of life. For example, a small child could be allowed to eat a meal, and then observe the carbohydrate consumption and provide the appropriate insulin dose. This has obvious advantages over predetermining and injecting an insulin dose based on potential carbohydrate intake only to discover that the child does not wish to eat.

Glycemic Effect of Fat

Fat intake has little direct effect on postprandial glucose levels because the glycerol moiety of a triglyceride contributes only a small amount of glucose to the circulation. However, large amounts of dietary fat will delay gastric emptying and peak blood glucose rise *(39)*. Doubling fat intake (65 g) in a standard meal consumed by individuals with type 1 diabetes shifted the postprandial glucose response curve slightly to the right, prolonging glucose elevation by approx 20 mg/dL at hours 3–5. A high-fat meal may require an adjustment in insulin dose that will include either the substitution of short-acting regular insulin for rapid-acting insulin or injecting rapid-acting insulin after the meal. Repeated experience and trial and error is the only real way to develop such a guideline. If the fat content of meals is fairly consistent from day to day, meal insulin requirements should not be affected.

Total dietary fat intake in type 1 diabetes should be driven by serum lipid and body weight goals. As a rule, general guidelines for lowering cholesterol, total fat, and saturated fat are sufficient to maintain a healthy fat intake unless LDL cholesterol is elevated. However, individuals in the DCCT gained weight as glycemic control improved. This well-accepted phenomenon results from reduced glucosuria, improved metabolism, and, potentially, an enhanced ability to eat ad libitum with flexible insulin dosing schedules. Although adjusting insulin to carbohydrate intake can improve blood glucose control, total calories, and, particularly, fat calories associated with sweets can increase and need to be considered if weight is to remain stable.

Glycemic Effect of Protein

Protein is absorbed as amino acids and transported directly into the portal blood system. Some amino acids are metabolized immediately in the liver but most enter the plasma as free amino acids and are transported to muscle and other tissue. Protein is not converted immediately into glucose and, as a result, does not immediately raise postprandial blood glucose levels. Consuming as much as 9 oz of protein in a mixed meal elevated postprandial blood glucose levels only slightly at 3–5 h after eating in persons with type 1 diabetes when compared to a standard meal with 3–4 oz of protein *(39)*. Plasma glucagon levels appear to be stimulated by protein consumption in type 1 diabetes and mirror the delayed glucose elevation *(40)*. Thus, increased hepatic glucose output, secondary to elevations in glucagon, during the latter half of the postprandial period appear responsible for the effect of protein when consumed along with carbohydrates. This attribute has led to the assumption that protein is required at every meal and in bedtime snacks to prolong the blood glucose response and prevent nighttime hypoglycemia. Little evidence exists to support or refute this practice. Adding 2 oz of turkey protein to an evening carbohydrate snack (15 g) in a crossover study resulted in slightly fewer hypoglycemic episodes and an insignificant rise in fasting blood glucose the following day *(41)*. Adding protein to carbohydrates when treating hypoglycemia does not appear to provide benefit. One study in type 1 diabetes illustrated that 15 g of carbohydrate with or without 1 oz of turkey produced identical blood glucose elevations over 180 min when treating hypoglycemia *(42)*.

PROTEIN AND RENAL FUNCTION

Persons with type 1 diabetes may attempt to substitute protein for carbohydrates to attenuate postprandial glucose response. A large cross-sectional study in type 1 diabetes found that protein intakes greater than 20% of total energy intake were associated with higher albumin excretions than <20% dietary protein *(43)*. Concern over the role protein intake plays in renal function suggests that consuming more than 20% protein in the diet is unwise. Furthermore, it is difficult to control total fat and saturated fat intake on a high-protein diet because saturated fat and cholesterol predominate in animal foods. Average protein consumption for most individuals is approx 10–20% of total calories, which coincides with recommended intake in diabetes *(2)*. Attempts to reduce albuminuria with protein restriction have shown that even small reductions in protein intake reduce the rate of decline of glomerular filtration rate and albuminuria in persons with type 1 diabetes *(44)*. Most studies find that it is not feasible to reduce intake to less than 0.7 g/kg body weight. The United States Department of Agriculture (USDA) Food Guide Pyramid recommendation of 150–210 g of animal protein per day (5–7 oz—with 1 oz approximately equal to 30 g) is adequate for most individuals with diabetes. This level can be reduced to 0.8–1.0 g/kg once microalbuminuria is present and 0.8 g/kg in overt nephropathy.

NUTRIENTS AND CARDIOVASCULAR RISK FACTORS

With the advent of the DCCT and a focus on intensive blood glucose control, the glycemic effect of the diet has been the central focus in the nutritional management of diabetes. Clearly, optimizing blood glucose levels is paramount to preventing the microvascular and macrovascular complications of diabetes, yet the risk of cardiovascular disease in diabetes is great. Elevated triglycerides, low high-density lipoprotein (HDL), and elevated LDL levels are common in untreated type 1 diabetes but normalize with intensive glucose control. Normal LDL concentrations generally characterize treated type 1 diabetes; however, the DCCT demonstrated that intensive control can improve atherogenic risk by producing a shift in LDL particle size from small, dense to fewer large buoyant particles *(45)*.

Individuals with type 1 diabetes respond to lipid lowering as well as persons without diabetes; therefore, the National Cholesterol Education Program (NCEP) and ADA nutrition guidelines for altering dietary fat intake seem prudent (*see* Table 1). Dietary fat, however, is not the only nutrient impacting cardiovascular risk. Dietary fiber has shown a slight correlation with serum cholesterol levels and reduced cardiovascular disease risk in type 1 diabetes, although the effect was confounded by a lower fat intake in the populations consuming more fiber *(46)*. Furthermore, the authors could not rule out other mechanisms of protection such as concomitant increases in antioxidants or factors influencing hemostasis or blood pressure.

Dietary Fat

Dietary fatty acids can have either a positive or negative effect on lipid levels. Few studies have been performed in type 1 diabetes; therefore, any effects of dietary fat must be extrapolated from studies in the general population. Saturated fat (SFA) and cholesterol intakes are the principal determinants of serum cholesterol. *Trans* fatty acids, produced during partial hydrogenation of unsaturated fat, are considered metabolically equivalent to saturated fats (i.e., raising serum cholesterol levels) *(47)*. The ADA and NCEP recommend that the combination of SFA and trans fatty acids not exceed 10% of calories. Replacing SFA with polyunsaturated fat (PUFA) of the omega-6 variety (safflower, corn, soy oils) reduces total and LDL cholesterol but may have little effect on serum triglycerides or HDL cholesterol *(48)*; nor are there epidemiological data to suggest that omega-6 PUFAs have a direct effect on reducing cardiovascular risk in individuals with or without diabetes. In contrast, omega-3 fatty acids, a form of PUFA found in cold-water fish oils, offer risk-reducing benefits by lowering triglycerides and decreasing thrombogenic factors *(49,50)*. Two to three 4-oz servings of fish each week is recommended to provide beneficial effects.

Studies in the general population support that substituting monounsaturated fat (MUFA) for SFA is equally as effective as a substituting carbohydrate for lowering total LDL levels *(51)*. An additional benefit of a slightly higher MUFA intake is that HDL levels are consistently maintained and not reduced, as they are on a low-fat/high-carbohydrate diet *(52)*. For this reason, substituting MUFA is often preferred over substituting with carbohydrate in type 2 diabetes. Although it is tempting to imply benefits in type 1 diabetes when insulin is replaced physiologically and control is optimal, there are no studies specifically examining the effect of MUFAs in type 1 diabetes. MUFA is at the heart of the Mediterranean diet promoted by some as preferable to PUFAs. Because there is no negative effect to increasing MUFA consumption within the normal range of fat intake, these fats can be encouraged. Cultural differences and food preferences may make this easier in some individuals than others.

Fat Replacers

Fat replacers or substitutes derived from modified proteins or carbohydrates were introduced into the market to assist in efforts to decrease total fat intake. Although this is theoretically possible, few studies have documented a health benefit. Most have been behavioral studies identifying that total fat, saturated fat, and dietary cholesterol intake can be reduced with the use of these products *(53)*. However, little change in energy intake or body weight has been reported. Persons with diabetes using large amounts of carbohydrate-based fat substitutes (salad dressings) must consider that fat has been replaced by carbohydrates and count the carbohydrates if amounts are above 5 g per serving.

Alcohol

Alcohol need not be restricted in individuals with type 1 diabetes as long as it is limited to no more than one daily serving for women and two for men. Alcohol in these amounts has little effect on glycemic control but does potentiate the glucose-lowering effect of insulin by reducing hepatic glucose production. Because patients with type 1 diabetes take insulin, they should take care to consume alcohol with food to prevent hypoglycemia. Moderate alcohol consumption has been associated with reduced cardiovascular disease risk in the general population, suggesting that alcohol may, in fact, be beneficial to some individuals at high risk *(54)*.

Micronutrients

Vitamins, minerals, and other compounds known as phytochemicals play a crucial role in metabolism, acting as coenzymes and cofactors in such diabetes-related metabolic pathways as carbohydrate, lipid, and homocysteine metabolism. Some of these same compounds act as antioxidants, controlling oxidative damage from free radicals produced during metabolism. The study of these vitamins and minerals and recommendations for consumption have gone beyond early concerns for diseases of deficiency to how these compounds influence the development and progression of chronic disease and genetic pathways.

MINERALS

Minerals such as calcium, potassium, and magnesium are involved in intracellular messaging systems, including insulin signaling. Serum magnesium levels have been found to be low in poorly controlled diabetes and low levels are associated with hypertension, cardiac arrhythmias, congestive heart failure, and insulin resistance. Magnesium deficiency is thought to be secondary to chronic glycosuria, but this is not a consistent finding. Magnesium can be easily acquired from natural foods, yet supplementation has been found useful, albeit in studies of individuals with type 2 diabetes *(55)*. Persons at high risk for magnesium deficiency (ketoacidosis, pregnancy, ethanol abuse) should be assessed for low serum levels and may benefit from supplementation until the hypomagnesemia is resolved *(55)*.

Chromium is known to be a potent potentiator of insulin activity by enhancing sensitivity in myocytes and activating insulin receptor kinase. Although most of the studies with chromium supplementation are conducted in type 2 diabetes, studies in type 1 diabetes show a beneficial effect of 200 μg chromium on reducing insulin dose by as much as 30% *(56)*. Total cholesterol and LDL cholesterol levels have been shown to improve with supplementation in insulin-resistant individuals; however, more research in humans is needed. No single food source is plentiful in chromium, yet deficiencies are rare with adequate intakes of 20–30 μg/d. Serious side effects from supplementation up to 1000 μg/d have not been identified *(57)*. A prudent clinical approach is to evaluate improvements in insulin activity, requirements, or serum lipid levels.

The daily recommended calcium intake of 1000–1500 mg in women is based on the desire to prevent osteoporosis *(2)*. These values are valid during pregnancy as well, because maternal hormones increase calcium absorption and utilization. Type 1 diabetes that is poorly controlled may or may not increase requirements for calcium.

VITAMINS AND ANTIOXIDANTS

Because women with type 1 diabetes are at increased risk of neural tube defects and can be of child-bearing age, it is important that they consume 400 μg of folic acid from a supplement, in addition to natural foods, to reduce the risk of neural tube defects *(58)*. Folate or folic acid (synthetic form) is involved in the formation of methionine from homocysteine. A folate deficiency results in hyperhomocysteinemia—a risk factor for atherosclerotic vascular disease *(59)*. Although the mechanism for how hyperhomocysteinemia increases cardiovacular risk is not known, it can be corrected with supplementation up to 400 μg *(59)*. Studies performed in the general population and in persons with type 2 diabetes have not used cardiovascular events as end points; furthermore, studies in type 1 diabetes are lacking, making it very unclear if there is any true benefit to supplementation with intent to reduce cardiovascular disease.

Diabetes and the resulting hyperglycemia is considered to be a highly oxidative state. Glucose can combine with oxygen to produce free radicals capable of causing damage to lipids and proteins. Furthermore, sorbitol and fructose produced in non-insulin-dependent tissues such as the eyes, kidneys, and nerves result in free-radical formation. As a result, several studies are examining the effect of specific antioxidants, such as vitamin E, on the development of the chronic complications of diabetes, including cardiovascular disease. Data are lacking to make any clinical suggestions in others such as selenium and alpha-lipoic acid. Randomized clinical trials with vitamin E have been performed in type 1 diabetes. Retinal blood flow and creatinine clearance improved with 1800 IU vitamin E per day for 4 mo *(60)*. Supplementation with 400 IU/d for 8 wk did not reduce oxidized LDL *(61)*; however, C-reactive protein levels have been decreased with 800 IU/d *(62)*. In contrast, the Heart Outcomes Prevention Evaluation (HOPE) study, a large randomized placebo-controlled trial, found no beneficial effect on cardiovascular outcomes or mortality in people with diabetes consuming 400 IU vitamin E/d for 4.5 yr *(63)*. Supplementation longer than 5 yr or earlier in the disease process needs to be evaluated prior to coming to any conclusions. No significant side effects from as high as 3200 IU/d of vitamin E have been observed.

Studies using supplementation of individual micronutrients and phytochemicals are far from conclusive but hold promise for the future. Interestingly, the consumption of these nutrients in real foods continues to yield the most consistent health results, suggesting that dietary patterns are very important. Shifting the balance of nutrients may, indeed, shift metabolism in a direction that could have more negative than positive effects. The Dietary Approaches to Stop Hypertension (DASH) study examined three dietary patterns on blood pressure when body weight, physical activity, and sodium intake were held constant *(64)*. The diet highest in fruits, vegetables, and low-fat dairy products in conjunction with the lowest total fat, SFA, and cholesterol intake produced the most consistent blood-pressure-lowering effect in both normal and hypertensive individuals. Sodium restriction in a subset of subjects was beneficial primarily in subjects who were hypertensive, female, and African-American.

CALORIC INTAKE

Energy intake is generally episodic, varying in carbohydrate, protein, and fat intake from meal to meal and day to day. Daily caloric or energy requirement is determined by daily energy expenditure. This is represented by the sum of calories required to meet the needs for resting metabolic rate (RMR), the thermic effect of food (TEF), and the thermic effect of physical activity or exercise (TEE). Resting metabolic rate comprises 60–75% of daily caloric needs and is dependent on age, gender, body composition, and genetics. An approximate 2–3% drop in RMR occurs for every decade, accounting for the greater caloric needs per kilogram body weight in infants, children, and adolescents. Men have a higher RMR and require more calories than women because of their larger size and greater muscle mass. The TEF (i.e., the amount of calories required to absorb, metabolize, and store nutrients) is fairly stable at 10% of daily need. Physical activity, however, varies considerably from individual to individual and from day to day and can influence caloric needs in the range of 150–3000 kcal/d. A very active athletic 16-yr-old could require up to 6000 kcal each day, whereas his/her sedentary counterpart may need less than the recommended caloric level, which is based on light to moderate physical activity (*see* Table 2).

Estimating caloric requirements is not easy or precise, yet guidelines have been recommended based on WHO calculations and modified for US populations (*see* Table 2). These should be used only as guidelines and are subject to variability resulting from genetic and ethnic differences as well as concurrent medical conditions. The recommendations for adults, for example, are the same for all individuals over 51 yr of age despite the fact that a 51-yr-old is very different than an 85-yr-old, with or without a medical condition such as heart failure.

A dietary assessment to evaluate usual intake can be combined with the caloric recommendations to arrive at a personalized meal plan. The meal plan is then evaluated by monitoring desired outcomes in terms of blood sugar and lipid levels but also growth and body weight. Infants and small children may need specific caloric prescriptions to achieve normal growth and development, however, in general, most individuals with type 1 diabetes inherently adjust their food intake to meet energy needs. As a result, carbohydrate may be the only nutrient requiring modification and monitoring. For example, a carbohydrate-counting plan outlining specific carbohydrate goals may be accompanied by general guidelines for reducing SFA and consuming moderate amounts of protein.

The increasing incidence of obesity in children and adults in the United States, coupled with the definite tendency to experience weight gain with intensive glucose management, may require greater attention to caloric intake. An analysis of weight gain in DCCT subjects identified that, on average, adult subjects achieving a mean HbA1c of 7.2% gained 4.8 kg more during a 6-yr follow-up than their conventionally controlled counterparts *(65)*. The rate of increase was greatest in the first year of intensive therapy and slowed thereafter and only age was consistently associated with major weight gain. Despite the benefits of improved glycemic control, care should be taken to reduce weight gain and maintain a healthy weight because the physical and health consequences of excessive weight gain remain to be quantified. Caloric requirements can be influenced by factors that are specific to stages in the life span of an individual (*see* Table 3), and although it is not known how these may be altered by diabetes, they should be considered when evaluating caloric needs.

Table 3
Specific Nutrition Considerations Through the Life Span

Age	*Concern*
Infant	Support growth and development.
Low birth weight	Requires approx 120 kcal/kg to continue intrauterine growth rate.
Children	Finicky eating is natural but can be used to exert control over parents/caregivers. • Recognize individual meals and single-day intake may not be balanced, but over several days, intake will balance. • Provide items from major food groups at meals and snacks. • Limit between-meal intake. • Monitor eating away from home.
Adolescents	Use food to experiment, gain control, and establish themselves as individuals. • Strict vegetarianism increases risk of poor quality and quantity of protein and inadequate calcium, iron, zinc, vitamin D, and B_{12}. • Obesity from overeating and underactivity. • Girls peak caloric need at menarche (approx 12-yr-old). • Boys peak caloric need during growth spurt until 16-yr-old. • Eating disorders if dissatisfied with body weight, fear of weight gain; leads to obsessive dieting and omitting insulin doses.
Elderly	Dehydration risk increases accounting for 7% of hospitalizations. • Increased need for water and liquids, particularly with hyperglycemia.

SUMMARY

Nutritional management of type 1 diabetes is dictated by prioritizing interventions that yield optimal metabolic outcomes and enhanced quality of life. The USDA Food Guide Pyramid continues to be the basis for a healthy diet providing vitamins, minerals, phytonutients, and fiber. Blood glucose control is best achieved with careful attention to adequately covering carbohydrate intake with insulin, generally utilizing carbohydrate-counting techniques. Although individuals with well-controlled type 1 diabetes generally have normal serum lipid levels, a low-fat and low-cholesterol diet substituting MUFAs or carbohydrates for SFA is prudent and beneficial. Protein intake should be moderate and include fish on a regular basis.

REFERENCES

1. American Diabetes Association. Standards of Medical Care for Patients with Diabetes Mellitus. Diabetes Care 2002;25:S33–S49.
2. American Diabetes Association. Evidence-Based Nutrition Principles and Recommendations for the Treatment and Prevention of Diabetes and Related Complications. Diabetes Care 2002;25:S50–S60.
3. American Diabetes Association. Postprandial Blood Glucose, Consensus Statement. Diabetes Care 2001;24:775–778.
4. Nuttall FQ, Gannon MC. Plasma glucose and insulin response to macronutrients in nondiabetic and NIDDM patients. Diabetes Care 1991;14:824–838.
5. Rabasa-Lhoret R, Garon J, Langelier H, et al. The effects of meal carbohydrate content on insulin requirements in type 1 diabetic patients treated intensively with the basal bolus (ultralent-regular) insulin regimen. Diabetes Care 1999;22:667–673.

6. Heinemann L, Heise T, Wahl LCh, et al. Prandial glycemia after a carbohydrate-rich meal in type 1 diabetic patients: using the rapid acting insulin analogue[Lys(B28), Pro(B29)] human insulin. Diabet Med 1996;13:625–629.
7. Ahren JA, Gatcomb PM, Held NA, et al. Exaggerated hyperglycemia after a pizza meal in well-controlled diabetes. Diabetes Care 1993;16:578–580.
8. Fraser RJ, Horowitz M, Maddox AF, et al. Hyperglycaemia slows gastric emptying rate in type 1 (insulin-dependent) diabetes mellitus. Diabetologia 1990;33:675–668.
9. Schvarcz E, Palmer M, Aman J, Berne C. Hypoglycemia increases the gastric emptying rate in healthy subjects. Diabetes Care 1995;18:674–676.
10. Liljberg H, Bjorck ME. Delayed gastric emptying rate as a potential mechanism for lowered glycemia after eating sourdough bread: studies in humans and rats using test products with added organic acids or an organic salt. Am J Clin Nutr 1996;64:886–893.
11. Jenkins DJA, Wolever TMS, Buckley G, et al. Low glycemic index starchy foods in the diabetic diet. Am J Clin Nutr 1988;48:248–254.
12. Venhaus A, Chanteleau E. Self-selected unrefined and refined carbohydrate diets do not affect metabolic control in pump-treated diabetic patients. Diabetologia 1988;31:153–157.
13. Hughes TA, Atchison J, Hazewlrig JB, Boshell BR. Glycemic responses in insulin-dependent diabetic patients: effect of food composition. Am J Clin Nutr 1989;49:658–666.
14. Report of a Joint FAO/WHO Expert Consultation: carbohydrates. In: Human Nutrition. Food and Agriculture Organization of the United Nations and World Health Organization, Rome, 1998.
15. Behall KM, Howe JC. Effect of long-term amylose vs amylopectin starch on metabolic variables in human subjects. Am J Clin Nutr 1995;61:334–340.
16. Jarvi A, Karlstrom B, Granfeldt Y, Bjorck I, Vessby B. The influence of food structure on postprandial metabolism in patients with NIDDM. Am J Clin Nutr 1995;61:837–842.
17. Raben A, Tagliabue A, Christensen NJ, et al. Resistant starch: the effect on postprandial glycemia, hormonal response, and satiety. Am J Clin Nutr 1994;60:544–551.
18. Kaufman FR, Halvorson M, Kaufman ND. A randomized blinded trial of uncoooked cornstarch to diminish nocturnal hypoglycemia at diabetes camp. Diabetes Res Clin Pract 1995;30:205–209.
19. Vaaler S, Hanssen KF, Aagenaes O. Effect of different kinds of fibre on postprandial blood glucose in insulin-dependent diabetics. Acta Med Scand 1980;15:972–978.
20. Riccardi G, Rivellese A, Pacioni D, et al. Separate influence of dietary carbohydrate and fibre on the metabolic control in diabetes. Diabetologia 1984;26:116–121.
21. Giacco R, Parillo M, Rivellese A, et al. Long-term dietary treatment with increased amounts of fiber-rich low-glycemic index natural foods improves blood glucose control and reduces the number of hypoglycemic events in type 1 diabetic patients. Diabetes Care 2000;23:1461–1466.
22. Lafrance L, Rabasa-Lhoret R, Poisson D, et al. The effects of different glycemic index foods and dietary fibre intake on glycaemic control in type 1 diabetic patients on intensive insulin therapy. Diabet Med 1998;15:972–978.
23. Expert Panel on Detection, Evaluation, and Treatment of High Blood Cholesterol in Adults. Executive summary of the Third Report of the National Cholesterol Education Program (NCEP) Expert Panel on Detection, Evaluation, and Treatment of High Blood Cholesterol in Adults (Adult treatment Panel III). JAMA 2001;285:2486–2497.
24. Bantle JP, Laine DC, Castle GW, et al. Postprandial glucose and insulin responses to meals containing different carbohydrates in normal and diabetic subjects. N Engl J Med 1983;309:7–12.
25. Nuttall FQ, Gannon MC. Sucrose and disease. Diabetes Care 1981;4:305–310.
26. Cryer PE, Fisher JN, Shamoon H. Hypoglycemia (technical review). Diabetes Care 1995;17:734–755.
27. Slama G, Traynard P-Y, Desplanque N, et al. The search for the optimized treatment of hypoglycemia: carbohydrates in tablets, solution, or gel in the correction of insulin reactions. Arch Intern Med 1990;150:589–593.
28. Brodows RG, Williams C, Amatruda JM. Treatment of insulin reactions in diabetics. JAMA 1984;252:3378–3381.
29. Bantle JP, Raatz SK, Thomas W, Georgopoulos A. Effects of dietary fructose on plasma lipids in healthy subjects. Am J Clin Nutr 2000;72:1128–1134.
30. Akgun S, Ertel NH. A comparison of carbohydrate metabolism after sucrose, sorbitol, and fructose meals in normal and diabetic subjects. Diabetes Care 1980;3:582–585.
31. Payne ML, Craig WJ, Williams AC. Sorbitol is a possible risk factor for diarrhea in young children. J Am Diet Assoc 1997;97:532–534.

32. Collier GR, Giudici S, Kalmusky J, et al. Low glycaemic index starchy foods improve glucose control and lower serum cholesterol In diabetic children. Diabet Nutr Metab 1988;1:11–19.
33. Fontvieille AM, Acosta M, Rizkalla SW, et al. A moderate switch from high to low glycaemic index foods for 3 weeks improves the metabolic control of type 1 (IDDM) diabetic subjects. Diabet Nutr Metab 1988;1:139–143.
34. Calle-Pascual AL, Gomez V, Leon E, Bordiu E. Foods with a low glycemic index do not improve glycemic control of both type 1 and type 2 diabetic patients after one month of therapy. Diabetes Metab 1988;14:629–633.
35. Gilbertson H, Brand-Miller J, Thorburn A, et al. The effect of flexible low glycemic index dietary advice versus measured carbohydrate exchange diets on glycemic control in children with type 1 diabetes. Diabetes Care 2001;24:1137–1143.
36. Gillespie S, Kulkarni K, Daly A. Using carbohydrate counting in diabetes clinical practice. J Am Diet Assoc 1998;98:897–899.
37. Delahanty LM, Halford BN. The role of diet behaviors in achieving improved glycemic control in intensively treated patients in the Diabetes Control and Complications Trial. Diabetes Care 1993;16:1453–1458.
38. Strachan MWJ, Frier BM. Optimal time of administration of insulin lispro. Diabetes Care 1998;21:26–31.
39. Peters AL, Davidson MB. Protein and fat effects on glucose responses and insulin requirements in subjects with insulin-dependent diabetes. Am J Clin Nutr 1993;58:555–560.
40. Nordt TK, Besenthal I, Eggstein M, Jakober B. Influence of breakfasts with different nutrient contents on glucose, C peptide, insulin, glucagon, triglycerides, and GIP in non-insulin-dependent diabetics. Am J Clin Nutr 1991;53:155–160.
41. Beebe CA, Hess A. Glycemic effect of protein added to an evening snack in type 1 diabetes, in press.
42. Gray RO, Butler PC, Beers TR, et al. Comparison of the ability of bread versus bread plus meat to treat and prevent subsequent hypoglycemia in patients with insulin-dependent diabetes. J Clin Endocrinol Metab 1996;81:1508–1511.
43. Toeller M, Buyken A, Heitkamp G, et al. and the EURODIAB IDDM Complications Study. Protein intake and urinary albumin excretion rates in the EURODIAB IDDM Complications study. Diabetologia 1997;40:1219–1226.
44. Pedrini MT, Levey AS, Lau J, Chalmers TC, Wang Ph. The effect of dietary protein restriction on the progression of diabetic and nondiabetic renal diseases: a meta analysis. Ann Intern Med 1996;124:627–632.
45. American Diabetes Association Position Statement: Management of Dyslipidemia in Adults with Diabetes. Diabetes Care 2001;24:S58–S61.
46. Toeller M, Buyken A, Heitkamp G, et al. Fiber intake, serum cholesterol levels, and cardiovascular disease in European individuals with type 1 diabetes. Diabetes Care 1999;22(Suppl):B21–B26.
47. Ascherio A, Katan MB, Zock PL, Stampfer MJ, Willett WC. Trans fatty acids and coronary heart disease. N Engl J Med 1999;340:1994–1998.
48. Mattson FH, Grundy SM. Comparison of effects of dietary saturated, monounsaturated and polyunsaturated fatty acids on plasma lipids and lipoproteins in man. J Lipid Res 1985;26:194–202.
49. Philipson BE, Rothrock DW, Conner WE, Harris WS, Illingworth DR. Reduction of plasma lipids, lipoproteins, and apoproteins by dietary fish oils in patients with hypertriglyceridemia. N Engl J Med 1985;312:1210–1216.
50. Leaf A, Weber PC. Cardiovascular effects of n-3 fatty acids. N Engl J Med 1988;318:549–557.
51. Mensink RP, Katan MB. Effect of monounsaturated fatty acids vs. complex carbohydrates on high-density lipoproteins in healthy men and women. Lancet 1987;1:122–125.
52. Mensink RP, Katan MB. Effect of dietary fatty acids on serum lipids and lipoproteins—a meta analysis of 27 trials. Arterioscler Thromb 1992;12:911–919.
53. Warshaw H, Franz M, Powers MA, Wheeler M. Fat replacers: their use in foods and role in diabetes medical nutrition therapy. (technical review). Diabetes Care 1996;19:1294–1301.
54. Ajani UA, Gaziano M, Lotufo PA, et al. Alcohol consumption and risk of coronary heart disease by diabetes status. Circulation 2000;102:500–505.
55. American Diabetes Association. Magnesium supplementation in the treatment of diabetes (Consensus Statement). Diabetes Care 1992;15:1065–1067.
56. Ravina A, Slezak L, Rubal A, et al. Clinical use of the trace element chromium(III) in the treatment of diabetes mellitus. J Trace Elements Exp Med 1995;8:183–190.
57. Anderson RA. Chromium in the prevention and control of diabetes. Diabetes Metab 2000;26:22–27.

58. Institute of Medicine. Folate. In: Dietary Reference Intakes. Standing Committee on the Scientific Evaluation of Dietary Reference Intakes, Food and Nutrition Board. National Academy Press, Washington, DC, 1998, p. 8–68.
59. Brattstrom LE. Vitamins as homocysteine lowering agents. J Nutr 1996;126:1276S–1280S.
60. Bursell SE, Clermont AC, Aiello LP, et al. High dose vitamin E supplementation normalizes retinal blood flow and creatinine clearance in patients with type 1 diabetes. Diabetes Care 1999;22:1245–1251.
61. Astley S, Langrish-Smith A, Southern S, Sampson M. Vitamin E supplementation and oxidative damage to DNA and plasma LDL in type 1 diabetes. Diabetes Care 1999;22:1626–1631.
62. Upritchard JE, Sutherland WHF, Mann JI. Effect of supplementation with tomato juice, vitamin E, and vitamin C on LDL oxidation and products of inflammatory activity in type 2 diabetes. Diabetes Care 2000;23:733–738.
63. Yusuf S, Dagenais G, Pogue J, et al. Vitamin E supplementation and cardiovascular events in high-risk patients. The Heart Outcomes Prevention Evaluation Study Investigators. N Engl J Med 2000;342:154–160.
64. Appel LJ, Moore TJ, Obarzanek E, et al. A clinical trial of the effects of dietary patterns on blood pressure. N Engl J Med 1997;336:1117–1124.
65. The DCCT Research Group. Influence of intensive diabetes treatment on body weight and composition of adults with type 1 diabetes in the Diabetes Control and Complications Trial. Diabetes Care 2001;24:1711–1721.

III

Special Management Issues in Type 1 Diabetes

15 Special Problems and Management of the Child Less Than 5 Years of Age

Nadia Tubiana-Rufi, MD
and Paul Czernichow, MD

CONTENTS

INTRODUCTION

Diabetes in a child less than 5 yr old is characterized by unstable glycemic control, frequent and asymptomatic hypoglycemia, and greater risk of severe hypoglycemia. Management of diabetes in young children is complicated by special age-related problems, including difficulties in administering and adjusting small doses of insulin and unpredictable behavior pattern or day-to-day variations in diet and physical activities. The inability of the young child to detect and communicate the symptoms of hypoglycemia could lead to delay in the treatment and contribute to the high risk of severe hypoglycemic episodes at this age. Evidence for neurocognitive and intellectual dysfunction subsequent to recurrent or severe hypoglycemia in early childhood explains the attitude of pediatricians to be prudent and not to attempt too strict metabolic control in children less than 5 yr of age. A multidisciplinary approach by a specialized team available for frequent contacts and that gives children and parents an adapted continuing education and support is necessary. In case of severe hypoglycemia despite a well-conducted conventional therapy, a more physiological way of insulin treatment, such as continuous subcutaneous insulin infusion (CSII) has been shown to be well-tolerated by young children and allows achievement of good metabolic control without severe hypoglycemia under the supervision of a specialized team.

From: *Contemporary Endocrinology: Type 1 Diabetes: Etiology and Treatment*
Edited by: M. A. Sperling © Humana Press Inc., Totowa, NJ

CHARACTERISTICS OF TYPE 1 DIABETES IN YOUNG CHILDREN

Epidemiology

Diabetes is less frequent in preschool children than in older ages. In a large survey in Europe, age-specific incidence was compared among 3 age groups in more than 3000 cases during 1989–1990 *(1)*. Eighteen percent of the cases were observed in children younger than 4 yr, 34% between 5 and 9 yr, and 48% in children aged 10–14 yr. Similar results have been obtained in North America *(2)*.

The incidence of insulin-dependent diabetes mellitus (IDDM) in childhood has increased in several countries from which the epidemiological data have been collected over an adequate period of time *(2,3)*. This rise in incidence has been observed in all age groups. Pediatricians are particularly concerned by the rising incidence in children aged under 5. In England, for example, the reported incidence in preschool children increased form 4.2 to 9.9/100,000 per year between 1973–1974 and 1988 *(4)*. In another study performed in the same country, this trend continued with an annual increase of 4% in the same age group from 1985–1996 *(5)*. The EURODIAB collaborative group established a prospective, geographically defined register of new cases in 1988 *(6)*. During the period 1989–1994, the annual rate of increase in incidence was 3.6%. This increase was observed in all countries, but as shown in Fig. 1, there was an impressive heterogeneity in the trend of incidence between age groups. The rate of annual increase varied from 6.5% for the preschool children to 3.2% for 5- to 9-yr-olds and 2.6% for 10- to 14-yr-olds. This rapid change in incidence favors a major role for an as yet undefined environmental factor that triggers this disease.

Etiology and Immunogenetics

There is no evidence that the etiology of IDDM before age 5 is different from the disease observed later in childhood. There are, however, some subtle differences in immunogenetic markers. Young children are more often positive for diabetes-related autoantibodies. This has been clearly shown by Komulainen et al. *(7)* in Finland when the islet cell autoantibody (ICA), insulin autoantibody (IAA), antibodies against GAD (GADA), and IA-2 antibodies were detected in a large population of 800 children with IDDM at diagnosis. The percentage of children who tested positive for all four antibodies were 53.1% in the very young children less than 2 yr, 42.0% in the age group between 2.0 and 4.9 yr, and 26.9% in the oldest group. Moreover the titers of antibodies were also different among the age groups, the youngest children having the highest serum level of IAA and ICA.

Some subtle differences in the HLA-DQ B genotypes have also been described in this population. For example, children before the age of 2 yr carried the high-risk genotype DQB1*02/*0302 more often than the older children *(7)*.

Altogether these differences are minor and do not suggest that the etiology of IDDM observed at this very young age is different from that seen in older children.

Clinical Presentation of Type 1 Diabetes

Young children presented more frequently with diabetic ketoacidosis (DKA) at diagnosis than older children *(8–10)*. The more severe metabolic deterioration at diagnosis of diabetes in children than in adults is probably related to a faster process of β-cell destruction *(10)*. Furthermore, the process of β-cell destruction may be faster in early childhood than later in childhood. This suggestion was supported by the findings of

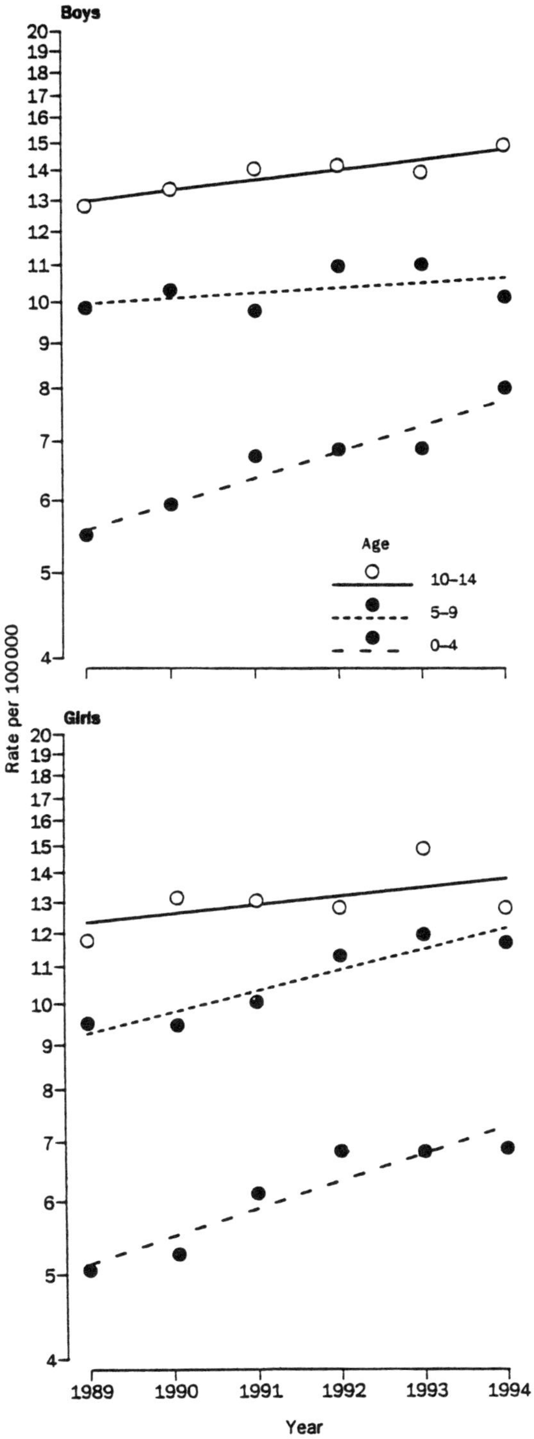

Fig. 1. Trends in childhood diabetes incidence in Europe during 1989–1994 by age group and sex. (From ref. *6*, with permission of the Lancet Ltd.)

two recent studies *(7,11)*. The last study showed that serum C-peptide concentrations at the time of diagnosis were significantly lower in very young children less than 2 yr old in comparison with children 2–4.9 and 5–15 yr old. At the same time, HbA1c was highest in children diagnosed after 5 yr of age, indicating a longer duration of the preceding period of hyperglycemia. In very young children, the severe clinical condition at diagnosis could also be explained by a delay in diagnosis of diabetes because of the difficulties for parents and physicians in identifing diabetes symptoms. Acute infections, more frequently observed at this age, may also mask the symptoms and contribute to delay in the diagnosis of diabetes *(7)*.

The remission rate is lower in young children than in older ones *(12)*. Komulainen et al. *(7)* showed that at 6 mo of follow-up, none of the children diagnosed before the age of 2 yr but 27% of the children aged 2–4.9 yr and 37% of those diagnosed after 5 yr of age ($p < 0.001$) were in partial remission. At the same time of follow-up, younger children also presented with significantly higher HbA1c levels, which were partly explained by their decrease in endogenous insulin secretion.

Blood Glucose Control

High Risk of Hypoglycemia

A major characteristic of metabolic control in type 1 preschool children is the unstable glycemic control with its accompanying risk of severe hypoglycemia. An international cross-sectional study of around 3000 children and adolescents has shown that the highest rate of severe hypoglycemia (60 episodes), resulting in unconsciousness or seizures, was observed in the younger children, aged less than 5 yr compared to the older children (10–20 episodes per 100 patients-years) *(13)*. In this study, the only variables with a significant effect on the incidence of severe hypoglycemia were age, which led to a decrease of 8.4% per year, and HbA1c, which led to a decrease by 21% for each increase of HbA1c by 1%. Nocturnal hypoglycemia events are also more frequent in young children than in older, as reported in two recent studies *(14,15)*. Thus, the frequency of nocturnal hypoglycemia was twice as high in children aged under 5 yr than in children aged 5–9 yr, respectively: 57% vs 28% *(14)*. These studies showed that young age was a major risk factor of nocturnal hypoglycemia and that this risk decreased with age. Furthermore, the lack of symptoms of nocturnal hypoglycemia was demonstrated in two-thirds of the children aged under 5 yr. Our study showed that in a large number of diabetic children *(15,16)*, the closer one monitors, the more frequent were the episodes of nocturnal hypoglycemia: 23% when testing blood glucose (BG) at midnight vs 47% when BG levels were measured hourly. This study also found that nocturnal hypoglycemia was frequently asymptomatic and of long duration (3–9 h in 30% of the cases), a finding confirmed in a smaller group of children studied at home *(17)*. Unawareness of hypoglycemia also does exist in children and is associated with a higher rate of severe hypoglycemia in younger than in older children *(18)*. Finally, all studies identified an alarming prevalence of unpredictable asymptomatic nocturnal hypoglycemia in young children, even under conventional insulin therapy.

Causes of Glycemic Control Instability/Hypoglycemia

Although factors related to the unpredictability of behaviors in the young child are of importance for their glycemic instability (*see* the subsection Specific Difficulties of Management) the reasons for the greater vulnerability of the young child to more severe and more frequent episodes of nocturnal hypoglycemia remain to be defined

(19). However, tolerance to fasting has been demonstrated to be lower in normal young children than in older ones *(20)*. Furthermore, few studies have been performed in diabetic children to explore their counterregulation during hypoglycemia. Those studies have shown contradictory results resulting from different methods *(21–23)*. Recently, a study *(24)* has been designed in order to understand reasons why nocturnal hypoglycemia is frequent, profound, prolonged, and asymptomatic in diabetic children *(14,15,17)* even in patients with a good awareness of hypoglycemia during waking hours. This study showed that although those nocturnal hypoglycemic episodes may be precipitated by overinsulinization during the early part of the night, their prolonged nature may result from defective nocturnal counterregulation. The authors concluded that these data provide strong evidence that intensification of insulin therapy may be especially hazardous in this age group.

Figure 2A shows the instability of blood glucose control in a 4-yr-old diabetic child and Table 1 summarizes the multiple factors potentially related to the instability of glycemic control and frequency of hypoglycemia in young children with type 1 diabetes.

NEUROPSYCHOLOGICAL CONSEQUENCES OF HYPOGLYCEMIA

In young children, severe and recurrent hypoglycemias are of major concern because they may impair normal brain development. When tested during adolescence, patients who presented with early-onset diabetes and/or a history of severe hypoglycemia showed global or selective neuropsychological dysfunction such as impairment of visual–spatial skills, psychomotor efficiency, attention, or memory *(28–32)*. As early as 2 yr after disease onset, evidence exists for mild neuropsychological dysfunction *(33)*. Onset of diabetes early in life (before 5 yr of age) predicted negative changes in neuropsychological performances over the first 2 yr of the disease *(34)*. Recent data suggest that school-aged children treated with intensive therapy had a threefold increase in the rate of severe hypoglycemia than conventionally treated children and may have an increased risk for memory problems *(35)*. Thus, until we know more about long-term outcome, neuropsychological impairments subsequent to severe hypoglycemia episodes must be taken into account when formulating specific objectives of metabolic control and therapeutic strategies for young children.

Specific Difficulties of Management

IDENTIFICATION AND TREATMENT OF HYPOGLYCEMIA

Young children are highly dependent on their parents or caregivers. They cannot self-regulate or communicate the need for assistance in case of hypoglycemia. Ross et al. found that the symptoms of hypoglycemia in type 1 diabetic patients vary with age *(36)*. They showed that behavioral symptoms are a valuable index of hypoglycemia in the younger age group and must be included in the initial education of parents and adult caregivers. This problem of recognition and treatment of hypoglycemia is a cause of major stress for parents when their child is not under their own supervision.

DAILY LIFE

Parents of infants and young children report frequent difficulties managing diabetes in their daily life, such as the necessity to wake up their child at a regular time in the morning to inject the insulin dose, the difficulty of respecting a delay between injection of regular insulin and the following meal, and hyperglycemia in the afternoon when the child sleeps after lunch. The major difficulties are caused by day-to-day variations in

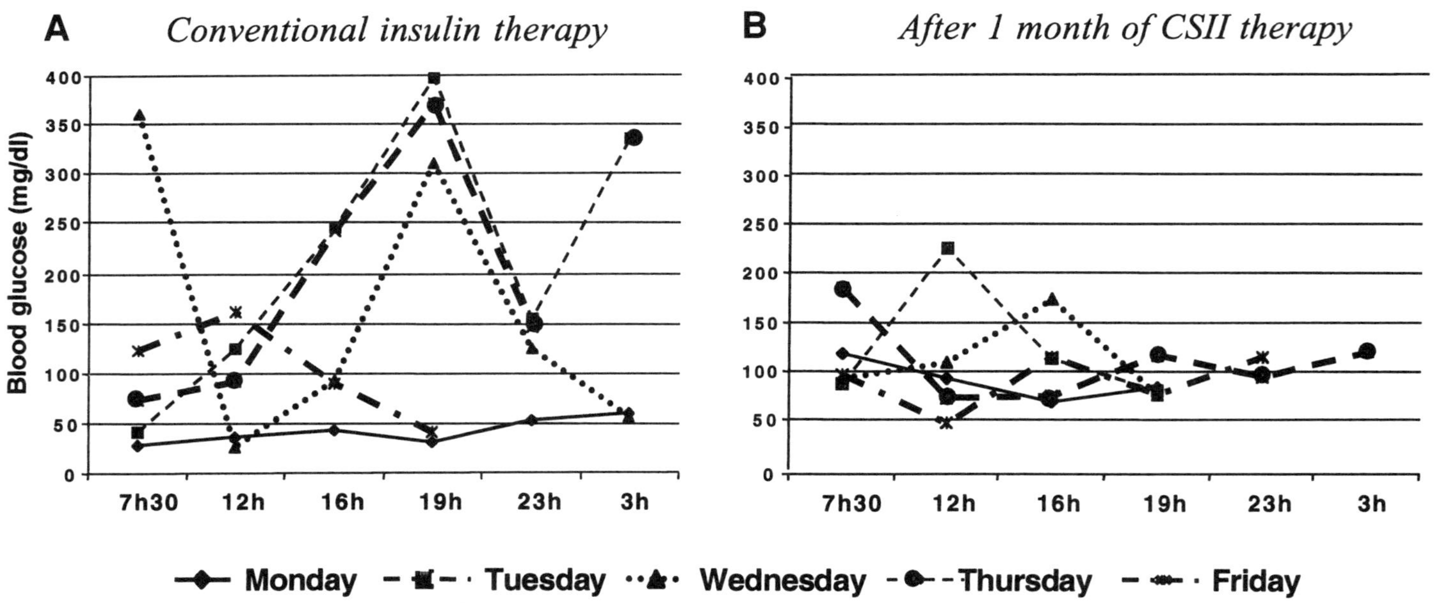

Fig. 2. Home blood glucose monitoring during 5 consecutive days under conventional therapy **(A)** compared to continuous subcutaneous insulin infusion (CSII) therapy **(B)** in a 4-yr-old diabetic boy. This figure illustrates the blood glucose instability observed in young diabetic children and the dramatic effect of CSII treatment on the blood glucose stability.

Table 1
Factors Related to Instability of Diabetes in Young Type 1 Diabetic Children

Metabolic and hormonal factors	
	Low residual insulin secretion *(7,11)*
	Low fasting tolerance in normal young children (defect of gluconeogenesis) *(20)*
	Defective nocturnal counterregulation *(24)*
	Impaired awareness of hypoglycemia *(18)*
Child behaviors	
	Lack of recognition of symptoms of hypoglycemia
	Inability to communicate the symptoms of hypoglycemia
	Unpredictability of meal intake
	Unpredictability of physical activities
Parent behaviors	
	Fear of hypoglycemia *(25)*
	Parents' adherence to diabetes regimen
Insulin therapy	
	Unphysiologic hyperinsulinemia (conventional therapy)
	Inaccuracy of low doses of insulin *(26)*
	Inadequacy of insulin dose changes
	Intramuscular injections *(27)*

Note: References are given in parentheses.

food intake. The lack of appetite or food refusals are particularly stressful for parents of the young diabetic child because they dread the occurrence of severe hypoglycemia. Physical activity is unpredictable and varied among seasons. The impact of physical exercise at this age may be very important for glycemic control. Close supervision by educated adults is needed in order to give appropriate additional snacks.

Acute intercurrent infectious illnesses are common in young children and could cause considerable deterioration in metabolic control. Sick-day management must be under the tight supervision of parents, with the help of a specialized team, in order to prevent both the risk of severe hypoglycemia and the risk of DKA.

Fear of insulin injections is frequent at this age. Some parents of young diabetic children describe true "battles" at each injection that considerably affect the relationship between parents and child. Health care providers must keep in mind that at this age, the child views an injection as an attack against his or her body *(37)*. It should be noted that pain has recently been reduced in children by using ultrashort needles (5 mm), which make the injection easier and less stressful, as reported by the parents *(38)*.

Small Doses of Insulin

The insulin dose changes are limited to a 0.5-U change when using pens. The precision of those changes with insulin syringes is highly questionable. It must, however, be noted that half-unit variations may represent an important percentage for a given dosage in young children. Furthermore, the inaccuracy of small-insulin-dose administration has been demonstrated, which consistently led to an overadministration of insulin *(26)*. To reduce variability in administered insulin, it is recommended that one parent or caretaker delivers the morning dose, and the other the evening dose. It is therefore possible that variations in small-dose delivery in young children contribute to blood glucose variability.

Age-Related Psychosocial Difficulties

Diabetes at this age can considerably affect the family members—parents and siblings—and family functioning. Very little data on psychosocial problems/adjustment in this age group are available in the literature, which focused on school-aged children and adolescents. There is a real need for study cohorts of young children at diagnosis of diabetes. When studying our data in a cohort of 165 children and adolescents, we did not find any relation between the young age at diagnosis and family functioning (Family Adaptability and Cohesion Scales [FACES] III scale) *(39)* or psychological problems (Achenbach scale) *(40)*. However, we have found consequences on socioeconomic condition of the family: The mothers had more frequently left their employment or reduced their work time after the diagnosis of diabetes when children were aged <6 yr at diagnosis compared to older children *(41)*. In this cohort, no difference in the divorce rate by age at diagnosis was observed.

Fear of hypoglycemia is common in parents of diabetic children, especially if they had experienced a seizure or loss of consciousness, and may lead them to maintain elevated blood glucose values to avoid hypoglycemia. This behavior is more frequent in parents of young children than in parents of older children *(25)*.

Long-Term Complications

Because of the long duration of diabetes, young children are at higher risk of developing long-term diabetic complications later in their life. However, a question of importance for this specific age group remains controversial in the literature: Did the years before puberty contribute less to the development of microvascular complications than postpubertal duration of diabetes *(42)*? Donaghue et al. *(43)* indicated that microvascular complications do occur in the prepubertal years, but a subanalysis in children under the age of 5 suggested that diabetes in children under the age of 5 does not contribute to microvascular disease.

TREATMENT OBJECTIVES

Theoretically, the treatment objectives are the same as in older diabetic children. However, achieving those goals, such as good control without an increased risk of severe or frequent hypoglycemia by currently available means, remains a challenge in young children, in whom it has been described as "the Scylla and Charybdis" of glucose control *(19)*. The patient consistently "navigates" between the high risk of severe hypoglycemia and its neurocognitive effects, on one hand, and the risks of short- or long-term hyperglycemia, on the other hand. That is why in children less than 5 yr of age, strict metabolic control is not desirable, if attempting it is associated with frequent documented hypoglycemia. In most of the young children, it seems difficult for the physician to obtain HbA1c values below 8% without an increase risk of hypoglycemia *(16)*. However, in our experience, a more physiological way of insulin treatment such as CSII is both well tolerated by young children and permits achievment of good metabolic control without severe hypoglycemia, when managed under the supervision of a specialized team.

TREATMENT MEANS AND STRATEGY

Management of Ketoacidosis

Young age (<5 yr) is a risk factor for cerebral edema, the major complication of DKA. Management of DKA in young children must be very prudent and take into account all factors that could minimize the risk of this dreadful complication by avoiding hyperhydration (<4 $L/m^2/24$ h) and hyponatremia and by obtaining a slow decrease in blood glucose level and in plasma osmolarity *(44)*.

Insulin Treatment

Conventional Insulin Therapy

In most preschool children, the usual treatment consists of two to three injections per day of mixed short- and intermediate-acting insulins. It must be noted that the superiority of multiple injections has not been demonstrated in children *(13)*. Therefore, treatment should be tailored to the individual child's needs, which must be evaluated by a competent multidisciplinary team *(45)*.

In young children, frequent blood glucose monitoring (BGM) is critical in order to navigate within acceptable targets of glycemic control by minimizing the risk of severe or frequent hypoglycemia. Usually five to six BGMs per day and two urine tests per day for urine glucose and ketone bodies are performed by parents or caregivers. Measurement of blood glucose level at the "parents' bedtime" must be encouraged in order to detect asymptomatic hypoglycemia or to give a snack when BG is below a specified level *(15)*. Nocturnal hypoglycemia should be suspected in children under conventional therapy with frequent fasting BG values below 120 mg/dL *(15)*. It must be noted that systematic carbohydrate intake at supper did not consistently prevent nocturnal hypoglycemia *(14)*.

Needle length has to be carefully considered in young children, as their role in the risk of hypoglycemia has been shown. Alternating intramuscular and subcutaneous injections can occur from one day to another and from one injection site to another, leading to variations in glucose control and increased risk of hypoglycemia. By using ultrasonography to visualize the injection site, we demonstrated that short needles significantly reduce the risk of intramuscular insulin injection in children *(27)*.

Short-Acting Insulin Analogs

Despite progress in the last decade, subcutaneous insulin therapy in children remains unphysiological. The so-called short-acting insulin, when compared with physiological insulin release, is characterized by a late or delayed peak and by too long a duration of action. Recently, the development of short-acting analogs such as lispro (Humalog®, Lilly) has been found to be safe in children and adolescents, to improve their postprandial blood glucose levels and to reduce the risk of nocturnal hypoglycemia *(27,46,47)*. A randomized crossover study comparing Humalog to regular insulin in preschool and school-aged diabetic children under conventional insulin therapy has demonstrated that postprandial administration of insulin lispro can accomplish glucose control comparable to preprandial human regular insulin *(48)*. This therapeutic option is very useful in management of diabetes in young children, allowing the parents to better adjust insulin administration according to their child's food intake (e.g., in sick-day management).

Insulin Pump Therapy

The best way to avoid hypoglycemia is to use insulin replacement regimen that minimizes the unphysiologic hyperinsulinemia, especially during the night. In our experience, the only present therapeutic method of achieving and maintaining good glucose control without frequent or severe hypoglycemia in young children is to use CSII therapy. CSII is a feasible and well-tolerated method of insulin therapy in young children *(49,50)*. In a previous study *(50)*, we have compared conventional insulin therapy to CSII in two groups of diabetic children aged below 6 yr (respectively $n = 17$, age = 5.1 yr vs $n = 10$,

Table 2
Comparison of the Frequency of Severe Hypoglycemia in Diabetic Children Aged Less than 6 Years Treated by Conventional and Continuous Subcutaneous Insulin Infusion (CSII) Therapy

		CSII therapy	
	Before CSII	*During CSII*	*Conventional insulin therapy*
No. of children	6	10	17
No. of severe episodes of hypoglycemia (SH)	11*	0	10*
No. of children with SH	3	0	6*

$* p < 0.05$.
Source: ref. *50*.

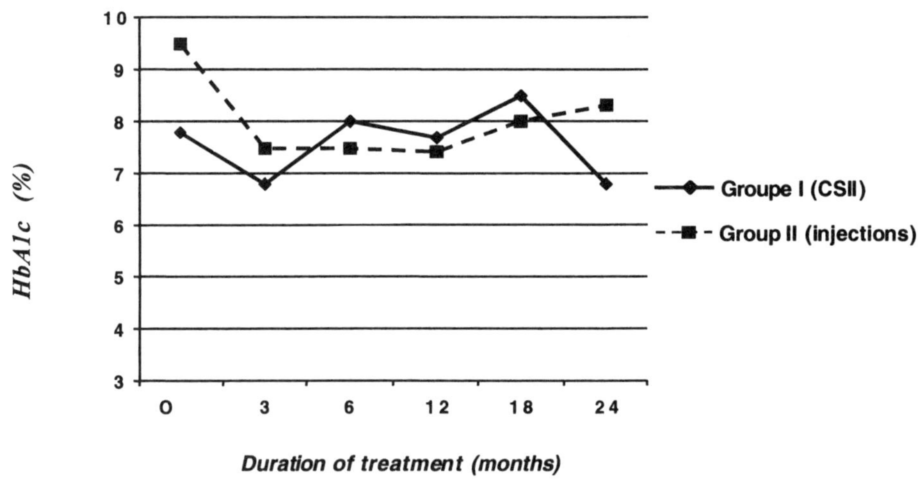

Fig. 3. Comparison of mean HbA1c levels in two groups of young diabetic children treated with conventional therapy (•, n=17) and with CSII (◆, n = 10) during a 24-mo follow-up. (From ref. *50*.)

age = 3.7 yr) during a mean treatment period of 2 yr. Mean insulin doses and HbA1c levels measured at 3, 6, 12, 18, and 24 mo did not differ significantly between the two groups. The most impressive results were related to the frequency of severe hypoglycemia in those very young diabetic children (*see* Table 2). In the group treated with twice-daily injections, the number of severe hypoglycemia episodes was 10, compared to none in the group under pump therapy. It must be noted that this result was obtained without an increase of HbA1c levels, which remained at 8% (*see* Fig. 3). The disappearance of severe hypoglycemia was shown when examining the subgroup of children who were treated first by conventional therapy (11 episodes) and thereafter by CSII (0 episodes) (*see* Table 2). Parents of children treated with the pump were very satisfied (9/10) mainly because of a more flexible lifestyle for their children and themselves and because of a major reduction of their anxiety (disappearance of severe hypoglycemia). Advantages of pump therapy in young children are summarized in Table 3 and shown in Fig. 2B.

Limits of pump therapy are well known. The risk of DKA as a result of obstruction of catheters must be prevented by specific education of the parents; skin tolerance has

Table 3
Advantages of Insulin Pump Therapy in Young Children by Comparison with Conventional Therapy

More physiological regimen
Adjustment of each premeal insulin dose (boluses)
Nocturnal basal rate
More accurate
Accuracy of low doses
Adequacy of insulin dose changes (e.g., 0.1 U or 0.2 U)
More comfortable
Children: injection every 3 d vs twice a day
Parents: less anxiety (reduction of hypoglycemia)
Children and parents: flexibility of the treatment (timing of meals, sleeping)
Easier management
Common infectious illnesses
Episodes of hyperglycemia with ketonuria
Food refusals

considerably improved by using Teflon catheters, which are also very convenient, allowing the disconnection for bath or swimming. Education of parents and supervision by a specialized pediatric diabetes team are the keys of the success of this treatment. Under these conditions, CSII can be recommended in young diabetic children in case of failure of a well-conducted trial of conventional insulin therapy (severe hypoglycemia despite intensification of education and use of lispro analogs). Recently, the use of lispro analogs in pump therapy has brought further progress in terms of comfort in daily life and metabolic effects in adults, as well as in young children *(51,52)*.

Diet

The diet recommendations for diabetic children aim at ensuring normal growth and optimal nutrition, achieving good glycemic control by coordination among insulin treatment, diet, and exercise, reducing risk factors for long-term complications and preserving the psychosocial dimension of meals. Little is know about dietary intake of young diabetic children. The recommendations for dietary intake in children with IDDM were well met in two groups of around 30 young diabetic children aged less than 6 yr at diagnosis *(53,54)*. However, protein intake was slightly higher than recommended in the Finish study, as well as in our inquiry in France (unpublished data). The recommended diet for diabetic child would also be beneficial for other members of the family. Similar food choices among family members would help the child with diabetes to adopt long-term good nutritional habits.

Education and Psychosocial Support

As glycemic control is very unstable in young children, expertise in insulin management is required from their parents. In young children, predictions of the insulin doses are challenging. Certain factors influencing the variability of blood glucose control are unpredictable, such as meal size or change in physical activities, whereas other factors can be managed, such as injection technique and time of injection. A specialized multidisciplinary pediatric diabetes team including a pediatric diabetologist, dietician, nurse educator, psychologist, and social worker is needed to give adequate and continuing counseling and education to parents and caregivers of young children. Frequent contacts between the family and the pediatric team is a key to achieve good metabolic control without acute complications. A 24-h telephone hotline will help to minimize acute metabolic complications or hospitalizations. It must be noted that the expertise in the management of young diabetic children requires a sufficient number of patients in order to give age-group-adapted education and support for parents and children. Education must continue throughout childhood and adolescence, with guidance adapted to cognitive and psycho-affective levels of the family members. This enables a gradual transfer of some responsibilities of care to the child. Adapted education may also be given to the young children by using appropriate pedagogic tools. Our team contributed to the development and multicenter evaluation of an educational game specifically dedicated to the recognition and communication of symptoms of hypoglycemia in preschool diabetic children (Hypopuzzle®).

Group discussions among parents of preschool children facilitate concrete solutions of individual specific daily difficulties and provide psychological support. Parents are encouraged to join regional Diabetic Patients Association.

FUTURE PERSPECTIVES FOR YOUNG CHILDREN WITH TYPE 1 DIABETES

Frequent daily BGM is necessary in young children because hypoglycemic episodes, especially nocturnal ones, are asymptomatic and difficult to detect, predict, and prevent. Nocturnal glucose sensors detecting hypoglycemia with an alarm are urgently needed for young diabetic children. These techniques seem to be close to becoming clinically applicable. The ultimate resolution of the difficult problems in managing diabetes in a preschool child will require closed-loop devices or cure via islet transplantation in the future.

CONCLUSION

The incidence of IDDM in children is increasing and this increase is particularly evident in very young children. This is of major concern for health professionals because treatment at this age is difficult. More than in any other age group, appropriate management requires the resources and utilization of a multidisciplinary diabetes team. Whether modern technology will help these children in the future remains to be determined and evaluated. Although there is concern about the risk of long-term vascular complications from hyperglycemia, hypoglycemia is also a major concern, as is the psychological vulnerability of the young child. All of these factors should be carefully considered in formulating a treatment protocol and therapeutic targets.

REFERENCES

1. Lévy-Marchal C, Patterson C, Green A, et al. Variation by age group and seasonality at diagnosis of childhood IDDM in Europe. Diabetologia 1995;38:823–830.
2. Diabetes Epidemiology Research International Group. Secular trends in incidence of childhood IDDM in 10 countries. Diabetes 1990;39:858–864.
3. Bingley PJ, Gale EAM. Rising incidence of IDDM in Europe. Diabetes Care 1989;12:289–295.
4. Metcalfe MA, Baum JD. Incidence of insulin-dependent diabetes in children under 15 years in the British Isles during 1988. Br Med J 1991;302:443–447.

5. Gardner SG, Bingley PJ, Sawtell PA, et al. Rising incidence of insulin dependent diabetes in children aged under 5 years in the Oxford region: time trend analysis. Br Med J 1997;315:713–717.
6. EURODIAB ACE Study Group. Variation and trends in incidence of childhood diabetes in Europe. Lancet 2000;355:873–876.
7. Komulainen J, Kulmala P, Savola K, et al. Clinical, autoimmune, and genetic characteristics of very young children with type 1 diabetes. Diabetes Care 1999;22:1950–1955.
8. Levy-Marchal C, Papoz L, de Beaufort C, Doutreix J, Froment V, Voirin J, et al. Clinical and laboratory findings of type 1 diabetic children at the time of diagnosis. Diabet Med 1992;9:279–284.
9. Tubiana-Rufi N, Habita C, Czernichow P. Etude critique de l'acidocétose diabétique de l'enfant. Description initiale et évolution au cours des 24 premières heures. Arch Fr Pediatr 1992;49:175–180.
10. Karjaleinen J, Salmela P, Ilonen J, Surcel HM, Knip M. A comparison of childhood and adult type 1 diabetes mellitus. N Engl J Med 1989;320:881–886.
11. Forsander G, Persson B, Sundelin J, Berglund E, Snellman K, Hellström R. Metabolic control in children with insulin-dpendent diabetes mellitus 5 y after diagnosis. Early detection of patients at risk for poor metabolic control. Acta Paediatr 1998;87:857–864.
12. Wallensteen M, Dahlquist G, Persson B, Landin-Olssonn M, Lernmark A, Sundkvist G, et al. Factors influencing the magnitude, duration and rate of B-cell function in type 1 (insulin-dependent) diabetic children followed for two years from their clinical diagnosis. Diabetologia 1988;31:664–669.
13. Mortensen HB, Hougaard P, for the Hvidore Study Group on Childhood Diabetes. Comparison of metabolic control in a cross-sectional study of 2873 children and adolescents with IDDM from 18 countries. Diabetes Care 1997;20:714–720.
14. Porter PA, Keating B, Byrne G, Jones TW. Incidence and predictive criteria of nocturnal hypoglycemia in young children with insulin-dependent diabetes mellitus. J Pediatr 1997;131:2–4.
15. Beregszaszi M, Tubiana-Rufi N, Benali K, Noel M, Bloch J, Czernichow P. Nocturnal hypoglycemia in children and adolescents with insulin-dependent diabetes mellitus: prevalence and risk factors. J Pediatr 1997;131:27–33.
16. Santiago J. Nocturnal hypoglycemia in children with diabetes: an important problem revisited. J Pediatr 1997;131:2–4.
17. Matyka KA, Wigg L, Pramming S, Stores G, Dunger DB. Cognitive function and mood after profound nocturnal hypoglycemia in prepubertal children with conventional insulin treatment for diabetes. Arch Dis Child 1999;81:138–142.
18. Barkai L, Vamosi I, Lukacs K. Prospective assessment of severe hypoglycemia in diabetic children and adolescents with impaired and normal awareness of hypoglycemia. Diabetologia 1998;41:898–903.
19. Sperling MA. The Scylla and Charybdis of blood glucose control in children with diabetes mellitus. J Pediatr 1997;130:339–341.
20. Chaussain J-L, Geaorges P, Calzada L, Job J-C. Glycemic response to 24-hour fast in normal children: III. Influence of age. J Pediatr 1977;91:711–714.
21. Brambilla P, Bougneres PF, Santiago JV, Chaussain JL, Pouplard A, Castano L. Glucose counterregulation in pre-school-age diabetic children with recurrent hypoglycemia during conventional treatment. Diabetes 1987;36:300–304
22. Amiel SA, Simonson DC, Sherwin RS, Lauritano AA, Tamborlane WV. Exaggerated epinephrine responses to hypoglycemia in normal and insulin-dependent diabetic children. J Pediatr 1987;110:32–37.
23. Hoffman RP, Singer-Granik C, Drash AL, Becker DJ. Plasma catecholamines responses to hypoglycemia in children and adolescents with IDDM. Diabetes Care 1991;2:1–8.
24. Matyka K, Crowne EC, Havel PJ, Macdonald IA, Matthews DM, Dunger DB. Counterregulation during spontaneous nocturnal hypoglycemia in prepubertal children with type 1 diabetes. Diabetes Care 1999;22:1144–1150.
25. Marrero DG, Guare JC, Vandagriff JL, Fineberg NS. Fear of hypoglycemia in the parents of children and adolescents with diabetes: maladaptive or healthy response. Diabetes Educ 1997;23:281–286.
26. Silva SR, Clark L, Goodman SN, Plotnick LP. Can caretakers of children with IDDM accurately measure small insulin doses and dose changes? Diabetes Care 1996;19:56–59.
27. Tubiana-Rufi N, Belarbi N, Du Pasquier-Fediaevsky L, Polak M, Kakou B, Leridon L, et al. Short needles (8 mm) reduce the risk of intramuscular injections in children with type 1 diabetes. Diabetes Care 1999;22:1621–1625.
28. Ryan C, Vega A, Drash A. Cognitive deficits in adolescents who developed diabetes early in life. Pediatrics 1985;75:921–927.
29. Rovet JF, Ehrlich RM, Hoppe M. Intellectual deficits associated with early onset of insulin-dependent diabetes mellitus in children. Diabetes Care 1987;10:510–515.

30. Golden MP, Ingersoll GM, Brack CJ, Russel BA, Wright JC, Huberty TJ. Longitudinal relationship of asymptomatic hypoglycemia to cognitive function in IDDM. Diabetes Care 1989;12:89–93.
31. Rovet J, Alvarez M. Attentional functioning in children and adolescents with IDDM. Diabetes Care 1997;20:803–810.
32. Bjorgaas M, Gimse R, Vik T, Sand T. Cognitive function in type 1 diabetic children with and without episodes of severe hypoglycemia. Acta Paediatr 1997;86:148–153.
33. Northam EA, Anderson PJ, Werther GA, Warne GL, Adler RG, Andrewes D. Neuropsychological complications of IDDM in children 2 years after disease onset. Diabetes Care 1998;21:379–384.
34. Northam EA, Anderson PJ, Werther GA, Warne GL, Andrewes D. Predictors of change in the neuropsychological profiles of children with type 1 diabetes 2 years after disease onset. Diabetes Care 1999;22:1438–1444.
35. Hershey T, Bhargava N, Sadler M, White NH, Craft S. Conventional versus intensive diabetes therapy in children with type 1 diabetes. Effects on memory and motor speed. Diabetes Care 1999;22:1318–1324.
36. Ross LA, McCrimmon RJ, Frier BM, Kelnar CJH, Deary IJ. Hypoglycaemic symptoms reported by children with type 1 diabetes mellitus and by their parents. Diabet Med 1998;15:836–843.
37. Kassiou K, Tsamasiros J. Family management of insulin-dependent diabetes mellitus: a practical problem-solving approach. Acta Paediatr 1999;427:47–51.
38. Tubiana-Rufi N. Role of short needles in pediatrics. In Report of the Second Injection Technique Event (SITE), May 2000, Barcelona, Spain. Pract Diabetes Int 2002;19:17–22.
39. Tubiana-Rufi N, Moret L, Czernichow P, Chwalow J, and the PEDIAB Collaborative Group. The associations of poor adherence and acute metabolic disorders with low levels of cohesion and adaptability in families with diabetic children. Acta Paediatr 1998;87:741–746.
40. Castro D, Tubiana-Rufi N, Moret L, Fombonne E, and the PEDIAB Collaborative Group. Psychological adjustment in a French cohort of type 1 diabetic children. Diabetes Metab 2000;26:29–34.
41. Tubiana-Rufi N, Moret L, Chwalow J, Czernichow P, et le Groupe Collaboratif PEDIAB. Description de l'état de santé et des facteurs liés au contrôle glycémique chez 165 enfants atteints de diabète insulinodépendant, âgés de 7 à 13 ans. Arch Ped 1994;1:982–990.
42. Kostraba JN, Dorman JS, Orchard TJ, Becker DJ, Ohki Y, Ellis D, et al. Contribution of diabetes duration before puberty to development of microvascular complications in IDDM subjects. Diabetes Care 1989;12:686–693.
43. Donaghue KC, Fung ATW, Hing S, Fairchild J, King J, Chan A, et al. The effect of prepubertal diabetes duration on diabetes. Microvascular complications in early and late adolescence. Diabetes Care 1997;20:77–80.
44. Duck SC, Wyatt DT. Factors associated with brain herniation in the treatment of diabetic ketoacidosis. J Pediatr 1988;113:10–14.
45. Becker D. Individualized insulin therapy in children and adolescents with type 1 diabetes. Acta Paediatr 1998;425(Suppl):20–24.
46. Holcombe J, Zalani S, Arora V, Headlee S, Gill A. Comparative study of insulin lispro and regular insulin in 481 adolescents with type 1 diabetes. Diabetes 1997;46(Suppl 1):A1253.
47. Holcombe J, Zalani S, Arora V, Headlee S, Gill A. Insulin lispro (LP) results in less nocturnal hypoglycemia compared with regular human insulin in adolescents with type 1 diabetes. Diabetes 1997;46(Suppl 1):A402.
48. Holcombe J, Brunelle R, Zalani S, Deeb LC. Comparative study of insulin lispro and regular insulin in prepubertal children with type 1 diabetes. Diabetes 1998;47(Suppl 1):A96.
49. Joseph MG, Ginies JL, Chomienne F, Limal JM. Traitement du diabète insulinodépendant par pompe à insuline chez l'enfant d'âge inférieur à 7 ans. Arch Pédiatr 1992;49:505–510.
50. Tubiana-Rufi N, de Lonlay P, Bloch J, Czernichow P. Disappearance of severe hypoglycemia in infants and young children with continuous subcutaneous insulin infusion therapy. Arch Pediatr 1996;3:969–976.
51. Melki V, Renard E, Lassmann-Vague V, et al. Improvement of HbA1c and blood glucose stability in IDDM patients treated with lispro insulin analog in external pumps. Diabetes Care 1999;21:977–982.
52. Tubiana-Rufi N, Coutant R, Bloch J, Munz-Licha G, Delcroix C, Limal JM, et al. Efficacy and tolerability of insulin lispro in young diabetic children treated with CSII. Diabetologia 2000;43(Suppl 1):A199 (762).
53. Randecker GA, Smiciklas-Wright H, MCKenzie JM, Shannon BM, Mitchell DC, Becker DJ, et al. The dietary intake of children with IDDM. Diabetes Care 1996;19:1370–1374.
54. Virtanen SM, Ylönen K, Räsänen L, Ala-Venna E, Mäenpää J, Äkerblom HK. Two year prospective dietary survey of newly diagnosed children with diabetes aged less than 6 years. Arch Dis Child 2000;82:21–26.

16 The Preadolescent Child with Type 1 Diabetes

William V. Tamborlane, MD,
Elizabeth A. Boland, MSN, APRN, PNP, CDE,
and Margaret Grey, DRPH, FAAN, CDE

CONTENTS

INTRODUCTION

Results of the Diabetes Control and Complications Trial (DCCT) indicate that most patients with type 1 diabetes should receive intensive treatments aimed at lowering glucose and glycosylated hemoglobin levels as close to normal as possible and as soon as possible in order to prevent and delay the development of microvascular complications of the disease *(1–3).* Among the pediatric age groups, the preadolescent child with type 1 diabetes is an ideal candidate for such therapy. Compared to infants and toddlers, preadolescents eat more predictably, can recognize and report hypoglycemic symptoms, are less vulnerable to the potential adverse effects of hypoglycemia on cognitive development *(4),* and can actively participate in their own treatment. Compared to adolescents, preadolescents are much more insulin sensitive *(5),* are less conflicted by dependence/independence struggles, and, consequently, are more responsive to parental guidance of treatment. Moreover, maladaptive adolescent behaviors around

From: *Contemporary Endocrinology: Type 1 Diabetes: Etiology and Treatment*
Edited by: M. A. Sperling © Humana Press Inc., Totowa, NJ

drugs, alcohol, and sexual activity have not yet emerged as important lifestyle issues in most preadolescents.

GOALS OF TREATMENT

The traditional goals of the treatment of preadolescent children with diabetes were to use insulin, diet, and exercise to minimize symptoms of hypoglycemia and hyperglycemia and promote normal growth and development and to use intensive education and psychosocial support to maximize independence and self-management in order to reduce the adverse psychosocial effects of this chronic disease *(6)*. Since the results of the DCCT were published, additional primary aims of therapy are to lower blood glucose and glycosylated hemoglobin values to as close to normal as possible. In preadolescents, achievement of such stringent treatment goals is best accomplished with a multidisciplinary team of clinicians to provide ongoing education and support of aggressive self-management efforts on the part of parents and patients. Matching the treatment to the patient (rather than vice versa) by taking a flexible and varied approach to insulin replacement, diet and exercise are critically important.

It is recognized that intensive treatment places extra burdens on patients and families and that practical considerations such as acceptability of and compliance to the treatment regimens must be balanced appropriately in order to obtain all of these aims of therapy. Nevertheless, recent data suggest that an intensive approach to diabetes education and aggressive self-management by patients and families may reduce rather than increase the adverse psychosocial effects of this chronic illness *(7)*.

INSULIN REPLACEMENT

Initiation of insulin treatment can be accomplished either in the inpatient or outpatient setting. Many youngsters require hospital admission because of vomiting, dehydration and/or moderate to severe ketoacidosis. In preteens who are not ill at presentation, admission to the hospital may also provide the child and parent with a safe and supportive environment in which to adjust to the shock of the diagnosis. Outpatient management in a comprehensive day treatment program staffed by individuals knowledgeable in the care of children with diabetes can also provide a supportive environment to initiate therapy *(8)* and such programs are becoming more widely available.

Once so simple, the choice of types of insulin and insulin regiments has become much more complicated. To the standard human regular, neutral protamine Hagedorn (NPH), lente, and ultralente insulins have been added new insulin analogs. Lispro and aspart insulin are produced by amino acid substitutions near the C-terminal end of the β-chain. These substitutions do not affect the biologic actions of insulin but result in more rapid absorption than regular insulin following subcutaneous injection. The sharper peak and shorter duration of these insulins vs regular insulin may be of particular advantage in teenagers who require large premeal bolus doses of rapid-action insulin. Glargine is the first soluble long-acting insulin. Soluble in the acid pH in which it is packaged, this insulin precipitates in the neutral pH of the extracellular fluid of the subcutaneous tissue. There are fixed mixtures of both human insulin and human insulin analogs, and inhaled insulin preparations are currently under study *(9)*. A sampling of

Table 1
Conventional and Unconventional Insulin Regimens

Doses	*Breakfast*	*Lunch/afternoon snack*	*Dinner*	*Bedtime*
Two	R + I		R + I	
	R + I + L		R + I + L	
	I + L		I + L	
Three	R + I ± L		R	I + R
	R + I	R	R + I ± L	
Four	R	R	R	I ± R

Note: R, rapid acting (regular, lispro, aspart) insulin; I, intermediate acting (NPH, lente) insulin; L, long-acting (ultralente, glargine).

the variety of conventional and unconventional insulin regimens that can be employed is given in Table 1.

Although many clinicians start insulin treatment with three or more daily injections, we begin most newly diagnosed preadolescent children on two injections of insulin per day using mixtures of human lente and lispro insulins. Each dose is given as two-thirds lente and one-third lispro insulin. The rationale for using two rather than three or more injections at onset of diabetes is that with aggressive control of blood levels, most children enter a "honeymoon" or partial remission period after a few weeks of therapy. This remission period is a result of increased insulin secretion by residual β-cells and improved insulin sensitivity with normalization of blood glucose levels *(10)*. To achieve these effects, we start each patient on a total daily dose of at least 1 U/kg body weight per day. Even more important, each component of the insulin regimen is adjusted on the basis of fingerstick blood glucose levels measured at least four times a day. The goal is to obtain premeal blood glucose values within the normal range and this is achieved via daily telephone contacts with the family for at least the first 3 wk of treatment. The DCCT data indicate that strict control of diabetes also serves to prolong the period of residual β-cell function in patients with type 1 diabetes *(11)*.

During the "honeymoon," insulin requirements rapidly decrease. Commonly, the doses of rapid-acting insulin are sharply reduced or discontinued during this time; many children are well managed with two injections of intermediate-acting insulin and some may not even require an evening injection. In the absence of symptomatic hypoglycemia, however, we try not to lower the total daily dose of insulin below 0.20–0.25 U/kg body weight per day, as these are doses currently being safely employed even in prediabetic children in the Diabetes Prevention Trial-1 (DPT-1) study *(12)*.

A major reason why the two daily injections regimen is effective during the honeymoon phase is that endogenous insulin secretion provides much of the overnight basal insulin requirements, leading to normal fasting blood glucose values. Thus, increased and more labile prebreakfast glucose levels often herald the loss of the relatively small amount of residual endogenous insulin secretion that is required for overnight glucose control. When residual β-cell function wanes, problems with the two-injection regimen become apparent. One problem is that the peak of the predinner intermediate-acting insulin may coincide with the time of minimal insulin requirements (i.e., midnight to 4 AM). Subsequently, insulin levels fall off when basal requirements are increasing (i.e., 4 AM to 8 AM). Increasing the presupper dose of intermediate-acting insulin to lower fasting glucose values often leads to hypoglycemia in the middle of the night without correcting hyperglycemia before breakfast. Patients are especially vulnerable to hypoglycemia in the middle of the night because the normal plasma epinephrine response to low blood glucose levels is markedly blunted during deep sleep *(13)*. Another problem with the conventional two-injection regimen is high presupper glucose levels, despite normal or low prelunch and mid-afternoon values. This is, in part, the result of eating an afternoon snack when the effects of the prebreakfast dose of intermediate acting insulin are waning.

One way to deal with these problems without increasing the number of injections is to add ultralente insulin to the prebreakfast and presupper mixtures of lispro and lente. With this combination in the morning, lispro covers breakfast, lente covers lunch, and ultralente covers the late afternoon period. With the presupper dose, lispro covers supper, lente covers the bedtime snack and part of the overnight period, and ultralente helps limit the prebreakfast rise in plasma glucose. However, when strict control cannot be achieved with two daily injections, we do not hesitate to switch to a regimen involving three or more daily injections. A common approach to the problem in the overnight period is to use a three-injection regimen; lispro and lente at breakfast, lispro only at dinner, and lente at bedtime. In youngsters who go to bed early, we recommend that the parents give the third shot at their bedtime (i.e., 10:00 PM to 11:00 PM). Lispro can also be added to the bedtime dose, especially if glucose levels are elevated. For patients with elevated presupper glucose levels, a prelunch dose of regular or a preafternoon snack dose of lispro can be added. Such extra doses of insulin can be facilitated by the use of insulin pens, which are small, light, and easy to use. Only a small number of our preadolescent patients are using a regimen of four or more injections of rapid-acting insulin before meals and intermediate insulin at bedtime.

Over the past few years, there has been a rediscovery of the effectiveness of insulin pump therapy in the management of young patients with diabetes *(14)*. Indeed, we are much more likely to turn to this method of insulin replacement rather than more frequent injections in preadolescents who are coming out of their honeymoon phase of diabetes. As illustrated in Fig. 1, the ability to achieve strict diabetes control with pump therapy in preadolescents with diabetes is quite remarkable.

With insulin pump treatment, small amounts of rapid-acting insulin are infused as a basal rate and larger bolus doses are given at each meal or snack. Although it is not yet labeled by the Food and Drug Administration (FDA) for use in pumps, lispro insulin appears to have advantages over regular insulin in pump therapy *(15)*. The pumps are battery powered and about the size of a beeper. The "basal" rate can be programmed to change each hour of the day, but it is unusual to need more than five or six basal rates. Varying the basal rate can be particularly helpful in regulating overnight blood glucose levels, as it can be lowered for the early part of the night to prevent hypoglycemia and increased in the hours before dawn to keep glucose from rising. However, younger children seem to need a higher basal rate during the night, perhaps because of earlier nocturnal peaks of growth hormone in this age group.

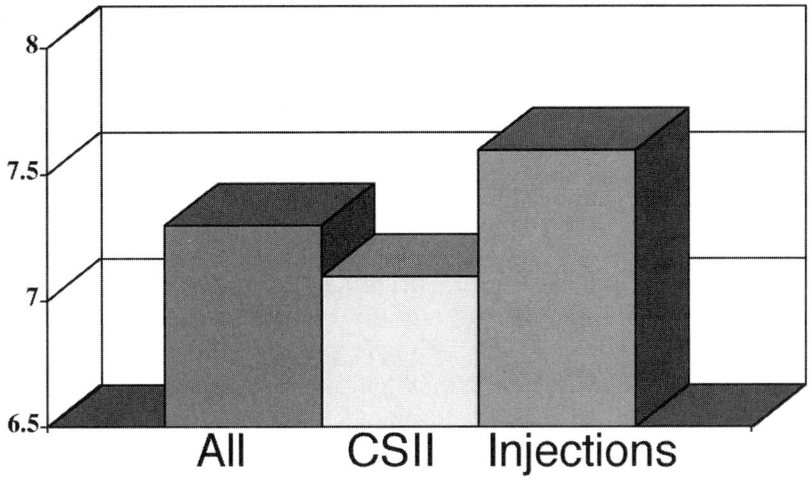

Fig. 1. Most recent mean HbA1c levels through 11/1/2002 in children 6–12 yr of age enrolled in the Yale Children's Diabetes Clinic. CSII, continuous subcutaneous insulin infusion.

Bolus doses are given before meals based on glucose level, exercise, and food intake. Pump treatment can be especially useful in youngsters who are picky eaters. In this setting, part of the usual premeal bolus can be given prior to the meal and the rest given at the end of the meal, depending on the actual amount of carbohydrate intake. Indeed, most children and parents are encouraged to use carbohydrate counting (*see* the Diet section) as a means to adjust premeal bolus doses. Pump therapy also enhances flexibility in children with variable exercise and meal routines.

The pump employs a reservoir (syringe) to hold the insulin and the infusion set, which consists of tubing with a small plastic catheter at the end. The insertion site can be the abdomen or hip area, except in the young child in whom there may not be sufficient subcutaneous tissue in the abdomen. Our patients are encouraged to change their catheters every other day. Because only a rapid-acting insulin is used in this pump, the child and parent must understand that the insulin infusion should not be discontinued for more than 4 h at a time.

Although there have been many failed attempts at finding alternatives to insulin injections *(16),* use of aerosolized preparations for inhaled insulin delivery is currently under active investigation. Preliminary studies in adults have been promising enough *(9)* that phase III studies are already underway in preadolescents as well as adolescents with type 1 diabetes. As with pump therapy, inhaled insulin allows the patients to take premeal boluses of insulin with each meal and snack without having to take extra insulin injections. However, one or more injections of intermediate or long-acting insulin are still needed for basal insulin replacement.

MONITORING GLUCOSE CONTROL

Insulin replacement in children is a special challenge because insulin requirements increase as weight and calorie intake increase and as residual endogenous secretion declines. Regular self-monitoring of blood glucose (SMBG) allows the family and clinicians to keep up with the child's steadily increasing insulin needs. We request that blood glucose levels be checked at least four times per day (before each meal and at bedtime) and most families with children in the preadolescent age group comply with this request. The most important component of SMBG is the interpretation of the results. The parent or child must be taught what the target value is and what the relationship is among diet, exercise, and insulin. If the parent and/or child grasp these concepts, they will make accurate adjustments aimed at achieving target goals. If they are unable to make accurate adjustments, they should be given guidelines of when to call the diabetes service for help. Day-to-day adjustments in the doses of rapid-acting insulin can be made based on the premeal blood glucose value, amount of carbohydrate in the meal, and the amount of anticipated exercise. In addition, patients and parents should be taught to look for repetitive patterns of hypoglycemia or hyperglycemia, in order to make ongoing changes in their usual insulin doses. To facilitate identification of trends, families are encouraged to maintain either a handwritten or computer-generated record of each glucose value in a spreadsheet format.

Self-monitoring of blood glucose is subject to a variety of problems, especially making up false numbers *(17)*. These issues must be addressed with the child and family. They must understand the reason for the tests and that they are only used to make proper adjustments to keep them healthy. Elevated glucose levels are not an indication of worsening of diabetes or that they have been cheating on their diet. Instead, we emphasize that the tests are being done primarily to determine when they have outgrown their current dose of insulin.

Even when performed correctly, four blood tests daily give only a limited glimpse of wide fluctuations in blood glucose that occur during a 24-h period in children with diabetes. Consequently, the recent introduction of continuous glucose monitoring systems has the potential to be the most important advance in assessing diabetes control in the past 20 yr. In intensively treated children and adolescents with type 1 diabetes, preliminary results in a relatively small number of children suggest that continuous glucose monitoring will provide a wealth of data regarding postprandial glycemic excursions and asymptomatic nocturnal hypoglycemia that were unavailable from capillary blood glucose measurements *(18)*. The wealth of data generated by the continuous glucose monitoring system is illustrated in Fig. 2. We anticipate that these technological breakthroughs will have a great impact on diabetes management over the next few years. Continuous monitoring of nocturnal glucose levels is likely to be particularly useful in programming overnight basal rates in pump-treated patients.

GLYCOSYLATED HEMOGLOBIN

A variety of methods are available for assaying glycosylated hemoglobin. The most widely accepted is the HbA1c method. A simple method that can be performed in the office in 6 min (Bayer DCA 2000) offers the opportunity to make immediate changes in the insulin regimen while the patient is being seen. The goal of treatment is to achieve HbA1c levels as close to normal as possible. Based on DCCT results *(2)*, our general goal of therapy is to try to keep all patients under 8.0%. HbA1c levels are determined at least every 3 mo.

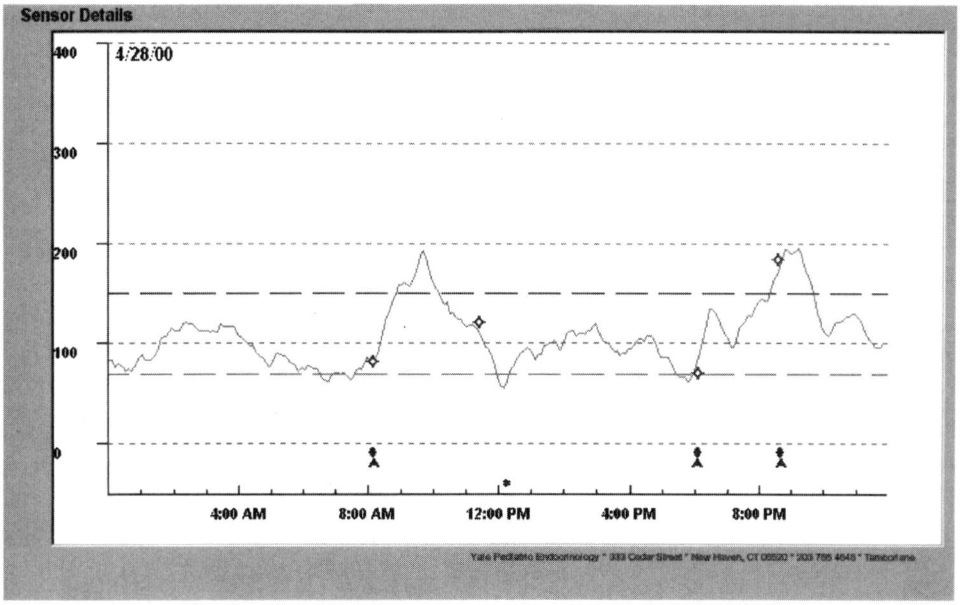

Fig. 2. The 24-h MiniMed Continuous Glucose Monitoring System results in an 11-yr-old with type 1 diabetes on insulin pump therapy who wore the sensor for 3 d on 3 successive months. Trackings demonstrate excellent glycemic control without hypoglycemia and is consistent with her HbA1c level of 5.8% (normal < 6.3%). Event markers are entered into the monitor by the patient to indicate time of insulin dose (▼), meal (•), hypoglycemic symptoms (*), and fingerstick blood glucose level (◇). A small adjustment was made in the premeal insulin-to-carbohydrate ratio based on these readings.

DIET

Diet guidance for children with diabetes is best provided by a nutritionist who is an integral part of the treatment team and comfortable working with children. In addition to helping achieve optimal glucose levels and normal growth and development, nutritional management of diabetes is aimed at reducing the risk for other diseases such as obesity, high blood cholesterol, or high blood pressure. Underlying all of these is the establishment of sound eating patterns that include balanced, nutritious foods and consistent timing of food intake *(19)*.

The American Diabetes Association dietary guidelines are used for dietary counseling. In addition to incorporating sound nutritional principles concerning the fat, fiber, and carbohydrate content, the importance of consistency in meal size and regularity in the timing of meals is emphasized. The prohibition of simple sugar in the diet has been de-emphasized, but it should still comprise no more than 10% of total carbohydrate intake. The success of the nutritional program may ultimately depend on the degree to which the meal planning is individualized and tailored to well-established eating patterns in the family. Moreover, flexibility can be enhanced if blood glucose monitoring results are used to evaluate the impact of change in dietary intake. As with other aspects of the treatment regimen, we preach consistency and teach how to adjust for deviations from the prescribed diet.

Carbohydrate counting is an increasingly popular way to increase flexibility in food intake that is commonly used by patients using insulin pumps or multiple daily injections. The amount of insulin that is needed for each gram or serving of carbohydrate is used to calculate the amount of regular or lispro to be taken, depending on the amount of carbohydrate in the meal. With instructions on how to use nutritional labels on food packages, even children can become expert at counting carbohydrates. An even simpler method is to vary the dose of regular or lispro by 1 or 2 U if it is a small, regular, or large meal. Some foods, like pizza, which cause a prolonged increase in blood glucose levels, may require an increase in the amount of intermediate-acting insulin or a temporary change in overnight basal rates in pump-treated patients.

EXERCISE

Regular exercise and active participation in organized sports have positive implications concerning the psychosocial and physical well-being of our patients. Parents and patients should be advised that different types of exercise may have different effects on blood glucose levels. For example, sports that involve short bursts of intensive exercise may increase rather than decrease blood glucose levels *(20)*. On the other hand, long-distance running and other prolonged activities are more likely to lower blood glucose levels. Parents also need to be warned that a long bout of exercise during the day may lead to hypoglycemia while the child is sleeping during the night, which may require a reduction in the dose of intermediate or long-acting insulin.

OUTPATIENT CARE

Children and adolescents with type 1 diabetes should be routinely cared for by a diabetes center that uses a multidisciplinary team knowledgeable about and experienced in the management of young patients. This team should ideally consist of pediatric diabetologists, diabetes nurse specialists, nutritionists, and social workers or psychologists.

In newly diagnosed patients, the first few weeks are critically important in the process of teaching self-management skills to the parent and child. In this age group, the parent is usually in daily contact with the diabetes clinical nurse specialist. Glucose levels, adjustment to diabetes, diet, and exercise are reviewed. The timing of the phone calls should be prearranged and ideally made to the same clinician. After making the insulin adjustment for the day, the rationale should be explained to the parent. Usually within 3 wk, the parents are feeling more confident and many are ready to attempt to make their own adjustments.

Once stabilized, regular follow-up visits on a two- to three-monthly basis are recommended for most patients *(21)*. The main purpose of these visits is to ensure that the patient is achieving primary treatment goals. In addition to serial measurements of height and weight, particular attention should be paid to monitoring of blood pressure and examinations of the optic fundus, thyroid, and subcutaneous injection sites. Routine outpatient visits provide an opportunity to review glucose monitoring, to adjust the

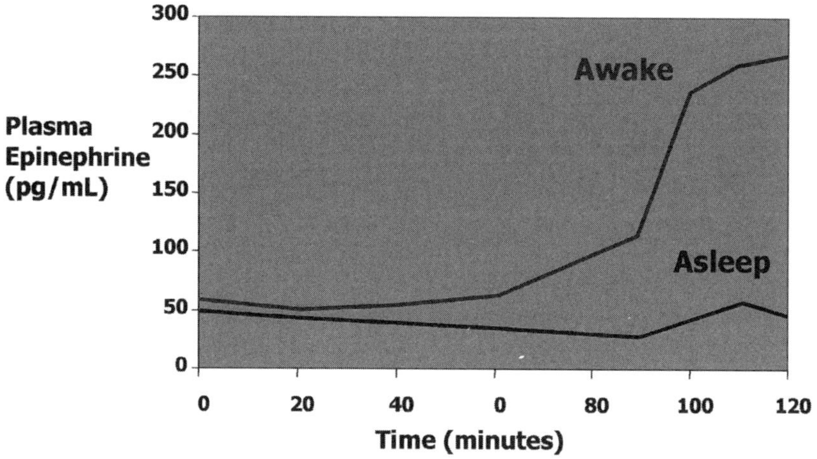

Fig. 3. The effect of deep sleep on plasma epinephrine responses during a hypoglycemic clamp study in which plasma glucose was lowered from 90 to 50 mg/dL in adolescents with type 1 diabetes mellitus. In contrast to the vigorous epinephrine responses observed when the youngsters were awake during the night or day, the rise in plasma epinephrine was virtually abolished during sleep. (*$p < 0.01$ vs awake studies). (Data from ref. *13*).

treatment regimen, and to assess child and family adjustment. Follow-up advice and support should be given by the nutritionist, diabetes nurse specialist, and psychologist or social worker. Use of the telephone, fax, or e-mail should be encouraged for adjustments in the treatment regimen between office visits.

HYPOGLYCEMIA

Severe hypoglycemia is a common problem in patients striving for strict glycemic control with intensive-treatment regimens. In the DCCT, the risk of severe hypoglycemia was threefold higher in intensively treated than in conventionally treated patients, and being an adolescent was an independent risk factor for a severe hypoglycemic event, as mentioned earlier *(2)*. The majority of severe hypoglycemic events occur overnight, in part, because of sleep-induced defects in counterregulatory hormone responses to hypoglycemia *(13)*. The failure of hypoglycemia to elicit an epinephrine response to hypoglycemia during deep sleep is shown in Fig. 3.

Monitoring glucose is critical in order to detect asymptomatic hypoglycemia, especially in the young child with diabetes. The older child is usually aware of symptoms such as weakness, shakiness, hunger, or a headache and is encouraged to treat these symptoms as soon as they occur. The older child who can accurately recognize symptoms is taught to immediately treat with 15 g of carbohydrate (e.g., three to four glucose tablets, 4 oz of juice, or 15 g of a glucose gel) without waiting to check a glucose level. Each episode should be assessed in order to make proper adjustments if a cause can be identified. Every family should have a glucagon emergency kit at home in order to treat severe hypoglycemia.

SICK-DAY RULES

Children with intercurrent illnesses, such as infections or vomiting, should be closely monitored for elevations in blood glucose levels and ketonuria. On sick days, blood glucose levels should be checked every 2 h and the urine should be checked for ketones with every void. Supplemental doses of short-acting insulin (0.1–0.3 U/kg) should be given every 2–4 h for elevations in glucose and ketones. Because of its more rapid absorption, lispro will lower plasma glucose faster than regular insulin *(22)*. If the morning dose has not been given and the child has a modestly elevated glucose level (150–250 mg/dL), small doses of NPH can be given to avoid a too rapid fall in plasma glucose levels. This works especially well in young children whose glucose levels fall quickly with rapid-acting insulin. Adequate fluid intake is essential to prevent dehydration. Fluids such as flat soda, clear soups, popsicles, and gelatin water are recommended to provide some electrolyte and carbohydrate replacement. If vomiting is persistent and ketones remain moderate or high after several supplemental insulin doses, arrangements should be made for parenteral hydration and evaluation in the emergency department.

Children receiving ultralente insulin seem to be prone to the development of hypoglycemia and ketonuria during episodes of gastroenteritis. If the child is unable to retain oral carbohydrate, then small doses of glucagon (i.e., 0.1–0.2 mg), given subcutaneously every 2–4 h, can be used to maintain normal blood glucose levels.

BEHAVIORAL AND PSYCHOSOCIAL ASPECTS OF TREATMENT

Between the ages of 7 and 11, the child is better able to think, learn, remember, listen, and communicate compared to younger children *(23)*. Cognitive processes are becoming more logical and less egocentric. They are learning concrete cognitive operations—they now understand rules and follow them closely. They are able to deal with symbols and begin to master classifications. As children deal with the challenges of school, they begin to turn their attention away from the home environment, and the peer group becomes more important. Each of these skills may affect the adaptation to diabetes.

In general, the majority of children will do well, but diabetes may serve as a risk factor for the development of psychosocial difficulties in a relatively small percentage of children, often estimated at approx 10–20% *(24)*. In most studies of overall adjustment, however, children with diabetes were found to score within the normal range or similarly to age- and gender-matched controls in such areas as behavior *(25)*, temperament *(26)*, and self-competence and self-esteem *(27,28)*. In those who do demonstrate psychosocial difficulties in the school-age years, children tend to be more depressed, withdrawn, and quiet, and their metabolic control may also be compromised *(27)*.

The psychosocial impact of the new diagnosis of diabetes in school-aged children has been fairly well characterized *(28)*. Mild depression and anxiety are commonly reported by school-aged children during the first few months of diabetes, but these symptoms usually resolve within 6 mo after diagnosis *(28)*. It is not uncommon, however, to have a recurrence of depressive symptoms during the second or third years of diabetes duration, which may coincide with the end of the honeymoon period *(27)*. The realization that the disease will not go away and that it is getting harder to manage may adversely affect the youngster's sense of well-being. Such problems are important clinically because preadolescents with adjustment problems are more likely to use avoidance behaviors regarding self-care of their diabetes *(29)*.

Another factor associated with regimen adherence is the involvement of the family. Earlier approaches to diabetes management advocated early transition of care responsibilities to children with diabetes. In 1987, Fonagy et al. *(30)* studied factors associated with poorer metabolic control and found that a child's early and independent participation in the diabetes regimen was significantly associated with poorer control. Thus, although school-age children with diabetes can begin to assume some of the tasks of daily diabetes management, they will still need significant assistance from their families for management decisions *(31)*. Current recommendations for care emphasize shared care responsibilities between parents and children.

It is important to recognize that the diagnosis of diabetes can have adverse effects on parents and on family functioning. Although concerns may be transient *(32,33)*, it is not uncommon for parents of school-aged children to be concerned about their abilities to cope with the burdens of therapy. Clinicians need to be aware of these concerns and provide appropriate support and counseling. It is also important to note that such parental distress may be associated with the child's adjustment *(34)*.

School-age children with diabetes can begin to assume some of the daily diabetes management tasks, such as insulin injections and blood glucose testing. However, they will still need significant assistance from their families for management decisions. It is important to encourage school-aged children to attend school regularly and to participate in school activities and sports to facilitate the development of normal peer relationships. Children with diabetes often feel that they are different from their peers because of the diabetes and may be at risk for difficulties with social competence *(35)*.

REFERENCES

1. DCCT Research Group. The effects of intensive diabetes treatment on the development and progression of long-term complications in insulin-dependent diabetes mellitus. The Diabetes Control and Complications Trial. N Engl J Med 1993;329:977–986.
2. The DCCT Research Group. The effect of intensive diabetes treatment on the development and progression of long-term complications in adolescents with insulin-dependent diabetes mellitus: the Diabetes Control and Complications Trial. J Pediatr 1994;125:177–188.
3. DCCT Research Group. Prolonged effect of intensive therapy on the risk of advanced complications in the Epidemiology of Diabetes Intervention and Complications (EDIC) follow-up of the DCCT cohort. N Engl J Med 2000;342:381–389.
4. Ryan C, Vega A, Drash A. Cognitive deficits in adolescents who developed diabetes early in life. Pediatrics 1983;75:921–927.
5. Amiel SA, Sherwin RS, Simonson DC, Lauritano AA, Tamborlane WV. Impaired insulin action in puberty: a contributing factor to poor glycemic control in adolescents with diabetes. N Engl J Med 1986:315:215–219.
6. Etzwiler DD. Patient education and management: a team approach. In: Rifkin H, Porte D, eds. Ellenberg and Rifkin's Diabetes Mellitus. Theory and Practice. Elsevier, New York, 1990, pp. 942–948.
7. Grey M, Boland EA, Davidson M, Li J, Tamborlane W. Coping skills training for youth on intensive therapy has long lasting effects on metabolic control and quality of life. J Pediatr 2000;137:107–114.

8. Dougherty G, Schiffrin A, White D, Soderstrom I, Sufrategui M. Home-based management can achieve intensification cost-effectively in type I diabetes. Pediatrics 1999;103:122–128.
9. Patton JW, Bukar J, Magarajan. Inhaled insulin. Adv Drug Deliv Rev 1999;36:235–247.
10. Yki-Jarvinen H, Koivisto VA. Natural course of insulin resistance in type I diabetes. N Engl J Med 1986;315:224–230.
11. The DCCT Research Group. The effect of intensive diabetes treatment in the DCCT on residual insulin secretion in IDDM. Ann Intern Med 1998;128:517–523.
12. Schatz DA, Rogers DG, Brouhard BH. Prevention of insulin-dependent diabetes mellitus: an overview of three trials. [review]. Cleve Clin J Med 1996;63:270–274.
13. Jones TW, Porter P, David EA, et al. Suppressed epinephrine responses during sleep: a contributing factor to the risk of nocturnal hypoglycemia in insulin-dependent diabetes. N Engl J Med 199;338:1657–1662.
14. Boland EA, Grey M, Fredrickson L, Tamborlane WV. CSII: a "new" way to achieve strict metabolic control, decrease severe hypoglycemia and enhance coping in adolescents with type I diabetes. Diabetes Care 1999;22:1779–1894.
15. Zinman B, Tildesley H, Chiasson TJ, Tsue E, Strack T. Insulin lispro in CSII: results of a double-blind crossover study [published erratum appears in Diabetes 1997, July 46:1239]. Diabetes 1997;46:440–443.
16. Moses AC, Gordon GS, Carey MC, Flier JS. Insulin administration intranasally as an insulin-bile salt aerosol. Effectiveness and reproducibility in normal and diabetic subjects. Diabetes 1983;32:1040–1047.
17. Mazze RS, Shamoon H, Pasmantier R, et al. Reliability of blood glucose monitoring by patients with diabetes mellitus. Am J Med 1984;77:211–217.
18. Boland EA, DeLucia M, Brandt C, Grey MJ, Tamborlane WV. Limitations of conventional methods of self blood glucose monitoring: lessons learned from three days of continuous glucose monitoring in pediatric patients with type I diabetes. Diabetes 2000:49(Suppl 1):A98.
19. Tamborlane WV, Held N. Diabetes. In: Tamborlane WV, ed. Yale Guide to Children's Nutrition. Yale University Press, New Haven, CT, 1997, pp. 161–169.
20. Mitchell TH, Abraham G, Schiffrin A, Leiter LA, Marls EB. Hyperglycemia after intensive exercise in IDDM subjects during continuous subcutaneous insulin infusion. Diabetes Care 1988;11:311–317.
21. American Diabetes Association. Clinical Practice Recommendations, 1992–1993. Diabetes Care 1993;16(Suppl 2):1–113.
22. Attia N, Jones TW, Holcombe J, Tamborlane WV. Comparison of human regular insulin and lispro insulin after interruption of CSII and in the treatment of acutely decompensated IDDM. Diabetes Care 1998;21:817–821.
23. Piaget J. The Origins of Intelligence in Children. International Universities, New York, 1952.
24. Bennett DS. Depression among children with chronic medical problems: A meta-analysis. J Pediatr Psychol 1994;19:149–169.
25. Jacobson AM, Hauser ST, Lavori P, Wolfdorf JI, Herskovitz RD, Miley JE, et al. Adherence among children and adolescents with insulin-dependent diabetes mellitus over a four-year longitudinal follow-up: 1. The influence of patient coping and adjustment. J Pediatr Psychol 1990;15:511–526.
26. Weissberg-Benchell J, Glasgow A. The role of temperament in children with insulin-dependent diabetes mellitus. J Pediatr Psychol 1997;22:795–809.
27. Grey M, Cameron ME, Lipman TH, Thurber FW. Psychosocial status of children with diabetes over the first two years. Diabetes Care 1995;18:1330–1336.
28. Kovacs M, Iyengar S, Goldston D, Stewart J, Obrosky DS, Marsh J. Psychological functioning of children with insulin-dependent diabetes mellitus: a longitudinal study. J Pediatr Psychol 1990;15:619–632.
29. Grey M, Cameron ME, Thurber FW. Coping and adaptation in children and adolescents with diabetes. Nurs Res 1991;40:144–149.
30. Fonagy P, Moran GS, Lindsay MKM, Kurtz AB, Brown R. Psychological adjustment and diabetic control. Arch Dis Child 1987;62:1009–1013.
31. Follansbee DS. Assuming responsibility for diabetes management. What age? What price? Diabetes Educ 1989;15(4):347–353.
32. Hodges LC, Parker J. Concerns of parents with diabetic children. Pediatr Nurs 1987;13:22–24, 68.
33. Kovacs M, Finkelstein R, Feinberg TL, Crouse-Novak M, Paulauskas S, Pollock M. Initial psychologic responses of parents to the diagnosis of insulin-dependent diabetes mellitus in their children. Diabetes Care 1985;8:568–575.

34. Chaney JM, Mullins LL, Frank RG, Peterson L, Mace LD, Kashani JH, et al. Transactional patterns of child, mother, and father adjustment in insulin-dependent diabetes mellitus. J Pediatr Psychol 1997;22:229–244.
35. Nassau JH, Drotar D. Social competence in children with IDDM and asthma: child, teacher, and parent reports of children's social adjustment, social performance, and social skills. J Pediatr Psychol 1995;20:187–204.

17 The Adolescent with Type 1 Diabetes

George A. Werther, MD, MSc,
Fergus J. Cameron, MD,
and John M. Court, MBBS

CONTENTS

INTRODUCTION

Adolescence is a challenging and complex stage in human development, involving major physical, hormonal, emotional, and psychological changes, which affect both the young person involved and members of his or her family. The burden of having to deal with a chronic disease such as diabetes at this time of life adds further to the potential for instability and turmoil. Diabetes is almost always insulin dependent or type 1 at this age, although type 2 is now increasingly recognized in adolescence, particularly in African and native American and similar racial groups *(1)*.

Diabetes affects most aspects of adolescence, including the physiologic processes of growth and puberty, and the emotional and social transitions into adulthood. Conversely, the various physiological, psychological, and behavioral changes of adolescence have significant impact on diabetes and its management. These include the effects of rapid growth and sexual development with their associated hormonal changes, the various behaviors associated with the growing independence from parents and associated potential conflicts, and experimentation with alcohol and drugs and other rebellious behaviors. Diabetes in the adolescent also has a number of comorbidities, both organic and psychosocial, some peculiar to this stage of development. It is also the period when the vascular complications of diabetes have their genesis and may first appear.

From: *Contemporary Endocrinology: Type 1 Diabetes: Etiology and Treatment*
Edited by: M. A. Sperling © Humana Press Inc., Totowa, NJ

The management of diabetes in the adolescent is thus highly challenging, requiring awareness of, and attention to, all of these components of the adolescent and his or her diabetes. This requires a multidisciplinary approach, involving a pediatric diabetologist, nurse-educator, dietician, social worker, psychologist, youth workers, peer group support, and others. In this chapter, we will review the current knowledge and understanding of diabetes in adolescence, dealing with both the underlying mechanisms and dynamics, as well as practical approaches to management.

GROWTH, PUBERTY, AND DIABETES: INSULIN DEFICIENCY AND RESISTANCE

Physical growth and development is a major feature distinguishing the child and adolescent from the mature adult. The major pathologic cause of impaired growth and maturation is inadequate nutritional supply to growing tissues, providing the basis of growth failure in most chronic diseases of childhood *(2)*. Diabetes may be considered an example of cellular malnutrition, whereby relative insulin deficiency leads to suboptimal or, frankly, inadequate nutrient supply to the tissues. Whereas, in childhood, the gross effect is impaired linear growth, in adolescence, an added effect is delayed or slowed pubertal development, similar to that seen in eating disorders *(3)*. The degree of impaired growth and pubertal development relates to the inadequacy of diabetic control over time, the most extreme example being Mauriac's syndrome, the triad of growth failure, hepatomegaly, and obesity, first described in the 1930s *(4)*. There have been many subsequent reports of delayed growth and puberty in adolescents with poorly controlled diabetes *(3,5–7)*.

The interaction among growth, puberty, and diabetes is complex, with studies reaching differing conclusions, both about the events themselves and about the mechanisms involved. If diabetes is diagnosed before puberty, linear growth prior to diagnosis has been variously described as being reduced, increased, or unchanged *(8–11)*. Following diagnosis, linear growth prior to puberty may be impaired, especially if diabetic control is poor *(5,11,12)*. This inverse relationship between growth and poor diabetic control is more marked during puberty, such that the pubertal growth spurt may be impaired as well as the onset of puberty and menarche being delayed *(6,7,13–17)*. Following menarche, menstrual dysfunction is more common, including secondary amenorrhoea and irregular cycles, as well as polycystic ovary syndrome *(15,18)*. Improved diabetic control, involving more adequate insulinization, often leads to restoration of linear growth *(19)* and restoration of regular menstrual cycles *(18)*.

A contrasting but frequent observation, particularly among adolescent girls with diabetes, is a tendency for excessive weight gain *(20,21)*, which may be related to a combination of overinsulinization and dietary excess, especially involving fat and carbohydrates. Eating disorders are certainly more common among adolescent girls with diabetes *(22)*, but estrogen–regulated fat deposition may play a role.

Another important but easily overlooked cause of adolescent growth failure or delayed puberty in adolescents with diabetes is hypothyroidism resulting from Hashimoto's thyroiditis. Although only a small proportion of affected children, mostly girls, develop hypothyroidism, up to 10% of children and adolescents with diabetes develop a goiter and antithyroid antibodies *(23)*. Similarly, celiac disease affects up to 5% of diabetic children and adolescents, often only presenting with growth failure or nonspecific gastrointestinal symptoms, and diagnosed by screening for endomysial and antigliadin antibodies *(24,25)*.

The pubertal growth spurt is induced by sex hormones in both boys and girls, leading to increased amplitude of growth hormone (GH) pulses, and a rise in circulating insulinlike growth factor-1 (IGF-1) *(26)*. Both the sex hormones and GH contribute to insulin resistance *(27)* and worsening glycemic control *(28)*, such that insulin requirements rise during puberty from less than 1 U/kg/d to over 1.5 U/kg/d *(29)*. Insulin also plays an important anabolic role during puberty. Failure to adequately increase insulin doses during this period has adverse effects on diabetic control, leading to the impairment of growth and pubertal development, as described earlier. Clearly, there are other well-recognized factors interfering with diabetic control during adolescence, including poor compliance with diet and insulin regimens and emotional and social stresses. However, inadequate insulin dosage during this period of increased insulin resistance and rapid growth is often overlooked as a cause of poor diabetic control, marked by rising glycosylated hemoglobin levels, leading to impaired growth *(14,17)*.

The GH/IGF axis, which plays a central role in the growth acceleration of puberty, can be significantly disordered in the diabetic adolescent with poor diabetic control, contributing to both growth impairment and greater insulin resistance *(30)*. Circulating GH is significantly elevated in adolescents with diabetes and is thought to contribute to both increased insulin resistance and the "dawn phenomenon" of rising early morning blood glucose *(30)*. There is also a dissociation of GH and IGF-1 levels, so that in contrast to GH, IGF-1 levels are depressed in diabetic adolescents with poor control. This hepatic insensitivity to GH is thought to result from reduced expression of the GH receptor in the liver and is reflected by low circulating GH-binding protein (BP), representing the extracellular domain of the GH receptor *(31)*. GH receptor expression is regulated by insulin, so that adequate insulinization reverses the apparent GH resistance and low IGF-1, providing a mechanism for restoration of linear growth *(31,32)*. The other important components of the IGF system are the IGFBPs, which regulate IGF availability for its receptors. GH regulates the major carrier of circulating IGF-1, IGFBP-3; it may be suppressed in poorly controlled diabetic adolescents, further accounting for low circulating IGF-1 *(33)*. In contrast, IGFBP-1, which shows diurnal variation, is negatively regulated by insulin, so that it is markedly elevated when diabetic control is poor at times of inadequate insulinization, such as prior to the morning insulin injection *(33,34)*. IGFBP-1 is thought to function as a "counterregulatory" hormone, rapidly binding free IGF-1, which has insulinlike effects when it is in excess. Persistently elevated IGFBP-1 levels would therefore further reduce IGF-1 availability, thus contributing to growth failure.

PSYCHOSOCIAL ISSUES

Adolescence is an often untidy, poorly defined rite of passage characterized by exploratory, iconoclastic, sexual, and risk-taking behavior. Underpinning the apparent turmoil of adolescence is a fundamental paradox—the need to identify self while conforming to a peer group *(35,36)*. This process has been described as a task of establishing a balance between intimacy and autonomy *(37)*. Although this paradox continues to some extent throughout adult life, it is during adolescence that it is most intense. Resolution is potentially hampered by conflict with parents, social and academic pressures, and the pubertally induced evanescent nature of "self." Sexual, cognitive, and physical maturation fundamentally change one's sense of identity throughout this period, rendering ephemeral the adolescent's point of relativity with the rest of the world. It is not surprising that, during this period, psychopathology is more likely to occur than at any other age during life. The prevalence of eating disorders, depression, suicide, and schizophrenia during adolescence are witness to this *(37)*.

Psychosocial and Physical Developmental Tasks Faced by the Adolescent with Diabetes

The psychosocial and physical developmental tasks of adolescence can be summarized as the development of an intact, independent psyche (including sexual identity), the establishment of good peer relationships, the evolution of abstract thought processes, and the completion of physical growth and reproductive capability. Adolescents encounter and resolve these challenges not in an orderly sequential manner, but in a simultaneous and often random fashion. Accusations of adolescents "behaving out of character," "thinking with their hormones," or "justifying the inexcusable" are frequently made by those responsible for their care. Behaviors that give rise to such accusations are a direct consequence of the concomitant nature of the emotional, cognitive, and physical changes that occur during this period. Adolescent actions can also be impulsive and seemingly without regard to consequence. None more so than physical risk-taking and recreational drug use. The former of these (more often seen in males) may result in significant injury or, more tragically, deaths associated with distinctly adolescent activities such as "train-surfing," "car joy-riding," or graffiti writing in hazardous environments *(38,39)*. Recreational drug use is correspondingly often impulsive. Physical morbidity, psychopathology, and mortality may arise in this context through accidental overdose, ingestion of unknown and multiple agents, infection, and the combination of an altered sensorium with risk-laden activity. When emerging sexual interest is added to this mix, unwanted teenage pregnancy and sexually transmitted disease often ensue.

Chronic disease, such as diabetes, during adolescence mitigates against untroubled passage through this period. The additional specific tasks faced by an adolescent with diabetes are as follows: the shift of responsibility for disease control from caregiver to self; the maintenance of good metabolic control in the face of the endocrine vagaries of puberty; the incorporation of an increasingly less regimented lifestyle into their diabetes control; and the maintenance of an active, "normal" lifestyle. Diabetic adolescents also encounter the reality of the risks of diabetes-related complications with the clinical advent of regular complication screening.

Impact of Diabetes on Behavior, Cognition, and Quality of Life

In many respects, diabetes can act as an obstruction to adolescent passage. Diabetes is a potent touchstone for areas of potential conflict with parents and caregivers (such as the locus of control issues) *(40,41)*. Diabetes may also increase the risk and likelihood of risk-taking behaviors *(42)* and may interfere with conformity to a peer group *(43)*. In some cases, diabetes also impedes physical and sexual maturation *(44)*. Poorly controlled diabetes is associated with subtle neuropsychological deficits that can impact on academic achievement and ultimately reduce career options and lifestyle choices *(45,46)*. There is evidence that the deterioration seen in both psychological well-being and metabolic control during adolescence are linked, with noncompliance with the treatment regimen acting as a mediating variable *(47,48)*. It is not surprising, therefore, that the convergence of diabetes and adolescence is frequently associated with conflict and a subsequent deterioration in diabetic control *(49–51)*. In a retrospective, longitudinal study of 118 adolescent 18-yr-olds with type 1 diabetes, studied at three-monthly intervals between 8 and 18 yr, we found a significant deterioration in metabolic control throughout the period of adolescence *(52)*. This deterioration was most marked for females. Quality of life may also deteriorate during this time *(53)*. Using the Child Health Questionnaire (CHQ), we surveyed 71 adolescents (12–18 yr of age). The CHQ is a parent/self-report tool that quantifies disease impact upon general health, psychosocial health, and family cohesion. Parents reported that for adolescents aged 12–18 yr, general health was markedly lower, parental impact (in terms of time and emotion) was high, and family activities mean scores were moderately lower. Adolescents with diabetes, unlike younger children, were reported by their parents as having poorer emotional and behavioral outcomes and poorer self-esteem outcomes than the nondiabetic adolescents. Interestingly, although parents reported a significantly lower quality of life for their adolescent offspring, the adolescents with diabetes rated themselves similar to adolescents without diabetes. This may be the result of adolescents with diabetes genuinely perceiving their health to be similar to that of their peers. Alternatively, even when health concerns are present, this form of adolescent self-report may not be the ideal way of describing their impact. Finally, adolescents may not wish to report themselves to be different.

Support Strategies

Clinical strategies aimed at improving diabetic control throughout adolescence have focused largely upon psychosocial support rather than clinical care. There is some evidence, however, that diabetic control is unlikely to improve from late childhood to late adolescence, and we have advocated that diabetic control needs to be optimal prior to the advent of adolescence *(52)*. Furthermore, research in our clinic has supported the notion that early adjustment to insulin-dependent diabetes mellitus (IDDM) is predictive of longer-term outcome, with early psychological difficulties leading to ongoing maladjustment, reduced treatment compliance, and poorer health outcome *(45)*. Early intervention is best done through identifying and addressing latent family and interpersonal issues that may be contributory to subsequent deterioration of an adolescent's psyche and their diabetes control. Such issues include parenting skills, communication, social skills, cognitive ability, self-esteem, and incipient psychopathology. Early identification of children "at risk" of moving along the trajectory of psychological maladjustment → reduced treatment compliance → poor metabolic control is required. Such research is imperative because, in our experience, it is much more difficult to address issues such as these once an "adolescent crisis" has precipitated itself. In the absence of this research and once adolescence has ensued, the most effective strategies appear to be orientated around peer-support models *(54)*. Positive role modeling, diabetes camps, buddy systems, and peer counseling are approaches that are gaining increasing usage within diabetes clinics that deal with adolescents *(54,55)*. Techniques that foster resiliency life skills are also garnering interest from clinicians who deal with adolescents and chronic disease, although specific diabetes research in this field is lacking.

ADHERENCE

Compliance with medical advice and adherence to a treatment regimen tend to diminish during adolescence as teenagers adjust their priorities toward the competing demands of their social life and an erratic lifestyle *(56–59)*. They may increasingly resent parental supervision of their diabetes care and, in so doing, resent the imposition and constraints of their diabetes treatment.

The extent that this may impact on health and diabetes control will vary from one child to another and may be manifest as an increased risk of severe hypoglycemia, deteriorating HbA1c levels, and episodes of ketoacidosis. A reluctance to do more than a minimum of blood glucose tests, erratic meals, and missed insulin doses are common *(60)* and may all contribute to this. The adolescent may feel that the less attention that is paid to diabetes management, the less intrusive it is on their life. Parental anxiety and threats or discipline tend to make matters worse, as the adolescent is already well aware of the long-term consequences of poor control, is abundantly reminded of parental concerns, and resents interference in their task of maintaining the complex balance of keeping healthy and growing up in conformity with their social environment.

There are a number of risk factors associated with poor adherence, particularly emotional disturbance and including family dysfunction *(61–64)*, poor school performance, and difficult peer relationships. The relationship between depression and diabetes control is less clear. Emotional disturbance has been linked previously with overzealous attention to diabetes care *(65)*, but it might be expected that psychiatric illness, especially depression, would reduce motivation to comply with good care. A recent study has found that depression is important to psychological adaptation and metabolic control in children with diabetes mellitus *(66)*. Poor adherence has been linked with "learned helplessness" *(67)*. The question of the relationship between psychiatric illness and diabetic adherence and control is unresolved *(68)*.

Education about diabetes and its management had been widely advocated as the answer to poor adherence. Unfortunately, there is little evidence to suggest a relationship between knowledge and health behavior *(69)*; health beliefs and attitudes and conflicting priorities are major determinants in influencing adherence *(70)*.

Perhaps the most helpful thing for a health care professional to do is to maintain a comfortable and mutually respectful relationship with an adolescent who is having trouble adhering to a diabetic regimen, providing family support, and encouraging attempts and small gains that the adolescent makes as he or she proceeds toward adult responsibility.

DRUGS

Adolescents with diabetes live in the same social environment and are subject to the same risks as their nondiabetic teenaged peers. Thus, the risk of drug use in adolescents with diabetes will reflect the common use of drugs in the community.

The effects of drugs, both the perceived advantages and the harmful effects, will be those that any young person will experience. The added risk related to diabetes will depend on four factors.

Interaction Between Drug Effects and Body Metabolism

Adolescents are liable to binge drink, with occasional bouts of heavy drinking with friends and at parties *(71)*. Their capacity to consume large amounts of alcohol, together with the lack of responsibility for their own health and safety that may accompany intoxication, may impact acutely on those with diabetes. Alcohol, in excess and in the absence of accompanying carbohydrate in some form, may lead to hypoglycemia through impaired release of hepatic glucose *(72,73)*. As many young adolescents do have alcohol and those with diabetes may choose to use a sugar-free mix, this is a potential risk. It is likely to be compounded by omitting normal diet at a party or when out drinking with friends.

A more common adverse sequel to a bout of drinking for a young diabetic, however, is ketoacidosis, precipitated by omission of an insulin injection and vomiting as a result of intoxication and associated with dehydration *(74)*.

Acute use of amphetamines, particularly the analog 3,4-methylenedioxymethamphetamine (MDMA, "Ecstasy"), before an all-night dance party is also likely to lead to hypoglycemia if followed by sustained levels of high physical activity *(75)*. There is also a risk of dehydration, which, if combined with missed insulin doses, may precipitate ketoacidosis. Methamphetamine ("Speed," "Ice," "Crank") leads to loss of appetite *(76)*, and chronic abuse of the drug can lead to long periods of missed meals and weight loss, impulsivity *(77)* with missed insulin doses, and deteriorating metabolic control.

Effects of Drugs on Motivation to Maintain Diabetes Control

Occasional use of drugs may have little or no lasting effect on behavior in most young people. Continuing use of cannabis, however, is associated with loss of motivation *(78,79)*. This is likely to be most noticeable on school and sporting achievement, but will be reflected in other aspects of a young person's life, including health care. Thus, the heavy or daily user of cannabis is likely to neglect any active responsibility in maintaining good glycaemic control—failing to do blood tests or adjust insulin.

Cannabis use is likely to lead to erratic eating, with increased snacking while intoxicated and subsequent loss of appetite when coming down from the effect *(80)*. Most regular users of cannabis have poor nutrition and poor weight gain. A further risk to diabetes health is the physical inactivity associated with chronic abuse. This is not only because of the sedative effect of tetrahydrocannabinol (THC) but also to the loss of motivation to become fit or to participate in sports.

Heroin use, particularly if there is addiction, will override all aspects of health—particularly good nutrition and active care of diabetes. Acquiring the money to buy the drug and the effects of the drug itself will inevitably take precedence over the needs for good glycaemic control.

Confusion Between Hypoglycemia and Intoxication

Intoxication in young people, whether from alcohol or drugs, is so common in many societies that people not knowing the youth with diabetes (and even those that do) may assume that he or she is intoxicated if they are showing dysfunctional behavior or diminished consciousness. This is particularly a risk if the young person has had some alcohol or is thought to use hallucinogenic or sedative drugs such as cannabis or LSD. Friends or family may let them "sleep it off," endangering them further if, in fact, they are hypoglycemic.

This risk further reinforces the advice to young diabetics that they should inform their friends about their diabetes and what to do if they may be hypoglycemic.

Added Risk Factors from Drugs with Respect to Microvascular or Macrovascular Disease

Most young people who decide to smoke cigarets or marijuana are only marginally influenced in their decision to do so by the knowledge of their harmful effects. Smoking, in particular, has been well established as being associated with an increased risk of macrovascular disease, in general *(81)*, and diabetic nephropathy, in particular *(82)*. The contributory role of smoking to diabetic retinopathy remains controversial *(83–86)*. Diabetic youth need to know the additional risk factor smoking provides to the long- term complications of diabetes and should have the opportunity to freely discuss these issues.

SPECIAL REQUIREMENTS FOR EDUCATION

All families with a child with diabetes need to have the basic information to manage their diabetes and to cope with any emergency or unusual situation. This information is provided through the process of education and often by highly trained diabetes educators. There are particular problems with relying on the provision of knowledge to adolescents, however, as knowledge does not relate well to health behavior at this age. A further problem is that education may have been given to the family when diabetes was first diagnosed, and if this was some years previously, it is probable that the adolescent has little memory of any formal teaching at that time and little inclination to learn now.

Most adolescents learn in a social environment. Adolescents may learn best through peer influence, both in taking responsibility and in acquiring knowledge *(87,88)*. Ideally, there should be a variety of opportunities for learning at this age, expanding the normal formal diabetes education at the clinic to include opportunities for teenagers to meet together to discuss problems and experience. In our institution, there are several peer-based support networks for adolescents with diabetes. These range from evening programs ("Me and My Diabetes"), to chronic illness support networks ("ChIPS" [Chronic Illness Peer Support]) and social groups ("The Injectors") *(54)*. Diabetes camps are also especially appropriate for adolescents, providing the opportunity to learn from their own and from each other's mistakes and to develop more positive attitudes toward diabetes care *(89,90)*. Unfortunately, only a proportion of adolescents are willing or able to attend camp, and often those who would most benefit are those who choose not to go *(91)*. The same is probably true for other voluntary peer-group programs.

There have been studies, both in diabetes and in other chronic illness, that have shown the value of group programs that involve families, including both parents, in parallel with adolescent peer groups *(87,88)*. These may be particularly helpful if directed to bringing about change in attitudes toward self-care and responsible diabetes control. The involvement of parents may help ensure that their teenage children actually attend, as well as helping parents develop a different role in the care of a young person seeking some degree of autonomy.

Perhaps the most helpful strategy for most adolescents, however, is to ensure that information is provided when they are most accessible and most likely to want it. This may be after some emergency or illness that perhaps could have been averted by specific strategies or decisions about diabetes management. It is helpful to avoid judgmental response to mistakes, but, rather, use them for learning.

Teenagers may not pay much attention when they come with their mother to a clinic visit or doctor's appointment, but they may ask questions if given a chance and then is the time to respond. Sometimes an adolescent will ask a question at the end of a consultation when there is little time to spend answering it, yet there may not be another opportunity.

TRANSITION TO ADULT CARE

The Process of Transition and the Eventual Transfer to Adult Care

In due course, the adolescent with diabetes who has been cared for in a pediatric environment, whether privately by a pediatric endocrinologist or in a pediatric clinic, must transfer care to an adult environment. The question of when and how will depend on a number of factors, including the perceived readiness of the young person, the availability of appropriate adult services, and the general policy of a hospital or clinic service. Most studies have suggested that from an adolescent's point of view, it is better to make the change at the end of adolescence when the young person has achieved some degree of autonomy and self-reliance *(92)*.

The act of transfer then becomes the logical end point of a process of transition that allows the young person to take responsibility for their care and for parents to relinquish their overriding role in their care. It may reasonably be seen as the pediatric physician's and pediatric nurse's task, in the later teenage years, to engage the family in this transition process and thus facilitate transfer.

This transition from the concept of parent dependence to autonomy, although probably never complete while the young person still lives at home and is financially and physically dependent, relates to all aspects of family interaction. It depends on the style of family functioning and the ability of the child's mother to trust her teenager and the extent it is reasonable for her to do so. The role of the physician is to facilitate that process and to encourage the young person to take responsibility.

The first step is increasingly to direct the consultation to the teenager. This may be by directing discussion and advice directly to the adolescent rather than the parent, which tends to occur during childhood. Parents, who regard themselves as principal carers, may feel threatened by this and express this by saying that their child will not tell the doctor about problems and difficulties, especially those of noncompliance. Thus, at this stage of transition, the needs of parents to relinquish control may be paramount.

Eventually, the adolescent should be able to consult with his/her doctor alone. This will prepare both them and their parents for an adult service, where parental involvement would usually be seen as inappropriate.

BARRIERS TO SUCCESSFUL TRANSFER

The pediatric endocrinologist is responsible for ensuring that the transfer is achieved. It may be helpful to recognize that there may be barriers to this being made successfully. These include the firm bond that may have developed between pediatric physician or service and the adolescent, which both the doctor and the teenager may find difficult to break, especially if this comes at a time when the adolescent is also moving away from home.

An adult service and an adult endocrinologist may seem less friendly than a pediatric setting. The pediatric approach may have allowed development of a warm relationship in which to give advice and care. The adult approach may be to offer advice and leave it to the patient, with little patience on behalf of the doctor if the advice is not followed. An adult diabetes clinic will usually serve an older population, mainly with NIDDM and many with obvious complications of diabetes. In many cases, there will be a large patient load and less consultation time for the young adult to develop a trusting relationship with his or her doctor. The adolescent should be prepared for this.

An ideal situation, which occurs in some centers, is for an adult service to provide a young adults' clinic to serve the younger adult-age group. Not only will the approach be closer in concept to a pediatric one, but the young diabetic may have the chance to have a more age-appropriate introduction to the process of adult responsibility.

The adverse result of not making appropriate or effective transfer to adult care is the risk that the young adult may be lost to ongoing specialist care, especially if he or she does not feel comfortable with the adult environment.

CONCLUSION

The psychosocial mores of adolescence are frequently forgotten or repressed by those who have passed through it. As a consequence, "mistakes of history" are often repeated by adult caregivers of adolescents. Clinicians may be expert in their field of clinical medicine, however, the temporal, transient and ephemeral nature of adolescence mitigates against expertise in the "experience" of adolescence *per se*. Therefore, as clinicians that care for adolescents with chronic disease, our role should be not to analyze and comprehend, but to be guiding and supportive. The goal of adulthood will arrive with or without our input, and the most we can hope to achieve is disease control within the context of an emerging and mature partnership.

REFERENCES

1. Dabelea D, Pettitt DJ, Jones KL, Arslanian SA. Type 2 diabetes mellitus in minority children and adolescents. An emerging problem. Endocrinol Metab Clin North Am 1999;28:709–729.
2. Werther GA. Non-endocrine causes of growth failure. In: Hintz RL, Rosenfeld RG, eds. Contemporary Issues in Endocrinology and Metabolism. Vol. 4: Growth Abnormalities. Churchill Livingstone, New York, 1987, pp. 81–107.
3. Rogers D. Puberty and insulin dependent diabetes mellitus. Clin Pediatr 1992;31:168–173.
4. Mauriac P. Hepatomegalies de l'enfance avec troubles de la croissance et du metabolisms des glucides. Paris Med 1934;2:525–528.
5. Jivani S, Rayner P. Does control influence the growth of diabetic children? Arch Dis Child 1973;48:109–115.
6. Herber S, Dunsmore I. Does control affect growth in diabetes mellitus? Acta Paediatr Scand 1988;77:303–305.
7. Stewart-Brown S, Lee T, Savage D. Pubertal growth in diabetics. Arch Dis Child 1985;60:768–769.
8. Hoskins P, Leslie R, Pyke D. Height at diagnosis of diabetes in children: a study in identical twins. Br Med J 1985;290:278–280.
9. Leslie R, Lo S, Millward A, Honour J, Pyke D. Decreased growth velocity before IDDM onset. Diabetes 1991;40:211–216.
10. Emmerson A, Savage D. Height at diagnosis in diabetes. Eur J Pediatr 1988;147:319–320.
11. Brown M, Ahmed M, Clayton K, Dunger D. Growth during childhood and final height in type I diabetes. Diabet Med 1994;11:182–187.
12. Thon A, Heinze E, Feilen K-D, et al. Development of height and weight in children with diabetes mellitus: report on two prospective multicentre studies, one cross sectional, one longitudinal. Eur J Paediatr 1992;151:258–262.

13. Rogers D, Sherman L, Gabbay K. Effect of puberty on insulin-like growth factor I and HBA1 in type I diabetes. Diabetes Care 1991;14:1031–1035.
14. Connors MH . Growth in the diabetic child. [review]. Pediatr Clin N Am 1997;44:301–306.
15. Kjaer K, Hagen C, Sando S, Eshoj O. Epidemiology of menarche and menstrual disturbances in an unselected group of women with insulin-dependent diabetes mellitus compared to controls. J Clin Endocrinol Metab 1992;75:524–529.
16. Schriock E, Winter R, Trasiman H. Diabetes mellitus and its effects on menarche. J Adolesc Health Care 1984;5:101–104.
17. Clarson C, Daneman D, Ehrlich R. The relationship of metabolic control to growth and pubertal development in children with insulin-dependent diabetes. Diabetes Res 1985;2:237–241.
18. Adcock C, Perry L, Lindsell D. Menstrual irregularities are more common in adolescents with type I diabetes: association with poor glycemic control and weight gain. Diabet Med 1994;11:465–470.
19. Rudolf M, Sherwin R, Markowitz R, et al. Effect of intensive insulin treatment on linear growth in the young diabetic adolescent. J Pediatr 1982;101:333–339.
20. Gregory J, Wilson A, Greene S. Body fat and overweight among children and adolescents with diabetes mellitus. Diabet Med 1992;9:344–348.
21. Domargard A, Sarnblad S, Kroon M, Karlsson I, Skeppner G, Aman J. Increased prevalence of overweight in adolescent girls with type 1 diabetes mellitus. Acta Paediatr 1999;88:1223–1228.
22. Peveler R, Fairburn E, Boller I. Eating disorders in adolescents with insulin-dependent diabetes mellitus: a controlled study. Diabetes Care 1992;15:1–5.
23. Court S, Parkin J. Hypothyroidism and growth failure in diabetes mellitus. Arch Dis Child 1982;57:622–624.
24. Maki M, Hallstrom O, Huupponen T. Increased prevalence of celiac disease in diabetes. Arch Dis Child 1984;59:739–742.
25. Barera G, Bianchi C, Calisti C. Screening of diabetic children for coeliac disease with antigliadin antibodies and HLA typing. Arch Dis Child 1991;66:491–494.
26. Devesa J, Lois N, Arce V, Diaz MJ, Lima L, Tresguerres JA. The role of sexual steroids in the modulation of growth hormone (GH) secretion in humans. J Steroid Biochem Mol Biol 1991;40(1–3):165–73.
27. Bloch C, Clemons P, Sperling M. Puberty decreases insulin sensitivity. J Pediatr 1987;110:481–487.
28. Amiel S, Sherwin R, Simonson D, Lauritano A, Tamborlane W. Impaired insulin action in puberty. A contributing factor to poor glycemic control in adolescents with diabetes. N Engl J Med 1986;315:215–219.
29. Kerouz N, el Hayek R, Langhough R, MacDonald MJ. Insulin doses in children using conventional therapy for insulin dependent diabetes. Diabetes Res Clin Pract 1995;29:113–120.
30. Dunger D, Cheetham T. Growth hormone insulin-like growth factor axis in insulin-dependent diabetes mellitus. Horm Res 1996;46:2–6.
31. Menon R, Arslanian S, May B, Cutfield W, Sperling M. Diminished growth hormone-binding protein in children with insulin-dependent diabetes mellitus. J Clin Endocrinol Metab 1992;74:934–938.
32. Clayton K, Holly J, Carlsson L, et al. Loss of the normal relationships between growth hormone, growth hormone-binding protein and insulin-like growth factor I in adolescents with insulin dependent diabetes mellitus. Clin Endocrinol 1994;41:517–524.
33. Batch J, Baxter R, Werther G. Abnormal regulation of insulin-like growth factor binding proteins in adolescents with insulin-dependent diabetes mellitus. J Clin Endocrinol Metab 1991;73:964–968.
34. Holly J, Dunger D, Edge J, Smith C, Chard T, Was J. Insulin-like growth factor binding protein-1 levels in diabetic adolescents and their relationship to metabolic control. Diabet Med 1990;7:618–623.
35. Erikson E. Childhood and Society. Norton, New York, 1959.
36. Seltzer VC. Adolescent Social Development: Dynamic Functional Interaction. Heath, Lexington, MA, 1982.
37. Thomas AM, Hauser ST. Psychosocial challenges and issues. In: Werther GA, Court JM, eds. Diabetes and the Adolescent. Miranova, Melbourne, 1998, pp. 35–55.
38. Strauch H, Wirth I, Geserick G. Fatal accidents due to train surfing in Berlin. Forensic Sci Int 1998;94:119–127.
39. Marshall C, Boyd KT, Moran CG. Injuries related to car crime: the joy-riding epidemic. Injury 1996;27:79–80.
40. Hauenstein E, Martin R, Snyder A, Clarke W. Stress in parents of children with diabetes mellitus. Diabetes Care 1989;12:18–23.
41. Schafer L, McCaul K, Glasgow R. Supportive and non-supportive family behaviours: relationships to adherence and metabolic control in persons with type 1 diabetes. Diabetes Care 1986,9:179–185.

42. Patterson JM, Garwick AW. Coping with chronic illness. A family systems perspective on living with diabetes In: Werther GA, Court JM, eds. Diabetes and the Adolescent. Miranova, Melbourne, 1998, pp. 3–35.
43. Jacobsen A, Hauser S, Wertlieb D, Wolsdorf J, Orleans J, Vieyra M. Psychological adjustment of children with recently diagnosed diabetes mellitus. Diabetes Care 1986;9:323–329.
44. Batch JA. Growth and puberty. In: Werther GA, Court JM, eds. Diabetes and the Adolescent. Miranova, Melbourne, 1998, pp. 93–112.
45. Northam EA, Anderson PJ, Werther GA, Warne GL, Adler RG, Andrewes D. Neuropsychological complications of IDDM in children with 2 years after disease onset. Diabetes Care 1998,21:379–384.
46. Northam EA, Anderson PJ, Werther GA, Warne GL, Andrewes D. Predictors of change in the neuropsychological profiles of children with type 1 diabetes 2 years after disease onset. Diabetes Care 1999;22:1438–1444.
47. Becker DJ. Management of insulin-dependent diabetes mellitus in children and adolescents. Curr Opin Pediatr 1991;3:710–723.
48. Hanson CL, Henggeler SW, Harris MA, Mitchell KA, Carle DL, Burghen GA. Associations between family members' perceptions of the health care system and the health of youths with insulin-dependent diabetes mellitus. J Pediatr Psychol 1988;13:543–554.
49. Vanelli M, Chiarelli F, Chiari G, Tumini S, Costi G, di Ricco L, et al. Metabolic control in children and adolescents with diabetes: experience of two Italian Regional Centers. J Pediatr Endocrinol Metab 1999;12:403–409.
50. Mortensen HB, Robertson KJ, Aanstoot HJ, Danne T, Holl RW, Hougaard P, et al. Insulin management and metabolic control of type 1 diabetes mellitus in childhood and adolescence in 18 countries. Hvidore Study Group on Childhood Diabetes. Diabet Med 1998;15:752–759.
51. Anderson B, Ho J, Brackett J, Finkelstein D, Laffel L. Parental involvement in diabetes management tasks: relationships to blood glucose monitoring adherence and metabolic control in young adolescents with insulin-dependent diabetes mellitus. J Pediatr 1997;130:257–265.
52. Dabaghdao P, Vidmar S, Cameron FJ. Deteriorating diabetic control through adolescence-do the origins lie in childhood. Diabet Med 2001;18:889–894.
53. Wake M, Hesketh K, Cameron FJ. The functional health status of children with diabetes. Diabet Med 2000;17:700–707.
54. Olsson C, Toumborurou J, Bowes G, Walsh B. Therapeutic peer support. In: Werther GA, Court JM, eds. Diabetes and the Adolescent. Miranova, Melbourne, 1998, pp. 217–230.
55. Court JM. Camping for youth with diabetes. In: Werther GA, Court JM, eds. Diabetes and the Adolescent. Miranova, Melbourne, 1998, pp. 271–280.
56. Cerkoney KA, Hart LK. The relationship between the health belief model and compliance of persons with diabetes mellitus. Diabetes Care 1980;3:594–598.
57. LaGreca A, Auslander W, Greco P, Spetter D, Fisher E, Santiago J. I get by with a little help from my family and friends: Adolescents' support for diabetes care. J Pediatr Psychol 1995;20:449–476.
58. Bryden KS, Neil A, Mayou RA, Peveler RC, Fairburn CG, Dunger DB. Eating habits, body weight, and insulin misuse. A longitudinal study of teenagers and young adults with type 1 diabetes. Diabetes Care 1999;22:1956–1960.
59. Du Pasquier-Fediaevsky L, Tubiana-Rufi N. Discordance between physician and adolescent assessments of adherence to treatment: influence of HbA1c level. The PEDIAB Collaborative Group. Diabetes Care 1999;22:1445–1449.
60. Kyngas H. Compliance of adolescents with diabetes. J Pediatr Nurs 2000;15:260–267.
61. Hanson CL, Henggeler SW, Burghen GA. Model associations between psychosocial variables and health-outcome measures of adolescents with IDDM. Diabetes Care 1987;10:752–758.
62. Hanson CL, DeGuire MJ, Schinkel AM, Henggler SW, Burghen GA. Comparing social learning and family systems correlates of adaptation in youths with IDDM. J Pediatr Psychol 1992;17:555–572.
63. Hanson CL, DeGuire MJ, Schinkel AM, Kolterman O. Empirical validation for a family-centered model of care. Diabetes Care 1995;18:1347–1356.
64. Hauser ST, Jacobson AM, Lavori P, et al. Adherence among children and adolescents with insulin-dependent diabetes mellitus over a four-year longitudinal follow-up. II. Immediate and long-term linkages with the family milieu. J Pediatr Psychol 1990;15:527–542.
65. Fonagy P, Moran GS, Lindsay LKM, et al. Psychological adjustment and diabetic control. Arch Dis Child 1987;62:1009–1113.
66. Lernmark B, Persson B, Fisher L, Rydelius P. Symptoms of depression are important to psychological adaptation and metabolic control in children with diabetes mellitus. Diabet Med 1999;16:14–22.

67. Kuttner MJ, Delamater AM, Santiago JV. Learned helplessness in diabetic youths. J Pediatr Psychol 1990;15:581–594.
68. Blanz BJ, Rensch-Riemann BS, Fritz-Sigmund DI, Schmidt MH. IDDM is a risk factor for adolescent psychiatric disorders. Diabetes Care 1993;16:1579–1587.
69. Ingersoll GM, Orr DP, Herrold AJ, et al. Cognitive maturity and self-management among adolescents with insulin-dependent diabetes mellitus. J Pediatr 1986;108:620–623.
70. Charron-Prochownik D, Becker D. Factors affecting adherence. In: Werther GA, Court JM, eds. Diabetes and the Adolescent. Miranova, Melbourne, 1998, pp. 57–67.
71. Johnson PB, Boles SM, Vaughan R, Kleber HD. The co-occurrence of smoking and binge drinking in adolescence. Addict Behav 2000;25:779–783.
72. Kriesberg RA, Owen W, Siegal AM. Ethanol-induced hyperlacticacidemia: inhibition of lactate utilization. J Clin Invest 1971;50:166–174.
73. Lecavalier L, Bolli G, Cryer P, et al. Contributions of gluconeogenesis and glycogenolysis during glucose counterregulation in normal humans. Am J Physiol 1989;256:E844–E851.
74. Court JM, Clarke C. The affect of alcohol, drugs and smoking. In: Werther GA, Court JM, eds. Diabetes and the Adolescent. Miranova, Melbourne, 1998, pp. 351–356.
75. Montgomery H, Myerson S. 3,4-Methylenedioxymethamphetamine (MDMA, or "ecstasy") and associated hypoglycemia. Am J Emerg Med 1997;15:218.
76. Bray GA. Use and abuse of appetite-suppressant drugs in the treatment of obesity. Ann Intern Med 1993;119:707–713.
77. Morgan MJ. Recreational use of "ecstasy" (MDMA) is associated with elevated impulsivity. Neuropsychopharmacology 1998;19:252–264.
78. Schwartz RH. Marijuana: an overview. Pediatr Clin North Am 1987;34:305–317.
79. Tunving K. Psychiatric aspects of cannabis use in adolescents and young adults. Pediatrician 1987;14:83–91.
80. Mohs ME, Watson RR, Leonard-Green T. Nutritional effects of marijuana, heroin, cocaine, and nicotine. J Am Diet Assoc 1990;90:1261–1267.
81. Haire-Joshu D, Glasgow RE, Tibbs TL. Smoking and diabetes. Diabetes Care 1999;22:1887–1898.
82. Ritz E, Ogata H, Orth SR. Smoking: a factor promoting onset and progression of diabetic nephropathy. Diabetes Metab 2000;26(Suppl 4):54–63.
83. Mulhauser I. Smoking and diabetes. Diabet Med 1990;7:10–15.
84. Grunwald JE, Brucker AJ, Grunwald SE, Riva CE. Retinal hemodynamics in proliferative diabetic retinopathy. A laser doppler velocimetry study. Invest Ophthalmol Vis Sci 1993;34:66–71.
85. Marshall G, Garg SK, Jackson WE, Holmes DL, Chase HP. Factors influencing the onset and progression of diabetic retinopathy in subjects with insulin-dependent diabetes mellitus. Ophthalmology 1993;100:1133–1139.
86. Chaturvedi N, Stephenson JM, Fuller JH. The relationship between smoking and microvascular complications in the EURODIAB IDDM Complications Study. Diabetes Care 1995;18:785–792.
87. Anderson BJ, Wolf FM, Burkhart MT, Cornell RG, Bacon GE. Effects of peer-group intervention on metabolic control of adolescents with IDDM. Diabetes Care 1989;12:179–183.
88. Misuraca A, Capobianco S, Lioniello M, Duval LM. Diabetic adolescents re-train young diabetics. J Pediatr Endocrinol Metab 1995;8(Suppl):227.
89. Thompson C, Greene SA, Newton RW. Camps for diabetic children and teenagers. In: Kelnar CJH, ed. Childhood and Adolescent Diabetes, Chapman & Hall Medical, Cambridge 1994, pp. 483–492.
90. Kida K, Nakamura K, Ito T, Kaino Y, Hirai H. The roles of local and international diabetes youth camps in diabetes education. In: Baba S, Kaneko T, eds. Diabetes 1994. Excerpta Medica Elsevier Science, Amsterdam, 1995, pp. 890–900.
91. Court JM. Camping for youth with diabetes. In: Werther GA, Court JM, eds. Diabetes and the Adolescent. Miranova, Melbourne, 1998, pp. 271–280.
92. Court JM. Outpatient based transition services for youth. Pediatrician 1991;18:150–156.

18 Hypoglycemia in Type 1 Diabetes

Stephanie A. Amiel, BSc, MD, FRCP,
and Krystyna Matyka, MRCP, MD

CONTENTS

INTRODUCTION

Although the introduction of insulin therapy was life-saving for patients with type 1 diabetes, problems of iatrogenic hypoglycemia were noticeable from the outset. In an article from 1923, describing the early experiences of using the new pancreatic extract, Banting et al. reports *(1):*

> *In giving a dose (of insulin), therefore, to render the patient sugar-free it sometimes happens that the blood sugar falls well below the normal level, and this sudden hypoglycemia is accompanied by a characteristic train of symptoms.*

Episodes of hypoglycemia continue to be a daily threat to all patients with type 1 diabetes mellitus and can lead to a significant reduction in quality of life.

PREVALENCE

Hypoglycemia is usually classified in one of two ways. Biochemical hypoglycemia is defined as a value falling below a predetermined blood glucose concentration *(2)* and depends on a blood sample being taken and assayed. The defining blood glucose concentration is controversial. Field used a venous plasma glucose concentration of 2.8 mmmol/L (1 mmol/L = 18 mg/dL) or less to define hypoglycemia and Marks used 2.2 mmol/L for people under 60 yr of age, but these concentrations were chosen to be unequivocally abnormal, in order to define patients with spontaneous pathological hypoglycemia as might occur with an insulin- or IGF (insulinlike growth factor)-

From: *Contemporary Endocrinology: Type 1 Diabetes: Etiology and Treatment*
Edited by: M. A. Sperling © Humana Press Inc., Totowa, NJ

secreting tumor *(3,4)*. In diabetes, glucose concentrations associated with physiological responses may be more appropriately used to define hypoglycemia. This may be as high as the glucose concentration at which endogenous insulin secretion starts to fall, but, by consensus, it is usually taken as a plasma glucose of ≤3.5 mmol/L. Symptomatic hypoglycemia is defined by patient description and is based on the reporting of symptoms, which are assessed according to an established hypoglycemia symptom hierarchy (e.g., *see* ref. 5). Symptomatic hypoglycemia is often further subdivided based on the severity of symptoms into mild (self-recognized and self-treated, without significant disruption to normal activity) or severe. Some classifications include a "moderate" class, in which the hypoglycemia and its treatment are less than severe but cause significant disruption of normal activity, but this is very subjective and often this class is not included. Definitions of severe hypoglycemia vary from an episode leading to mild alterations in central nervous system function to an episode involving coma and/or convulsions. In adults, the need for assistance from another person is a prerequisite and some definitions require the administration of parenteral therapy, but in pediatrics, this may not be so useful an indication of severity, as young children may require help to treat hypoglycemia of a minor degree.

A classification based purely on symptomatology will exclude episodes that go unnoticed, particularly those occurring during sleep, and does not demand confirmation of the presence of hypoglycemia with a documented low blood glucose concentration.

Given the difficulties of definition, it is not surprising that studies examining the prevalence of hypoglycemia have found widely varying rates. This is compounded by the fact that hypoglycemia is notoriously underreported, as episodes, particularly mild ones, are quickly forgotten. As a result, most studies have concentrated on reporting of severe episodes only, although these can also be overlooked.

Estimates of prevalence of severe hypoglycemia, occurring either during the day or during the night, vary from 18.7 to 280 episodes per 100 patient-years in studies of adults *(6–9)* and from 3.6 to 85.7 episodes per 100 patient-years in children *(10–13)*. This includes all definitions of severe hypoglycemia. In studies of nocturnal hypoglycemia, biochemical definitions are always used, but these have varied from 2.0 to 3.0 mmol/L in adult studies and from 3.0 to 3.9 mmol/L in pediatric studies. The prevalence of nocturnal hypoglycemia has varied from 10% to 55% in both adult *(14–17)* and pediatric reports *(18–22)*.

GLUCOSE HOMEOSTASIS

Plasma glucose concentrations are normally maintained within a narrow range reflecting a balance between glucose production and glucose utilization. Postprandially, glucose is derived from carbohydrate sources in the diet, whereas in the fasting state, glucose is released from the liver, initially through glycogenolysis and, with more prolonged fasting, through gluconeogenesis. The kidney may also contribute to overall endogenous glucose production during the postabsorptive state. The kidney has been shown to release glucose in response to both hypoglycemia *(23)* and catecholamines *(24)*, as well as being insulin sensitive *(25)*. In the anhepatic phase of surgery for liver transplantation, the kidney is the only source of sustained glucose production *(26)*. However, its overall contribution to endogenous glucose production in health is still not clear.

The mechanisms of glucose homeostasis are controlled by a complex interaction of hormonal and metabolic regulatory processes that act to maintain a constant supply of circulating glucose, vital for the brain, which can neither store nor synthesize much of this substrate. Insulin is an essential hormone in the maintenance of this glucose balance. Portal venous insulin stimulates glycogen synthesis and suppresses gluconeogenesis, with the effect of decreasing hepatic glucose output. Insulin also has effects on peripheral tissues, with an increase in glucose uptake by adipose tissue and muscle. Decreased hepatic glucose production and an increase in peripheral glucose uptake results in a net decrease in circulating glucose concentrations. One of the earliest responses to a fall in circulating glucose concentration is the curtailment of pancreatic insulin secretion. The inability of the insulin-treated diabetic individual to do this modulating of insulin concentration is the main cause of hypoglycemia in the treatment of type 1 diabetes.

Normally, the effects of insulin are balanced by counterregulatory hormones that oppose the action of insulin and hence prevent a significant fall in glucose. The most important of these hormones is glucagon, which is released from the α-cells of the pancreas immediately when glucose falls below a threshold of 3.6–3.8 mmol/L. Glucagon acts primarily to restore glucose concentrations by increasing glycogenolysis and gluconeogenesis. The mechanism of control of glucagon secretion is still debated *(27)*. Three potential mechanisms may act individually, or in concert. There may be direct effects of glucopenia and hyperinsulinemia or an indirect stimulatory effect via activation of the sympathetic and parasympathetic nervous systems *(27)*. The evidence suggests a major role for falling insulin concentrations within the pancreas in the α-cell response to acute hypoglycemia. Thus, C-peptide-negative diabetic patients have defective glucagon responses specifically to hypoglycemia *(28)*—the second major cause of hypoglycemia in children with type 1 diabetes *(29)*.

Release of catecholamines from the adrenal medulla during hypoglycemia is probably under neural control *(30)*. Catecholamines increase hepatic glucose output by a direct effect on the liver and by stimulating lipolysis, providing a substrate for gluconeogenesis *(31)*. Norepinephrine, released through stimulation of the parasympathetic nervous system, can stimulate hepatic glycogenolysis but has a more potent effect on lipolysis *(32)*. Peripheral glucose uptake is diminished through a direct effect of catecholamines on muscle and adipose tissue *(33)* but also through the provision of alternative substrate in the form of nonesterified fatty acids, glycerol, and ketones. Defects in this third defense against hypoglycemia occur in significant numbers of diabetic patients, further increasing their risk of severe episodes, with loss of cognitive function *(34)*

Growth hormone (GH) and cortisol are also important but work over a much longer time scale. The control of GH secretion during hypoglycemia is incompletely understood, but is probably mediated by secretion of GH releasing hormone (GHRH) from the hypothalamus, which, in turn, stimulates GH release from pituitary somatotrophs—with a 30- to 60-min time lag *(35)*. Reductions in somatostatin and activation of the autonomic nervous system may also play a role (36–39). GH promotes hepatic glucose production and provides substrates for gluconeogenesis by stimulating lipolysis and ketogenesis (40–42).

Adrenocorticotrophic hormone (ACTH) is released from the hypothalamus in response to hypoglycemia by a complex activation of stimulatory and inhibitory pathways *(35)*. The plasma ACTH concentration peaks approx 45 min after the hypoglycemic

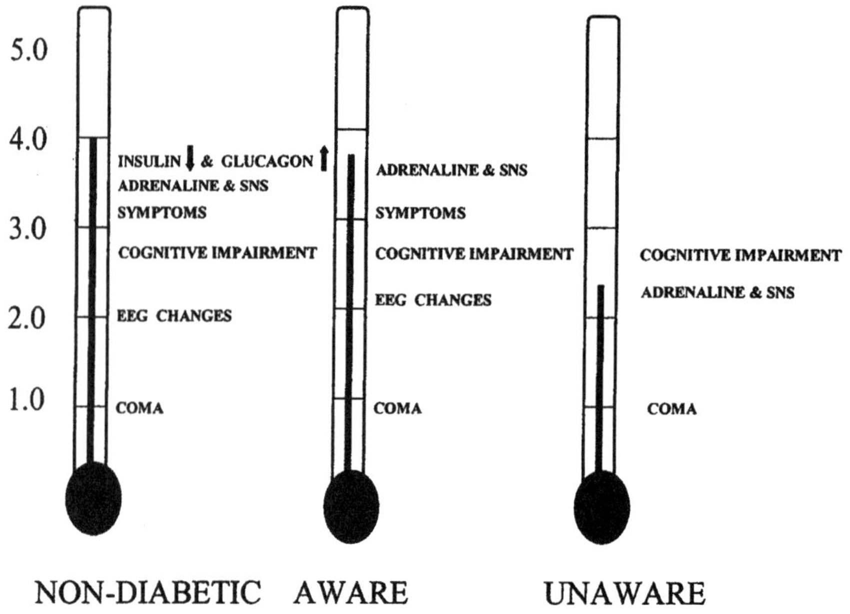

Fig. 1. Schematic representation of counterregulatory responses in healthy diabetic people (left), people with type 1 diabetes and good awareness of hypoglycemia (center), and those with hypoglycaemia unawareness (right). Sympathetic nervous system (SNS) represents sympathetic activation.

nadir *(43)* and stimulates a rise in plasma cortisol within 30 min, with a peak response achieved after 60–90 min *(44)*. Nevertheless, the effects of cortisol on glucose metabolism generally take several hours to become evident *(45)*. Cortisol augments glucose production during protracted hypoglycemia by stimulating gluconeogenesis *(46)*. It also decreases peripheral glucose utilization and increases plasma free fatty acid and ketone concentrations *(46)*.

Glucagon is the most important hormone during hypoglycemia (*see* Fig. 1). Epinephrine is less important in the hierarchy of hormones, but it becomes crucial for effective glucoregulation in the presence of deficient glucagon release *(47)*. GH and cortisol become more important if hypoglycemia is prolonged *(46,48)*.

There are few studies of glucose counterregulation in the pediatric literature *(49–54)*. These studies have confirmed that glucagon responses during hypoglycemia are also lost in children with diabetes soon after diagnosis. This was even the case in a study of very young children, aged 18–57 mo, who had the shortest duration of diabetes *(50)*. Epinephrine responses have been found to be more variable, although the majority suggest that children have exaggerated epinephrine responses during hypoglycemia and this has been postulated as a reason for the glycemic lability that can be observed during childhood *(49,53)* (*see* Fig. 2). Although this exaggerated response is likely to be associated with initiation of responses at a higher glucose level during hypoglycemia than in adults *(53)*, the main cause of elevated and exaggerated responses to acute hypoglycemia is likely to be poor glycemic control, with counterregulatory systems accustomed to a higher blood glucose, in general, and therefore responding to “hypoglycemia” at relatively high glucose levels. More recently, adolescents were found to have blunted epinephrine responses during hypoglycemia *(54)*.

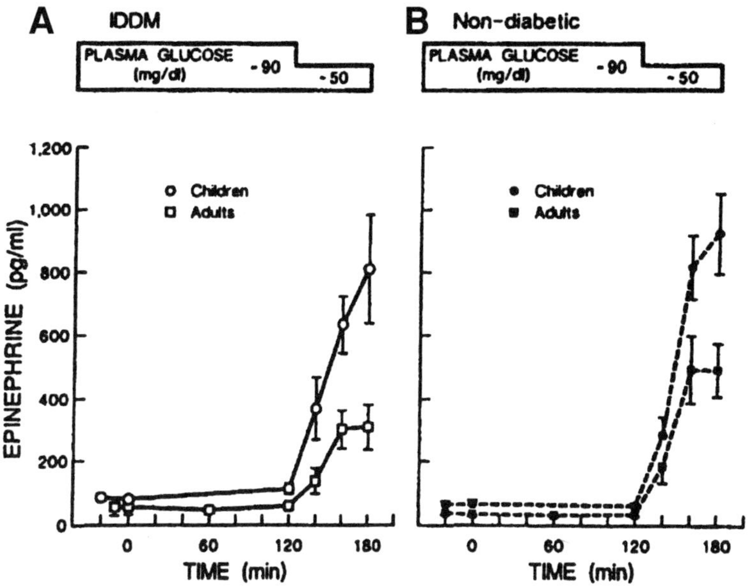

Fig. 2. Mean (± SEM) plasma epinephrine concentrations during sequential euglycemic–hypoglycemic clamp study in 16 children and 11 adults with insulin-dependent diabetes **(A)** and in 14 children and eight adults without diabetes **(B)**. (Reproduced with permission from ref. *49.*)

The reason for the discrepant results compared to the earlier studies may be the result of differences in the techniques of inducing experimental hypoglycemia.

CLINICAL FEATURES

The classical symptoms of hypoglycemia, as seen in adults, are classified into two distinct stages. As glucose concentration falls, a neurohumoral response is provoked that acts both to restore glucose concentrations to normal and to alert the individual to the falling glucose (*see* previous section). This response is partly responsible for the classical autonomic symptoms of hypoglycemia *(5)*. These symptoms warn the individual that the glucose concentration is low and that appropriate action should be taken: in experimentally induced, controlled hypoglycemia, neurohumoral responses usually occur in healthy men at an arterialized plasma glucose of 3.6 mmol/L *(55)* and are more vigorous than in women *(56)*. If glucose concentrations fall further, neuroglycopenia results, usually at a glucose concentration of about 2.8 mmol/L, and it is at this stage that the individual is less likely to be able to manage the episode of hypoglycemia themselves and will require outside assistance. If action is not taken at this stage and glucose concentration falls further, coma or convulsion can ensue. In experimentally induced hypoglycemia, it has been shown that, at any given glucose concentration, the onset of the different components of the responses also occurs in a temporal hierarchy, with immediate onset and resolution of symptoms, delayed onset and quick recovery of catecholamine responses, and immediate onset but delayed recovery of congitive dysfunction *(57)*.

Symptoms of hypoglycemia in childhood may be different. They have been shown not to cosegregate into autonomic and neuroglycopenic categories, and behavioral symptoms are more prominent than those reported in adults *(58)*. The most common presenting symptoms are neuroglycopenic or nonspecific behavioral indicators and

Table 1
Symptoms and Signs of Hypoglycemia in Children

Neuroglycopenic and autonomic	*Behavioral*
Reported by the children	
Weakness	Headache
Trembling	Argumentative
Dizziness	Aggressive
Poor concentration	Irritability
Hunger	Naughty
Sweating	
Confusion	
Blurred vision	
Slurred speech	Nausea
Double vision	Nightmares
Observed by parents	
As above plus	
Pallor	
Sleepiness	
Convulsions	

Source: ref. *58,* with permission.

appear to be different in different age groups of children. Those children less than 6 yr of age are likely to have fewer autonomic symptoms than adolescents (*see* Table 1) *(59).* Because young children are less able to express themselves, signs of hypoglycemia, observed by parents and carers, assume much greater importance than in adults. Other reasons for the discrepancies between children and adults are unclear.

RISK FACTORS

Insulin

Plasma concentrations of insulin in healthy individuals fluctuate from minute to minute, depending on food and exercise. Insulin administration, which fails to mimic the normal pattern of insulin secretion, will predispose to hypoglycemia. In normal physiology, portal concentrations of insulin are up to twofold greater than peripheral concentrations. Exogenous insulin replacement occurs via the peripheral subcutaneous tissues, leading to peripheral hyperinsulinaemia and low portal concentrations of insulin, which do not fluctuate in response to changes in circulating glucose concentrations. This mismatch of insulin delivery and insulin requirements is particularly evident in adolescents whose insulin requirements can be as high as 1.5–2 U/kg/d, reflecting the insulin resistance during this period of rapid growth and development *(60,61).* The need for large doses of insulin, coupled with the imperfections of exogenous insulins in terms of pharmacodynamics and route of administration, can result in an increased risk of intermittent hypoglycemia even when glycemic control is poor *(11).*

Diet

Although little work has been done looking at the effect of diet on rates of hypoglycemia, a number of studies examining the frequency of hypoglycemia have cited missed meals as a significant risk factor for the occurrence of severe hypoglycemia *(59,62,63)*. The question in reverse, as to whether dietary modifications can decrease the likelihood of hypoglycemia, has been addressed and will be discussed later. It is worth noting that in one study of 139 children with type 1 diabetes, 44% of hypoglycemic episodes were thought to be attributable to a missed meal or snack *(64)*.

The effect of alcohol on glycemic control varies between individuals. The oxidation of ethanol by the liver leads to an increase in NADH : NAD ratio, which impairs gluconeogenesis. In the early postabsorptive state, glucose concentrations are maintained by glycogen breakdown in the liver, but as the fast becomes prolonged, gluconeogenesis becomes more important. Individuals with type 1 diabetes are at risk of hypoglycemia for over 12 h following alcohol ingestion, which is, in part, the result of problems of gluconeogenesis, but cannot be entirely explained by this. Furthermore, alcohol ingestion can cause cognitive deficits, which can lead to mistakes regarding insulin administration and food consumption as well as decreased awareness of hypoglycemia *(65)*.

Exercise

Day-to-day differences in level of activity are likely to account for a large proportion of the intraindividual variance in glucose concentrations, particularly in children. The increased need for metabolic fuel in the exercising muscle is met partly by an increase in the uptake and utilization of glucose *(66,67)*. In addition to the acute effects of exercise to increase muscle glucose uptake, the period after exercise is characterized by elevated rates of basal and insulin-stimulated glucose uptake as depleted muscle glycogen is replaced *(68)*. The degree of glycogen depletion resulting from the antecedent exercise is an important factor in determining the rate and duration of the increase in muscle glucose uptake after exercise *(69)*, during which time the muscle is also more sensitive to the actions of insulin *(70)*. The precise mechanism for this increased sensitivity is unclear, but hypoglycemia can occur up to 24 h after vigorous or prolonged exercise.

As early as 1926, it was found that exercise could potentiate the hypoglycemic effect of insulin in patients with type 1 diabetes *(71)*. However, there appears to be no systematic study of the role of exercise in the development of hypoglycemia, particularly nocturnal episodes. Only a few studies, examining the frequency and predisposing factors for hypoglycemia, have shown unplanned exercise to be an important contributory factor in childhood *(59,62,64)*.

Sleep

The night is a particularly problematic time for people with type 1 diabetes, even those with poor glycemic control *(14)*. In the Diabetes Control and Complications Trial (DCCT), over 50 % of severe episodes of hypoglycemia occurred during sleep in both the intensively treated and conventionally treated cohorts *(6)*. Nocturnal hypoglycemia is discussed in detail later.

Age and Duration of Diabetes

Young children are more at risk of severe hypoglycemia, particularly those aged less than 5 yr, possibly as a result of differences in symptomatic awareness *(59)*. Duration of diabetes has also been associated with increased risk of severe hypoglycemia, as has the absence of C-peptide secretion *(29)*. The former may relate to loss of the counter-regulatory response and the latter to a higher requirement of insulin.

Hypoglycemia Unawareness

In diabetes, the best defense against a severe episode of hypoglycemia is the early subjective recognition of a low glucose concentration, prior to the onset of neuroglycopenia with so much congitive impairment that the individual is incapable of reacting in an appropriate way. For people with long-duration diabetes and for those aiming for tight glycemic control (*see* following subsection), hypoglycemia unawareness can become a clinical problem, as the inability to detect falling glucose concentrations is blunted or even lost. This predisposes the individual to unpredictable episodes of hypoglycemia that can be severe. Diabetic patients reporting themselves as unaware or only partially aware of their own hypoglycemia are three times more likely to experience severe hypoglycemic episodes *(9)* and patients with a history of recurrent severe hypoglycemia demonstrate defective counterregulation when challenged with intravenous insulin infusions in a laboratory setting *(34)*. The etiology of hypoglycemia unawareness is uncertain. However, there is a growing body of evidence to implicate hypoglycemia itself as a cause of reduced awareness of subsequent episodes. It has been shown experimentally that even one episode of hypoglycemia can blunt counterregulatory hormone responses to subsequent hypoglycemia in individuals both with and without type 1 diabetes. The degree of hypoglycemia in these experimental studies needed to induce defective responses to a subsequent hypoglycemic challenge is not great and includes 2 h of exposure to arterialized plasma glucose concentrations of 2.8 mmol/L *(72,73)*. Minor defects in counterregulatory hormone responses to subsequent hypoglycemia have been seen with exposure to 2 h at 3.9 mmol/L in healthy adult volunteers *(74)*. Under these conditions, release of counterregulatory hormones is diminished and occurs at lower glucose concentrations than in individuals not exposed to such antecedent hypoglycemia. Normally, autonomic symptoms occur at a glucose concentration of around 3.2 mmol/L and impaired congitive performance at around 2.8 mmol/L. In the hypoglycemia-unaware individual or the individual exposed to antecedent hypoglycemia, the arterialized plasma glucose concentration triggering symptomatic responses can be lowered to as little as 2.1 mmol/L with a less dramatic effect on the reduction in glucose concentration required for significant impairment of cognitive performance *(75–77)*. If the sympatho-adrenal response is not triggered until a lower concentration of glucose, significant cortical neuroglycopenia can ensue before the individual becomes aware of the feeling of a low glucose.

Most compelling as evidence that defective responses to hypoglycemia are induced and sustained by antedent exposure to low blood glucose concentrations are the data showing restoration of symptomatic and counterregulatory hormonal responses to acute hypoglycemia by avoidance of exposure to blood glucose concentrations of less than 3 mmol/L on home glucose monitoring *(76,77)*.

There is also evidence that patients with recurrent severe hypoglycemia may be less sensitive to adrenergic stimulation than normal *(78,79)*. This, too, may be reversible by scrupulous avoidance of hypoglycemia *(80)*.

The mechanisms whereby hypoglycemia begets subsequent hypoglycemia unresponsiveness are not clear. The cortisol responses to the initial hypoglycemia have been implicated *(81)* and there are suggestions that changes in brain glucose metabolism may occur in response to hypoglycemia exposure *(82)*.

Intensive Insulin Therapy

Intensification of insulin therapy commonly leads to a significant increase in the risk of severe hypoglycemia. In the intensively treated cohort of the DCCT, the risk of a first episode of severe hypoglycemia, defined as an episode requiring another person's assistance, increased by 27% for a 10% lowering in monthly HbA1c value *(6)*. This risk was almost twofold greater in the adolescents taking part in the DCCT, despite the fact that they did not achieve the same degree of tight glycemic control as their adult counterparts *(11)*. It is likely that most intensifications of insulin therapy for diabetes increase the frequency of exposure to mild hypoglycemia in daily life *(83)* and that this may create hypoglycemia unawareness as described earlier in the chapter, with its attendent increased risk of severe hypoglycemia.

Young children seem to be at particular risk of severe hypoglycemia, which increases with intensification of insulin treatment *(12,13,63)*. In a study examining the effect of an improvement in mean HbA1c over a 4-yr period, rates of severe hypoglycemia increased dramatically. This effect was most obvious in those children less than 6 yr of age in whom there was a fourfold increase in severe hypoglycemia in the fourth year of the study *(13)*. Nevertheless, conventional therapy also carries high risk of hypoglycemia in children, perhaps especially at night.

NOCTURNAL HYPOGLYCEMIA

Nocturnal hypoglycemia may be considered as the submerged part of the iceberg that constitutes hypoglycemia in insulin therapy. In a study of nocturnal glucose control in young children, episodes of hypoglycemia were observed in 45% of patients studied. The median glucose nadir was 1.9 mmol/L (range: 1.1–3.3) and the median duration of hypoglycemia was 270 min (range: 30–630) *(22)*. There are a number of risk factors for hypoglycemia that are specific to the night. First, the overnight period represents the longest time without food and glucose concentrations are maintained by mobilization of liver glycogen stores and, subsequently, through gluconeogenesis. Adults with diabetes studied during the course of a day during which three mixed meals were ingested were shown to synthesize only one-third of the amount of glycogen that was synthesized by nondiabetic controls *(84)*. This may be, in part, the result of an imbalance in the portal glucagon : insulin ratio, as rates of hepatic glycogen synthesis could be enhanced almost to those of nondiabetic subjects by increasing portal insulin during a hyperinsulinaemic hyperglycaemic clamp *(85)*. It is possible that because mobilization of hepatic glycogen is the main mechanism of preventing hypoglycemia, decreased hepatic glycogen stores might be an important predisposing factor for the development of severe hypoglycemia in patients with type 1 diabetes, particularly overnight.

Second, the problems of mimicking background insulin requirements are exacerbated during the night. Insulin requirements vary from a nadir between 2400 and 0300 to a peak between 0400 and 0800. This so-called "dawn phenomenon" is the result of decreases in intrahepatic and extrahepatic insulin sensitivity, probably as a result of overnight GH secretion *(86)* and is particularly marked during adolescence. Current insulin replacement regimens lead to overinsulinization in the early part of the night, leading to the risk of hypoglycemia at this time. Then, in the early hours of the morning, insulin concentrations are waning at a time when insulin resistance is at its greatest (*see* Fig. 3). This may be a particular problem with conventional, nonintensified twice-daily insulin injection therapy, with the evening intermediate-acting insulin given at the time of the evening meal. In adults, delaying the evening injection of the intermediate-acting insulin to bedtime has recently been shown to benefit fasting glucose concentration and reduce risk of nocturnal hypoglycemia *(88)*.

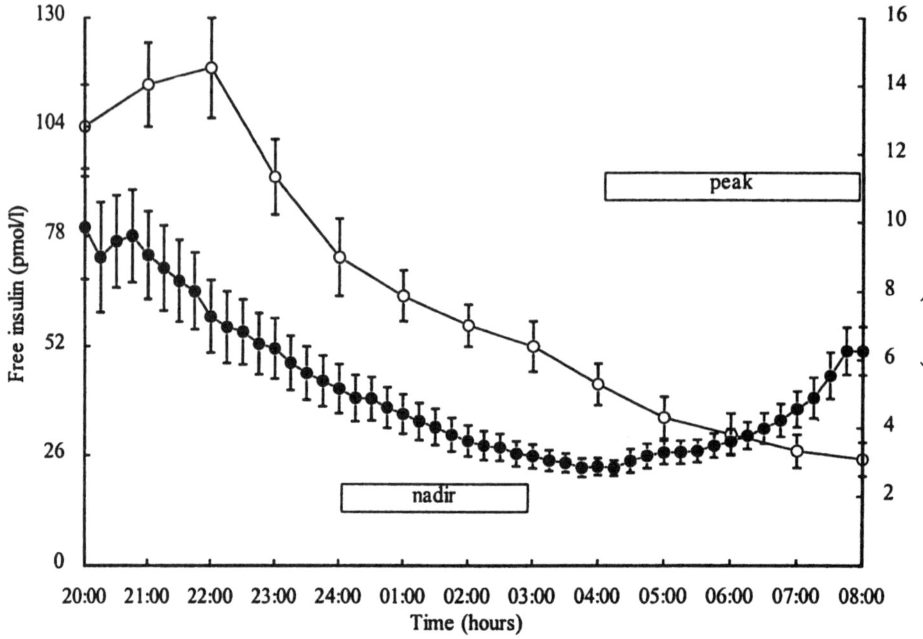

Fig. 3. Glucose (●) and insulin (○) profiles of 16 children taking part in a study of overnight hypoglycemia who had one night of hypoglycaemia and one night without hypoglycaemia for comparison. Data are from the nonhypoglycemic night. Text boxes highlight time of "nadir" and "peak" in insulin resistance overnight. [Data from children taking part in a study of overnight hypoglycemia performed by one of the authors *(87)*.]

Third, the main defense against a severe episode of hypoglycemia is the adequate early subjective recognition of falling glucose concentrations. The great majority of episodes of nocturnal hypoglycemia, even when mild, are asymptomatic *(22)*. The precise reason for this lack of awareness is unclear, as even those with good awareness of hypoglycemia during the day will sleep through hypoglycemia at night. However, there was strong evidence for reduced counterregulatory hormone responses during these spontaneous nocturnal hypoglycemic episodes. Epinephrine responses were blunted and there were no significant increments in either glucagon or cortisol concentrations *(87)*. A few studies have looked for differences between daytime and nighttime counterregulation. No differences were found in early studies, but the stage of sleep during which hypoglycemia was induced was not considered *(89)*. A study examining counterregulatory hormone responses during hypoglycemia induced during slow wave sleep (SWS) in a group of adolescents demonstrated that peak epinephrine responses were significantly lower when hypoglycemia was induced during SWS than when the subjects were awake either during the day or during the night *(90)*. The possibility that counterregulation may be entrained to the sleep stage, reflecting altered cerebral metabolism at different times of the night, deserves further evaluation.

A possible explanation is that cerebral metabolism may be protected during different stages of sleep. Studies of normal sleep in adults have shown that during SWS, cerebral glucose metabolism is decreased, and during rapid eye movement sleep (REM), it is similar to, or even greater, than that seen when the individual is awake *(91,92)*. Therefore, hypoglycemia occurring during SWS may cause less metabolic stress than hypoglycemia occurring at any other time.

Finally, lifestyle can influence nighttime hypoglycemia. In young children, unplanned exercise during the day may lead to delayed hypoglycemia overnight *(59,62)*. In adolescents and adults, alcohol will play an important role in the risk of nocturnal hypoglycemia.

CONSEQUENCES OF HYPOGLYCEMIA

In 1923, Banting et al. reported that "up to the present time no serious mishap has occurred as a result of these hypoglycemic reactions, but while this is so it is felt that hypoglycemia constitutes a real source of danger" *(1)*. Subsequently, much information has been gathered regarding the potential consequences of severe hypoglycaemia, as outlined next.

Defective Counterregulation

As described earlier, impaired hormonal responses to a decrease in blood glucose have been found to occur in adults with type 1 diabetes and manifest as either a diminished hormonal response and/or an altered glucose threshold for hormone release; these defects can be induced by exposure to antecedent hypoglycemia *(73)* and reversed by its elimination *(76,77)*. Defects in counterregulation have been found to occur after only one night of hypoglycemia *(93)*. This leads to delayed glucose recovery, which can result in an increased risk of severe episodes of hypoglycemia resulting in coma or convulsions *(94)*.

Cognitive Function

There have been increasing concerns that recurrent hypoglycemia could affect cognitive function. Glucose has a dual role for normal brain function: as the major metabolic fuel and as a precursor of essential macromolecules during the rapid phase of brain growth *(95)*. There is no doubt that profound and prolonged hypoglycemia can cause catastrophic cerebral damage as occurs in young children from a variety of causes *(96)*. Patients with type 1 diabetes may be at even greater risk, as the hyperinsulinemia that accompanies hypoglycemia also inhibits mobilization of alternative substrates for metabolism, a situation analogous to the hyperinsulinemia/hypoglycemia syndrome of infancy.

Subacute Effects of Hypoglycemia

COGNTIVE EFFECTS AND MOOD

Most research of the acute effects of hypoglycemia on cognitive performance has been performed in adults both with and without diabetes. A variety of neuropsychological tests have been used to assess cognition in these acute situations and there has been considerable variation among study results, depending on glucose nadir achieved and tests employed. The limitation of all of these studies is the difficulty in interpreting psychological test results. Although decrements may be demonstrated, the meaning of these in terms of brain processes is not unequivocal, and it is not clear to what extent they represent abilities that are important in everyday functioning *(97)*.

There is a distinct hierarchy of glycemic thresholds with cerebral dysfunction occurring at a lower glucose threshold than either release of counterregulatory hormones or symptom generation *(98)*. Studies have shown that cognitive function consistently deteriorates at a glucose concentration of about 2.8 mmol/L in adults both with and without type 1 diabetes *(99–101)* but it can occur at a higher glucose concentration, which may indicate that some tests are more sensitive than others in the detection of cognitive dysfunction provoked during hypoglycemia *(99,102)*. Simple motor tasks are relatively unaffected by even marked experimental hypoglycemia *(99,103)*. The functions of attention and vigilance seem to be more susceptible and can be assessed by study of reaction times. Reaction times were prolonged in both diabetic and nondiabetic individuals at a blood glucose of 2.8–3.2 mmol/L *(75,104)*. In a study comparing responses during hypoglycemia between older, 60–70 yr, and younger men, reaction time deteriorated at a higher glucose, 3.0 vs 2.6 mmol/L, and to a greater degree *(55)*.

In addition, the impairment can be multimodal. Simple psychomotor function may be preserved, but more complex tasks may be detrimentally affected *(103,105)*. Subjects may lose volitional control during hypoglycemia, which may magnify any other cognitive impairment that is present *(102)*. Deterioration of cognitive performance at a given glucose concentration may precede generation of symptoms in time *(57)*, although in a gradual fall of blood glucose concentrations, this effect is likely to be overridden by the fact that symptoms are generated at lesser degrees of hypoglycemia. Recovery of cognitive impairment following hypoglycemia may be delayed for up to 1 h *(57,106,107)*. This is important when considering the performance of tasks involving complex skills, such as driving, after apparent recovery from hypoglycemia. In adults, there are concerns that recurrent severe hypoglycemia, from which apparent complete recovery occurs at the time, may have a cumulative effect particularly on memory, but whether this is because memory is poorly formed during a hypoglycemic episode or because of structural damage to memory circuits caused by hypoglycemia is not known.

Although it is difficult to extrapolate from experimental changes in neuropsychological assessment to performance of the day-to-day routines, it is probable that normal functioning will be impaired. Children, who spend the majority of their day at school assimilating information, could be seriously compromised if they regularly experienced episodes of hypoglycemia during class time. There is some evidence that suggests that children may be particularly susceptible to even mild episodes of hypoglycemia: Studies examining p300 evoked potentials and electroencephalogram (EEG) changes have found a deterioration in children at a higher glucose concentration than that found in adults *(108,109)*.

The effect of nocturnal hypoglycemia on cognitive function has been little studied. Neuropsychological performance could be affected by a direct effect of hypoglycemia itself but also by disturbing sleep; a wide range of adverse effects on cognition, mood, and behavior have been reported in both adults and children in relation to reduced duration of sleep, impaired quality of sleep, and timing of the sleep disturbance in relation to the sleep–wake cycle *(110,111)*. The few studies of nocturnal hypoglycemia in adults and adolescents with type 1 diabetes have shown no deleterious effect on overall sleep physiology *(112–114)*. Studies of cognitive function following a night of hypoglycemia have found no significant deterioration in either children or adults *(22,115,116)*. However, detrimental effects on mood the following day have been observed *(22,116)*. The potential effects of lowered mood on subsequent neurocognitive performance remain to be evaluated.

Hypoglycemic Hemiplegia

This is a rare complication of acute hypoglycemia in which the patient recovers from the hypoglycemia with a hemiparesis that may last for several hours, usually less than 24. In children, the syndrome is slightly different than in adults, occurring with equal frequency on the right and left sides, and where neuroimaging has been performed, it is rare to find any abnormality. There is no evidence of severe sequalae *(117)*. Anecdotally, lesser degrees of neurological dysfunction may persist in the hours after recovery from profound hypoglycemia, presumably similar to the well-described postictal state.

Permanent Effects of Hypoglycemia

The long-term risk of recurrent severe episodes of hypoglycemia, involving coma or convulsions, on the development of permanent cognitive impairment remains controversial. Increased cortical atrophy was found in a small group of type 1 diabetic patients with recurrent hypoglycemia compared with a group without such a history *(118)* and there have been concerns that adults experiencing more than five episodes of severe hypoglycemia are in danger of permanent cognitive dysfunction *(119),* but this has remained controversial. Langan and colleagues found increased deterioration in measures of current IQ vs "premorbid" IQ, as measured by reading skills in diabetic patients with more exposure to severe hypoglycemia *(120);* another group later found the association only in patients with neuropathy and complications more related to chronic hyperglycemia *(121)*. Sachon et al. found performance on some cognitive tasks to be less effective in diabetes *per se,* rather than just in association with severe hypoglycemia, whereas others were less well performed only in the patients with severe hypoglycemia *(122)*. Reassuringly, neither the DCCT nor the earlier Stockholm studies found untoward neuropsychological effects of recurrent severe hypoglycemia in their cohort of patients on intensified therapy, despite their higher incidence of severe hypoglycemia *(123,124)*. There were concerns that because neither group lacked severe hypoglycemia and the follow-up was only a median of 6.5 yr, small changes that might have become clinically more significant over time may have been missed. However, analysis has found no difference in cognitive performance in the DCCT patients who had less than one, one to four, or more than four episodes of severe hypoglycemia at 7 yr of follow-up *(125)*.

There continue to be concerns about young children with type 1 diabetes, particularly those diagnosed less than 5 yr of age in whom defects in tests of cognitive function have consistently been found *(126–131)*. In one small study, intensified insulin therapy was associated with a three-fold increase in severe hypoglycemia and the children on that therapy showed a selective relative memory defect, although the diabetic children on conventional therapy shared impaired performance of a motor task *(132)*. It is likely that the developing brain is more susceptible to damage during episodes of metabolic derangement. Deficiencies have been found in a number of cognitive domains but especially those that are more likely to be those originating in the frontal lobe. Not all of these studies have found a link with prior episodes of severe hypoglycemia, although more recent investigations have shown links between hypoglycemia and cognitive impairment. Of more concern was the finding of a correlation between visuospatial problems and episodes of asymptomatic (biochemical) hypoglycemia *(127)*. In one of the few longitudinal studies, Northam and her colleagues have assessed neuropsychological performance in a group of children with newly diagnosed diabetes *(130)*. They were aged from 3 to 14 yr of age and were examined at 3 mo and 2 yr following diagnosis. The results were compared with those from a group of age- and sex-matched "community" controls. Performance scores in a number of cognitive domains were found to be similar in the two groups at baseline but, by 2 yr, children with diabetes had poorer information processing speed, poorer acquisition of new knowledge, and poorer conceptual reasoning abilities. These defects were again more prominent in those with early-onset disease but not restricted to these children. They were related to a prior history of severe hypoglycemia but also with a persistently raised HbA1c over the 2 study years, suggesting that chronic hyperglycemia may also affect cognitive function *(130)*. There are two possible confounding factors: One is that in many studies, reduced cognitive impairment is associated not just with early-onset diabetes but also with severe hypoglycemia complicated by seizure *(129)*, and in a further study from the same group, earlier seizures were the most significant association *(131)*.

Dead in Bed

It has been well established that adolescents and young adults are at a small but significant risk of sudden unexpected death, the so-called "dead-in-bed" syndrome. A recent study from the United Kingdom examining the cause of death in people with type 1 diabetes dying before the age of 20 yr, has suggested that "dead in bed" accounted for up to 11% of all diabetes-related deaths and is restricted to the adolescent age group *(133)*. A similar study from Sweden found that "dead in bed" could account for 25% of deaths in young people with type 1 diabetes *(134)*. The precise mechanism is not known, but a ventricular arrhythmia has been postulated as a possible cause in view of the suddenness and unpredictability of the circumstances.

A number of studies have suggested that subclinical autonomic neuropathy may be common even in young people with type 1 diabetes. Heart rate variability has been shown to be decreased in young children with type 1 diabetes and there is a significant negative correlation with age with pubertal subjects being most at risk *(135,136)*. This suggests an imbalance between sympathetic and parasympathetic tone, with an increase in sympathetic activity that has been found to be a predictor for increased mortality in patients following myocardial infarction *(137)*. As sympathetic predominance increases, the QT interval increases. The QT interval also increases during hypoglycemia, either as a direct effect on the myocardium or possibly the result of catecholamines released during counterregulation *(138)*. Thus, it is conceivable that a fatal ventricular arrhythmia can occur during an episode of nocturnal hypoglycemia in a susceptible individual, such as an adolescent. Why the syndrome appears to occur only at night needs to be clarified.

Fear of Hypoglycemia

There is no doubt that patients worry about the prospect of a severe episode of hypoglycemia *(139)*. It has also been shown that parents of children and spouses of adults with type 1 diabetes also worry about hypoglycemia *(140–142)*. Although there is little evidence that this leads to hypoglycemia-avoiding behavior, such as relaxing glycemic control or increasing snacks, the adverse effects on quality of life should not be underestimated *(139)*.

PREVENTION

There is a tendency to associate severe hypoglycemia with intensified insulin therapy, but it must be remembered that the studies documenting frequent nocturnal hypoglycaemia, especially, were conducted in children on conventional therapy. However, there is little doubt that in children and adolescents with diabetes, lower HbA1c and/or current methods of applying intensfied control increase the risk significantly *(64,132,143)*. The question arises as to whether hypoglycemia, both during the day and at night, can be avoided without compromising overall glycemic control?

Avoidance of Daytime Hypoglycemia

Good hypoglycemia awareness is the best defense against a severe episode of hypoglycemia. Hypoglycemia awareness can be recovered by strict avoidance of hypoglycemia *(77)*. Intensive patient education can lead to improved self-management behavior and, thus, it is likely that some episodes of hypoglycemia may be avoided by a rigorous educational approach *(144)*. One group was able to reduce HbA1c concentrations with a positive decrement in episodic severe hypoglycemia by virtue of a structured intensive teaching program, focusing on patient insulin adjustment *(145)*.

Regular snacking between meals may be necessary to reduce hypoglycemic excursions after meals, while allowing sufficient prandial insulin to be given to control the immediate postprandial blood glucose concentrations and maintain a near-normal HbA1c *(146)*. There is also some early evidence to indicate that replacement of basal insulin by twice-daily isophane insulin may be beneficial, at least in adults, perhaps by reducing the dependency on the meal insulin boluses to provide background between meals. There is some evidence that replacing insulin by continuous subcutaneous insulin infusion (CSII) rather than intermittent injection therapy may reduce rates of hypoglycemia for a given HbA1c, but the evidence is clouded by patient self-selection for CSII therapy *(147)* or general diabetes re-education at the time of starting the new therapy *(148)*.

Recently, successful islet cell transplants have been performed in a small number of patients with extremely problematic hypoglycemia with complete palliation *(149)*. Long-term results of these studies will be eagerly awaited.

Avoidance of Nocturnal Hypoglycemia

Most of the studies investigating hypoglycemia prevention have focused on nocturnal hypoglycemia. There have been a number of studies examining the effect of dietary intervention on the prevalence of nocturnal hypoglycemia. Most of these studies have involved the manipulation of the bedtime snack with uncooked cornstarch being used to provide part of the carbohydrate load. The beneficial effects have been variable. Some studies found a decrease in the rate of nocturnal hypoglycemia, but these studies only looked at one or two glucose concentrations overnight *(150,151)* or relied on self-reporting of overnight hypoglycemia *(152)*. Other studies have found cornstarch to be less useful, although glucose concentrations did fall more slowly following a cornstarch snack *(22,153)*. In one of these studies, hypoglycemia was avoided at the expense of hyperglycemia *(22)*. The role of dietary fiber has also been examined with no beneficial effects on rates of hypoglycemia found *(154)*. One study has found that α-glucosidase inhibitors given to patients with type 1 diabetes do have a beneficial effect on decreasing the frequency of nocturnal hypoglycemia, but there do not appear to have been any further studies *(155)*. Attention to reduced evening intermediate-acting insulins after unusual duration or intensity of exercise is critical.

Probably the best approach to the avoidance of nocturnal hypoglycemia is insulin manipulation. Splitting the evening dose of insulin such that soluble insulin is given with the evening meal and intermediate-acting insulin before bedtime may decrease the frequency of nocturnal hypoglycemia. In this way, the peak action of isophane insulin is delayed until after the time of maximum insulin sensitivity overnight, between midnight and 3 AM. The use of subcutaneous insulin infusion both continuously and just for the overnight period have also been found to be beneficial for both adults and children, presumably by replacing insulin in a more physiological way *(147,156,157)*. The new analog insulins have also been shown to be of some benefit. Rapid-acting insulins can decrease nocturnal hypoglycemia, possibly by causing less overinsulinization in the early part of the night, but often at the expense of hyperglycemia in the earlier part of the night *(158–160)*. The novel long-acting insulins, which have a peakless action profile over 24 h, may also be of use, but there is less published work in this area at the time of writing and none in children *(161)*.

CONCLUSION

There are many unresolved questions regarding the etiology, sequelae, and prevention of this common acute complication of the treatment of type 1 diabetes. Definitions of good glycemic control that do not include a statement about absence of problematic hypoglycemia are incomplete and inadequate. The benefits of long-term good glycemic control cannot be gainsaid, but further progress in the application of intensified diabetes therapy needs to be made before it can be safely applied to all patients with type 1 diabetes. Avoidance of severe hypoglycemia remains an important goal for all patients, and perhaps especially for those under 6 yr of age.

REFERENCES

1. Banting FG, Campbell WR, Fletcher AA. Further clinical experience with insulin (pancreatic extracts) in the treatment of diabetes mellitus. Br Med J 1923;1:8–12.
2. Pramming S, Thorsteinsson B, Bendtson I, Binder C. The relationship between symptomatic and biochemical hypoglycaemia in insulin-dependent diabetic patients. J Intern Med 1990;228:641–646.
3. Field JB. Hypoglycemia. Definition, clinical presentations, classification, and laboratory tests. Endocrinol Metab Clin North Am 1989;18:27–43.
4. Marks V. The measurement of blood glucose and the definition of hypoglycemia. Horm Metab Res 1976;6(Suppl):1–6.
5. Deary IJ, Hepburn DA, MacLeod KM, Frier BM. Partitioning the symptoms of hypoglycaemia using multi-sample confirmatory factor analysis. Diabetologia 1993;36:771–777.
6. The Diabetes Control and Complications Trial Research Group. Hypoglycemia in the Diabetes Control and Complications Trial. Diabetes 1997;46:271–286.
7. Pramming S, Thorsteinsson B, Bendtson I, Binder C. Symptomatic hypoglycaemia in 411 type 1 diabetic patients. Diabet Med 1991;8:217–222.
8. MacLeod KM, Hepburn DA, Frier BM. Frequency and morbidity of severe hypoglycaemia in insulin-treated diabetic patients. Diabet Med 1993;10:238–245.
9. Gold AE, MacLeod KM, Frier BM. Frequency of severe hypoglycemia in patients with type I diabetes with impaired awareness of hypoglycemia. Diabetes Care 1994;17:697–703.
10. Goldstein D, England J, Hess R, Rawlings S, Walker B. A prospective study of symptomatic hypoglycemia in young diabetic patients. Diabetes Care 1981;4:601–605.

11. The Diabetes Control and Complications Trial Research Group. Effect of intensive diabetes treatment on the development and progression of long-term complications in adolescents with insulin-dependent diabetes mellitus: Diabetes Control and Complications Trial. J Pediatr 1994;125:177–188.
12. Mortensen HB, Hougaard P, for the Hvidore Study Group on Childhood Diabetes. Comparison of metabolic control in a cross-sectional study of 2873 children and adolescents with IDDM from 18 countries. Diabetes Care 1997;20:714–720.
13. Davis EA, Keating B, Byrne GC, Russell, Jones TW. Impact of improved glycaemic control on rates of hypoglycaemia in IDDM. Arch Dis Child 1998;78:111–115.
14. Gale EAM, Tatersall RB. Unrecognised nocturnal hypoglycaemia in insulin-treated diabetics. Lancet 1979;i:1049–1052.
15. Pramming S, Thorsteinsson B, Bendtson I, Ronn B, Binder C. Nocturnal hypoglycaemia in patients receiving treatment with insulin. Br Med J 1985;291:376–379.
16. Bendtson I, Gade J, Rosenfalck AM, Thomsen CE, Wildschiodtz G, Binder C. Nocturnal EEG registration in type 1 (insulin-dependent) patients with hypoglycemia. Diabetologia 1991;34:750–756.
17. George E, Bedford C, Peacey SR, Hardisty CA, Heller SR. Further evidence for a high incidence of nocturnal hypoglycaemia in IDDM: no effect of dose for dose transfer between human and porcine insulins. Diabet Med 1997;14:442–448.
18. Whincup G, Milner RDG. Prediction and management of nocturnal hypoglycaemia in diabetes. Arch Dis Child 1987;62:333–337.
19. Beregszaszi M, Tubiana-Rufi N, Benali K, Noel M, Bloch J, Czernichow P. Nocturnal hypoglycemia in children and adolescents with insulin-dependent diabetes mellitus: Prevalence and risk factors. J Pediatr 1997;131:27–33.
20. Porter PA, Keating B, Byrne G, Jones TW. Incidence and predictive criteria of nocturnal hypoglycemia in young children with insulin-dependent diabetes mellitus. J Pediatr 1997;130:366–372.
21. Lopez MJ, Oyarzabal M, Barrio R, Hermoso F, Lopez JP, Rodriguez M, et al. Nocturnal hypoglycaemia in IDDM patients younger than 18 years. Diabet Med 1997;14:772–777.
22. Matyka KA, Wiggs L, Pramming S, Stores G, Dunger DB. Cognitive function and mood following profound nocturnal hypoglycaemia during conventional therapy of diabetes. Arch Dis Child 1999;81: 138–142.
23. Meyer C, Dostou JM, Gerich J. Role of the human kidney in glucose counterregulation. Diabetes 1999;48:943–948.
24. Stumvoll M, Chintalapudi U, Periello G, Gutierrez O, Gerich J. Uptake and release of glucose by the human kidney: postabsorptive rates and responses to epinephrine. J Clin Invest 1995;96:2528–2533.
25. Cersosimo E, Judd RL, Miles JM. Insulin regulation of renal glucose metabolism in conscious dogs. J Clin Invest 1994;93:2584–2589.
26. Joseph SE, Heaton N, Potter D, Pernet A, Umpleby MA, Amiel SA. Renal glucose production compensates for the liver during the anhepatic phase of liver transplantation. Diabetes 2000;49:450–456.
27. Taborsky GJ, Ahren B, Havel PJ. Autonomic mediation of glucagon secretion during hypoglycemia. Implications for impaired α-cell responses in type 1 diabetes. Diabetes 1998;47:995–1005.
28. Landstedt-Hallin L, Adamson U, Lins PE. Oral glibenclamide suppresses glucagon secretion during insulin-induced hypoglycemia in patients with type 2 diabetes. J Clin Endocrinol Metab 1999;84:3140–3145.
29. Egger M, Gschwend S, Smith GD, Zuppinger K. Increasing incidence of hypoglycemic coma in children with IDDM. Diabetes Care 1991;14:1001–1005.
30. Mathias CJ, Frankel HL, Turner RC, Christensen NJ. Physiological responses to insulin hypoglycaemia in spinal man. Paraplegia 1979;17:319–326.
31. Frizzell RT, Campbell PJ, Cherrington AD. Gluconeogenesis and hypoglycemia. Diabetes Metab Rev 1988;4:51–70.
32. Cryer PE. Catecholamines, pheochromocytoma, and diabetes. Diabetes Rev 1993;1:309–317.
33. Clutter WE, Rizza RA, Gerich JE, Cryer PE. Regulation of glucose metabolism by sympathochromaffin catecholamines. Diabetes Metab Rev 1988;4:1–15.
34. Ryder RE, Owens DR, Hayes TM, Ghatei MA, Bloom SR. Unawareness of hypoglycaemia and inadequate hypoglycaemic counterregulation: no causal relation with diabetic autonomic neuropathy. Br Med J 1990;301:783–787.
35. Thompson CJ, Bayliss PH. Endocrine changes during insulin-induced hypoglycaemia. In: Frier B, and Fisher BM, eds. Hypoglycaemia in Clinical Diabetes. Edward Arnold, London 1993, pp. 116–132.

36. Blackgard WG, Hiedingsfelder SA. Adrenergic receptor control mechanism for growth hormone secretion. J Clin Invest 1968;47:1407–1414.
37. Tatar P, Vigas M. Role of α1- and α2-adrenergic receptors in the growth hormone and prolactin response to insulin-induced hypoglycemia in man. Neuroendocrinology 1984;39:275–280.
38. Evans PJ, Dieguez C, Foord SM, Peters JR, Hall R, Scanlon MF. The effect of cholinergic blockade on the growth hormone and prolactin response to insulin hypoglycaemia. Clin Endocrinol 1985;22:733–737.
39. Cordido F, Dieguez C, Casanueva FF. Effect of central cholinergic neurotransmission enhancement by pyridostigmine on the growth hormone secretion elicited by clonidine, arginine or hypoglycaemia in normal and obese subjects. J Clin Endocrinol Metab 1990;70:1361–1370.
40. Metcalfe P, Johnston DG, Nosadini R, Orksov H, Alberti KGMM. Metabolic effects of acute and prolonged growth hormone excess in normal and insulin deficient man. Diabetologia 1981;20:123–128.
41. Bratush-Marrain PR, Smith D, De Fronzo RA. The effect of growth hormone on glucose metabolism and insulin secretion in man. J Clin Endocrinol Metab 1982;55:1648–1658.
42. Sherwin RS, Shulman GA, Hendler R, Walesky M, Belous A, Tamborlane WV. Effect of growth hormone on oral glucose tolerance and circulating metabolic fuels in man. Diabetologia 1983;24:155–161.
43. Donald RA. Plasma immunoreactive corticotrophin and cortisol response to insulin hypoglycemia in normal subjects and subjects with pituitary disease. J Clin Endocrinol Metab 1971;32:225–231.
44. Fish HR, Chernow B, O'Brian JT. Endocrine and neurophysiologic responses of the pituitary to insulin-induced hypoglycemia; a review. Metabolism 1986;35:763–780.
45. Baxter J, Forsham J. Tissue effects of glucocorticoids. Am J Med 1972;53:573–589.
46. DeFeo P, Perriello G, Torlone E, Ventura MM, Fanelli C, Santeusanio F, et al. Contribution of cortisol to glucose counterregulation in humans. Am J Physiol 1989;257:E35–E42.
47. Rizza RA, Cryer PE, Gerich JE. Role of glucagon, catecholamines, and growth hormone in human glucose counterregulation. Effects of somatostatin and combined α- and β-adrenergic blockade on plasma glucose recovery and glucose flux rates after insulin-induced hypoglycemia. J Clin Invest 1979;64:62–71.
48. DeFeo P, Perriello G, Torlone E, Ventura MM, Santeusanio F, Brunetti P, et al. Demonstration of a role for growth hormone in glucose counterregulation. Am J Physiol 1989;256:E835–E843.
49. Amiel SA, Simonson DC, Sherwin RS, Lauritano AA, Tamborlane WV. Exaggerated epinephrine responses to hypoglycemia in normal and insulin-dependent diabetic children. J Pediatr 1987;110:832–837.
50. Brambilla P, Bougneres PF, Santiago JV, Chaussin JL, Pouplard A, Castano L. Glucose counterregulation in pre-school-age children with recurrent hypoglycemia during conventional treatment. Diabetes 1987;36:300–304.
51. Singer-Granick C, Hoffman RP, Kerensky K, Drash AL, Becker DJ. Glucagon responses to hypoglycemia in children and adolescents with IDDM. Diabetes Care 1988;11:643–649.
52. Hoffman RP, Singer-Granick C, Drash AL, Becker DJ. Plasma catecholamine responses to hypoglycemia in children and adolescents with IDDM. Diabetes Care 1991;14:81–88.
53. Jones TW, Boulware SD, Kraemer DT, Caprio S, Sherwin RS, Tamborlane WV. Independent effects of youth and poor diabetes control on responses to hypoglycemia in children. Diabetes 1991;40:358–363.
54. Bjorgaas M, Vik T, Sand T, Birkeland K, Sager G, Vea H, et al. Counterregulatory and symptom responses to hypoglycaemia in diabetic children. Diabet Med 1997;14:433–441.
55. Matyka K, Evans M, Lomas J, Cranston I, Macdonald I, Amiel SA. Altered hierarchy of protective responses against severe hypoglycemia in normal aging in healthy men. Diabetes Care 1997;20:135–141.
56. Amiel SA, Maran A, Powrie JK, Umpleby AM, Macdonald IA. Gender differences in counterregulation to hypoglycaemia. Diabetologia 1993;36:460–464.
57. Evans M, Pernet A, Lomas J, Jones J, Amiel SA. Delay in onset of awareness of acute hypoglycemia and of restoration of cognitive performance during recovery. Diabetes Care 2000;23:893–897.
58. McCrimmon RJ, Gold AE, Deary IJ, Kelnar CJ, Frier BM. Symptoms of hypoglycemia in children with IDDM. Diabetes Care 1995;18:858–861.
59. Tupola S, Rajantie J. Documented symptomatic hypoglycaemia in children and adolescents using multiple daily injection therapy. Diabet Med 1998;15:492–496.
60. Amiel SA, Sherwin RS, Simonson DC, Lauritano AA, Tamborlane WV. Impaired insulin action in puberty: a contributor to poor diabetic control during adolescence. N Engl J Med 1986;315:215–219.

61. Dunger DB. Diabetes in puberty. Arch Dis Child 1992;67:569–570.
62. Daneman D, Frank M, Perlman K, Tamm J, Ehrlich R. Severe hypoglycemia in children with insulin-dependent diabetes mellitus: frequency and predisposing factors. J Pediatr 1989;5:681–685.
63. Davis EA, Keating B, Byrne GC, Russell M, Jones TW. Hypoglycemia: incidence and clinical predictors in a large population based sample of children and adolescents with IDDM. Diabetes Care 1997;20:20–25.
64. Shehadeh N, Kassem J, Tchaban I, Ravid S, Shahar E, Naveh T, et al. High incidence of hypoglycemic episodes with neurologic manifestations in children with insulin dependent diabetes mellitus. J Pediatr Endocrinol Metab 1998;11:183–187.
65. Kerr D, Macdonald IA, Heller SR, Tattersall RB. Alcohol causes hypoglycaemic unawareness in healthy volunteers and patients with type 1 (insulin-dependent) diabetes. Diabetologia 1990;33: 216–221.
66. Richter EA. Glucose utilization. In: Rowell LB, Shepherd JT, eds. Exercise: Regulation and Integration of Multiple Systems. Oxford University Press, New York, 1996, pp. 912–951.
67. Holloszy JO, Hansen PA. Regulation of glucose transport into skeletal muscle. Rev Physiol Biochem Pharmacol 1996;128:99–193.
68. Ivy JL, Holloszy JO. Persistent increase in glucose uptake by rat skeletal muscle following exercise. Am J Physiol 1981;241:C200–C203.
69. Cartee GD, Young DA, Sleeper MD, Zierath J, Wallberg-Henriksson H, Holloszy JO. Prolonged increase in insulin-stimulated glucose transport in muscle after exercise. Am J Physiol 1989;256:E494–E499.
70. Mikines KJ, Sonne B, Farrell PA, Tronier B, Galbo H. Effect of physical exercise on sensitivity and responsiveness to insulin in humans. Am J Physiol 1988;254:E248–E259.
71. Lawrence RD. The effects of exercise on insulin action in diabetes. Br Med J 1926;1:648–652.
72. George E, Marques JL, Harris ND, Macdonald IA, Hardisty CA, Heller SR. Preservation of physiological responses to hypoglycemia 2 days after antecedent hypoglycemia in patients with IDDM. Diabetes Care 1997;20:1293–1298.
73. Ovalle F, Fanelli CG, Paramore DS, Hershey T, Craft S, Cryer PE. Brief twice-weekly episodes of hypoglycemia reduce detection of clinical hypoglycemia in type 1 diabetes mellitus. Diabetes 1998;47:1472–1479.
74. Davis SN, Shavers C, Mosqueda-Garcia R, Costa F. Effects of differing antecedent hypoglycemia on subsequent counterregulation in normal humans. Diabetes 1997;46:1328–1335.
75. Maran A, Lomas J, Macdonald IA, Amiel SA. Lack of preservation of higher brain function during hypoglycaemia in patients with intensively-treated IDDM. Diabetologia 1995;38:1412–1418.
76. Fanelli CG, Epifano L, Rambotti AM, Pampenelli S, Vincenzo A, Modarelli F, et al. Meticulous prevention of hypoglycemia normalizes the glycemic thresholds and magnitude of most of neuroendocrine resposes to, symptoms of, and cognitive function during hypoglycemia in intensively treated patients with short-term IDDM. Diabetes 1993;42:1683–1689.
77. Cranston I, Lomas J, Maran A, Macdonald I, Amiel SA. Restoration of hypoglycaemia awareness in patients with long-duration insulin-dependent diabetes. Lancet. 1994;344:283–287.
78. Berlin I, Grimaldi A, Landault C, Zoghbi F, Thervet F, Puech AJ, et al. Lack of hypoglycemic symptoms and decreased beta-adrenergic sensitivity in insulin-dependent diabetic patients. J Clin Endocrinol Metab 1988;66:273–278.
79. Fritsche A, Stumvoll M, Grub M, Sieslack S, Renn W, Schmulling RM, et al. Effect of hypoglycemia on beta-adrenergic sensitivity in normal and type 1 diabetic subjects. Diabetes Care 1998;21:1505–1510.
80. Fritsche A, Stumvoll M, Haring HU, Gerich JE Reversal of hypoglycemia unawareness in a long-term type 1 diabetic patient by improvement of beta-adrenergic sensitivity after prevention of hypoglycemia. J Clin Endocrinol Metab 2000;85:523–525.
81. Davis SN, Shavers C, Costa F, Mosqueda-Garcia R. Role of cortisol in the pathogenesis of deficient counterregulation after antecedent hypoglycemia in normal humans. J Clin Invest 1996;98:680–691.
82. Boyle PJ, Kempers SF, O'Connor AM, Nagy RJ. Brain glucose uptake and unawareness of hypoglycemia in patients with insulin-dependent diabetes mellitus. N Engl J Med 1995;333:1726–1731.
83. Lager I, Atvall S, Blohme G, Smith U. Altered recognition of hypoglycaemic symptoms in type 1 diabetes during intensified control with continuous subcutaneous insulin infusion. Diabet Med 1986;3:322–325.
84. Hwang J-H, Perseghin G, Rothman DL, Cline GW, Magnusson I, Petersen KF, et al. Impaired net hepatic glycogen synthesis in insulin-dependent diabetic subjects during mixed meal ingestion. J Clin Invest 1995;95:783–787.

85. Cline GW, Rothman DL, Magnusson I, Katz LD, Shulman GI. ^{13}C-nuclear magnetic resonance spectroscopy studies of hepatic glucose metabolism in normal subjects and subjects with insulin-dependent diabetes mellitus. J Clin Invest 1994;94:2369–2376.
86. Perriello G, De Feo P, Torlone E, Fanelli C, Santeusanio F, Brunetti P, et al. Nocturnal spikes of growth hormone secretion cause the dawn phenomenon in type 1 (insulin-dependent) diabetes mellitus by decreasing hepatic (and extrahepatic) sensitivity to insulin in the absence of insulin waning. Diabetologia 1990;33:52–59.
87. Matyka KA, Crowne EC, Havel PJ, Macdonald IA, Matthews D, Dunger DB. Counterregulation during spontaneous nocturnal hypoglycaemia in prepubertal children with insulin dependent diabetes mellitus. Diabetes Care 1999;22:1144–1150.
88. Fanelli CG, Pampanelli S, Porcellati F, et al. Administration of neutral protamine Hagedorn insulin at bedtime versus with dinner in type 1 diabetes mellitus to avoid nocturnal hypoglycemia and improve control. A randomized, controlled trial. Ann Intern Med 2002;136:504–514.
89. Bendtson I, Rosenfalck AM, Binder C. Nocturnal versus diurnal counterregulation to hypoglycemia in type 1 (insulin-dependent) diabetic patients. Acta Endocrinol 1993;128:109–115.
90. Jones TW, Porter P, Sherwin RS, Davis EA, O'Leary P, Frazer F, et al. Decreased epinephrine responses to hypoglycemia during sleep. N Engl J Med 1998;338:1657–1662.
91. Sawaya R, Ingvar DH. Cerebral blood flow and metabolism in sleep. Acta Neurol Scand 1989:80;481–491.
92. Maquet P, Dive D, Salmon E, Sadzot B, Franco G, Poirrier R, et al. Cerebral glucose utilization during the sleep–wake cycle in man determined by positron emission tomography and ^{18}F-2-fluoro-2-deoxy-D-glucose method. Brain Res 1990;513:136–143.
93. Veneman T, Mitrakou A, Mokan M, Cryer P, Gerich J. Induction of hypoglycemia unawareness by asymptomatic nocturnal hypoglycemia. Diabetes 1993;42:1233–1237.
94. Boden G, Reichard GA, Hoeldtke RD, Rezvani I, Owen OE. Severe insulin induced hypoglycemia associated with deficiencies in the release of counterregulatory hormones. N Engl J Med 1981;305:1200–1205.
95. Glazer RI, Weber G. Incorporation of [6-^{3}H] glucose into lipid, protein, RNA and DNA slices of differentiating rat cerebral cortex. J Neurochem 1971;18:1569–1576.
96. Lucas A, Morley R, Cole TJ. Adverse neurodevelopmental outcome of moderate neonatal hypoglycaemia. Br Med J 1988;297:1304–1308.
97. Anastasi A. Validity: basic concepts. In: Psychological Testing, 6th ed. Macmillan, New York. 1988, pp. 139–164.
98. Mitrakou A, Ryan C, Veneman T, Evron W, Jensen T, Cryer P, et al. Hierarchy of glycemic thresholds for activation of counterregulatory hormone secretion, initiation of symptoms and onset of cerebral dysfunction in normal humans. Am J Physiol 1991;260:E67–E74.
99. Hoffman RG, Speelman DJ, Hinnen DA, Conley KL, Guthrie RA, Knapp RK. Changes in cortical functioning with acute hypoglycemia and hyperglycemia in type 1 diabetes. Diabetes Care 1989;12:193–197.
100. Widom B, Simonson DC. Glycemic control and neuropsychologic function during hypoglycemia in patients with insulin-dependent diabetes mellitus. Ann Intern Med 1990;112:904–912.
101. Kerr D, Macdonald IA, Tatersall RB. Patients with type 1 diabetes adapt acutely to sustained mild hypoglycaemia. Diabet Med 1991;8:123–128.
102. Pramming S, Thorsteinsson B, Theilgaard A, Pinner EM, Binder C. Cognitive function during hypoglycaemia in type 1 diabetes mellitus. Br Med J 1986;292:647–650.
103. Holmes CS, Koepke KM, Thompson RG. Simple versus complex performance impairments at three blood glucose levels. Psychoneuroendocrinology 1986;11:353–357.
104. Heller SR, Macdonald IA, Herbert M, Tattersall RB. Influence of sympathetic nervous system on hypoglycaemic warning symptoms. Lancet 1987;2:359–363.
105. Holmes CS. Metabolic control and auditory information processing at altered glucose levels in insulin-dependent diabetes. Brain Cogn 1987;6:161–174.
106. Blackman JD, Towle VL, Lewis GF, Spire J-P, Polonsky KS. Hypoglycemic thresholds for cognitive dysfunction in humans. Diabetes 1990;39:828–835.
107. Herold KC, Polonsky KS, Cohen RM, Levy J, Douglas F. Variable deterioration in cortical function during insulin induced hypoglycemia. Diabetes 1985;34:677–685.
108. Jones TW, Borg WP, Boulware SD, McCarthy G, Sherwin RS, Tamborlane WV. Enhanced adrenomedullary response and increased susceptibility to neuroglycopenia: mechanisms underlying the adverse effects of sugar ingestion in healthy children. J Pediatr 1995:126;171–177.

109. Bjorgaas M, Sand T, Vik T, Jorde R. Quantitative EEG during controlled hypoglycaemia in diabetic and non-diabetic children. Diabet Med 1998;15:30–37.
110. Bonnet MH. Effect of sleep disruption on sleep, performance, and mood. Sleep 1985;8:11–19.
111. Stores G. Children's sleep disorders: modern approaches, developmental effects, and children at special risk. Dev Med Child Neurol 1999;41:568–573.
112. Bendtson I, Gade J, Thomsen CE, Rosenfalck A, Wildschiodtz G. Sleep disturbances in IDDM patients with nocturnal hypoglycemia. Sleep 1992;15:74–81.
113. Porter P, Byrne G, Stick S, Jones TW. Nocturnal hypoglycaemia and sleep disturbances in young teenagers with insulin dependent diabetes mellitus. Arch Dis Child 1996;75:120–123.
114. Matyka KA, Crawford C, Wiggs L, Dunger DB, Stores G. Alterations in sleep physiology in young children with insulin dependent diabetes mellitus: relationship to nocturnal hypoglycemia. J Pediatr 2000;137:233–238.
115. Bendtson I, Gade J, Theilgaard A, Binder C. Cognitive function in type 1 (insulin-dependent) diabetic patients after nocturnal hypoglycaemia. Diabetologia 1992;35:898–903.
116. King P, Kong M-F, Parkin H, Macdonald IA, Tatersall RB. Well-being, cerebral function, and physical fatigue after nocturnal hypoglycemia in IDDM. Diabetes Care 1998;21:341–345.
117. Pocecco M, Ronfani L. Transient focal neurologic deficits associated with hypoglycaemia in children with insulin-dependent diabetes mellitus. Italian Collaborative Paediatric Diabetologic Group. Acta Paediatr 1998;87:542–544.
118. Perros P, Deary IJ, Sellar RJ, Best JJ, Frier BM. Brain abnormalities demonstrated by magnetic resonance imaging in adult IDDM patients with and without a history of recurrent severe hypoglycemia. Diabetes Care 1997;20:1013–1018.
119. Wredling R, Levander S, Adamson U, Lins PE. Permanent neuropsychological impairment after recurrent episodes of severe hypoglycaemia in man. Diabetologia 1990;33:152–157.
120. Langan SJ, Deary IJ, Hepburn DA, Frier BM. Cumulative cognitive impairment following recurrent severe hypoglycaemia in adult patients with insulin-treated diabetes mellitus. Diabetologia 1991;34:337–344.
121. Ryan CM, Williams TM, Finegold DN, Orchard TJ. Cognitive dysfunction in adults with type 1 (insulin-dependent) diabetes mellitus of long duration: effects of recurrent hypoglycaemia and other chronic complications. Diabetologia 1993;36:329–334.
122. Sachon C, Grimaldi A, Digy JP, Pillon B, Dubois B, Thervet F. Cognitive function, insulin-dependent diabetes and hypoglycaemia. J Int Med 1992;231:471–475.
123. Reichard P, Berglund A, Britz A, Levander S, Rosenquist U. Hypoglycaemic episodes during intensified insulin treatment: increased frequency but no effect on cognitive function. J Intern Med 1991;229:9–16.
124. The Diabetes Control and Complications Trial Research Group. Effects of intensive therapy on neuropsychological function in adults in the Diabetes Control and Complications Trial. Ann Intern Med 1996;124:379–388.
125. Austin EJ, Deary IJ. Effects of repeated hypoglycemia on cognitive function. Diabetes Care 1999;22:1273–1277.
126. Ryan C, Vega A, Drash A. Cognitive deficits in adolescents who developed diabetes early in life. Pediatrics 1985;75:921–927.
127. Golden MP, Ingersoll GM, Brack CJ, Russell BA, Wright JC, Huberty TJ. Longitudinal relationship of asymptomatic hypoglycemia to cognitive function in IDDM. Diabetes Care 1989;12:89–93.
128. Bjorgraas M, Gimse R, Vik T, Sand T. Cognitive function in type 1 diabetic children with and without episodes of severe hypoglycaemia. Acta Paediatr 1997;86:148–153.
129. Rovet J, Alvarez M. Attentional functioning in children and adolescents with IDDM. Diabetes Care 1997;20:803–810.
130. Northam EA, Anderson PJ, Werther GA, Warne GL, Andrewes D. Predictors of change in the neuropsychological profiles of children with type 1 diabetes 2 years after disease onset. Diabetes Care 1999;22:1438–1444.
131. Rovet JF, Ehrlich RM. The effect of hypoglycemic seizures on cognitive function in children with diabetes: a seven year prospective study. J Pediatr 1999;134:503–506.
132. Hershey T, Bhargava N, Sadler M, White NH, Craft S. Conventional versus intensive diabetes therapy in children with type 1 diabetes—effects on memory and motor speed. Diabetes Care 1999;22:1318–1324.
133. Edge JA, Ford-Adams ME, Dunger DB. Causes of death in children with insulin dependent diabetes 1990–1996. Arch Dis Child 1999;81:318–323.

134. Sartor G, Dahlquist G. Short-term mortality in childhood onset insulin-dependent diabetes mellitus:a high frequency of unexpected deaths in bed. Diabet Med 1995;12:607–611.
135. Massin MM, Derkenne B, Tallsund M, Rocour-Brumioul D, Ernould C, Lebrethon M, et al. Cardiac autonomic dysfunction in diabetic children. Diabetes Care 1999;22:1845–1850.
136. Rollins MD, Jenkins JG, Carson DJ, McClure BG, Mitchell RH, Imam SZ. Power spectral analysis of the electrocardiogram in diabetic children. Diabetologia 1992;35:452–455.
137. Singh N, Mironov D, Armstrong PW, Ross AM, Langer A. Heart rate assessment early after acute myocardial infarction. Circulation 1996;93:1388–1395.
138. Weston PJ, Gill GV. Is undetected autonomic dysfunction responsible for sudden death in type 1 diabetes mellitus? The "dead in bed" syndrome revisited. Diabet Med 1999;16:626–631.
139. Gold AE, Deary IJ, Frier BM. Hypoglycaemia and non-cognitive aspects of psychological function in insulin-dependent (type 1) diabetes mellitus (IDDM). Diabet Med 1997;14:111–118.
140. Clarke WL, Gonder-Frederick A, Snyder AL, Cox DJ. Maternal fear of hypoglycemia in their children with insulin dependent diabetes mellitus. J Pediatr Endocrinol Metab 1998;11:189–194.
141. Gonder-Frederick L, Cox D, Kovatchev B, Julian D, Clarke W. The psychosocial impact of severe hypoglycemic episodes on spouses of patients with IDDM. Diabetes Care 1997;20:1543–1546.
142. Marrero DG, Guare JC, Vandagriff JL, Fineberg NS. Fear of hypoglycemia in the parents of children and adolescents with diabetes: maladaptive or healthy response? Diabetes Educ 1997;23:281–286.
143. The Diabetes Control and Complications Trial Research Group. The effect of intensive treatment of diabetes on the development and progression of long-term complications in insulin-dependent diabetes mellitus. N Engl J Med 1993;329:977–986.
144. Cox D, Gonder-Frederick L, Polonsky W, Schlundt D, Julian D, Clarke W. A multicenter evaluation of blood glucose awareness training—II. Diabetes Care. 1995;18:523–528.
145. Jorgens V, Grusser M, Bott U, Muhlhauser I, Berger M. Effective and safe translation of intensified insulin therapy to general internal medicine departments. Diabetologia 1993;36:99–105.
146. Orre-Pettersson AC, Lindstrom T, Bergmark V, Arnqvist HJ. The snack is critical for the blood glucose profile during treatment with regular insulin preprandially. J Intern Med 1999;245:41–45.
147. Boland EA, Grey M, Oesterle A, Fredrickson L, Tamborlane WV. Continuous subcutaneous insulin infusion. A new way to lower risk of severe hypoglycemia, improve metabolic control, and enhance coping in adolescents with type 1 diabetes. Diabetes Care 1999;22:1779–1784.
148. Bode BW, Steed RD, Davidson PC. Reduction in severe hypoglycemia with long-term continuous subcutaneous insulin infusion in type I diabetes. Diabetes Care 1996;19:324–327.
149. Shapiro AMJ, Lakey JRT, Ryan EA, Korbutt GS, Toth E, Warnock GL, et al. Islet transplantation in seven patients with type 1 diabetes mellitus using a glucocorticoid-free immunosuppressive regimen. N Engl J Med 2000;343:230–238.
150. Kaufman FR, Halvorson M, Kaufman ND. A randomized, blinded trial of uncooked cornstarch to diminish nocturnal hypoglycemia at diabetes camp. Diabetes Res Clin Pract 1995;30:205–209.
151. Detlofson I, Kroon M, Aman J. Oral bedtime cornstarch supplementation reduces the risk for nocturnal hypoglycaemia in young children with type 1 diabetes. Acta Paediatr 1999;88:595–597.
152. Axelsen M, Wesslau C, Lonnroth P, Arvidsson Lenner R, Smith U. Bedtime uncooked cornstarch supplement prevents nocturnal hypoglycemia in intensively treated type 1 diabetes subjects. J Intern Med 1999;245:229–236.
153. Ververs MT, Rouwe C, Smit GP. Complex carbohydrates in the prevention of nocturnal hypoglycaemia in diabetic children. Eur J Clin Nutr 1993;47:268–273.
154. Buyken AE, Toeller M, Heitkamp G, Vitelli F, Stehle P, Scherbaum WA, et al. Relation of fibre intake to HbA1c and the prevalence of severe ketoacidosis and severe hypoglycaemia. EURODIAB IDDM Complications Study Group. Diabetologia 1998;41:882–890.
155. McCulloch DK, Kutrz AB, Tattersall RB. A new approach to the treatment of nocturnal hypoglycemia using alpha-glucosidase inhibition. Diabetes Care 1983;6:483–487.
156. Kanc K, Janssen MM, Keulen ET, Jacobs MA, Popp-Snijders C, Snoek FJ, et al. Substitution of night-time continuous subcutaneous insulin infusion therapy for bedtime NPH insulin in a multiple injection regimen improves counterregulatory hormonal responses and warning symptoms of hypoglycaemia in IDDM. Diabetologia 1998;41:322–329.
157. Kaufman FR, Halvorson MJ, Kim C. Use of insulin pump therapy at night only for pre-teen children with type 1 diabetes. Diabetes 1999;48:A12.
158. Ahmed AB, Home PD. The effect of the insulin analog lispro on night-time blood glucose control in type 1 diabetic patients. Diabetes Care 1998;21:32–37.

159. Heller SR, Amiel SA, Mansell P. Effect of the fast-acting insulin analog lispro on the risk of nocturnal hypoglycemia during intensified insulin therapy. U.K. Lispro Study Group. Diabetes Care 1999;22:1607–1611.
160. Mohn A, Matyka KA, Harris DA, Ross KM, Edge JA, Dunger DB. Lispro or regular insulin for multiple injection therapy in adolescence. Differences in free insulin and glucose levels overnight. Diabetes Care 1999;22:27–32.
161. Rosskamp RH, Park G. Long-acting insulin analogs. Diabetes Care 1999;22:B109–B113.

19 Pregnancy and Type 1 Diabetes

Erica M. Sommermann, BS,
Erin K. Van Meter, BA, *and Lois Jovanovic*, MD

CONTENTS

INTRODUCTION

Few diabetic women lived to childbearing age before the advent of insulin in 1922. Until then, less than 100 pregnancies were reported in diabetic women and most likely these women had type 2 and not type 1 diabetes. Even with this assumption, these cases of diabetes and pregnancy were associated with a greater than 90% infant mortality rate and a 30% maternal mortality rate *(1,2)*. As late as 1980, physicians were still counseling diabetic women to avoid pregnancy *(3)*. This philosophy was justified because of the poor obstetric history in 30–50% of diabetic women. Improved infant mortality rates finally occurred after 1980, when treatment strategies stressed better control of maternal plasma glucose levels and once self-blood glucose monitoring and hemoglobin A1c became available to enable better metabolic control in persons with diabetes *(3)*. As the pathophysiology of pregnancy complicated by diabetes has been elucidated and as management programs have achieved and maintained near normoglycemia throughout pregnancy complicated by type 1 diabetes, perinatal mortality rates have become comparable to those of the general population *(4)*.

From: *Contemporary Endocrinology: Type 1 Diabetes: Etiology and Treatment*
Edited by: M. A. Sperling © Humana Press Inc., Totowa, NJ

EFFECT OF HYPERGLYCEMIA ON THE FETUS AND THE MOTHER

Fetal Complications Secondary to Maternal Hyperglycemia

If the mother has hyperglycemia, the fetus will be exposed to either sustained hyperglycemia or intermittent periods of hyperglycemia. Both situations prematurely stimulate fetal insulin secretion. The Pedersen hypothesis links maternal hyperglycemia-induced fetal hyperinsulinemia to morbidity of the infant *(2)*. Fetal hyperinsulinemia may cause increased fetal body fat (macrosomia) and, therefore, a difficult delivery, or cause inhibition of pulmonary maturation of surfactant and, therefore, respiratory distress of the neonate. The fetus may also have decreased serum potassium levels caused by the elevated insulin and glucose levels and may, therefore, have cardiac arrhythmias. Neonatal hypoglycemia may cause permanent neurological damage. The maternal postprandial glucose level has been shown to be the most important variable to impact the subsequent risk of neonatal macrosomia *(5)*. When the postprandial glucose levels are maintained below 120 mg/dL 1 h after beginning the meal, the risk of macrosomia is minimized *(5)*.

There is an increased prevalence of congenital anomalies and spontaneous abortions in diabetic women who are in poor glycemic control during the period of fetal organogenesis, which is nearly complete by 7 wk postconception. A woman may not even know she is pregnant at this time. It is for this reason that prepregnancy counseling and planning is essential in diabetic women of childbearing age. Because organogenesis is complete so early on, if a woman presents to her health care team and announces that she has missed her period by only a few days, there is still a chance to prevent cardiac anomalies by swiftly normalizing the glucose levels. However, potential neural tube defects are probably already established by the time the menstrual period is missed.

Glycosylated hemoglobin (HbA1c) values provide the best assessment of the degree of chronic glycemic control, reflecting the average blood glucose concentration during the preceding 6–8 wk. As a result, measurement of HbA1c can, in early pregnancy, estimate the level of glycemic control during the period of fetal organogenesis. There are two important observations in this regard: (1) HbA1c values early in pregnancy are correlated with the rates of spontaneous abortion and major congenital malformations, and (2) normalizing blood glucose concentrations before and early in pregnancy can reduce the risks of spontaneous abortion and congenital malformations nearly to that of the general population *(6–12)*.

One report compared 110 women who were already 6–30 wk pregnant at the time of referral, with 84 women recruited before conception and then put on a daily glucose monitoring regimen *(13)*. The mean blood glucose concentration was between 60 and 140 mg/dL (3.3 and 7.8 mmol/L) in 50% of the latter women. The incidence of anomalies was 1.2% in the women recruited before conception vs 10.9% in those first seen during pregnancy. Very similar findings were noted in another study: 1.4% vs 10.4% incidence of congenital abnormalities *(14)*. Major congenital malformations, which either require surgical correction or significantly affect the health of the child, are more common in infants of poorly controlled diabetic mothers *(15)*.

The increased rate of spontaneous abortion in poorly controlled diabetic women is thought to be secondary to hyperglycemia, maternal vascular disease, including uteroplacental insufficiency, and, possibly, immunologic factors *(7,16)*. In addition, animal studies suggest that hyperglycemia regulates the expression of an apoptosis (programmed cell death) regulatory gene as early as the preimplantation blastocyst stage, resulting in increased DNA fragmentation *(17)*. These findings emphasize the importance of glycemic control at the earliest stages of conception.

Ideally, a diabetic woman would plan her pregnancy so that there is time to create an individualized algorithm of care. When a diabetic woman presents in her first few weeks of pregnancy, there is no time for individualization, and rather rigid protocols must be urgently instituted to provide optimal control within 24–48 h and maintain control thereafter.

Maternal Complications

Women with type 1 diabetes mellitus have a relatively high risk of developing diabetic complications before pregnancy because the onset of the disease occurred at a young age *(18)*. Complications include retinopathy, nephropathy, hypertension, impaired thyroid function, neuropathy, and atherosclerosis, in rare cases. In addition, hyperglycemia in the mother may lead to maternal complications, such as polyhydramnios, urinary tract infections, candidal vaginitis, recurrent spontaneous abortions, and infertility. Because these concomitant diseases affect growth and development of the fetus, it is all the more important to treat and control them. They can be minimized and prevented by tight glycemic control, maintaining HbA1c measurements under 5% in pregnant women. HbA1c values are generally lower in pregnancy because of active hemopoiesis and hemodilution from an expanded blood volume.

Retinopathy

Retinopathy, the growth and deterioration of blood vessels in the retina, leads to impaired vision and blindness. This disease is caused by poor blood circulation in the eye and the interplay of hypoxia with endothelial growth factors as a consequence of continually high blood glucose levels. Although pregnancy is not known to cause retinopathy, it can exacerbate pre-existing disease in the mother *(19)*. The study conducted by Merimee et al. *(20)* in ateliotic dwarfs who lack growth hormone (GH) indicated that the lack of GH may prevent diabetic retinopathy. The investigators did not observe any retinopathy in their study group of patients completely lacking GH. Human chorionic somatomammotropin (HCS), present in high concentrations during pregnancy, is known to have GH-like qualities and may also contribute to the acceleration of neovascularization noted in pregnant women *(21)*. Therefore, careful ophthalmic evaluation and monitoring is necessary before and during pregnancy to screen for any changes in the retina. After screening, proper treatment includes laser therapy for proliferative diabetic retinopathy as well as improving overall glycemic control. Because rapid return to optimal control can itself lead to progression of worsening in retinopathic changes in pregnant women *(22–25)*, it is imperative that an ophthalmologist examine the patient to be able to initiate laser therapy if retinopathy progresses *(18)*.

Nephropathy and Hypertension

Nephropathy and hypertension, common complications of poorly controlled diabetes, can be aggravated during pregnancy. Although the primary cause of nephropathy is a glomerular lesion, atherosclerosis, papillary necrosis, and urinary tract infections can also play contributing roles. Diabetic nephropathy during the first half of pregnancy

Table 1
Important Tests for Monitoring Concomitant Diseases and Glucose During Pregnancies Complicated by Type 1 Diabetes

Test	*Frequency*
Eye examination	Prior to conception and then once each trimester
Kidney function	Prior to conception and once each trimester
Thyroid function	Prior to conception and once each trimester
HbA1c	Prior to conception and once a month
Self-blood glucose monitoring	Premeals and 1-h postmeals Target: capillary whole blood glucose: Premeal < 90 mg/dL Postmeal < 120 mg/dL
Blood pressure and weight	Prior to conception and at each visit

is defined as consistent proteinuria over 300 mg/24 h without the presence of a urinary tract infection. Creatinine clearance should be considered in prepregnancy counseling, because levels lower than 50 mL/min indicate that hypertension may develop during pregnancy *(26)*. A creatinine clearance greater than 50 mL/min (normal: 120–170 mL/min), however, should pose no problems to the pregnancy as long as the mother keeps her blood glucose levels (*see* Table 1) and blood pressure (less than 120/80 mm Hg) in the normal ranges. In some cases, it is necessary to delay treatment of maternal nephropathy until after delivery in order to maintain normalcy in fetal development. The growing child may not be receiving sufficient amounts of nitrogen if the mother presents with low blood protein levels and proteinuria. Appropriate courses of action may include a high-protein diet for the mother or even intravenous protein supplementation in extreme cases. Although this high-protein supplementation may worsen renal disease in the mother, this treatment is justified in order to improve the protein status of the maternal–fetal interface.

Hypertension is associated with diabetic nephropathy and is dangerous in a pregnant woman to both her and the developing fetus. Hypertension should be well under control before considering pregnancy. Common antihypertensive agents such as angiotensin-converting enzyme inhibitors (ACE inhibitors), as well as other medications increasing insulin resistance, should be avoided during pregnancy, as they incur danger to the fetus. ACE inhibitors can, however, be used to treat proteinuria before the pregnancy and discontinued before conception without any negative effects *(27)*. Although the best treatment for hypertension is bed rest and restriction of sodium intake to under 4 g/d, other medications such as α-methyldopa and hydralazine may be used if the blood pressure rises above 130/90 mm Hg *(28)*. In addition, α-adrenergic receptor blockers and calcium channel blockers may also be used.

Thyroid Disease

Thyroid disease is autoimmune disease colinked with diabetes. Physiological stress from pregnancy brings out the tendency toward thyroid disease in diabetic women. Hypothyroidism may lead to gestational hypertension, which, in turn, causes increased incidence of pre-eclampsia and low birth weight *(29)*. Controlling maternal hypothyroidism should be a concern during pregnancy. A study by Haddow and colleagues *(30)* indicates that hypothyroidism in the mother can impair the intellectual development of the child. Therefore, we recommend periodical examinations to ensure normal thyroid function (*see* Table 1).

Hyperthyroidism is accompanied by an overall increase in metabolic activity. This hypermetabolic state becomes especially dangerous during pregnancy, because the mother cannot provide sufficient nourishment for both her child and herself. Fetal malnourishment resulting from hyperthyroidism increases the risk of fetal mortality and reduced birth weight *(31)*. Hyperthyroidism also increases insulin requirements and makes blood glucose control extremely difficult. Antithyroid drugs (ATDs) are the preferred treatment in pregnant women, as opposed to radiation or surgery *(32)*. Furthermore, use of propylthiouracil (PTU) is recommended over methimazole and carbimazole. Combined therapy of ATDs and levothyroxine is discouraged, as it will lead to hypothyroidism and goiter in the fetus *(32)*, because ATDs cross the placenta, whereas thyroxine crosses the placenta poorly, or not at all, remaining bound to the increased thyroxine-binding globulin produced in response to placental estrogen production *(33)*. Perhaps the most dangerous result, however, is the mother's increased level of IgG thyrotropin receptor antibodies (TRAb) that cross the placenta and affect fetal thyroid function in the same way that they affect maternal function (i.e., to stimulate synthesis and secretion of thyroid hormones) *(33)*. PTU, which crosses the placenta, provides both suppression of thyroid function and mild immunosuppression and, hence, is suitable for both mother and fetus. Physicians must monitor the thyroid function in pregnant women with diabetes very closely throughout the duration of the pregnancy, testing at least once each trimester (*see* Table 1). Because the use of prenatal vitamin pills is so standardized, the iodine content consumed may induce thyroid disease, regardless of the mother's preconception nutritional status. Physicians should be mindful of this possibility when caring for pregnant diabetic women, another indication for monitoring maternal thyroid function.

Neuropathy and Atherosclerosis

Pregnant women often experience increased swelling around the wrists and ankles because of the salt and water-retaining tendency of pregnancy-related hormones. Cases of carpal or tarsal tunnel syndrome can aggravate pre-existing background neuropathy into painful overt neuropathy in the hands and feet. Behavioral modification, such as sleeping with the hands and wrists curled to improve circulation and elevating the affected areas at night to drain fluids, can ameliorate the condition. If this proves ineffective, it may be necessary to surgically cut the carpal or tarsal sheaths.

Atherosclerosis is a complication of diabetes that rarely affects diabetic women in their childbearing years because its manifestation occurs 10–15 yr after diabetes onset. If nephropathy and hypertension are present in prepregnancy counseling and testing, however, the physician should assess cardiac function with an exercise stress test. If atherosclerotic heart disease is evident, pregnancy is not advised and, if attempted, could prove fatal to both mother and child *(34)*.

Infection

Special considerations in pregnancy include urinary tract infections, which are reported in as many as 20% of diabetic pregnancies *(35)*. Infection may lead to exaggerated hyperglycemia, which should be normalized to protect the fetus. The woman with diabetes is also subject to the adverse effects of maternal infection with herpes, toxoplasmosis, syphilis, and other infections associated with fetal morbidity and mortality. Antibiotic therapy should be used sparingly, because the fetal serum levels could be

Table 2
Classification of Risk Associated with Type 1 Diabetes During Pregnancy Based on Glycemic Control, Vascular Disease, and Type of Disease

Condition	*Risk classification*
Optimal glucose control[a]	
No vascular disease	Low
Vascular disease	
Retinopathy	Minimal
Neuropathy	Minimal
Nephropathy	Moderate
ASCVD[c]	High
Less than optimal glucose control[b]	
No vascular disease	High
Vascular disease	
Retinopathy	High
Neuropathy	High
Nephropathy	High
ASCVD	High

[a] Optimal glucose control is defined as fasting blood glucose (BG) concentration of 55–65 mg/dL, average BG level of 84 mg/dL, and 1-h postprandial BG value of <120 mg/dL *(5)*.

[b] Less than optimal glucose control status is diagnosed when patient fails to achieve optimal control.

[c] ASCVD, atherosclerotic cardiovascular disease.

significant. Antibiotics usually considered safe in pregnancy include penicillin and erythromycin. Tetracycline and sulfa drugs should be avoided because of their effects on tooth coloration and bilirubin metabolism, respectively.

RISK CLASSIFICATION BASED ON MATERNAL GLUCOSE LEVELS AND MATERNAL VASCULAR COMPLICATIONS

Classifications of pregestational diabetes have been formulated to help the physician predict the outcome of pregnancy for both the mother and child. The White classification categorized diabetic women based on the mode of therapy, duration, age at onset of diabetes, and the degree of vascular compromise of each patient at the beginning of the pregnancy *(1)*. This classification led to confusion, because the "B" determination was given to both the pregnancy-related diabetes (gestational diabetes), which necessitated insulin, and to the pregestational woman with fewer than 10 yr of insulin therapy. However, as the evidence mounts that maternal normoglycemia is necessary at the time of conception, during fetal organogenesis, and throughout gestation, newer classifications place more emphasis on maternal plasma glucose concentrations. Such a classification should include a statement about the control of the patient, with the category of either pregestational or gestational. Criteria for "good diabetic control" should be plasma glucose levels equal to nondiabetic pregnant women. This should include fasting blood glucose concentration of 55–65 mg/dL, average blood glucose level of 84 mg/dL, and 1-h postprandial blood glucose value of less than 120 mg/dL *(5)*. Table 2

Table 3
Diabetogenic Pregnancy-Related Hormones

Hormone	*Onset (in wk)*	*Peak (in wk)*	*Diabetogenic*[a]
Human chorionic gonadotropin (hCG)	2.3	10	0
17-Hydroxy-progesterone (17-OHP)	2.3	8	3
Estradiol (E_2)	3.3	26	1
Prolactin (PRL)	5	10	2
Human chorionic somatomammotropin (hCS)	6.5	26	4
Cortisol	7	26	5
Progesterone (P_4)	9.2	32	3

[a] Arbitrary scale indicating relative effect on insulin requirements (1 being low, 5 being high).

suggests a classification of type 1 diabetes and pregnancy based on both maternal glucose and maternal vascular status.

PATHOPHYSIOLOGY

Diabetogenic Pregnancy Hormones

The natural tendency of normal pregnancy hormones is to sustain elevated postprandial blood glucose levels to provide nourishment to the fetus. Table 3 outlines the sequential rise of these hormones. The first of these hormones, human chorionic gonadotropin (hCG), does not, itself, possess diabetogenic properties. It does, however, maintain the corpus luteum, which produces progesterone, a hormone with powerful anti-insulin properties. Estradiol has weaker diabetogenic traits. Its full effect is difficult to determine because it is released almost simultaneously with the very potent progesterone. The major diabetogenic hormones of the placenta are hCS, previously referred to as human placental lactogen (hPL), and progesterone. Also, serum maternal cortisol levels (both bound and free) are increased. At the elevated levels seen during gestation, prolactin also has a diabetogenic effect *(36)*.

In addition to the increasing anti-insulin hormones of pregnancy, there is also increased degradation of insulin in pregnancy caused by placental enzymes comparable to liver insulinases. The placenta also has membrane-associated insulin-degrading activity *(37)*. Concomitant with the hormonally induced insulin resistance and increased insulin degradation, the rate of disposal of insulin slows. The normal pancreas can adapt to these factors by increasing the insulin secretory capacity up to fourfold. If the pancreas fails to respond adequately to these alterations, gestational diabetes develops.

Insulin Requirements

Women with type 1 diabetes must increase their insulin dosage to compensate for these diabetogenic forces of normal pregnancy. Table 3 shows that insulin requirements increase until wk 32, at which time they stabilize until the end of term. The exact pattern of insulin dosage requirement, however, is still controversial. Many observers have detected a decline in insulin requirement in late first trimester of diabetic pregnancies *(38)*. Others have shown no changes *(39,40)* or an increase *(41–43)*.

Jovanovic et al. *(43)* have described the insulin requirements during pregnancy of a population of well-controlled type 1 diabetic women. They reported the first-trimester

Table 4
Initial Calculation of Insulin Therapy

	Fraction of total insulin dose[a]	
Time	*NPH*	*Regular*
Prebreakfast	5/18	2/9
Prelunch		1/6
Predinner		1/6
Bedtime	1/6	

[a] Total insulin = 0.7 U times present pregnant weight in kilograms for wk 1–18; 0.8 U times present pregnant weight in kilograms for wk 18–26; 0.9 U times present pregnant weight in kilograms for wk 26–36; 1.0 U times present pregnant weight in kilograms for wk 36–40.

insulin requirement to be 0.7 U/kg/d, and 0.8 U/kg/d by the second trimester. By term, the insulin requirement is 0.9–1.0 U/kg/d. The investigators also found that the anti-insulin antibody titer does not affect the insulin requirement or the ability to achieve normoglycemia *(44)*. In another report *(45)*, they showed that the mean insulin requirement during pregnancy was significantly ($p < 0.05$) lower in a group of diabetic women who received human insulin compared to animal insulin.

TREATMENT OF DIABETES DURING PREGNANCY

Insulin Therapy

The normal pancreas secretes 50% of the insulin as mealtime "boluses." This delivery may be mimicked by four injections a day of combinations of neutral protamine Hagedorn (NPH) and regular insulin (*see* Table 4); however, it is possible to decrease the number of injections to three a day if the patient is willing to time her lunch to coincide with the preprogrammed insulin mid-day peak. The total daily dose of insulin is based on the gestational week and the woman's current pregnant body weight. After the initial insulin calculation, the dose is adjusted for each woman until all the blood glucose levels before and after each meal are normal. Six or more glucose measurements each day may be required to optimize therapy (*see* Table 1).

The titration of insulin needs to blood glucose levels is based on frequent monitoring and ensures a smooth increase of insulin as the pregnancy progresses to a higher insulin requirement of up to 1.0 U/kg/24 h at term. Twin gestations will cause an approximate doubling of the insulin requirement throughout pregnancy. The outpatient visits should be frequent enough to provide the needed consultation, guidance, and emotional support to facilitate compliance. Moreover, tests and therapy should be appropriate for gestational age (*see* Table 1). The health care delivery team should put forth an extra effort during pregnancy. Each patient should have telephone access to the team on a 24-h basis for questions concerning therapy, and visits should be frequent (i.e., 2 wk apart). A blood sample to measure glycosylated hemoglobin (hemoglobin A1c), drawn at monthly intervals, helps to confirm that the home blood glucose diary reflects the real maternal blood glucose control. Memory chips in current glucose meters also facilitate documentation of the accuracy of home glucose measurements.

Rationale for the Use of Human Insulin During Pregnancy

Maternal anti-insulin antibodies may contribute to hyperinsulinemia *in utero* and thus potentiate the metabolic aberrations in the fetus. Although insulin does not cross the placenta, antibodies to insulin do cross the placenta and may bind fetal insulin; this necessitates the increased production of free insulin to reestablish normoglycemia. Thus, the anti-insulin antibodies may potentiate the effect of maternal hyperglycemia to produce fetal hyperinsulinemia. Human and highly purified insulins are significantly less immunogenic than mixed beef–pork insulins *(45)*. Human insulin treatment has been reported to achieve improved pregnancy and infant outcome compared to using highly purified animal insulins *(45)*. Recently, the insulin analog lispro (which has the amino acid sequence in the β-chain reversed at position B28, B29) has been reported to be more efficacious than human regular insulin to normalize the blood glucose levels in gestational diabetic women. This insulin rapidly lowered the postprandial glucose levels, resulting in lower glycosylated hemoglobin levels, with fewer hypoglycemic episodes, without increasing the anti-insulin antibody levels *(45)*. Although the safety and efficacy of insulin lispro in the treatment of type 1 and type 2 diabetic women throughout pregnancy is yet not reported, the following discussion helps the clinician decide if the newer insulin's benefit outweighs any risks.

Insulin Lispro Use During Pregnancy

Possible Effects on the Fetus

Diamond and Kormas first questioned the safety of using insulin lispro during pregnancy in a letter to *The New England Journal of Medicine* in 1997 *(46)*. They reported on two patients who used insulin lispro during pregnancies and deliveries. One of these pregnancies was terminated at 20 wk gestation and the second pregnancy resulted in a seemingly healthy infant after elective cesarean delivery, but who subsequently died unexpectedly 3 wk later. Both infants were discovered to have congenital abnormalities, which led the authors to question whether insulin lispro might have teritogenic effects on the fetus, in which case it should not be used during pregnancy. The report causes concerns about insulin lispro use during pregnancy, yet it does not provide conclusive evidence that insulin lispro is responsible for the malformations of the infants mentioned earlier. In fact, there is sufficient reason to doubt that insulin lispro is to blame in the above-described cases, as these isolated case reports were not part of a study and there was no control group. Therefore, the findings should stimulate the conduction of clinical trials testing the safety of insulin lispro during pregnancy, not as evidence that it is unsafe.

Despite the opinion of the authors that poor glycemic control was not responsible for the abnormalities of the infants in the above-described cases, there is insufficient evidence to support this claim. The letter reports that HbA1c levels were determined every 3 mo and that both women had values less than 7% at each test. However, an HbA1c of 7% may be associated with an increased risk of fetal malformations. Because organogenesis is complete within the first 7 wk of pregnancy *(12)* and women tend to improve their glycemic control as the pregnancy progresses, an HbA1c measured at 3 mo of pregnancy is a poor reflection of the mother's blood glucose levels at conception and during the critical first organogenic weeks of pregnancy.

The report also indicates that both women maintained a mean blood glucose level of less than 108 mg/dL. A pregnant woman's target blood glucose should be less than 90 fasting and less than 120 postprandial *(47)*. If the women measured their fasting blood glucose only, the reported mean is obviously too high. If postprandial measurements were also taken into account, the mean is still too high, although less so. According to our classification table (Table 2), these women would be categorized as being at high risk for fetal malformations.

Throughout pregnancy, the second mother was being treated for hypertension, and if the malformations were the result of a medication, perhaps it is unfair to single out insulin lispro. In spite of the medication history, the malformations reported are more indicative of poor glycemic control. Situs inversus, one of the abnormalities in the first infant, occurs almost exclusively in children of mothers with diabetes *(48)*.

During the initial clinical trials testing insulin lispro, pregnant women were excluded. However, some participants became pregnant unexpectedly during the trials and 19 infants were born by these mothers who were using insulin lispro. Of these births, one child had a right dysplastic kidney, but the other 18 were healthy *(49)*.

Jovanovic and associates *(50)* designed a controlled, randomized study in order to compare the immunologic effects of insulin lispro vs regular human insulin when used during gestational diabetes. A group of 42 women with gestational diabetes was randomly divided into 2 groups based on the type of insulin they would use during the study. The two groups showed similar results of rates of cesarean deliveries and length of pregnancy at delivery, and all of the infants born in both groups were healthy. When compared to the regular human insulin group, the insulin lispro group did not show a larger increase of lispro-specific antibodies or insulin-specific antibodies. Umbilical cord blood was analyzed for traces of insulin lispro, but none was found. This is true for the women who received their last dose of lispro hours prior to delivery and for the four women who received lispro during delivery. This outcome suggests that insulin lispro does not cross the placenta. Although these findings emanate from studies in gestational diabetes, there is no reasonable basis that a study done with pregnant type 1 women would generate different results. Insulin aspart and insulin glargine have not been studied in a large clinical trial in pregnancies complicated by type 1 diabetes.

Possible Effects of Lispro on the Mother

The safety of insulin lispro use in pregnant women was brought to the forefront again in 1999 *(51)*. Three instances were reported in which pregnant diabetic women with no previously detected background of diabetic retinopathy quickly developed proliferative diabetic retinopathy while using insulin lispro. Although the authors acknowledge that further research needs to be conducted in a controlled study, the report questioned whether insulin lispro could have some action that makes it responsible for the onset of retinopathy in the above cases. It should be noted, however, that all three women had at least three pre-existing risk factors for retinopathy development regardless of the type of insulin they used: pregnancy, "significant accelerated reduction of HbA1c," and diabetes duration of greater than 6 yr *(52)*. In addition, although the interaction between insulin lispro and the growth promoting factor IGF-1 is not fully understood *(51)*, it is not probable that different insulin types behave differently in this regard *(53)*. A report on 16 pregnant women with type 1 and type 2 diabetes who used insulin lispro and 21 who used regular insulin showed that in both groups combined, none of the 6 women with retinopathy at the beginning of pregnancy had further deterioration of the retina, and the other women had no signs of retinopathy at any time during or surrounding pregnancy *(53)*. There were no new cases of progression of

Table 5
Diet Calculation for Women 80% to 120% of Ideal Body Weight

Time	*Meal*	*Fraction (kcal/24 h)*	*% of daily carbohydrate allowed*
8:00 AM	Breakfast	2/18	10
10:30 AM	Snack	1/18	5
12:00 noon	Lunch	5/18	30
3:00 PM	Snack	2/18	10
5:00 PM	Dinner	5/18	30
8:00 PM	Snack	2/18	5
11:00 PM	Snack	1/18	10

retinopathy in either group. Thus, there is insufficient evidence to identify insulin lispro as responsible for retinal deterioration.

Dietary Prescription and Monitoring

The goal of dietary management for the type 1 diabetic woman is to maintain normoglycemia *(54)*. Moreover, in the type 1 diabetic woman, the food and the insulin must match. The diet shown in Table 5 demonstrates a frequent small-feedings schedule designed to avoid postprandial hyperglycemia and preprandial starvation ketosis, as well as to promote an average weight gain of 12.5 kg in accord with the Committee on Maternal Nutrition *(55)*. In the obese type 1 diabetic woman (>120% of ideal body weight), fewer calories per kilogram of total pregnant weight are needed to prevent ketosis yet provide sufficient nutrition for the fetus and mother (about 24 kcal/kg/24 h). Recently, it has been reported that when overfeeding of the pregnant woman completely suppresses ketone production, there is an increased risk of macrosomia *(56)*.

Glycosylated Hemoglobin Determinations

Glycosylated hemoglobin levels are not sensitive enough to detect minor elevations of glucose and cannot be used as a screening tool for gestational diabetes; however, the glycosylated hemoglobin levels can be used as a monitor of "control" *(6,54)*. Monthly determinations (*see* Table 1) can reinforce the patient's records and are useful when the patient sees her own trends compared with her starting glycosylated hemoglobin level. Treatment decisions should be based solely on the self-monitored glucose levels, complemented by double-checking of this value with a laboratory standard.

The best way to use glycosylated hemoglobin in pregnancy is to create "pregnancy norms." Because the mean plasma glucose level is about 20% lower in pregnancy, the glycosylated hemoglobin levels in normal pregnancy are about 20% lower than nonpregnant levels. Achieving a glycosylated hemoglobin within 6 standard deviations above the mean of nondiabetic women decreases the rates of retinopathy progression *(57)*, spontaneous abortion, and birth defects to near that of the general population *(9–11,57)*. Therefore, optimal therapy demands that normoglycemia be achieved before conception, because most of fetal organogenesis is complete by the seventh or eighth week of gestation *(12)*.

TIMING OF DELIVERY

When pregnancy is complicated by hyperglycemia, the risk of stillbirth increases as term approaches *(58)*. In an attempt to decrease these losses, obstetricians have delivered such pregnancies electively between 35 and 38 wk of gestation. However, this approach may have caused significant neonatal morbidity because of prematurity and hyaline membrane disease *(59)*.

Neonatal morbidity can be markedly reduced if delivery is delayed until pulmonary maturity is documented *(59)*. Eighty percent of preterm infants have some form of morbidity, compared with 40% of term infants *(60)*. Therefore, watchful waiting is warranted after the 36th wk of gestation and should be continued as long as maternal normoglycemia is maintained and as long as the fetus remains stable, as documented by antepartum heart rate testing every 2–3 d and daily fetal movement records. Because programs of normoglycemia are relatively new and because tools for fetal surveillance are improving rapidly, a protocol for optimal fetal surveillance remains to be worked out. At least two sonograms are useful during pregnancy (at 22 and 32 wk) to document gestational age and to diagnose defects *(61)*.

In pregnancies in which glucose control has been less than optimal, the lecithin/sphingomyelin (L/S) ratio of the amniotic fluid should be assessed at 36 or 37 wk of gestation; patients with documented good control do not need early delivery, and there is no need for an amniocentesis *(58)*. The presence of phosphatidylglycerol in the fluid indicates pulmonary maturity *(59,62)*. The fetus with documented pulmonary maturity and poor results on fetal surveillance protocols should be delivered immediately. In the pregnancy in which glucose control is documented to be normal by six daily blood glucose self-determinations and monthly normal glycosylated hemoglobin tests, the woman should be allowed to go to term, as long as the fetal surveillance tests are normal.

INSULIN AND GLUCOSE TREATMENT DURING LABOR

With improvement in antenatal care, intrapartum events play an increasingly crucial role in the outcome of pregnancy *(60,63)*. The artificial β-cell may be used to maintain normoglycemia during labor and delivery, but normoglycemia can be maintained easily by subcutaneous injections *(62,64)*. Before active labor, insulin is required and glucose infusion is not necessary to maintain a blood glucose level of 70–90 mg/dL. With the onset of active labor, insulin requirements decrease, often to zero, and glucose requirements are relatively consistent at 2.55 mg/kg/min. From these data, a protocol for supplying the glucose needs of labor has been developed.

In cases of the onset of active spontaneous labor, insulin is withheld and an intravenous dextrose infusion is begun at a rate of 2.55 mg/kg/min. If labor is latent, normal saline is usually sufficient to maintain normoglycemia until active labor begins, at which time, dextrose is infused at 2.55 mg/kg/min. Blood glucose is then monitored hourly, and if it is below 60 mg/dL, the infusion rate is doubled for the subsequent hour. If the blood glucose rises to more than 120 mg/dL, 2–4 U of regular insulin are given subcutaneously each hour until the blood glucose level is 70–90 mg/dL and is titrated to the target infusion rate of 2.55 mg/kg/min as active labor is achieved. In the case of an elective cesarean section, the bedtime dose of NPH insulin is repeated at 8 AM on the day of surgery and every 8 h if the surgery is delayed. A dextrose infusion may be started if the plasma glucose level falls below 60 mg/dL.

POSTPARTUM

Maternal insulin requirements usually drop precipitously postpartum and these requirements may be decreased for 48–96 h postpartum. Insulin requirements should be recalculated at 0.6 U/kg based on the postpartum weight and should be started when the 1-h postprandial plasma glucose value is above 150 mg/dL or the fasting glucose level is greater than 100 mg/dL. The postpartum caloric requirements are 25 kcal/kg/d, based on postpartum weight. For women who wish to breast feed, the calculation is 27 kcal/kg/d and insulin requirements are 0.6 U/kg/d. The insulin requirement during the night drops dramatically during lactation, owing to the glucose siphoning into the breast milk. Thus, the majority of the insulin requirement is needed during the daytime to cover the increased caloric needs of breast-feeding. Normoglycemia should especially be prescribed for nursing diabetic women, because hyperglycemia elevates milk glucose levels *(65)*.

NEONATAL CARE

If blood glucose concentration is normalized throughout pregnancy in a woman with diabetes, there is no evidence that excess attention need be paid to her offspring. However, if normal blood glucose level has not been documented throughout pregnancy, it is wise to monitor the neonate in an intensive care situation for at least 24 h postpartum. The blood glucose level should be monitored hourly for 6 h. If the neonate shows no signs of respiratory distress, hypocalcemia, or hyperbilirubinemia at 24 h after delivery, discharge to the normal nursery can be safely performed *(53)*.

CONCLUSION

With the advent of tools and techniques to maintain normoglycemia before, during, and between all pregnancies complicated by diabetes, infants of diabetic mothers now have the same chances of good health as those infants born to the nondiabetic woman. Animal and human studies clearly implicate glucose as the teratogen. In the Boston experience, hyperglycemia in the first trimester was associated with a 23% incidence of major malformations; in the East German experience, the malformation rate associated with a first-trimester elevated glycohemoglobin was 15.8% *(7,8)*. In this study, when the glucose was normalized before conception, the malformation rate dropped to 1.6%. These studies and others emphasize the need for preconceptional programs to achieve and maintain normoglycemia *(66,67)*.

The morbidity and subsequent development of the infant of the diabetic mother is associated with hyperglycemia *(68)*. Neonatal macrosomia, hyperinsulinemia, and hypoglycemia improve after maternal glucose is normalized. The authors' series of 53 infants born to 52 type 1 diabetic women who maintained normoglycemia yielded 53 normal infants *(69)*. Therefore, the goal for all pregnancies complicated by diabetes is to achieve and maintain normoglycemia.

REFERENCES

1. White P. Pregnancy and diabetes. In: Marble A, White P, Bradley RF, Krall LP, eds. Joslin's Diabetes Mellitus, 11th ed. Lea & Febiger, Philadelphia, 1971, p. 50.
2. Pedersen J. The pregnant diabetic and her newborn: problems and management. Williams & Wilkins, Baltimore, MD, 1967.
3. Jovanovic L, Peterson CM, Fuhrmann K, eds. Diabetes and Pregnancy: Teratology, Toxicology and Treatment. Praeger, Philadelphia, 1985.
4. Pedersen J, Pedersen LM. Diabetes mellitus and pregnancy: the hyperglycemia, hyperinsulinemia theory and the weight of the newborn baby. In: Rodriguez RR, Vallance-Owen J, eds. Proceedings of the 7th Congress of the International Diabetes Federation. Excerpta Medica, Amsterdam, 1971, p. 678.

5. Jovanovic-Peterson L, Peterson CM, Reed G, et al. Postprandial blood glucose levels predict birthweight: the Diabetes in Early Pregnancy Study. Am J Obstet Gynecol 1991;164:103.
6. Jovanovic L, Peterson CM. The clinical utility of glycosylated hemoglobin. Am J Med 1981;70:331.
7. Miller E, Hare JW, Clogerty JP, et al. Elevated maternal hemoglobin A_{1c} in early pregnancy and major congenital anomalies in infants of diabetic mothers. N Engl J Med 1981;304:1331.
8. Fuhrmann K, Ruher H, Semmler K, et al. Prevention of congenital malformations in infants of insulin dependent diabetic mothers. Diabetes Care 1983;6:219.
9. Mills JL, Simpson JL, Driscoll SG, et al. The National Institutes of Child Health and Human Development—Diabetes in Early Pregnancy Study: Incidence of spontaneous abortion among normal women and insulin dependent diabetic women whose pregnancies were identified within 21 days of conception. N Engl J Med 1988;319:1617.
10. Mills JL, Knopp RH, Simpson JL, et al. Lack of relation of increased malformation roles in infants of diabetic mothers to glycemic control during organogenesis. N Engl J Med 1988;318:671.
11. Kitzmiller JL, Gavin LA, Gin GD, et al. Preconceptional care of diabetes: glycemic control prevents congenital anomalies. JAMA 1991;265:731.
12. Mills JL, Baker L, Goldman A. Malformations in infants of diabetic mothers occur before the seventh gestational week: implications for treatment. Diabetes 1979;23:292.
13. Ylinen K, AuLa P, Stenman UH, et al. Risk of minor and major fetal malformations in diabetics with high hemoglobin A_{1c} values in early pregnancy. Br Med J 1984;289:345.
14. Steel JM, Johnstone FD, Hepburn DA, Smith AF. Can pre-pregnancy care of diabetic women reduce the risk of abnormal babies? Br Med J 1990;301:1070.
15. Cousins L. Etiology and prevention of congenital anomalies among infants of overt diabetic women. Clin Obstet Gynecol 1991;34:481.
16. Kitzmiller JL, Watt N, Driscoll SG. Decidual arteriopathy in hypertension and diabetes in pregnancy and immunofluorescent studies. Am J Obstet Gynecol 1981;141:773.
17. Moley KH, Chi MM, Knudson CM, et al. Hyperglycemia induces apoptosis in pre-implantation embryos through cell death effector pathways. Nat Med 1998;4:1421.
18. Healy K, Jovanovic-Peterson L, Peterson CM. Pancreatic disorders of pregnancy: pregestational diabetes. Endocrinol Metab Clin North Am 1995;24:73–101.
19. Elman KD, Welch RA, Frank RN. Diabetic retinopathy in pregnancy: a review. Obstet Gynecol 1990;75:119.
20. Merimee TJ, Zapf J, Froesch ER. Insulin like growth factors: studies in diabetics with and without retinopathy. N Eng J Med 1983;309:527.
21. Petersen LP, Kundu N. Endocrine assessment of high risk pregnancies. Obstet Gynecol Annu 1980;9:169.
22. Brinchmann-Hanson O, Dahl-Jorgensen K, Hanssen KF, et al. Effects of an intensified insulin treatment on various lesions of diabetic retinopathy. Am J Ophthalmol 1985;100:644.
23. Daneman D, Drash AL, Lobes LA, et al. Progressive retinopathy with improved control in diabetic dwarfism (Mauriac's syndrome). Diabetes Care 1981;4:360.
24. Lawson PM, Champion MC, Canny C, et al. Continuous subcutaneous insulin infusion (CSII) does not prevent progression of proliferative and preproliferative retinopathy. Br J Ophthalmol 1982;66:762.
25. Van Ballegooie E, Hooymans JMM, Timerman Z, et al. Rapid deterioration of diabetic retinopathy during treatment with continuous subcutaneous insulin infusion. Diabetes Care 1984;7:236.
26. Cunningham FG, Cox SM, Harstad TW, et al. Chronic renal disease and pregnancy outcome. Am J Obstet Gynecol 1990;163:453–459.
27. Hugo K, Jovanovic L. Diabetes in pregnancy. In: Leahy JL, Clark NG, Cefalu WT, eds. Medical Management of Diabetes Mellitus. Marcel Dekker, New York, 2000, pp. 183–200.
28. Peterson CM, Jovanovic-Peterson L. Prevalence of hypertension in diabetic patients. Diabetes Prof 1990;1–5.
29. Davis LE, Leveno KJ, Cunningham FG. Hypothyroidism complicating pregnancy. Obstet Gynecol 1988;72:108–112.
30. Haddow JE, Palomaki GE, Allan WC. Maternal thyroid deficiency during pregnancy and subsequent neuropsychological development of the child. N Engl J Med 1999;341:549–555.
31. Gonzalez-Jiminenez A, Fernandez-Soto ML, Escobar-Jiminez F, et al. Thyroid function parameters and TSH-receptor antibodies in healthy subjects and Graves' disease patients: a sequential study before, during and after pregnancy. Thyroidology 1993;5:13,029.
32. Fernandez-Soto ML, Jovanovic LG, Gonzalez-Jiminez A, et al. Thyroid function during pregnancy and the postpartum period: Iodine metabolism and disease states. Endocr Pract 1998;4:97–105.

33. Mestman JH, Goodwin TM, Montoro MM. Thyroid disorders of pregnancy. Endocrinol Metab Clin North Am 1995;24:41–71.
34. Hare JW. Diabetic neuropathy and coronary heart disease. In: Reece EA, Coustan DR, eds. Diabetes Mellitus in Pregnancy, Principles and Practice. Churchill Livingstone, New York, 1988, pp. 515–522.
35. Fuhrmann K. Outcome of normoglycemic diabetic pregnancies in Karlsburg. In: Jovanovic L, Peterson CM, Fuhrmann K, eds. Diabetes and Pregnancy: Teratology, Toxicology and Treatment. Praeger, Philadelphia, 1985, p. 168.
36. Josimovich JB. Placental lactogenic hormone. In: Mintz DH, ed. Endocrinology of Pregnancy. Harper & Row, New York, 1971, pp. 184–196.
37. Klopper A. The assessment of placental function in clinical practice. In: Klopper A, Diczfalusy E, eds. Foetus and Placenta. Blackwell Scientific, Oxford, 1969, p. 471.
38. Pederson J. Weight and length at birth of infants of diabetic mothers. Acta Endocrinol 1954;16:330–342.
39. Rayburn W, Piehl E, Lewis E, Schork A, Sereika S, Zabrensky K. Changes in insulin therapy during pregnancy. Am J Perinatol 1985;2:271–275.
40. Steel JM, Johnstone FD, Hume R, Mao JH. Insulin requirements during pregnancy in women with type 1 diabetes. Obstet Gynecol 1994;83(2):250–258.
41. McManus RM, Ryan EA. Insulin requirements in insulin-dependent and insulin-requiring GDM women during final month of pregnancy. Diabetes Care 1992;15:1323–1327.
42. Langer O, Anyaegbunam A, Brustman L, Guidetti D, Ley J, Mazze R. Pregestational diabetes: insulin requirements throughout pregnancy. Am J Obstet Gynecol 1988;159:616–621.
43. Jovanovic L, Druzin M, Peterson CM. The effect of euglycemia on the outcome of pregnancy in insulin-dependent diabetics as compared to normal controls. Am J Med 1981;71:921–927.
44. Jovanovic L, Mills JL, Peterson CM. Anti-insulin titers do not influence control or insulin requirements in early pregnancy. Diabetes Care 1984;7:68–71.
45. Jovanovic L, Kitzmiller JL, Peterson CM. Randomized trial of human versus animal species insulin in pregnancies complicated by diabetes. Am J Obstet 1992;167:1325–1330.
46. Diamond T, Kormas N. Possible adverse fetal effects of insulin lispro. N Engl J Med 1997;337:1009.
47. Jovanovic L. Role of diet and insulin treatment of diabetes in pregnancy. Clin Obstet Gynecol 2000;43:46.
48. Kucera J. Rate and type of congenital anomalies among offspring of diabetic mothers. J Reprod Med 1971;7:61.
49. Anderson J, Bastyr E, Wishner K. Response to Diamond and Kormas. N Engl J Med 1997;337:1009.
50. Jovanovic L, Illich S, Pettitt D, et al. Metabolic and immunologic effects of insulin lispro in gestational diabetes. Diabetes Care 1999;22:1422.
51. Kitzmiller J, Main E, Ward B, Theiss T, Peterson D. Insulin lispro and the development of proliferative diabetic retinopathy during pregnancy. Diabetes Care 1999;22:874.
52. Jovanovic L. Retinopathy risk: what is responsible? Hormones, hyperglycemia, or humalog? Diabetes Care 1999;22:846.
53. Bhattacharyya A, Vice P. Insulin lispro, pregnancy, and retinopathy. Diabetes Care 1999;22:2101.
54. Jovanovic L, Peterson CM, eds. Contemporary Issues in Nutrition: Diabetes Mellitus. Alan R Liss, New York, 1985.
55. Committee of Nutrition. Nutrition in Maternal Health Care. American College of Obstetricians and Gynecologists, Chicago, IL, 1974.
56. Jovanovic L, Metzger BE, Knopp RH, et al. The diabetes in early pregnancy study: beta-hydroxybutyrate levels in type 1 diabetic pregnancy compared with normal pregnancy. Diabetes Care 1998;21:1978–1984.
57. Chew EY, Mills JL, Metzger BE, et al. The Diabetes in Early Pregnancy Study: metabolic control and progression of retinopathy. Diabetes Care 1995;18:631–637.
58. Gabbe SG, Lowenson RI, Wu PY, Guerra G. Current patterns of neonatal morbidity and mortality in infants of diabetic mothers. Diabetes Care 1978;1:335.
59. Driscoll SG, Benirshke K, Curtis GW. Neonatal deaths among infants of diabetic mothers. Am J Dis Child 1961;100:818.
60. Kenny JD, Adams JM, Corbet AJ, Rudolph AJ. The role of acidosis at birth in the development of hyaline membrane disease. Pediatrics 1976;58:181.
61. Buchanan TA, Kjos, SL, Montoro MN, et al. Use of fetal ultrasound to select metabolic therapy for pregnancies complicated by mild gestational diabetes. Diabetes Care 1994;17:275.
62. Freeman RK. Obstetric management of the diabetic patients. Contemp Obstet Gynecol 1976;1:51.

63. Gurson CT, Etili L, Soyak S. Relation between endogenous lipoprotein lipase activity, free fatty acids, and glucose in plasma of women in labor and of their newborns. Arch Dis Child 1968;43:679.
64. Jovanovic L, Peterson CM. Glucose and insulin requirements during labor in insulin-dependent pregnant diabetic women. Am J Med 1983;75:607.
65. Jovanovic-Peterson L, Fuhrmann K, Hedden K, Walker L, Peterson CM. Maternal milk and plasma glucose and insulin levels: studies in normal and diabetic subjects. Am J Nutr 1989;8:125.
66. Janz NK, Herman WH, Becker MP. Diabetes and pregnancy: factors associated with seeking pre-conception care. Diabetes Care 1995;18:157.
67. Jovanovic L, Peterson CM, Fuhrmann K, eds. Diabetes in Pregnancy: Teratology, Toxicology and Treatment. Praeger, Philadelphia, 1985.
68. Petersen M, Pedersen SA, Greisen G, et al. Early growth delay in diabetic pregnancy: relation to psychomotor development at age 4. Br Med J 1988;296:598.
69. Jovanovic L, Peterson CM, Saxena BB, Dawood MY, Saudek CD. Feasibility of maintaining euglycemia in insulin-dependent diabetic women. Am J Med 1980;68:105–112.

20 Surgery for the Patient with Type 1 Diabetes

Adrian Vella, MD, MRCP (UK)
and Robert A. Rizza, MD

CONTENTS

Advances in the treatment of type 1 diabetes (T1DM) have allowed people with this disease to live longer. Aggressive treatment of complications and the widespread use of renal transplantation and coronary artery bypass grafting have substantially improved quality of life. Consequently, the number of people with T1DM who require elective and emergency surgery has increased.

Surgery and anesthesia affect glucose homeostasis in a variety of ways. Surgery leads to catabolism with hyperglycemia, a decrease in insulin action, and an increased risk of ketoacidosis. It is associated with an increased risk of infection and a period of starvation. The effects of these processes on glucose concentration can be dramatic if not compensated for by an increase in insulin secretion, as is indeed the case in T1DM.

Management of the surgical patient with T1DM is therefore complex and needs to take into account the nature and severity of the surgical intervention, as well as the presence of diabetic complications or other concurrent illnesses present in the patient undergoing the procedure. Preoperative stabilization of glucose concentrations is ideal but is not possible in emergency surgery and is becoming less practical in an environment of cost containment with increasing emphasis on shorter hospital stays.

Therefore, the goals of perioperative management of a person with T1DM is to minimize the risk of ketoacidosis, severe hyperglycemia, or hypoglycemia as well as to facilitate wound healing without prolonging hospitalization.

From: *Contemporary Endocrinology: Type 1 Diabetes: Etiology and Treatment*
Edited by: M. A. Sperling © Humana Press Inc., Totowa, NJ

METABOLIC CONSEQUENCES OF SURGERY IN TYPE 1 DIABETES

Surgery and, to a lesser extent, general anesthesia represent major stress with the release of adrenocorticotropic hormone (ACTH), cortisol, growth hormone, catecholamines, and glucagon. The magnitude of these counterregulatory responses is related to the severity of surgery *(1–3)* and the presence of complications such as sepsis.

In normal subjects, anabolism and catabolism are balanced by a complex interplay between the catabolic "stress" hormones and insulin, the major anabolic hormone. Despite adequate anesthesia, surgery alters carbohydrate metabolism, increases lipolysis, and causes catabolism of tissue protein *(4,5)*. In T1DM endogenous insulin secretion is minimal or absent and, therefore, surgical stress in the presence of a relative or absolute insulin deficiency can lead to unopposed catabolism and, potentially, ketoacidosis.

The loss of body nitrogen after surgery is considered to be a normal response to stress, with nitrogen losses being in proportion to the degree of trauma. Protein turnover as measured by ^{14}C-leucine flux before and after uncomplicated abdominal surgery consistently demonstrates a decreased flux after operation that is primarily the result of a decrease in protein synthesis with an unchanged rate of protein breakdown *(5–7)*.

Hyperglycemia attributed to the concomitant hypersecretion of catecholamines, glucagon, and cortisol has even been described in nondiabetic humans during periods of severe surgical or medical stress *(8–10)*. Routine abdominal surgery such as hysterectomy raises plasma epinephrine and norepinephrine concentrations threefold *(11)*. Elevation of these individual hormones does not cause marked alterations in fasting plasma glucose concentrations in normal subjects. However, a simultaneous infusion of all three hormones at concentrations that reproduce circulating levels occurring in major illness causes marked hyperglycemia in healthy volunteers *(12)*.

Increases in plasma epinephrine concentrations correlate with severity of stress *(13,14)* and can rise to concentrations that produce peripheral lipolysis, elevated plasma glucose and lactate, as well as inhibit insulin secretion in normal subjects *(15,16)*. During surgery in otherwise healthy patients, cortisol and growth hormone are also significantly elevated. Together with a decrease in insulin levels, this can result in mild hyperglycemia in the perioperative period *(17)*.

Epinephrine infusion produces a transient increase in endogenous glucose production (EGP) together with decreased peripheral glucose uptake. Epinephrine is an important hormonal signal for muscle glycogen mobilization and stimulates lipolysis *(18)*. Infusion of glucagon and epinephrine simultaneously has an additive, albeit transient, effect on EGP, but a sustained, additive, and negative effect on peripheral glucose uptake. When epinephrine, cortisol, and glucagon are infused together, there is a sustained and marked increase in EGP, with a concomitant decrease in peripheral glucose uptake *(12)*.

The decrease in insulin secretion produced by surgery in healthy humans is not accompanied by a parallel fall in glucagon concentrations. This leads to a fall in the insulin : glucagon ratio, which further favors hepatic glycogenolysis and gluconeogenesis. Plasma ACTH concentrations and, consequently, cortisol concentrations rise after patients are initially reversed from anesthesia, but these hormone concentrations gradually decrease during the recovery period to within the normal range by the morning of the first postoperative day *(19)*. Although epidural anesthesia is associated with a decreased hyperglycemic response to surgery *(20)*, this cannot be attributed to increased insulin secretion as compared with general anesthesia but rather to less counterregulatory stress hormone secretion *(21)*.

Surgery is associated with insulin resistance that persists for 2–3 wk after uncomplicated abdominal surgery *(22)*. However, postoperative insulin resistance can be overcome provided sufficient insulin is infused to maintain euglycemia *(23)*. Perioperative infusion of insulin and glucose maintains normal insulin sensitivity after uncomplicated abdominal surgery *(24)*. Surgery causes a decrease in insulin-stimulated translocation of glucose transporter (GLUT)-4 in skeletal muscle as well as defective nonoxidative glucose disposal at the level of glycogen synthesis *(25)*. Interestingly, preoperative oral or intravenous administration of carbohydrate reduces postoperative peripheral insulin resistance *(26,27)*. This is associated with increased postoperative glucose oxidation and decreased fatty acid oxidation *(28)*. Lipolysis can adversely affect insulin action by increasing the availability of nonesterified fatty acids (NEFAs) for participation in the glucose–fatty acid cycle. Plasma NEFAs are significantly elevated by surgical stress; administration of insulin does not suppress NEFA concentrations to the degree seen in unoperated subjects.

In rats undergoing laparotomy under ether anesthesia, neither glucose uptake nor lactate output is significantly increased compared to unoperated controls *(29)*. Although subsequent glucose administration causes hyperglycemia in the surgically stressed rat, hepatic glucose output suppresses to an equal degree as in the control unstressed animals. Surgical stress is associated with increased blood lactate concentrations and decreased peripheral glucose uptake. Pyruvate dehydrogenase (PDH) activity is markedly decreased by laparotomy and is not restored by the administration of glucose alone, but it is restored by the concurrent administration of glucose plus insulin. Inhibition of peripheral lipolysis by the addition of 5-methylpyrazole-3-carboxylic acid restores the response of PDH activity to insulin administration, suggesting a role of NEFA in the pathogenesis of decreased insulin action after surgery *(29)*.

EVALUATION OF PATIENTS WITH TYPE 1 DIABETES PRIOR TO SURGERY

The assessment of patients with T1DM prior to surgery centers on the preoperative optimization of glycemic control as well as identification and treatment of diabetic complications that may affect the surgical management as well as its successful outcome. The previous practice of routine preoperative admission is no longer tenable in current health care practice. However, outpatient assessment is not necessarily a poorer substitute.

The history provides essential information such as the presence of complications, duration of diabetes, adherence to treatment, and hypoglycemia unawareness. A complete and accurate drug history will allow the physician to rationalize management and decide which drugs need to be discontinued during hospitalization and which drugs may affect operative risk or mask the symptoms of hypoglycemia. Additional therapy such as β-blockade may be indicated perioperatively.

The goals of glycemic control at this time are to provide reasonable control of blood glucose and therefore prevent unrestrained catabolism and ketoacidosis while avoiding hypoglycemia, which may have disastrous consequences in the unconscious patient. Most patients with T1DM now use intensive insulin therapy with multiple daily injections

(MDI) or continuous subcutaneous infusion. Inspection of the patient's diabetic record (and glycosylated hemoglobin) allows assessment of the adequacy of insulin replacement in the fasting, nonexercising state and the frequency with which fasting blood glucose is in an acceptable range. Frequent glucose monitoring is especially important at this time.

Attention to the systems affected by diabetes is essential, most notably the circulatory and autonomic nervous systems. Autonomic neuropathy is associated with sudden death *(30)* in the perioperative setting as well as a greater need of intraoperative pressors *(31)* to maintain blood pressure. The presence of cardiac dysautonomia is associated with impaired cardiovascular responses to hypotension and anesthesia induction *(32)*.

Patients with T1DM are at increased risk of hypothyroidism and adrenal insufficiency, in isolation or as part of a polyglandular autoimmune endocrinopathy *(33–35)*. Recognition of either condition is important prior to operation.

Cardiac risk management prior to surgery is a controversial subject, especially in T1DM, where cardiovascular disease may be silent or present in an atypical manner. However, surgical risk can be stratified using established risk factors *(36,37)* to identify patients at high risk of perioperative cardiac events. Patients thus identified could subsequently undergo specific investigation as indicated. However, there is little consensus regarding the approach to adopt when severe, correctable coronary artery disease is identified.

Decreased cardiac morbidity can be achieved by prophylactic coronary artery bypass grafting (CABG), a procedure associated with significant morbidity and mortality *(38–40)*. There are little data regarding the value of percutaneous transluminal coronary angioplasty (PTCA) in this setting *(41)* and the long-term results of PTCA in patients with diabetes are disappointing *(42,43)*. Perioperative β-blockade significantly decreases the risk of cardiovascular events in high-risk patients *(44,45)* and may be the ideal intervention prior to elective surgery in the patient with T1DM at moderate to high risk of perioperative cardiovascular events.

MANAGEMENT OF PATIENTS WITH TYPE 1 DIABETES DURING SURGERY

Optimal management of diabetes during surgery requires reliable, frequent blood glucose monitoring as well as timely and appropriate insulin replacement to maintain blood glucose in an acceptable range while avoiding ketoacidosis. The actual regimen adopted depends on the nature of the surgical procedure, expected duration of fasting, as well as the pre-existing insulin regimen. For example, for a patient using an MDI program who is due to undergo cataract extraction, diabetes could be managed by continuing long-acting insulin preparations while omitting the shorter-acting preparations taken with meals. (*see* Table 1).

On the other hand, more complex strategies are necessary for operations requiring prolonged anesthesia and subsequent delay in oral intake. Ideally, care of patients with T1DM undergoing surgery should be supervised by a team with expertise in the management of T1DM *(46)*.

A "no insulin – no glucose" regimen enjoyed some currency because of the demonstration of minimal loss of glucose control in T1DM treated with this regimen *(47)*. However, although starvation may decrease blood glucose, ketone concentrations rise rapidly, as do NEFAs and other indices of catabolism *(48)*.

The introduction of continuous intravenous insulin therapy for the treatment of diabetic ketoacidosis *(49)* led to its application for the treatment of T1DM during surgery

Table 1
Management of Type 1 Diabetes Mellitus in the Patient Undergoing Elective Surgery

	Minor surgery	*Major surgery*
Laboratory investigation	Complete blood count + Glyco-Hb Na^+, K^+, and creatinine APTT/INR if indicated	Complete blood count + Glyco-Hb Na^+, K^+, and creatinine APTT/INR if indicated EKG/lipid profile indicated
Glycemic management	Establish intravenous access Glucose monitoring as indicated Omit short-acting insulin preparations Use basal insulin provided by long-acting insulin or CSII	Establish intravenous access Glucose monitoring as indicated Antibiotic prophylaxis as appropriate Use basal insulin replacement provided by long-acting insulin or CSII or intravenous insulin infusion if indicated Potassium replacement

APTT/INR, activated partial thromboplastin time/international normalized ratio; CSII, continuous subcutaneous insulin infusion.

and other diabetic emergencies *(50–52)*. Taitelman et al. demonstrated improved glycemic control with continuous intravenous insulin infusion, together with glucose over conventional subcutaneous administration of neutral protein Hagedorn (NPH) insulin *(52)*. Similarly, adoption of continuous intravenous insulin infusion for patients with T1DM undergoing renal transplant provided effective glycemic control as compared to patients treated with subcutaneous insulin *(53)*. In the operative setting, absorption of insulin from subcutaneous tissues is likely to be slow, erratic, and unpredictable, secondary to the poor perfusion of these regions in the patient undergoing surgery *(54)*.

The closed-loop "artificial β-cell" or Biostator™ is able to monitor blood glucose continuously and adjust insulin and/or glucose delivery to maintain blood glucose within preset limits. It has been used with some success in patients undergoing CABG *(55,56)*. However, the Biostator is expensive, complex, and labor intensive. It utilizes a double-lumen peripheral-venous sampling line, which is prone to disruption during procedures, leading to submaximal insulin delivery. Furthermore, conventional open-loop insulin delivery is associated with better intraoperative glycemic control in patients with T1DM *(57)*.

Simultaneous infusion of glucose, potassium, and insulin (GKI) has been advocated because of its simplicity and (theoretically) a decreased risk of hyperglycemia or hypoglycemia as compared to separate-line systems *(46,48,58,59)*. However, infusion of glucose and insulin in a fixed ratio does not allow flexibility in dose adjustment in patients who are hyperglycemic or have high insulin requirements preoperatively. Patients with underlying renal disease or who are receiving an angiotensin-converting enzyme inhibitor are at risk of hypercalemia when receiving intravenous potassium. Prolonged GKI infusion may cause dilutional hyponatremia requiring concomitant infusion of 0.9% saline in these situations.

Separate continuous insulin and glucose infusions are now the standard of therapy, coupled with frequent (hourly or two-hourly) monitoring of plasma glucose (*see* Table 2). Infusions are adjusted to allow adequate insulin infusion rates (preventing unrestrained

Table 2
Insulin Infusion Algorithm Utilized in the Management of Patients with Type 1 Diabetes Undergoing Surgery

Blood or plasma glucose (mg/dL)	*iv infusion rate (mL/h)*	*Insulin infusion rate (U/h)*
>400	8	8
351–400	6	6
301–350	4	4
250–300	3	3
200–249	2.5	2.5
150–199	2	2
120–149	1.5	1.5
100–119	1	1
70–99	0	0
<70	0	0

Note: The insulin administered consists of a standard solution of insulin (250 U of regular insulin in 250 mL of 0.45% sodium chloride) delivered by means of an infusion pump.

tissue catabolism and ketoacidosis) while maintaining plasma glucose in the 100- to 200-mg/dL (5.5–11.1 mmol/L) range.

Insulin infusion can be kept relatively constant once a proper "basal" rate has been determined by serial measurements of glucose concentrations. Subcutaneous injections of small doses of rapidly acting insulin can then be utilized to fine-tune glucose concentrations. Another approach is to continue long-acting insulin such as Ultralente™ while omitting short-acting insulin that is generally used with meal ingestion. Similarly, in the patients who receive two injections of NPH or Lente™ insulin, the dose can be reduced by approx 50% to create pseudobasal insulin coverage with regular insulin being given at regular intervals to maintain blood glucose in a (predetermined) goal range. The rationale for such programs is to ensure that adequate basal insulin concentrations are present at all times. If glucose concentrations rise or fall, then basal insulin coverage needs to be increased or decreased.

The principles of intravenous fluid management in the patient with T1DM are identical to those in the nondiabetic patient. Care must be taken to ensure adequate potassium replacement and to avoid lactate-containing intravenous fluids, as these could potentially raise blood glucose by conversion of lactate *(60)*.

A significant proportion of patients undergoing open-heart surgery have diabetes mellitus. The management of diabetes in this setting is complicated by the difficulties in achieving and maintaining reasonable glycemic control. These arise because of the severe degree of insulin resistance that occurs in this setting as well as the use of glucose containing "priming" solutions at induction of cardiac bypass *(61–65)*. A high intraoperative glucose load produces marked hyperglycemia during the hypothermic phase of CABG in nondiabetic humans *(66)*.

The insulin resistance during CABG has been attributed to the severe degree of trauma, the induction of hypothermia, as well as the effects of inotropes on glucose metabolism. Insulin requirements change rapidly and dramatically during open-heart surgery and are highest in the immediate postoperative period *(57,66)*. Intravenous

Table 3
Management of Type 1 Diabetes in the Patient Undergoing Unplanned Minor Surgery

Laboratory investigation
Complete blood count + Glyco-Hb
Na^+, K^+, and creatinine
APTT/INR if indicated
EKG if indicated
Glycemic management
Establish intravenous access
Establish last time of administration and nature of insulin administered
Glucose monitoring as indicated
Omit short-acting insulin preparations
Use basal insulin replacement provided by long-acting insulin or CSII or intravenous insulin infusion if indicated

APTT/INR, activated partial thromboplastin time/international normalized ratio; CSII, continuous subcutaneous insulin infusion.

insulin and frequent glucose monitoring are required in this setting to prevent uncontrolled hyperglycemia. Therapy with GKI is not appropriate in this setting.

Sternal wound infections and sternal dehiscence are more common in patients with diabetes. Dehiscence is more likely to occur in patients with diabetes who have undergone bilateral internal mammary artery bypass grafting *(67,68)*. Optimal glycemic control at the time of surgery should decrease the risk of sternal infection *(69,70)*.

MANAGEMENT OF PATIENTS WITH TYPE 1 DIABETES DURING EMERGENCY SURGERY

Patients with T1DM require emergency surgery with the same frequency as does the general population. Most surgery can be postponed long enough to optimize metabolic status prior to surgery, but this may not always be possible.

Rarely, ketoacidosis may present with abdominal pain that disappears with appropriate treatment *(71–73)*. Conversely, a silent intra-abdominal catastrophe may present with metabolic decompensation and should be considered in the differential diagnosis of unexplained ketoacidosis. A common error in the management of a patient with T1DM who is nauseated and has poor oral intake is to completely withhold insulin therapy. The adoption of MDI programs and increased patient and physician education should decrease the frequency with which this error is made.

Although there is no time for an extensive evaluation of the patient with T1DM prior to emergency surgery, a complete physical examination and history are essential. The insulin regimen followed by the patient is important in determining the subsequent management of the patient. Intravenous delivery of insulin will have to account for subcutaneous injection of insulin in the hours prior to the procedure (*see* Tables 3 and 4).

Appropriate laboratory investigation should include electrolytes, urea, and creatinine as well as measurement of plasma β-hydroxybutyrate and an assessment of acid–base status. An elevated serum amylase is commonly present in ketoacidosis and does not necessarily imply the presence of pancreatitis *(74,75)*. Infection and sepsis are potentially serious complications in people with T1DM and require careful evaluation. Early and appropriate intravenous antibiotic therapy may be life-saving in these settings (*see* Table 4).

Table 4
Management of Type 1 Diabetes in the Patient Undergoing Major Emergency Surgery

Laboratory investigation
Complete blood count + Glyco-Hb
Na^+, K^+, and creatinine
Serum lactate
Serum amylase
β-Hydroxybutyrate
Arterial blood gases if indicated
Blood cultures if indicated
APTT/INR if indicated
EKG if indicated
Glycemic management
Establish intravenous access
Establish last time of administration and nature of insulin administered
Glucose monitoring as indicated
Ensure adequate hydration and K^+ replacement
Intravenous insulin infusion at appropriate rates
Antibiotic therapy as appropriate

CONCLUSION

The management of patients with T1DM during surgery requires careful attention to detail and continuous monitoring by a multidisciplinary team experienced in the care of patients with T1DM. With appropriate insulin replacement as well as careful monitoring to avoid hyperglycemia or hypoglycemia, there is no reason why outcomes in patients with T1DM undergoing surgery should be any different from unselected patients undergoing identical surgical procedures.

REFERENCES

1. Chernow B, Alexander HR, Smallridge RC, et al. Hormonal responses to graded surgical stress. Arch Intern Med 1987;147(7):1273–1278.
2. Thorell A, Efendic S, Gutniak M, et al. Development of postoperative insulin resistance is associated with the magnitude of operation. Eur J Surg 1993;159(11–12):593–599.
3. Frayn KN, Little RA, Maycock PF, Stoner HB. The relationship of plasma catecholamines to acute metabolic and hormonal responses to injury in man. Circ Shock 1985;16(3):229–240.
4. Kaukinen S, Salmi J, Marttinen A, Koivula T. Postoperative hyperglycaemia—are the patients diabetic? Exp Clin Endocrinol 1992;100(3):85–89.
5. O'Keefe SJ, Sender PM, James WP. Proceedings of the Medical Research Society. "Catabolic" loss of body nitrogen in response to surgery. Lancet 1974;2(7888):1035–1038.
6. O'Keefe SJ, Sender PM, Clark CG, James WP. The dynamics of protein metabolism following operative trauma. Clin Sci Mol Med 1974;47(3):15P.
7. Barle H, Nyberg B, Ramel S, et al. Inhibition of liver protein synthesis during laparoscopic surgery. Am J Physiol 1999;277(4 Pt 1):E591–E596.
8. Batstone GF, Hinks L, Whitefoot R, Bloom S, Laing JE. Hormonal changes after thermal injury. J Endocrinol 1976;68(3):38P–39P.
9. Wilmore DW. Carbohydrate metabolism in trauma. Clin Endocrinol Metab 1976;5(3):731–745.
10. Willerson JT, Hutcheson DR, Leshin SJ, et al. Serum glucagon and insulin levels and their relationship to blood glucose values in patients with acute myocardial infarction and acute coronary insufficiency. Am J Med 1974;57(5):747–752.

11. Ratge D, Wiedemann A, Kohse KP, et al. Magnitude and kinetics of alterations in plasma catecholamines and leukocyte beta-adrenergic receptors in response to anaesthesia and surgery. J Clin Chem Clin Biochem 1990;28(6):391–398.
12. Shamoon H, Hendler R, Sherwin RS. Synergistic interactions among antiinsulin hormones in the pathogenesis of stress hyperglycemia in humans. J Clin Endocrinol Metab 1981;52(6):1235–1241.
13. Barton RN, Stoner HB, Watson SM. Relationships among plasma cortisol, adrenocorticotrophin, and severity of injury in recently injured patients. J Trauma 1987;27(4):384–392.
14. Stoner HB, Frayn KN, Barton RN, Threlfall CJ, Little RA. The relationships between plasma substrates and hormones and the severity of injury in 277 recently injured patients. Clin Sci 1979;56(6):563–573.
15. Galster AD, Clutter WE, Cryer PE, Collins JA, Bier DM. Epinephrine plasma thresholds for lipolytic effects in man: measurements of fatty acid transport with [l-^{13}C]palmitic acid. J Clin Invest 1981;67(6):1729–1738.
16. Clutter WE, Bier DM, Shah SD, Cryer PE. Epinephrine plasma metabolic clearance rates and physiologic thresholds for metabolic and hemodynamic actions in man. J Clin Invest 1980;66(1):94–101.
17. Goschke H, Bar E, Girard J, et al. Glucagon, insulin, cortisol, and growth hormone levels following major surgery: their relationship to glucose and free fatty acid elevations. Horm Metab Res 1978;10(6):465–470.
18. Frayn KN. Hormonal control of metabolism in trauma and sepsis. Clin Endocrinol 1986;24(5):577–599.
19. Udelsman R, Norton JA, Jelenich SE, et al. Responses of the hypothalamic–pituitary–adrenal and renin–angiotensin axes and the sympathetic system during controlled surgical and anesthetic stress. J Clin Endocrinol Metab 1987;64(5):986–994.
20. Brandt M, Kehlet H, Binder C, Hagen C, McNeilly AS. Effect of epidural analgesia on the glycoregulatory endocrine response to surgery. Clin Endocrinol 1976;5(2):107–114.
21. Brandt MR, Kehlet H, Faber O, Binder C. C-Peptide and insulin during blockade of the hyperglycaemic response to surgery by epidural analgesia. Clin Endocrinol 1977;6(2):167–170.
22. Thorell A, Efendic S, Gutniak M, et al. Insulin resistance after abdominal surgery. Br J Surg 1994;81(1):59–63.
23. Brandi LS, Frediani M, Oleggini M, et al. Insulin resistance after surgery: normalization by insulin treatment. Clin Sci 1990;79(5):443–450.
24. Nygren JO, Thorell A, Soop M, et al. Perioperative insulin and glucose infusion maintains normal insulin sensitivity after surgery. Am J Physiol 1998;275(1 Pt 1):E140–E148.
25. Thorell A, Nygren J, Hirshman MF, et al. Surgery-induced insulin resistance in human patients: relation to glucose transport and utilization. Am J Physiol 1999;276(4 Pt 1):E754–E761.
26. Nygren J, Soop M, Thorell A, et al. Preoperative oral carbohydrate administration reduces postoperative insulin resistance. Clin Nutr 1998;17(2):65–71.
27. Ljungqvist O, Thorell A, Gutniak M, et al. Glucose infusion instead of preoperative fasting reduces postoperative insulin resistance. J Am Coll Surgeons 1994;178(4):329–336.
28. Nygren J, Thorell A, Efendic S, Nair KS, Ljungqvist O. Site of insulin resistance after surgery: the contribution of hypocaloric nutrition and bed rest. Clin Sci 1997;93(2):137–146.
29. French TJ, Holness MJ, Goode AW, Sugden MC. Acute effects of surgery on carbohydrate production and utilization in the fed rat. Clin Sci 1988;74(1):107–112.
30. Page MM, Watkins PJ. Cardiorespiratory arrest and diabetic autonomic neuropathy. Lancet 1978;1(8054):14–16.
31. Burgos LG, Ebert TJ, Asiddao C, et al. Increased intraoperative cardiovascular morbidity in diabetics with autonomic neuropathy. Anesthesiology 1989;70(4):591–597.
32. Vohra A, Kumar S, Charlton AJ, et al. Effect of diabetes mellitus on the cardiovascular responses to induction of anaesthesia and tracheal intubation. Br J Anaesth 1993;71(2):258–261.
33. Baker JR Jr. Autoimmune endocrine disease. JAMA 1997;278(22):1931–1937.
34. Armstrong L, Bell PM. Addison's disease presenting as reduced insulin requirement in insulin dependent diabetes. Br Med J 1996;312(7046):1601–1602.
35. Leong KS, Wallymahmed M, Wilding J, MacFarlane I. Clinical presentation of thyroid dysfunction and Addison's disease in young adults with type 1 diabetes. Postgrad Med J 1999;75(886):467–470.
36. Goldman L. Multifactorial index of cardiac risk in noncardiac surgery: ten-year status report. J Cardiothorac Anesth 1987;1(3):237–244.
37. Eagle KA, Coley CM, Newell JB, et al. Combining clinical and thallium data optimizes preoperative assessment of cardiac risk before major vascular surgery. Ann Intern Med 1989;110(11):859–866.
38. Hertzer NR, Beven EG, Young JR, et al. Coronary artery disease in peripheral vascular patients. A classification of 1000 coronary angiograms and results of surgical management. Ann Surg 1984;199(2):223–233.

39. Reul GJ Jr, Cooley DA, Duncan JM, et al. The effect of coronary bypass on the outcome of peripheral vascular operations in 1093 patients. J Vasc Surg 1986;3(5):788–798.
40. Foster ED, Davis KB, Carpenter JA, Abele S, Fray D. Risk of noncardiac operation in patients with defined coronary disease: the Coronary Artery Surgery Study (CASS) registry experience. Ann Thorac Surg 1986;41(1):42–50.
41. Huber KC, Evans MA, Bresnahan JF, et al. Outcome of noncardiac operations in patients with severe coronary artery disease successfully treated preoperatively with coronary angioplasty. Mayo Clin Proc 1992;67(1):15–21.
42. The Bypass Angioplasty Revascularization Investigation (BARI) Investigators. Comparison of coronary bypass surgery with angioplasty in patients with multivessel disease. N Engl J Med 1996;335(4):217–225.
43. Influence of diabetes on 5-year mortality and morbidity in a randomized trial comparing CABG and PTCA in patients with multivessel disease: the Bypass Angioplasty Revascularization Investigation (BARI). Circulation 1997;96(6):1761–1769.
44. Mangano DT, Layug EL, Wallace A, Tateo I. Effect of atenolol on mortality and cardiovascular morbidity after noncardiac surgery. Multicenter Study of Perioperative Ischemia Research Group. N Engl J Med 1996;335(23):1713–1720.
45. Poldermans D, Boersma E, Bax JJ, et al. The effect of bisoprolol on perioperative mortality and myocardial infarction in high-risk patients undergoing vascular surgery. Dutch Echocardiographic Cardiac Risk Evaluation Applying Stress Echocardiography Study Group. N Engl J Med 1999;341(24):1789–1794.
46. Thai AC, Husband DJ, Gill GV, Alberti KG. Management of diabetes during surgery. A retrospective study of 112 cases. Diabete Metab 1984;10(2):65–70.
47. Sato T, Hoshi H, Kumon T, et al. Managing diabetic surgical patients with glucose-free saline and insulin. Diabetes Res Clin Pract 1988;5(3):191–195.
48. Alberti KG, Thomas DJ. The management of diabetes during surgery. Br J Anaesth 1979;51(7):693–710.
49. Page MM, Alberti KG, Greenwood R, et al. Treatment of diabetic coma with continuous low-dose infusion of insulin. Br Med J 1974;2(921):687–690.
50. Barnett AH, Robinson MH, Harrison JH, Watkins PJ. Mini-Pump: method of diabetic control during minor surgery under general anaesthesia. Br Med J 1980;280(6207):78–79.
51. Leslie RD, Mackay JD. Intravenous insulin infusion in diabetic emergencies. Br Med J 1978;2(6148):1343–1344.
52. Taitelman U, Reece EA, Bessman AN. Insulin in the management of the diabetic surgical patient: continuous intravenous infusion vs subcutaneous administration. JAMA 1977;237(7):658–660.
53. Meyer EJ, Lorenzi M, Bohannon NV, et al. Diabetic management by insulin infusion during major surgery. Am J Surg 1979;137(3):323–327.
54. Pezzarossa A, Taddei F, Cimicchi MC, et al. Perioperative management of diabetic subjects. Subcutaneous versus intravenous insulin administration during glucose–potassium infusion. Diabetes Care 1988;11(1):52–58.
55. Kuntschen FR, Galletti PM, Hahn C, et al. Alterations of insulin and glucose metabolism during cardiopulmonary bypass under normothermia. J Thorac Cardiovasc Surg 1985;89(1):97–106.
56. Kuntschen F, Galletti PM, Hahn C. Blood glucose control by closed loop insulin delivery during coronary artery bypass surgery. Trans Am Soc Artif Intern Organs 1981;27:241–245.
57. Elliott MJ, Gill GV, Home PD, et al. A comparison of two regimens for the management of diabetes during open-heart surgery. Anesthesiology 1984;60(4):364–368.
58. Husband DJ, Thai AC, Alberti KG. Management of diabetes during surgery with glucose–insulin–potassium infusion. Diabet Med 1986;3(1):69–74.
59. Walts LF, Miller J, Davidson MB, Brown J. Perioperative management of diabetes mellitus. Anesthesiology 1981;55(2):104–109.
60. Thomas DJ, Alberti KG. Hyperglycaemic effects of Hartmann's solution during surgery in patients with maturity onset diabetes. Br J Anaesth 1978;50(2):185–188.
61. Thomas DJ, Hinds CJ, Rees GM. The management of insulin dependent diabetes during cardiopulmonary bypass and general surgery. Anaesthesia 1983;38(11):1047–1052.
62. Gill GV, Sherif IH, Alberti KG. Management of diabetes during open heart surgery. Br J Surg 1981;68(3):171–172.
63. Ekroth R, Berggren H, Bjorntorp P, et al. Effect of valvular aortic stenosis on insulin sensitivity. Scand J Thorac Cardiovasc Surg 1982;16(2):141–144.

64. Stephens JW, Krause AH, Peterson CA, et al. The effect of glucose priming solutions in diabetic patients undergoing coronary artery bypass grafting. Ann Thorac Surg 1988;45(5):544–547.
65. Crock PA, Ley CJ, Martin IK, Alford FP, Best JD. Hormonal and metabolic changes during hypothermic coronary artery bypass surgery in diabetic and non-diabetic subjects. Diabet Med 1988;5(1):47–52.
66. Werb MR, Zinman B, Teasdale SJ, et al. Hormonal and metabolic responses during coronary artery bypass surgery: role of infused glucose. J Clin Endocrinol Metab 1989;69(5):1010–1018.
67. Stahle E, Tammelin A, Bergstrom R, et al. Sternal wound complications—incidence, microbiology and risk factors. Eur J Cardio-Thorac Surg 1997;11(6):1146–1153.
68. Loop FD, Lytle BW, Cosgrove DM, et al. J. Maxwell Chamberlain Memorial Paper. Sternal wound complications after isolated coronary artery bypass grafting: early and late mortality, morbidity, and cost of care. Ann Thorac Surg 1990;49(2):179–186.
69. Furnary AP, Zerr KJ, Grunkemeier GL, Starr A. Continuous intravenous insulin infusion reduces the incidence of deep sternal wound infection in diabetic patients after cardiac surgical procedures. Ann Thorac Surg 1999;67(2):352–360.
70. Zerr KJ, Furnary AP, Grunkemeier GL, et al. Glucose control lowers the risk of wound infection in diabetics after open heart operations. Ann Thorac Surg 1997;63(2):356–361.
71. Rajasoorya C, Wong SF, Chew LS. Diabetic ketoacidosis—a study of 33 episodes. Singapore Med J 1993;34(5):381–384.
72. Campbell IW, Duncan LJ, Innes JA, MacCuish AC, Munro JF. Abdominal pain in diabetic metabolic decompensation. Clinical Significance. JAMA 1975;233(2):166–168.
73. Knight AH, Williams DN, Ellis G, Goldberg DM. Significance of hyperamylasaemia and abdominal pain in diabetic ketoacidosis. Br Med J 1973;3(872):128–131.
74. Moller-Petersen J, Andersen PT, Hjorne N, Ditzel J. Hyperamylasemia, specific pancreatic enzymes, and hypoxanthine during recovery from diabetic ketoacidosis. Clin Chem 1985;31(12):2001–2004.
75. Goldberg DM, Spooner RJ, Knight AH. Proceedings of the Association of Clinical Pathologists, 91st General Meeting. Serum amylase and related enzymes in diabetic ketoacidosis. J Clin Pathol 1973;26(12):985.

IV Long-Term Complications of Type 1 Diabetes

21 Biochemistry and Molecular Biology of Diabetic Complications

Kenya Sakamoto, MD, PhD
and Michael Brownlee, MD

CONTENTS

INTRODUCTION

Type 1 diabetes is, by far, the most common serious metabolic disorder in children. Type 1 diabetes is characterized by hyperglycemia, an absolute lack of insulin, and the development of diabetes-specific microvascular pathology in the retina, renal glomerulus, peripheral nerve, and macrovascular changes in the arteries. As a consequence of this microvascular pathology, diabetes is now the leading cause of new blindness in people age 20–74 yr and the leading cause of end-stage renal disease. Patients with diabetes are the fastest growing group of recipients for renal dialysis and transplantation. The life expectancy for patients with diabetic end-stage renal failure is only 3 or 4 yr. Over 60% of patients with diabetes are affected by neuropathy, which includes distal symmetrical polyneuropathy, mononeuropathies, and a variety of autonomic neuropathies causing erectile dysfunction, urinary incontinence, gastroparesis, and nocturnal diarrhea. Accelerated lower extremity arterial disease in conjunction with neuropathy makes diabetes account for 50% of all nontraumatic amputations in the United States. The risk for developing cardiovascular complications is increased twofold to sixfold in subjects with diabetes *(1)*. Life expectancy is about 7–10 yr shorter than for people without diabetes *(2)*.

Epidemiological studies show a strong relationship between glycemia and diabetic complications in type 1 diabetes *(3)*. There is a continuous, although not linear, rela-

From: *Contemporary Endocrinology: Type 1 Diabetes: Etiology and Treatment*
Edited by: M. A. Sperling © Humana Press Inc., Totowa, NJ

tionship between level of glycemia and the risk of development and progression of complications *(4,5)*. This chapter integrates the vast amount of data about specific mechanisms by which hyperglycemia may damage diabetic blood vessels into a coherent, unified perspective. After discussing each known major mechanism of hyperglycemia-induced vascular damage, recent data are presented showing that these different pathogenic mechanisms all reflect a single hyperglycemia-induced process. The chapter concludes with a brief consideration of the prospects for mechanism-based pharmacologic intervention.

SHARED PATHOPHYSIOLOGIC FEATURES OF DIABETIC COMPLICATIONS

In the retina, glomerulus, vasa nervorum, and artery, diabetes-specific vascular disease is characterized by similar pathophysiologic features.

Requirement for Intracellular Hyperglycemia

Clinical and animal model data indicate that chronic hyperglycemia is the central initiating factor for all types of diabetic microvascular disease. Duration and magnitude of hyperglycemia are both strongly correlated with the extent and rate of progression of diabetic microvascular disease. In the Diabetes Control and Complications Trial (DCCT), for example, type 1 diabetic patients whose intensive insulin therapy resulted in HbA1c levels 2% lower than those receiving conventional insulin therapy had a 76% lower incidence of retinopathy, a 54% lower incidence of nephropathy, and a 60% reduction in neuropathy *(3)*. Similarly, several studies have shown that glycohemoglobin A1 is an independent risk factor for cardiovascular disease *(6,7)* in type 1 diabetes. Intimal-medial thickness (IMT) of the carotid artery, which is strongly correlated with coronary heart disease (CHD), was demonstrated to be increased in type 1 diabetes *(8,9)*.

Although all cells in a person with diabetes are exposed to elevated levels of plasma glucose, hyperglycemic damage is limited to those cell types, such as endothelial cells, that develop intracellular hyperglycemia. Endothelial cells develop intracellular hyperglycemia because, unlike most other cells, they are unable to downregulate glucose transport when exposed to extracellular hyperglycemia. As illustrated in Fig. 1, vascular smooth muscle cells, which are not damaged by hyperglycemia, show an inverse relationship between extracellular glucose concentration and subsequent rate of glucose transport measured as 2-deoxyglucose uptake (Fig. 1A). In contrast, vascular endothelial cells show no significant change in subsequent rate of glucose transport after exposure to elevated glucose concentrations (Fig. 1B) *(10)*. That intracellular hyperglycemia is necessary and sufficient for the development of diabetic pathology is demonstrated by the fact that overexpression of the glucose transporter (GLUT)-1 glucose transporter in mesangial cells cultured in a normal glucose milieu mimics the diabetic phenotype, inducing the same increases in collagen type IV, collagen type I, and fibronectin gene expression as diabetic hyperglycemia *(11)*.

Abnormal Endothelial Cell Function

Early in the course of diabetes, before structural changes are evident, hyperglycemia causes abnormalities in blood flow and vascular permeability in the retina, glomerulus, peripheral nerve vasa nervorum *(12,13)*, and arterial endothelium *(14)*. The increase in blood flow and intracapillary pressure is thought to reflect hyperglycemia-induced

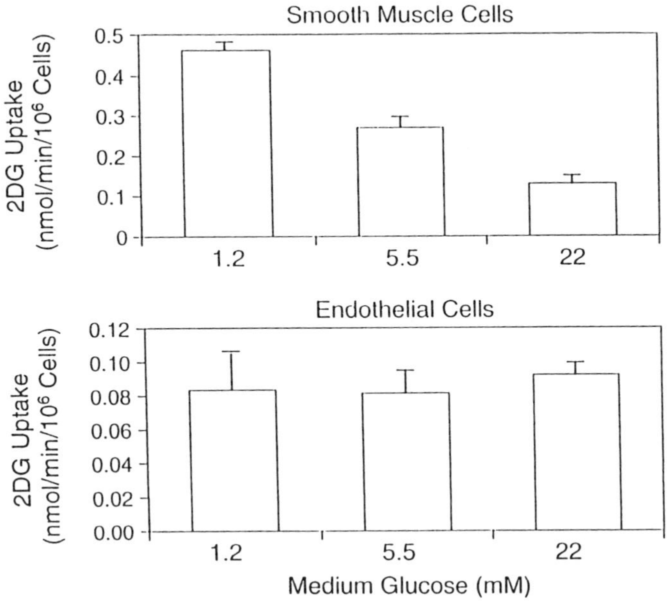

Fig. 1. Lack of downregulation of glucose transport in cells affected by diabetic complications. **(A)** 2-deoxyglucose uptake in vascular smooth muscle cells pre-exposed to either 1.2, 5.5, or 22 m*M* glucose; **(B)** 2-deoxyglucose uptake in vascular endothelial cells pre-exposed to either 1.2, 5.5, or 22 m*M* glucose (Reproduced with permission from ref. *10.*)

decreased nitric oxide production on the efferent side of capillary beds and, possibly, an increased sensitivity to angiotensin II. As a consequence of increased intracapillary pressure and endothelial cell dysfunction, retinal capillaries exhibit increased leakage of fluorescein and glomerular capillaries have an elevated albumin excretion rate. Comparable changes occur in the vasa vasorum of the peripheral nerve and arterial endothelium *(15).* Early in the course of diabetes, increased permeability is reversible, but as time progresses, it becomes irreversible.

Increased Vessel Wall Protein Accumulation

The common pathophysiologic feature of diabetic microvascular disease is progressive narrowing and eventual occlusion of vascular lumina, which results in inadequate perfusion and function of the affected tissues. Early hyperglycemia-induced microvascular hypertension and increased vascular permeability contribute to irreversible microvessel occlusion by three processes. The first is an abnormal leakage of periodic acid–Schiff (PAS)-positive, carbohydrate-containing plasma proteins, which are deposited in the capillary wall and may stimulate perivascular cells such as pericytes and mesangial cells to elaborate growth factors and extracellular matrix. The second is extravasation of growth factors such as transforming growth factor-β_1 (TGF-β_1), which directly stimulate overproduction of extracellular matrix components *(16).* The third pathologic process is hypertension-induced stimulation of pathologic gene expression by endothelial cells and supporting cells, which include growth factors, growth factor receptors, extracellular matrix components, and adhesion molecules that can activate circulating leukocytes *(17).* The observation that unilateral reduction in the severity of diabetic microvascular disease occurs on the side with ophthalmic or renal artery stenosis is consistent with this concept *(18,19)*. Similar changes may account for intimal-medial thickening in diabetic arteries.

Features of Diabetic Macrovascular Disease

Unlike microvascular disease, which occurs only in patients with diabetes, macrovascular disease resembles that in subjects without diabetes. However, subjects with diabetes have more rapidly progressive and extensive cardiovascular disease, with a greater incidence of multivessel disease and a greater number of diseased vessel segments than nondiabetic persons *(20)*. In both subjects with and without diabetes, atherosclerosis begins with endothelial dysfunction that results from injury caused by many factors, including hyperglycemia *(21)*. Endothelial injury increases the adhesiveness of the endothelium with respect to leukocytes and platelets, as well as its permeability to lipoproteins and other plasma constituents. A number of studies have shown that elevated glucose levels and/or glucose-derived advanced glycation end products (AGEs) induce the expression of monocyte chemotactic protein 1 (MCP-1) *(22)* and adhesion molecules such as intercellular adhesion molecule-1 (ICAM-1) and vascular-cell adhesion molecule-1 (VCAM-1) in vascular cells *(23–28)*. These specific molecules induce the adherence, migration, and accumulation of monocytes and T-cells on the endothelium and stimulate the infiltration of these cells into the subendothelial space. After infiltration, monocytes become macrophages and form foam cells. Progression beyond the first step of atherogenesis is associated with subsequent migration, lipid accumulation, and foam-cell formation of smooth muscle cells. The persistence of these changes causes more advanced, complex, lesions of atherosclerosis. These lesions are covered by a fibrous cap, which forms as a result of increased activity of platelet-derived growth factor, TGF-β , interleukin-1 (IL-1), tumor necrosis factor-α (TNF-α), osteopontin, and matrix metalloproteinases (MMPs). Rupture of this fibrous cap by MMPs and consequent thrombosis may lead to the acute coronary syndrome *(29–31)*. Hyperglycemia and/or hyperglycemia-induced AGEs have been shown to induce TGF-β *(32,33)*, IL-1 *(34,35)*, TNF-α *(36,37)*, osteopontin *(38)*, and MMP9 *(39)*.

MECHANISMS OF HYPERGLYCEMIA-INDUCED DAMAGE

Four major hypotheses about how hyperglycemia causes diabetic complications have generated a large amount of data, as well as several clinical trials based on specific inhibitors of these mechanisms. Until quite recently, there was no unifying hypothesis linking these four mechanisms.

Increased Polyol Pathway Flux

Aldose reductase is a cytosolic, monomeric oxidoreductase that catalyzes the NADPH-dependent reduction of a wide variety of carbonyl compounds, including glucose. Aldose reductase has a low affinity (high K_m) for glucose, and at the normal glucose concentrations found in nondiabetics, the metabolism of glucose by this pathway constitutes a very small percentage of total glucose utilization. However, in a hyperglycemic environment, increased intracellular glucose concentration (and possibly oxidant stress-induced aldose reductase activation) results in increased enzymatic conversion to the polyalcohol sorbitol. In the polyol pathway, sorbitol is oxidized to fructose by the enzyme sorbitol dehydrogenase (SDH), with NAD^+ reduced to NADH (*see* Fig. 2).

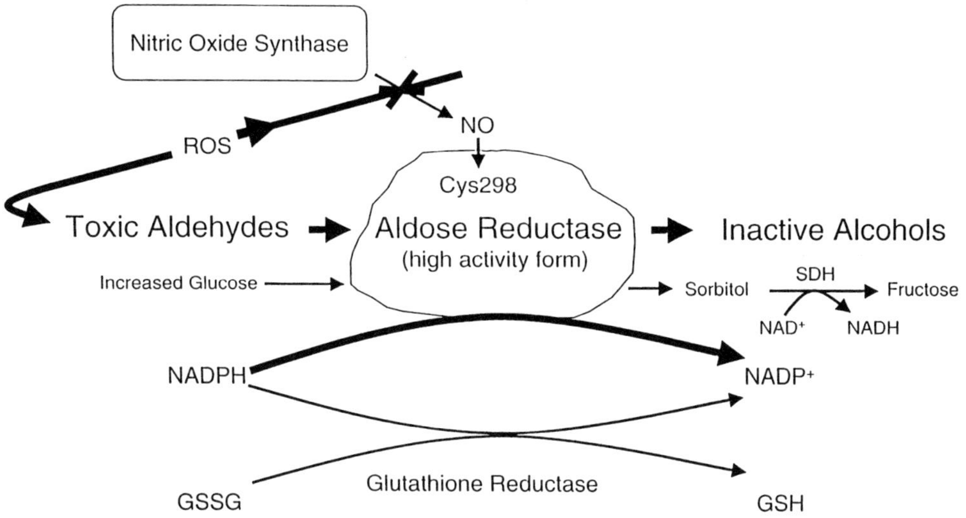

Fig. 2. Aldose reductase function and the polyol pathway. Aldose reductase reduces reactive oxygen species (ROS)-generated toxic aldehydes to inactive alcohols, and glucose to sorbitol, using NADPH as a cofactor. Sorbitol dehydrogenase oxidizes sorbitol to fructose using NAD^+ as a cofactor (*see* the text for details). Aldose reductase may be activated by ROS-induced reduction of nitric oxide modification of a cysteine residue in the enzyme's active site. (Adapted from ref. *40.*)

It has been proposed that reduction of glucose to sorbitol by NADPH consumes the cofactor NADPH. Because NADPH is required for regenerating reduced glutathione (GSH), this could induce or exacerbate intracellular oxidative stress. Less of the reduced GSH has, in fact, been found in the lens of transgenic mice that overexpress aldose reductase, and this is the most likely mechanism by which increased flux through the polyol pathway has deleterious consequences *(41)*.

Increased Intracellular AGE Formation

Advanced glycation and products are found in increased amounts in extracellular structures of diabetic retinal vessels *(42–44)* and renal glomeruli *(45–47)*. These AGEs were originally thought to arise from nonenzymatic reactions between extracellular proteins and glucose. However, the rate of AGE formation from glucose is orders of magnitude slower than the rate of AGE formation from glucose-derived dicarbonyl precursors generated intracellularly, and it now seems likely that intracellular hyperglycemia is the primary initiating event in the formation of both intracellular and extracellular AGEs *(48)*. AGEs can arise from intracellular autoxidation of glucose to glyoxal *(49)*, decomposition of the Amadori product to 3-deoxyglucosone (perhaps accelerated by an amadoriase), and fragmentation of glyceraldehyde-3-phosphate to methylglyoxal *(50)* (*see* Fig. 3). These reactive intracellular dicarbonyls react with amino groups of intracellular and extracellular proteins to form AGEs. Methylglyoxal and glyoxal are detoxified by the glyoxalase system *(50)*.

Intracellular production of AGE precursors damages target cells by three general mechanisms. First, intracellular proteins modified by AGEs have altered function. Second, extracellular matrix components modified by AGE precursors interact abnormally with other matrix components and with matrix receptors (integrins) on cells. Third,

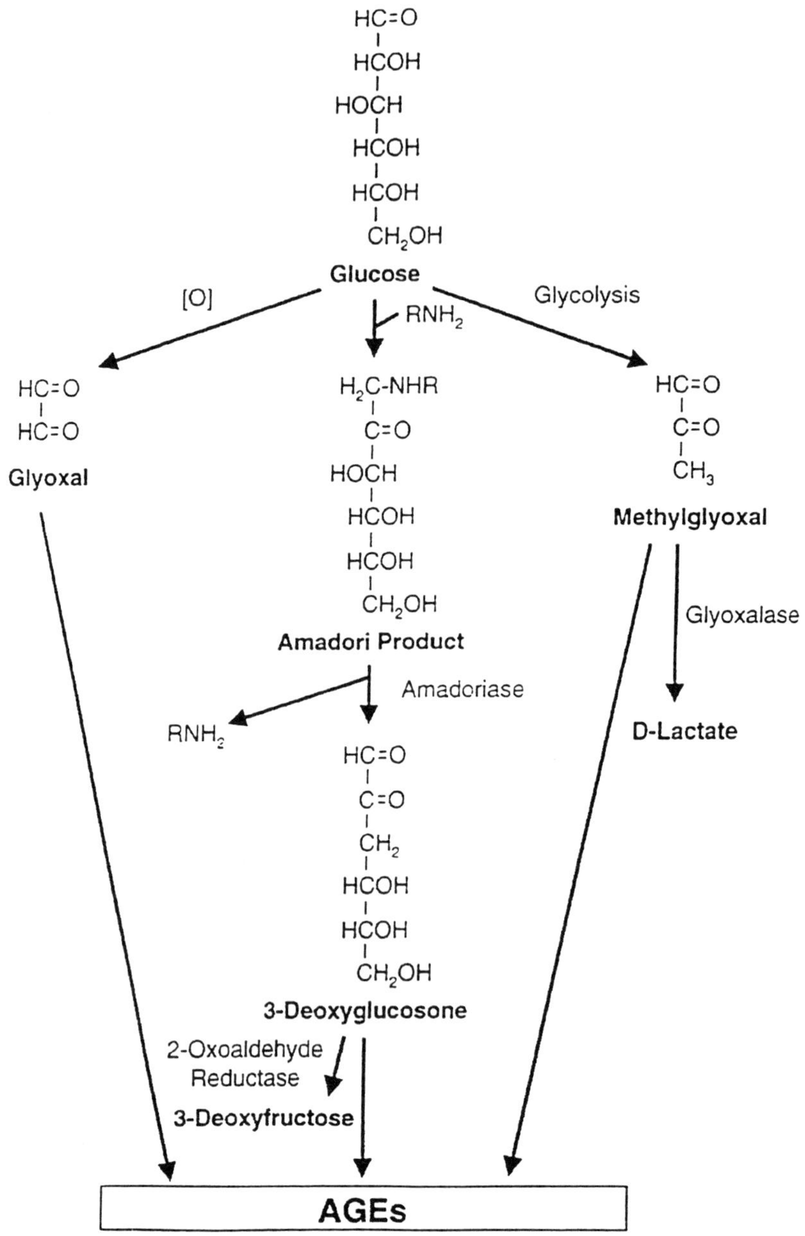

Fig. 3. Intracellular advanced glycation endproduct (AGE) formation. Potential pathways leading to the formation of AGEs inside cells (*see* the text for details). (Reproduced with permission from ref. *49.*)

plasma proteins modified by AGE precursors bind to AGE receptors on cells such as macrophages, inducing receptor-mediated reactive oxygen species production. This AGE receptor ligation activates the pleiotrophic transcription factor NF-κB, causing pathologic changes in gene expression *(51)*.

In endothelial cells, intracellular AGE formation occurs very quickly. Proteins involved in macromolecular endocytosis are modified by AGEs because the 2.2-fold increase in endocytosis induced by hyperglycemia is also prevented by overexpression of the methylglyoxal-detoxifying glyoxalase I *(52)*. Glyoxalase-I overexpression also completely prevents the fourfold hyperglycemia-induced increase in Muller cell expression of angiopoietin-2, a factor that has been implicated in both pericyte loss and capillary regression *(53–55)*.

Intracellular AGEs leak out of cells and alter the functional properties of several important matrix molecules. Collagen was the first matrix protein used to demonstrate that glucose-derived AGEs form covalent, intermolecular bonds. In vitro AGE formation on intact glomerular basement membrane increases its permeability to albumin in a manner that resembles the abnormal permeability of diabetic nephropathy *(56,57)*. AGE formation on extracellular matrix not only interferes with matrix–matrix interactions, it also interferes with matrix–cell interactions. For example, AGE modification of type IV collagen's cell-binding domains decrease endothelial cell adhesion *(58)*, and AGE modification of a six-amino-acid growth-promoting sequence in the A-chain of the laminin molecule markedly reduces neurite outgrowth *(59)*. AGE modification of vitronectin reduced cell attachment-promoting activity *(60)*.

Specific receptors for AGEs were first identified on monocytes and macrophages. Two AGE-binding proteins isolated from rat liver are both present on monocyte/macrophages. Antisera to either the 60-kDa or 90-kDa protein, recently identified as OST-48 and 80K-H, respectively *(61)*, block AGE binding *(62)*. AGE protein binding to this receptor stimulates macrophage production of IL-1, insulin-like growth factor-1 (IGF-1), TNF-α, TGF-β, macrophage colony-stimulating factor and, granulocyte/macrophage colony-stimulating factor at levels that have been shown to increase glomerular synthesis of type IV collagen and to stimulate proliferation and chemotaxis of both arterial smooth muscle cells and macrophages *(33–35,63–68)*. The macrophage scavenger receptor type II and galectin-3 have also been shown to recognize AGEs *(69–72)*.

Vascular endothelial cells also express AGE-specific receptors (RAGEs). A 35-kDa and a 46-kDa AGE-binding protein have been purified to homogeneity from endothelial cells *(73–75)*.

In endothelial cells, AGE binding to its receptor induces changes in gene expression that include alterations in thrombomodulin, tissue factor, and VCAM-1 *(25–28)*. These changes induce procoagulatory changes in the endothelial surface and increase the adhesion of inflammatory cells to the vessel wall. In addition, endothelial AGE-receptor-binding appears to mediate, in part, the hyperpermeability induced by diabetes, probably through the induction of vascular endothelial growth factor (VEGF) *(76–78)*.

Activation of Protein Kinase C

Protein kinase Cs (PKCs) are a family of at least 11 isoforms, 9 of which are activated by the lipid second-messenger diacylglycerol (DAG). Intracellular hyperglycemia increases DAG content in cultured microvascular cells and in the retina and renal glomeruli of diabetic animals *(79–81)*. Intracellular hyperglycemia appears to increase DAG content primarily by increasing its *de novo* synthesis from the glycolytic intermediate glyceraldehyde-3-phosphate via reduction to glycerol-3-phosphate and stepwise acylation *(80,82)*. Increased *de novo* synthesis of DAG activates PKC both in cultured vascular cells *(80,83–85)* and in the retina and glomeruli of diabetic animals *(80,81,83)*. Increased DAG primarily activates the β and δ isoforms of PKC, but increases in other isoforms have also been found, such as PKC-α and PKC-ε isoforms in the retina *(81)* and PKC-α and -δ in the glomerulus *(86,87)* of diabetic rats.

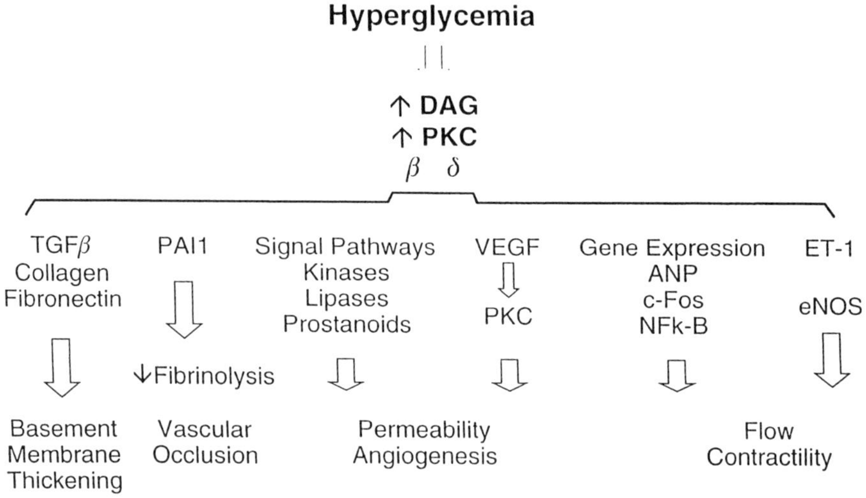

Fig. 4. Potential consequences of hyperglycemia-induced PKC activation. Hyperglycemia increases DAG content, which activates PKC, primarily the β and δ isoforms. Activated PKC has a number of pathogenic consequences that are described in the text. DAG, diacylglycerol; PKC, protein kinase C. (From ref. *86*.)

In early experimental diabetes, activation of PKC-β isoforms has been shown to mediate retinal and renal blood flow abnormalities *(88),* perhaps by depressing nitric oxide production and/or increasing endothelin-1 activity (*see* Fig. 4). Abnormal activation of PKC has been implicated in the decreased glomerular production of nitric oxide induced by experimental diabetes *(89)* and in the decreased smooth muscle cell nitric oxide production induced by hyperglycemia *(90)*. PKC activation also inhibits insulin-stimulated expression of endothelial nitric oxide synthase (eNOS) mRNA in cultured endothelial cells *(91)*. Hyperglycemia increases endothelin-1-stimulated mitogen-activated protein kinase (MAPK) activity in glomerular mesangial cells by activating PKC isoforms *(92)*. The increased endothelial cell permeability induced by high glucose in cultured cells is mediated by activation of PKC-α, however *(15)*. Activation of PKC by elevated glucose also induces expression of the permeability-enhancing factor VEGF in smooth muscle cells *(93)*.

In addition to affecting hyperglycemia-induced abnormalities of blood flow and permeability, activation of PKC contributes to increased microvascular matrix protein accumulation by inducing expression of TGF-β_1 , fibronectin, and α1(IV) collagen in both cultured mesangial cells *(94,95)* and in glomeruli of diabetic rats *(86)*. This effect appears to be mediated through PKC's inhibition of nitric oxide production *(96)*. Hyperglycemia-induced expression of laminin C1 in cultured mesangial cells is independent of PKC activation, however *(97)*. Hyperglycemia-induced activation of PKC has also been implicated in the overexpression of the fibrinolytic inhibitor plasminogen activator inhibitor-1 *(98),* and in the activation of the pleiotrophic transcription factor NF-κB in cultured endothelial cells and vascular smooth muscle cells *(99,100)*.

Increased Hexosamine Pathway Flux

A fourth hypothesis about how hyperglycemia causes diabetic complications has recently been formulated *(101,102),* in which glucose is shunted into the hexosamine pathway (*see* Fig. 5). In this pathway, fructose-6-phosphate is diverted from

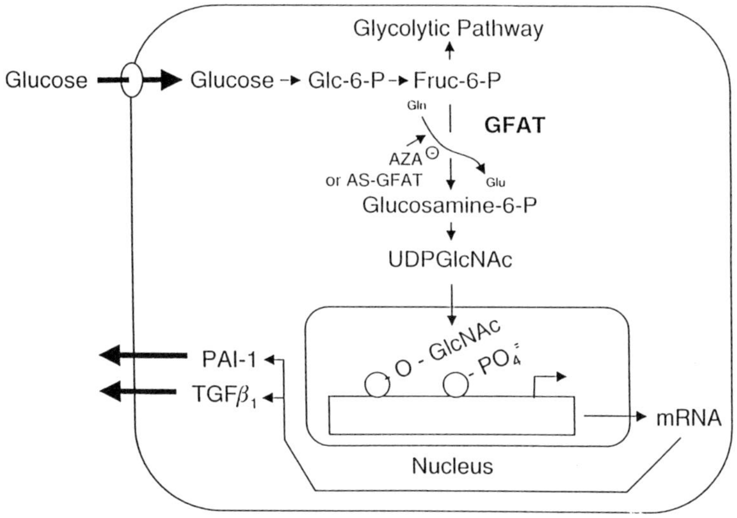

Fig. 5. Hyperglycemia increases hexosamine pathway flux. In this pathway, increased O-linked GlcNAc moieties on the transcription factor Sp1 increase its transactivating function and thus increase transcription of complications-associated genes (Reproduced with permission from ref. 103.)

glycolysis to provide substrates for reactions that require urine diphosphate (UDP)-*N*-acetylglucosamine, such as proteoglycan synthesis and the formation of O-linked glycoproteins. Inhibition of the rate-limiting enzyme in the conversion of glucose to glucosamine, glutamine : fructose-6-phosphate amidotransferase (GFAT), blocks hyperglycemia-induced increases in the transcription of TGF-α *(101)*, TGF-β_1 *(102)*, and plasminogen activator inhibitor-1 (PAI-1), by preventing O-linked *N*-acetylglucosamine (O-GlcNAc) modification of the transcriptional factor Sp1. This pathway has previously been shown to play an important role in hyperglycemia-induced and fat-induced insulin resistance *(103–105)*.

In addition to transcription factors, many other nuclear and cytoplasmic proteins are dynamically modified by O-GlcNAc moieties and may exhibit reciprocal modification by phosphorylation in a manner analogous to Sp1 *(106)*. Thus, activation of the hexosamine pathway by hyperglycemia may result in many changes in both gene expression and in protein function that, together, contribute to the pathogenesis of diabetic complications.

DIFFERENT PATHOGENIC MECHANISMS REFLECT A SINGLE HYPERGLYCEMIA-INDUCED PROCESS

Although specific inhibitors of aldose reductase activity, AGE formation, and PKC activation each ameliorate various diabetes-induced abnormalities in animal models, there has been no apparent common element linking the four mechanisms of hyperglycemia-induced damage discussed in the preceding section *(88,107–110)*. This issue has now been resolved by the recent discovery that each of the four different pathogenic mechanisms reflects a single hyperglycemia-induced process: overproduction of superoxide by the mitochondrial electron transport chain *(111,112)*.

Hyperglycemia increases reactive oxygen species (ROS) production inside cultured bovine aortic endothelial cells *(113)*. To understand how this occurs, a brief overview

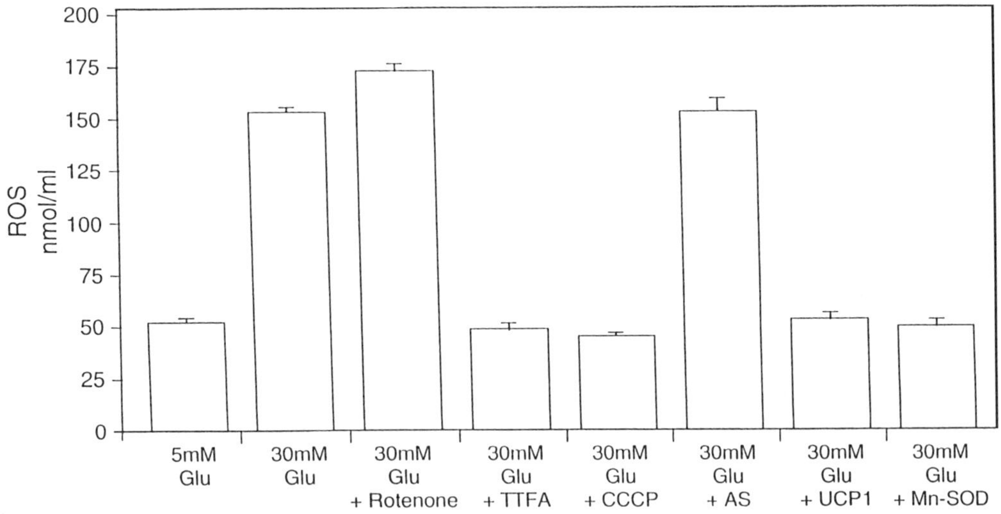

Fig. 6. Effect of agents that alter mitochondrial metabolism on hyperglycemia-induced ROS formation in bovine aortic endothelial cells. Cells were incubated in 5 m*M* glucose, 30 m*M* glucose alone, and 30 m*M* glucose plus either rotenone, thenoyltrifluoroacetone (TTFA), carbonyl cyanide *m*-chlorophenylhydrazone (CCCP), antisense, uncoupling protein-1 (UCP-1), or manganese superoxide dismutase (Mn-SOD) hemagglutinating virus of Japan (HVJ)-liposomes, and ROS were quantitated. (Reproduced with permission from ref. *111.*)

of glucose metabolism is helpful. Intracellular glucose oxidation begins with glycolysis in the cytoplasm, which generates NADH and pyruvate. Cytoplasmic NADH can donate reducing equivalents to the mitochondrial electron-transport chain via two shuttle systems, or it can reduce pyruvate to lactate, which exits the cell to provide substrate for hepatic gluconeogenesis. Pyruvate can also be transported into the mitochondria, where it is oxidized by the tricarboxylic acid (TCA) cycle to produce CO_2, H_2O, four molecules of NADH, and one molecule of $FADH_2$. Mitochondrial NADH and $FADH_2$ provide energy for ATP production via oxidative phosphorylation by the electron-transport chain.

Electron flow through the mitochondrial electron-transport chain is carried out by four inner-membrane-associated enzyme complexes, plus cytochrome-*c* and the mobile carrier ubiquinone *(114)*. NADH derived from both cytosolic glucose oxidation and mitochondrial TCA cycle activity donates electrons to NADH : ubiquinone oxidoreductase (complex I). Complex I ultimately transfers its electrons to ubiquinone. Ubiquinone can also be reduced by electrons donated from several $FADH_2$-containing dehydrogenases, including succinate : ubiquinone oxidoreductase (complex II) and glycerol-3-phosphate dehydrogenase. Electrons from reduced ubiquinone are then transferred to ubiquinol : cytochrome-*c* oxidoreductase (complex III) by the ubisemiquinone radical-generating Q cycle *(115)*. Electron transport then proceeds through cytochrome-*c*, cytochrome-*c* oxidase (complex IV), and, finally, molecular oxygen.

Electron transfer through complexes I, III, and IV generates a proton gradient that drives ATP synthase (complex V). When the electrochemical potential difference generated by this proton gradient is high, the life of superoxide-generating electron-transport intermediates such as ubisemiquinone is prolonged. There appears to be a threshold value above which superoxide production is markedly increased *(116)*.

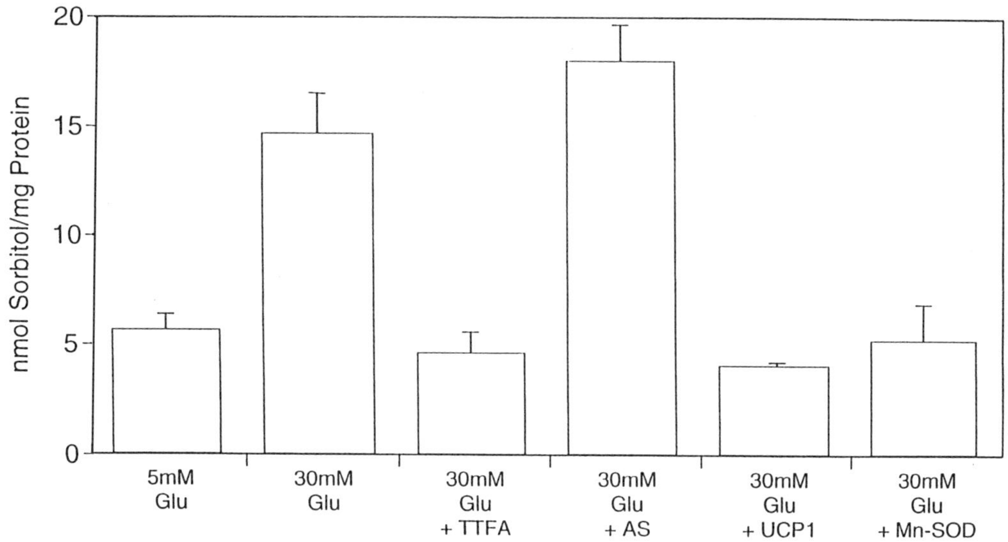

Fig. 7. Effect of agents that alter mitochondrial metabolism on hyperglycemia-induced sorbitol accumulation. Cells were incubated in 5 m*M* glucose, 30 m*M* glucose alone, and 30 m*M* glucose plus either TTFA, UCP-1, or Mn-SOD HVJ-liposomes, as indicated. (Reproduced with permission from ref. *111*.)

Using inhibitors of both the shuttle that transfers cytosolic NADH into mitochondria and the transporter that transfers cytolsolic pyruvate into the mitochondria, the TCA cycle was shown to the source of hyperglycemia-induced ROS in endothelial cells. Overexpression of uncoupling protein-1 (UCP-1), a specific protein uncoupler of oxidative phosphorylation capable of collapsing the proton electrochemical gradient *(117)*, prevented the effect of hyperglycemia (*see* Fig. 6). Antisense cDNA in the same gene transfer vector did not (*see* Fig. 6). These results demonstrate that hyperglycemia-induced intracellular ROS are produced by the proton electrochemical gradient generated by the mitochondrial electron-transport chain. Overexpression of manganese superoxide dismutase, the mitochondrial form of this antioxidant enzyme *(118)*, also prevented the effect of hyperglycemia (*see* Fig. 6). This result demonstrates that superoxide is the reactive oxygen radical produced by this mechanism.

The effect of hyperglycemia-induced mitochondrial superoxide overproduction on polyol pathway flux was evalulated after first determining that sorbitol in these cells was exclusively derived from aldose reductase activity. Sorbitol levels were 2.6-fold higher than baseline (5 m*M* glucose) when endothelial cells were incubated in 30 m*M* glucose (*see* Fig. 7). Hyperglycemia-induced sorbitol accumulation was completely prevented by UCP-1 and manganese superoxide dismutase (Mn-SOD) (*see* Fig. 7), indicating that mitochondrial superoxide overproduction stimulates aldose reductase activity.

Next, the effect of hyperglycemia-induced mitochondrial superoxide overproduction on intracellular AGE formation was determined. In bovine aortic endothelial cells, hyperglycemia increases intracellular AGEs primarily, if not exclusively, by increasing the formation of AGE-forming methylglyoxal *(52)*. Therefore, the effect of UCP-1 and Mn-SOD on hyperglycemia-induced formation of intracellular methylglyoxal-derived AGEs was examined (*see* Fig. 8). Each of these agents completely prevented

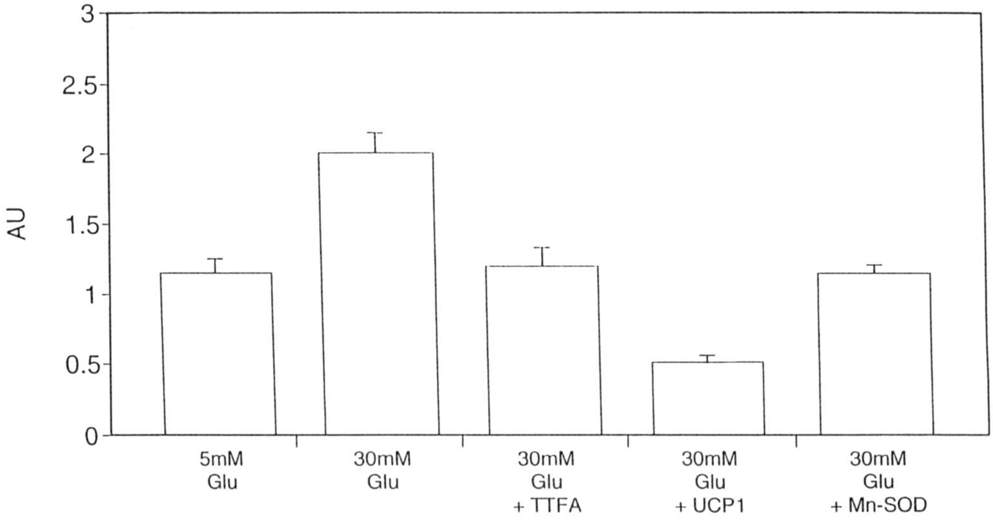

Fig. 8. Effect of agents that alter mitochondrial metabolism on hyperglycemia-induced intracellular AGE formation. Cells were incubated in 5 m*M* glucose, 30 m*M* glucose alone, and 30 m*M* glucose plus either TTFA, UCP-1, or Mn-SOD HVJ-liposomes, as indicated. (Reproduced with permission from ref. *111*.)

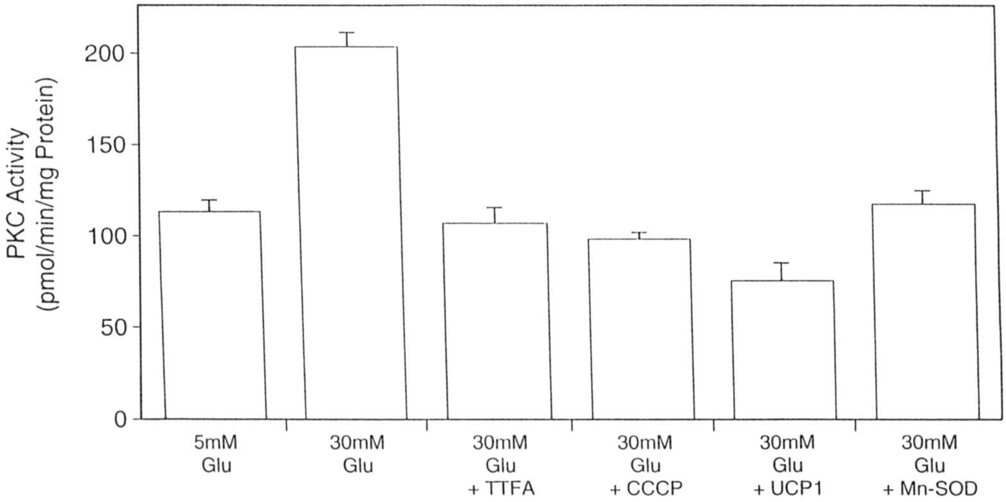

Fig. 9. Effect of agents that alter mitochondrial metabolism on hyperglycemia-induced PKC activation. Cells were incubated in 5 m*M* glucose, 30 m*M* glucose alone, and 30 m*M* glucose plus either TTFA, CCCP, UCP-1, or Mn-SOD HVJ-liposomes, as indicated, and PKC activity was determined in the membrane fraction. (Reproduced with permission from ref. *111*.)

hyperglycemia-induced formation of intracellular AGEs (*see* Fig. 8), indicating that mitochondrial superoxide initiates intracellular AGE formation.

The effect of UCP-1 and Mn-SOD on hyperglycemia-induced activation of PKC was also evaluated (*see* Fig. 9). Each of these agents completely inhibited PKC activation,

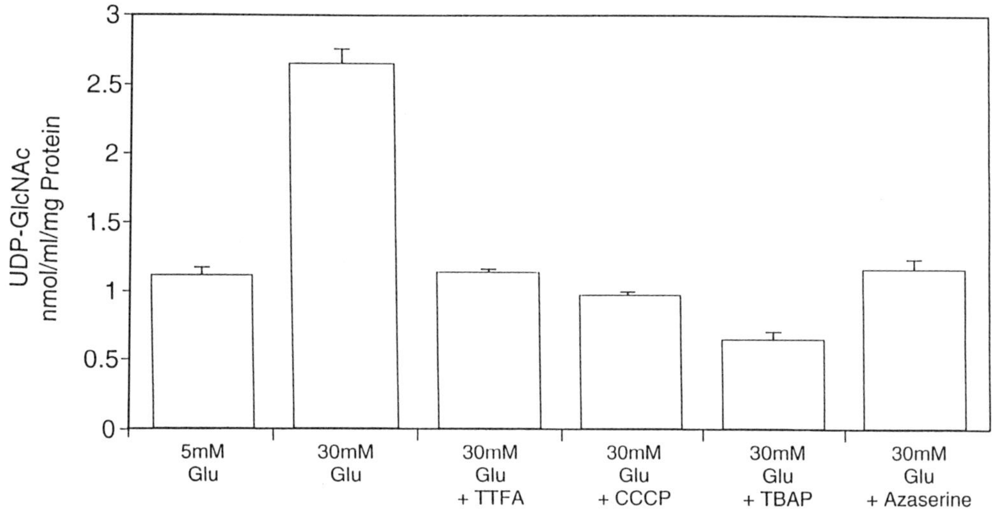

Fig. 10. Effect of agents that alter mitochondrial metabolism on hyperglycemia-induced hexosamine pathway activity. Cells were incubated in 5 m*M* glucose, 30 m*M* glucose alone, and 30 m*M* glucose plus either TTFA, CCCP, manganese(III) tetrakis(4-benzoic acid) porphyrin (TBAP), or azaserine as indicated, and UDP-GlcNAc concentration was determined. (Reproduced with permission from ref. *112.*)

suggesting that mitochondrial superoxide overproduction initiates the hyperglycemia-induced *de novo* synthesis of diacylglycerol that activates PKC *(119).*

Finally, the effect of hyperglycemia-induced mitochondrial superoxide overproduction on the hexosamine pathway was determined *(112).* Hyperglycemia induced an increase in hexosamine pathway activity that was completely prevented by UCP-1, Mn-SOD, and azaserine, an inhibitor of the rate-limiting enzyme in the hexosamine pathway (*see* Fig. 10).

Hyperglycemia-induced activation of the redox-sensitive pleiotrophic transcription factor NF-κB was also prevented by inhibition of mitochondrial superoxide overproduction *(111).*

FUTURE DRUGS TARGETS

The recent discovery that each of the four different pathogenic mechansisms discussed in this chapter reflects a single hyperglycemia-induced process *(111,112)* suggests that interrupting the overproduction of superoxide by the mitochondrial electron-transport chain would normalize polyol pathway flux, AGE formation, PKC activation, and hexosamine pathway flux, as well as a number of other hyperglycemia-induced mechanisms that remain to be discovered.

Novel compounds that act as superoxide dismutase/catalase mimetics already exist *(120,121),* and these compounds have been shown to normalize hyperglycemia-induced mitochondrial superoxide overproduction *(112).* Compounds that directly prevent hyperglycemia-induced mitochondrial superoxide overproduction may also hold promise. Drugs that normalize superoxide-induced triose phosphate accumulation are another logical therapeutic strategy. These and the other agents described in this section may have unique clinical efficacy in preventing the development and progression of diabetic complications.

REFERENCES

1. Ruderman NB, Williamson JR, Brownlee M. Glucose and diabetic vascular disease. FASEB J 1992;6:2905–2914.
2. Skyler J. Diabetic complications: the importance of glucose control. In: Brownlee, MB, King, GL eds. Endocrinol Metab Clin North Am. Volume 25. WB Saunders, Philadelphia, 1996, pp. 243–254.
3. The Diabetes Control and Complications Trial Research Group. The effect of intensive treatment of diabetes on the development and progression of long-term complications in insulin-dependent diabetes mellitus. N Engl J Med 1993;329:977–986.
4. Krolewski AS, Laffel LM, Krolewski M, Quinn M, Warram JH. Glycosylated hemoglobin and the risk of microalbuminuria in patients with insulin-dependent diabetes mellitus. N Engl J Med 1995;332:1251–1255.
5. The absence of a glycemic threshold for the development of long-term complications: the perspective of the Diabetes Control and Complications Trial. Diabetes 1996;45:1289–1298.
6. Ronald K. Hyperglycemia and microvascular and macrovascular disease in diabetes. Diabetes Care 1995;18:258–268.
7. Lehto S, Ronnemaa T, Pyorala K, Laakso M. Poor glycemic control predicts coronary heart disease events in patients with type I diabetes without nephropathy. Arterioscler Thromb Vasc Biol 1999;19:1014–1019.
8. Kawamori R, Yamasaki Y, Matsushima H, et al. Prevalence of carotid atherosclerosis in diabetic patients. Diabetes Care 1992;15:1290–1294.
9. Yamasaki Y, Kawamori R, Matsushima H, et al. Atherosclerosis in carotid artery of young type I diabetes patients monitored by ultrasound high-resolution B-mode imaging. Diabetes 1994;43:634–639.
10. Kaiser N, Feener EP, Boukobza-Vardi N, et al. Differential regulation of glucose transport and transporters by glucose in vascular endothelial and smooth muscle cells. Diabetes 1993;42:80–89.
11. Heilig CW, Concepcion LA, Riser BL, Freytag SO, Zhu M, Cortes P. Overexpression of glucose transporters in rat mesangial cells cultured in a normal glucose milieu mimics the diabetic phenotype. J Clin Invest 1995;96:1802–1814.
12. Shore AC, Tooke JE. Microvascular function and haemodynamic disturbances in diabetes mellitus and its complications. In: Pickup J, Williams G, eds. Textbook of Diabetes, Vo. 1, Blackwell Scientific, Oxford, 1997, pp. 43.1–43.13.
13. Kihara M, Schmelzer JD, Poduslo JF, Curran GL, Nickander KK, Low PA. Aminoguanidine effects on nerve blood flow, vascular permeability, electrophysiology, and oxygen free radicals. Proc Natl Acad Sci USA 1991;88:6107–6111.
14. Poston L, Taylor PD. Endothelium-mediated vascular function in insulin-dependent diabetes mellitus. Clin Sci 1995;88:245–255.
15. Hempal A, Maasch C, Heintze U, et al. High glucose concentrations increase endothelial cell permeability via activation of protein kinase C alpha. Circ Res 1997;81:363–371.
16. Kopp JB, Factor VM, Mozes M, et al. Transgenic mice with increased plasma levels of TGF-beta 1 develop progressive renal disease. Lab Invest 1996;74:991–1003.
17. Chien S, Li S, Shyy YJ. Effects of mechanical forces on signal transduction and gene expression in endothelial cells. Hypertension 1998;31:162–169.
18. Walker JD, Viberti GC. Pathophysiology of microvascular disease: an overview. In: Pickup J, Wiliams G, eds. Textbook of Diabetes, Vol. 2. Blackwell Scientific, Oxford, 1997, pp. 526–533.
19. Brownlee M. Advanced products of nonenzymatic glycosylation and the pathogenesis of diabetic complications. In: Rifkin H, Porte D, Jr., eds. Diabetes Mellitus, Theory and Practice. Elsevier, New York, 1990, pp. 279–291.
20. Granger CB, Califf RM, Young S, et al. Outcome of patients with diabetes mellitus and acute myocardial infarction treated with thrombolytic agents. The Thrombolysis and Angioplasty in Myocardial Infarction (TAMI) Study Group. J Am Coll Cardiol 1993;21:920–925.
21. Ross R. Atherosclerosis—an inflammatory disease. N Engl J Med 1999;340:115–126.
22. Sassy-Prigent C, Heudes D, Mandet C, et al. Early glomerular macrophage recruitment in streptozotocin-induced diabetic rats. Diabetes 2000;49:466–475.
23. Ceriello A, Falleti E, Motz E et al. Hyperglycemia-induced circulationg ICAM-1 increased in diabetes mellitus: the possible role of oxidative stress. Horm Metab Res 1998;30:146–149.
24. Kim JA, Berliner JA, Natarajan RD, Nadler JL. Evidence that glucose increases monocyte binding to human aortic endothelial cells. Diabetes 1994;43:1103–1107.

25. Vlassara H, Fuh H, Donnelly T, Cybulsky M. Advanced glycation endproducts promote adhesion molecule (VCAM-1, ICAM-1) expression and atheroma formation in normal rabbits. Mol Med 1995;1:447–456.
26. Schmidt AM, Hori O, Chen JX, et al. Advanced glycation endproducts interacting with their endothelial receptor induce expression of vascular cell adhesion molecule- 1 (VCAM-1) in cultured human endothelial cells and in mice: a potential mechanism for the accelerated vasculopathy of diabetes. J Clin Invest 1995;96:1395–1403.
27. Sengoelge G, Fodinger M, Skoupy S, et al. Endothelial cell adhesion molecule and PMNL response to inflammatory stimuli and AGE-modified fibronectin. Kidney Int 1998;54:1637–1651.
28. Schmidt AM, Crandall J, Hori O, et al. Elevated plasma levels of vascular cell adhesion molecule-1 (VCAM-1) in diabetic patients with microalbuminuria: a marker of vascular dysfunction and progressive vascular disease. Br J Haematol 1996;92:747–750.
29. Ross R. The pathogenesis of atherogenesis: a perspective for the 1990s. Nature 1993;362:801–809.
30. Falk E, Shan PK, Fuster V. Pathogenesis of plaque disruption. In: Fuster V, Ross R, Topo EJ, eds. Atherosclerosis and Coronary Artery Disease. Vol. 2. Lippincott-Raven, Philadelphia, 1996, pp. 492–510.
31. Davies MJ. A macro and micro view of coronary vascular insult in ischemic heart disease. Circulation 1990;82(Suppl II):II-38–II-46.
32. Ziyadeh FN, Sharma K, Ericksen M, Wolf G. Stimulation of collagen gene expression and protein synthesis in murine mesangial cells by high glucose is mediated by autocrine activation of transforming growth factor-beta. J Clin Invest 1994;93:536–542.
33. Higashi T, Sano H, Saishoji T, et al. The receptor for advanced glycation end products mediates the chemotaxis of rabbit smooth muscle cells. Diabetes 1997;46:463–472.
34. Westwood ME, Thornalley PJ. Induction of synthesis and secretion of interleukin 1 beta in the human monocytic THP-1 cells by human serum albumins modified with methylglyoxal and advanced glycation endproducts. Immunol Lett 1996;50:17–21.
35. Asakawa H, Miyagawa J, Hanafusa T, Kuwajima M, Matsuzawa Y. High glucose and hyperosmolarity increase secretion on interleukin-1 beta in cultured human aortic endothelial cells. J Diabetes Complic 1997;11:176–179.
36. Abordo EA, Thornalley PJ. Synthesis and secretion of tumor necrosis factor-alpha by human monocytic THP-1 cells and chemotaxis induced by human serum albumin derivatives modified with methylglyoxal and glucose-derived advanced glycation endproducts. Immunol Lett 1997;58:139–147.
37. Guha M, Bai W, Nadler JL, Natarajan R. Molecular mechanisms of tumor necrosis fctor alpha gene expression in monocytic cells via hyperglycemia-induced oxidant stress-dependent and -independent pathways. J Biol Chem 2000;275:17,728–17,739.
38. Takemoto M, Yokote K, Yamazaki M et al. Enhanced expression of osteopontin by high glucose in cultured rat aortic smooth muscle cells. Biochem Biophys Res Commun 1999;258:722–726.
39. Ebihara I, Nakamura T, Shimada N, Koide H. Increased plasma metalloproteinase-9 concentrations precede development of microalbumoinuria in non-insulin-dependent diabetes mellitus. Am J Kidney Dis 1998;32:544–550.
40. Brownlee M. Mechanisms of hyperglycemic damage in diabetes. In: Kahn CR, eds. Atlas of Clinical Endocrinology. Philadelphia, Blackwell Science, 1999, pp. 121–133.
41. Lee AY, Chung SS. Contributions of polyol pathway to oxidative stress in diabetic cataract. FASEB J 1999;13:23–30.
42. Hammes H-P, Martin S, Federlin K, et al. Aminoguanidine treatment inhibits the development of experimental diabetic retinopathy. Proc Natl Acad Sci USA 1991;88:11,555–11,559.
43. Stitt AW, Moore JE, Sharkey JA, et al. Advanced glycation end products in vitreous: structural and functional implications for diabetic vitreopathy. Invest Ophthalmol Vis Sci 1998;39:2517–2521.
44. Stitt AW, Li YM, Gardiner TA, et al. Advanced glycation end products (AGEs) co- localize with AGE receptors in the retinal vasculature of diabetic and of AGE- infused rats. Am J Pathol 1997;150:523–528.
45. Nishino T, Horri Y, Shikki H, et al. Immunohistochemical detection of advanced glycosylation end products within the vascular lesions and glomeruli in diabetic nephropathy. Hum Pathol 1995;26:308–312.
46. Horie K, Miyata T, Maeda K, et al. Immunohistochemical colocalization of glycoxidation products and lipid peroxidation products in diabetic renal glomerular lesions. Implication for glycoxidative stress in the pathogenesis of diabetic nephropathy. J Clin Invest 1997;100:2995–2999.
47. Niwa T, Katsuzaki T, Miyazaki S, et al. Immunohistochemical detection of imidazolone, a novel advanced glycation end product, in kidneys and aortas of diabetic patients. J Clin Invest 1997;99: 1272–1276.
48. Degenhardt TP, Thorpe SR, Baynes JW. Chemical modification of proteins by methylglyoxal. Cell Mol Biol 1998;44:1139–1145.

49. Wells-Knecht KJ, Zyzak DV, Litchfield JE, et al. Mechanism of autoxidative glycosylation: identification of glyoxal and arabinose as intermediates in the autoxidative modification of proteins by glucose. Biochemistry 1995;34:3702–3709.
50. Thornalley PJ. The glyoxalase system: new developments towards functional characterization of a metabolic pathway fundamental to biological life. Biochem J 1990;269:1–11.
51. Chang EY, Szallasi Z, Acs P, et al. Functional effects of overexpression of protein kinase C-alpha, -beta, -delta, -epsilon, and -eta in the mast cell line RBL-2H3. J Immunol 1997;1159:2624–2632.
52. Shinohara M, Thornalley PJ, Giardino I, et al. Overexpression of glyoxalase-I in bovine endothelial cells inhibits intracellular advanced glycation endproduct formation and prevents hyperglycemia-induced increases in macromolecular endocytosis. J Clin Invest 1998;101:1142–1147.
53. Maisonpierre PC, Suri C, Jones PF, et al. Angiopoietin-2, a natural antagonist for Tie2 that disrupts in vivo angiogenesis. Science 1997;277:55–60
54. Papapetropoulos A, Garcia-Cardena G, Dengler TJ, Maisonpierre PC, Yancopoulos GD, Sessa WC. Direct actions of angiopoietin-1 on human endothelium: evidence for network stabilization, cell survival, and interaction with other angiogenic growth factors. Lab Invest 1999;79:213–223.
55. Hanahan D. Signaling vascular morphogenesis and maintenance. Science 1997;277:48–50.
56. Cochrane SM, Robinson GB. In vitro glycation of a glomerular basement membrane alters its permeability: a possible mechanism in diabetic complications. FEBS Lett 1995;375:41–44.
57. Boyd-White J, Williams JC Jr. Effect of cross-linking on matrix permeability. A model for AGE-modified basement membranes. Diabetes 1996;45:348–353.
58. Haitoglou CS, Tsilibary EC, Brownlee M, Charonis AS. Altered cellular interactions between endothelial cells and nonenzymatically glucosylated laminin/type IV collagen. J Biol Chem 1992;267:12,404–12,407.
59. Federoff HJ, Lawrence D, Brownlee M. Nonenzymatic glycosylation of laminin and the laminin peptide CIKVAVS inhibits neurite outgrowth. Diabetes 1993;42:509–513.
60. Hammes HP, Weiss A, Hess S, et al. Modification of vitronectin by advanced glycation 325alters functional properties in vitro and in the diabetic retina. Lab Invest 1996;75:325–338.
61. Li YM, Mitsuhashi T, Wojciechowicz D, et al. Molecular identity and cellular distribution of advanced glycation endproduct receptors: relationship of p60 to OST- 48 and p90 to 80K-H membrane proteins. Proc Natl Acad Sci USA 1996;93:11047–11052.
62. Yang Z, Makita Z, Horii Y, et al. Two novel rat liver membrane proteins that bind advanced glycosylation endproducts: relationship to macrophage receptor for glucose-modified proteins. J Exp Med 1991;174:515–524.
63. Vlassara H, Brownlee M, Monogue K, et al. Cachectin/TNF and IL-1 induced by glucose-modified proteins: role in normal tissue remodeling. Science 1988;240:156–157.
64. Kirstein M, Aston C, Hintz R, Vlassara H. Receptor-specific induction of insulin-like growth factor I in human monocytes by advanced glycosylation end product-modified proteins. J Clin Invest 1992;90:439–446.
65. Yui S, Sasaki T, Araki N, et al. Induction of macrophage growth by advanced glycation end products of the Maillard reaction. J Immunol 1994;152:1943–1949.
66. Abordo EA, Westwood ME, Thornalley PJ. Synthesis and secretion of macrophage colony stimulating factor by mature human monocytes and human monocytic THP-1 cells induced by human serum albumin derivatives modified with methylglyoxal and glucose-derived advanced glycation endproducts. Immunol Lett 1996;53:7–13.
67. Webster L, Abordo EA, Thornalley PJ, Limb GA. Induction of TNF alpha and IL-beta mRNA in monocytes by methylglyoxal- and advanced glycated endproduct-modified human serum albumin. Biochem Soc Trans 1997;25:250S.
68. Pugliese G, Pricci F, Romeo G, et al. Upregulation of mesangial growth factor and extracellular matrix synthesis by advanced glycation end products via a receptor-mediated mechanism. Diabetes 1997;46:1881–1887.
69. Smedsrod B, Melkko J, Araki N, et al. Advanced glycation end products are eliminated by scavenger-receptor-mediated endocytosis in hepatic sinusoidal kupffer and endothelial cells. Biochem J 1997;322:567–573.
70. Horiuchi S, Higashi T, Ikeda K, et al. Advanced glycation end products and their recognition by macrophage and macrophage-derived cells. Diabetes 1996;45:S73–S76.
71. Sano H, Higashi T, Matsumoto K, et al. Insulin enhances macrophage scavenger receptor-mediated endocytic uptake of advanced glycation end products. J Biol Chem 1998;273:8630–8637.

72. Vlassara H, Li YM, Imani F, et al. Identification of galectin-3 as a high-affinity binding protein for advanced glycation end products (AGE): a new member of the AGE-receptor complex. Mol Med 1995;1:634–646.
73. Schmidt AM, Vianna M, Gerlach M, et al. Isolation and characterization of two binding proteins for advanced glycosylation end products from bovine lung which are present on the endothelial cell surface. J Biol Chem 1992;267:14,987–14,997.
74. Neeper M, Schmidt AM, Brett J, et al. Cloning and expression of RAGE: a cell surface receptor for advanced glycosylation end products of proteins. J Biol Chem 1992;267:14,998–15,004.
75. Schmidt AM, Mora R, Cao K, et al. The endothelial cell binding site for advanced glycation endproducts consists of A complex: an integral membrane protein and a lactoferrin-like polypeptide. J Biol Chem 1994;269:9882–9888.
76. Wautier JL, Zoukourian C, Chappey O, et al. Receptor-mediated endothelial cell dysfunction in diabetic vasculopathy: soluble receptor for advanced glycation end products blocks hyperpermeability in diabetic rats. J Clin Invest 1996;97:238–243.
77. Lu M, Kuroki M, Amano S, et al. Advanced glycation end products increase retinal vascular endothelial growth factor expression. J Clin Invest 1998;101:1219–1224.
78. Hirata C, Nakano K, Nakamura N, et al. Advanced glycation end products induce expression of vascular endothelial growth factor by retinal Muller cells. Biochem Biophys Res Commun 1997;236:712–715.
79. Inoguchi T, Battan R, Handler E, Sportsman JR, Heath W, King GL. Preferential elevation of protein kinase C isoform beta II anddiacylglycerol levels in the aorta and heart of diabetic rats: differential reversibility to glycemic control by islet cell transplantation. Proc Natl Acad Sci USA 1992;89: 11,059–11,063.
80. Craven PA, Davidson CM, DeRubertis FR. Increase in diacylglycerol mass in isolated glomeruli by glucose from denovo synthesis of glycerolipids. Diabetes 1990;39:667–674.
81. Shiba T, Inoguchi T, Sportsman JR, Heath WF, Bursell S, King GL Correlation of diacylglycerol level and protein kinase C activity in rat retina to retinal circulation. Am J Physiol 1993;265:E783–E793.
82. Inoguchi T, Xia P, Kunisaki M, Higashi S, Feener EP, King G. Insulin's effect on protein kinase C and diacylglycerol induced by diabetes and glucose in vascular tissues. Am J Physiol 1994;267:E369–E379.
83. Derubertis FR, Craven PA. Activation of protein kinase C in glomerular cells in diabetes. Mechanisms and potential links to the pathogenesis of diabetic glomerulopathy. Diabetes 1994;43:1–8.
84. Xia P, Inoguchi T, Kern TS, Engerman RL, Oates PJ, King GL. Characterization of the mechanism for the chronic activation of diacylglycerol-protein kinase C pathway in diabetes and hypergalactosemia. Diabetes 1994;43:1122–1129.
85. Ayo SH, Radnik R, Garoni JA, Troyer DA, Kreisberg JI. High glucose increases diacylglycerol mass and activates protein kinase C in mesangial cell cultures. Am J Physiol 1991;261:F571–F577.
86. Koya D, Jirousek MR, Lin YW, Ishii H, Kuboki K, King GL. Characterization of protein kinase C beta isoform activation on the gene expression of transforming growth factor-beta, extracellular matrix components, and prostanoids in the glomeruli of diabetic rats. J Clin Invest 1997;100:115–126.
87. Kikkawa R, Haneda M, Uzu T, Koya D, Sugimoto T, Shigeta Y. Translocation of protein kinase C alpha and zeta in rat glomerular mesangial cells cultured under high glucose conditions. Diabetologia 1994;37:838–841.
88. Ishii H, Jirousek MR, Koya D, et al. Amelioration of vascular dysfunctions in diabetic rats by an oral PKC beta inhibitor. Science 1996;272:728–731.
89. Craven PA, Studer RK, DeRubertis FR. Impaired nitric oxide-dependent cyclic guanosine monophosphategeneration in glomeruli from diabetic rats. Evidence for protein kinase C-mediated suppression of the cholinergic response. J Clin Invest 1994;93:311–320.
90. Ganz MB, Seftel A. Glucose-induced changes in protein kinase C and nitric oxide are prevented by vitamin E. Am J Physiol 2000;278:E146–E152.
91. Kuboki K, Jiang ZY, Takahara N, et al. Regulation of endothelial constitutive nitric oxide synthase gene expression in endothelial cells and in vivo: a specific vascular action of insulin. Circulation 2000;101:676–681.
92. Glogowski EA, Tsiani E, Zhou X, Fantus IG, Whiteside C. High glucose alters the response of mesangial cell protein kinase C isoforms to endothelin-1. Kidney Int 1999;55:486–499.
93. Williams B, Gallacher B, Patel H, Orme C. Glucose-induced protein kinase C activation regulates vascular permeability factor mRNA expression and peptide production by human vascular smooth muscle cells in vitro. Diabetes 1997;46:1497–1503.
94. Studer RK, Craven PA, DeRubertis FR. Role for protein kinase C in the mediation of increased fibronectin accumulation by mesangial cells grown in high-glucose medium. Diabetes 1993;42:118–126.

95. Pugliese G, Pricci F, Pugliese F, et al. Mechanisms of glucose-enhanced extracellular matrix accumulation in rat glomerular mesangial cells. Diabetes 1994;43:478–490.
96. Craven PA, Studer RK, Felder J, Phillips S, DeRubertis FR. Nitric oxide inhibition of transforming growth factor-beta and collagen synthesis in mesangial cells. Diabetes 1997;46:671–681.
97. Phillips SL, DeRubertis FR, Craven PA. Regulation of the laminin C1 promoter in cultured mesangial cells. Diabetes 1999;48:2083–2089.
98. Feener EP, Xia P, Inoguchi T, Shiba T, Kunisaki M, King GL. Role of protein kinase C in glucose- and angiotensin II-induced plasminogen activator inhibitor expression. Contrib Nephrol 1996;118:180–187.
99. Pieper GM, Riaz-ul-Haq J. Activation of nuclear factor-kappaB in cultured endothelial cells by increased glucose concentration: prevention by calphostin C. Cardiovasc Pharmacol 1997;30:528–532.
100. Yerneni KK, Bai W, Khan BV, Medford RM, Natarajan R. Hyperglycemia-induced activation of nuclear transcription factor kappaB in vascular smooth muscle cells. Diabetes 1999;48:855–864.
101. Sayeski PP, Kudlow JE. Glucose metabolism to glucosamine is necessary for glucose stimulation of transforming growth factor-alpha gene transcription. J Biol Chem 1996;271:15,237–15,243.
102. Kolm-Litty V, Sauer U, Nerlich A, Lehmann R, Schleicher ED. High glucose-induced transforming growth factor beta1 production is mediated by the hexosamine pathway in porcine glomerular mesangial cells. J Clin Invest 1998;101:160–169.
103. Marshall S, Bacote V, Traxinger RR. Discovery of a metabolic pathway mediating glucose-induced desensitization of the glucose transport system. Role of hexosamine biosynthesis in the induction of insulin resistance. J Biol Chem 1991;266:4706–4712.
104. Rossetti L, Hawkins M, Chen W, Gindi J, Barzilai N. In vivo glucosamine infusion induces insulin resistance in normoglycemic but not in hyperglycemic conscious rats. J Clin Invest 1995;96:132–140.
105. Hawkins M, Barzilai N, Liu R, Hu M, Chen W, Rossetti L. Role of the glucosamine pathway in fat-induced insulin resistance. J Clin Invest 1997;99:2173–2182.
106. Hart GW. Dynamic O-linked glycosylation of nuclear and cytoskeletal proteins. Annu Rev Biochem. 1997;66:315–335.
107. Engerman RL, Kern TS, Larson ME. Nerve conduction and aldose reductase inhibition during 5 years of diabetes or galactosaemia in dogs. Diabetologia 1994;37:141–144.
108. Sima AA, Prashar A, Zhang WX, Chakrabarti S, Greene DA. Preventive effect of long-term aldose reductase inhibition (ponalrestat) on nerve conduction and sural nerve structure in the spontaneously diabetic Bio-Breeding rat. J Clin Invest 1990;85:1410–1420.
109. Lee AY, Chung SK, Chung SS. Demonstration that polyol accumulation is responsible for diabetic cataract by the use of transgenic mice expressing the aldose reductase gene in the lens. Proc Natl Acad Sci USA 1995;92:2780–2784.
110. Brownlee M. Advanced protein glycosylation in diabetes and aging. Annu Rev Med 1995;46:223–234.
111. Nishikawa T, Edelstein D, Du XL, et al. Normalizing mitochondrial superoxide production blocks three pathways of hyperglycemic damage. Nature 2000;404:787–790.
112. Du XL, Edelstein D, Rossetti L, et al. Hyperglycemia-induced mitochondrial superoxide overproduction activates the hexosamine pathway and induces PAI-1 expression by increasing Sp1 glycosylation. Proc Natl Acad Sci USA, 2002;97:12,222–12,226.
113. Giardino I, Edelstein D, Brownlee M. BCL-2 expression or antioxidants prevent hyperglycemia-induced formation of intracellular advanced glycation endproducts in bovine endothelial cells. J Clin Invest 1996;97:1422–1428.
114. Wallace DC. Diseases of the mitochondrial DNA. Annu Rev Biochem 1992;61:1175–1212.
115. Trumpower BL. The protonmotive Q cycle. J Biol Chem 1990;265:11,409–11,412.
116. Korshunov SS, Skulachev VP, Starkov AA. High protonic potential actuates a mechanism of production of reactive oxygen species in mitochondria. FEBS Lett 1997;416:15–18.
117. Casteilla L, Blnodel O, Klaus S, et al. Stable expression of functional mitochondrial uncoupling protein in Chinese hamster ovary cells. Proc Natl Acad Sci USA 1990;87:5124–5128.
118. Manna SK, Zhang HJ, Yan T, et al. Overexpression manganese superoxide dismutase suppresses tumor necrosis factor-induced apoptotsis and activation of nuclear transcription factor-κB and activated protein-1. J Biol Chem 1998;273:13,245–13,254.
119. Koya D, King GL. Protein kinase C activation and the development of diabetic complications. Diabetes 1998;47:859–866.
120. Faulkner KM, Liochev SI. Fridovich I table Mn(III) porphyrins mimic superoxide dismutase in vitro and substitute for it in vivo. J Biol Chem 1994 269:23,471–23,476.
121. Doctrow SR, Huffman K, Marcus CB, et al. Salen–manganese complexes: combined superoxide dismutase/catalase mimics with broad pharmacological efficacy. Adv Pharmacol 1997;38:247–269.

22 The Eye
Diabetic Retinopathy/Ophthalmopathy

David Kent, MD, and Peter A. Campochiaro, MD

CONTENTS

EPIDEMIOLOGY

Diabetes accounts for 10% of blindness of all ages and an astonishing 20% of new blindness between the ages of 45 and 74 yr within the United States *(1)*. Considering the millions of people with undiagnosed diabetes and the increasing rate of development of type 2 diabetes in developed countries *(2,3)*, diabetic eye disease is a major public health problem. Unless new and more effective treatments are developed, it will continue to exact a huge toll on affected individuals during their most productive years at tremendous personal and societal cost. Furthermore, as the life span of people with diabetes increases, the visual disability arising from diabetes will have greater and greater impact on our society.

Around 10–15% of the total diabetic population have type 1 diabetes (defined as diabetes diagnosis at or before age 30) *(2)*. Diabetic retinopathy is seen in 13% of these patients with duration of disease less than 5 yr. This figure increases to 90% with disease duration of 10–15 yr. Proliferative diabetic retinopathy (PDR), which is defined by the presence of retinal neovascularization, is present in around 25% of those individuals with a duration of disease of 15 yr, whereas the prevalence of diabetic macular edema in type 1 diabetes is approx 20%.

Diabetes affects multiple ocular tissues, but it is its effect on the retina that has greatest significance because it is the source of almost all visual loss resulting from diabetes. Diabetic retinopathy is an insidious condition. Even patients with minimal or no symptoms can have severe sight-threatening disease. There are treatments that can

From: *Contemporary Endocrinology: Type 1 Diabetes: Etiology and Treatment*
Edited by: M. A. Sperling © Humana Press Inc., Totowa, NJ

be beneficial if provided at the appropriate stage of the disease; therefore, it is critical for diabetics to have regular eye examinations.

DIABETIC EYE DISEASE

Vision loss in diabetes mellitus is usually the result of diabetic retinopathy. A complication of severe diabetic retinopathy is neovascular glaucoma, which can lead to a blind painful eye if not treated expeditiously. Other less common causes of vision loss in diabetes are cataracts and, occasionally, keratopathy (corneal disease). Corneal disease stems from basement membrane thickening that makes the corneal epithelium less adherent, susceptible to injury, and slower to heal than the nondiabetic cornea. Diabetic papillopathy (swelling of the optic nerve) is an uncommon cause of vision loss that is usually transient, but sometimes permanent. Cranial nerve palsies are uncommon causes of diplopia (double vision) that occur more commonly in diabetics than nondiabetics.

DIABETIC RETINOPATHY

Pathophysiology

Hyperglycemia is the basic cause of diabetic retinopathy *(4,5)*. One possible reason for the susceptibility of the retina to hyperglycemia is that, opposed to many tissues in which the entry of glucose is controlled by insulin, glucose enters the retina by facilitated diffusion. Therefore, high serum glucose translates into high levels of glucose in the retina. There are several theories as to how high glucose causes damage to the retina, manifested primarily by damage to retinal blood vessels, but none of these have been sufficiently supported to gain prominence over the others. One theory suggests that excess glucose is metabolized by aldose reductase to sorbitol, and because sorbitol does not diffuse out of cells, it accumulates and causes damage *(6)*. Levels of sorbitol sufficient to cause hyperosmostic damage have been demonstrated in the lenses, but not the retinas of diabetic animals. It has been suggested that high sorbitol levels may decrease myoinositol levels, resulting in damage to cell membranes. Another theory is that high glucose results in nonenzymatic glycosylation of proteins that results in cellular dysfunction *(7)*. High glucose also results in selective activation of the β isoform of protein kinase C (PKC), which has also been suggested to cause cellular dysfunction *(8)*. Although it is clear that these changes occur, it is not yet clear whether they are causally related to subsequent structural changes or whether they are epiphenomena.

Most theories have assumed that retinal vascular cells, particularly pericytes, are preferentially susceptible to the damaging effects of high glucose, because pericyte dropout is a well-recognized pathologic feature. However, it has recently been demonstrated that apoptosis of retinal neurons and glia occurs early in diabetes, raising the possibility that this may somehow contribute to subsequent vascular damage *(9)*. Other early changes are increases in retinal blood flow and vascular permeability *(10,11)*, but, as with other early changes, it is not certain whether they play any role in the clinically significant changes that occur years later.

Evidence of damage to retinal vessels appears many years after the onset of hypergylcemia and is seen clinically by the presence of hemorrhages, microaneurysms, nerve fiber layer infarcts, venous beading, and intraretinal microvascular abnormalities

(IRMA). A diabetic who has some or all of these features is said to have background diabetic retinopathy (BDR) or nonproliferative diabetic retinopathy (NPDR) *(12)*. Leakiness of retinal vessels results in edema, which when located in the macula is referred to as diabetic macular edema (DME), a major cause of decreased vision *(13)*. Occlusion of blood vessels results in retinal ischemia. If the perifoveal capillaries become occluded, permanent visual loss can occur from ischemic damage to the macula (ischemic maculopathy). Recently, leukocytic plugging has been implicated in capillary occlusion in diabetes *(14)*.

The occurrence of large areas of capillary occlusion heralds the onset of PDR. Retinal ischemia occurs in other retinovascular diseases other than diabetic retinopathy, including branch vein occlusion, central vein occlusion, retinopathy of prematurity, and several others. These diseases are collectively called ischemic retinopathies. Retinal ischemia causes increased levels of hypoxia-inducible factor-1 (HIF-1) in the retina *(15)* and increased expression of genes that contain a HIF-1-binding site in their promoter region, including vascular endothelial growth factor (VEGF) and VEGF receptor-1 *(16–18)*. Increased VEGF signaling plays a central role in the development of retinal neovascularization (for review, *see* ref. *19*). Retinal neovascularization grows through the internal limiting membrane (ILM) of the retina onto the surface of the retina and into the vitreous. The new blood vessels leak and bleed resulting in vitreous hemorrhage. Glial cells and retinal pigmented epithelial (RPE) cells migrate onto the retinal surface and surround the neovascularization, forming sheets and bands of scar tissue. Contraction of the vitreous and scar tissue pulls on the retina, resulting in traction retinal detachment, and if the macula is involved, there is severe loss of vision. Unless the retina is surgically reattached in a timely fashion, the eye becomes permanently blind.

Genetic Component

Severe diabetic retinopathy tends to run in families *(20)* and there is concordance among identical twins indicating that diabetic retinopathy has a genetic component. Several candidate gene or case-control studies have reported that there are genetic variations that are associated with an increased *(21–25)* or decreased *(26)* risk of diabetic retinopathy. This suggests that diabetic retinopathy is a genetically complex trait, meaning that there are genetic variations that increase susceptibility and others that provide a protective effect. This is very complicated, because type 1 diabetes itself is a genetically complex trait *(27,28)*. Therefore, diabetic retinopathy is a complex genetic trait occurring in the setting of a systemic disease that is a complex genetic trait. Regardless of the complexity, the identification of the genetic variations that impact on features of diabetic retinopathy can provide new insights into the molecular mechanisms involved and provide the basis for new strategies for treatment.

Risk Factors for Diabetic Retinopathy

Glycemic Control

The association between blood glucose control and the complications of diabetes, including retinopathy, have been well documented in several observational studies *(29–31)*. These observations led investigators to speculate that a reduction in blood glucose might cause a corresponding reduction in the risk of progression of retinopathy, which led to the initiation of the Diabetes Control and Complication Trial (DCCT)

(5,32). In the DCCT, patients with type 1 diabetes were randomly assigned to either conventional or intensive insulin therapy. The trial demonstrated that subjects receiving the intensive regimen had a statistically significant reduction in the development and progression of diabetic retinopathy. In patients without retinopathy who received intensive treatment, the 3-yr risk of developing retinopathy was reduced by 75% when compared to the conventional group. Tight glycemic control was also shown to be beneficial in subjects with pre-existing retinopathy, in whom there was a 50% reduction in the rate of progression of retinopathy compared to controls. There was a 35–40% reduction in the risk of progression of retinopathy for every 10% decrease in HbA1C (e.g., from 10% to 9%). Intensive insulin treatment was also found to reduce the incidence of both nephropathy and neuropathy. It follows that both physicians and patients should closely follow the HbA1C level, because it provides a measure of recent glycemic control and, thereby, the risk of progression of retinopathy and other diabetic complications.

Although tight glycemic control is very important, development of other complementary approaches for prophylaxis are needed, because over the 9-yr course of the DCCT, the onset of retinopathy was delayed, but not prevented. Also, patients with pre-existent retinopathy frequently show transient accelerated progression of retinopathy when first converted from conventional to intensive management of blood glucose *(5,33)*. Also, tight control has its down side as well, because there was a twofold to threefold increase in severe hypoglycemia in the intensively managed group compared to the conventionally managed group.

Hypertension

The most meaningful data analyzing the effect of blood pressure control on the progression of NPDR comes from the United Kingdom Prospective Diabetes Study (UKPDS) *(34)*. It demonstrated that intensive control of blood pressure is associated with a 37% decrease in risk of progression of retinopathy and other microvascular complications. Although this study was carried out exclusively in subjects with type 2 diabetes, it is reasonable to extrapolate its findings to patients with type 1 diabetes. In another part of the study, β-blockers were found to be equally beneficial as angiotensin-converting enzyme (ACE) inhibitors, calling into question the previous suggestion that ACE inhibitors have a beneficial effect in type 1 diabetes that is independent of their effect on blood pressure *(35)*.

Elevated Serum Cholesterol/Triglycerides

Several studies have suggested that elevated serum lipids increase the risk of vision loss from diabetic retinopathy *(36–38)*. The Early Treatment Diabetic Retinopathy Study (ETDRS) and the Wisconsin Epidemiologic Study of Diabetic Retinopathy (WESDR) found that elevated levels of cholesterol were associated with increased severity of hard exudates, which was a significant risk factor for moderate vision loss independent of macular edema. The presence of hard exudate was the strongest risk factor for the development of submacular fibrosis, an important cause of permanent vision loss. The ETDRS also found that elevated serum triglycerides is associated with a greater risk of developing high-risk PDR *(39)*. Thus, it is imperative for ophthalmologists and diabetes specialists to carefully follow the patient's lipid profile and treat when necessary, to decrease the risk of visual morbidity as well as cardiovascular disease.

Other potential risk factors for progression of retinopathy include diabetic nephropathy, neuropathy, cardiovascular autonomic neuropathy, anemia, and decreasing hematocrit *(39–42)*.

Clinical Features of Diabetic Retinopathy

Retinal hemorrhages are a common feature of diabetic retinopathy and vary in their appearance based on their location within the retina. The superficial capillary bed is located in the nerve fiber layer and hemorrhages from superficial capillaries have a flame-shaped appearance as the blood spreads between nerve fibers that run parallel to the retinal surface. Hemorrhages occurring from the deep capillary beds, where the arrangement of cells is perpendicular and more compact, tend to be circular and called dot (small) or blot (larger) hemorrhages depending on their size (*see* Fig. 1). Loss of pericytes results in microaneursyms, small outpouchings of vessel walls that leak plasma into the surrounding retina, causing retinal edema. When the edema spreads into the macula, the center portion of the retina that is responsible for our best vision, it is referred to as macular edema. Macular edema is the most prevalent cause of visual loss in diabetics. As edema fluid diffuses away from the major sources of leakage, it is resorbed by more normal areas of the capillary bed. Poorly soluble serum lipoproteins frequently precipitate near sites of resorption, resulting in hard exudates (*see* Fig. 2).

Pericyte loss is initially followed by endothelial cell proliferation, which, along with leukostasis, may result in occlusion of capillaries. When capillary occlusion becomes widespread, there is retinal ischemia, which is often recognized clinically by its effects on adjacent larger vessels, including venous dilation, beading, reduplication, and loop formation (*see* Fig. 3). IRMAs (Figs. 3 and 4) probably represent new vessel formation that is within the retina; it is only when new vessels penetrate the internal limiting membrane and grow along the surface of the retina into the vitreous cavity that they are recognized as neovascularization (*see* Figs. 3 and 4). A cotton-wool spot (or soft exudate) is thought to develop as a result of obstruction of a retinal arteriole. The resultant focal hypoxia leads to blockage of axoplasmic flow in the nerve fiber layer that is clinically recognizable as a cotton-wool spot (*see* Fig. 4).

Neovascularization occurs at the border of the perfused and nonperfused retina. Some outflow of fluid from the eye occurs at the optic nerve, and when retinal ischemia becomes severe enough, vasoproliferative factors may become concentrated at the optic nerve, resulting in neovascularization at the disk (NVD) (*see* Fig. 5). Neovascularization that occurs elsewhere in the retina is called neovascularization elsewhere or NVE (*see* Figs. 3 and 4). Because NVD tends to be associated with more severe retinal ischemia than comparable sized areas of NVE, NVD is associated with a greater risk of visual loss. When retinal ischemia is extremely severe, vasoproliferative factors may become concentrated at the anterior outflow channels of the eye, resulting in neovascularization on the trabecular meshwork and the iris that make up the anterior chamber angle. This is referred to as neovascularization of the iris (NVI) or rubeosis. Blockage of outflow through the trabecular meshwork by new vessels results in neovascular glaucoma.

Vitreous hemorrhages seen in PDR arise secondary to NVD and/or NVE and occur anterior to the retina, in the vitreous cavity. They can be either diffuse, as a result of bleeding into the vitreous humor, or bow shaped, an appearance that arises from the accumulation of blood in the potential space between the retina and vitreous (*see* Fig. 6).

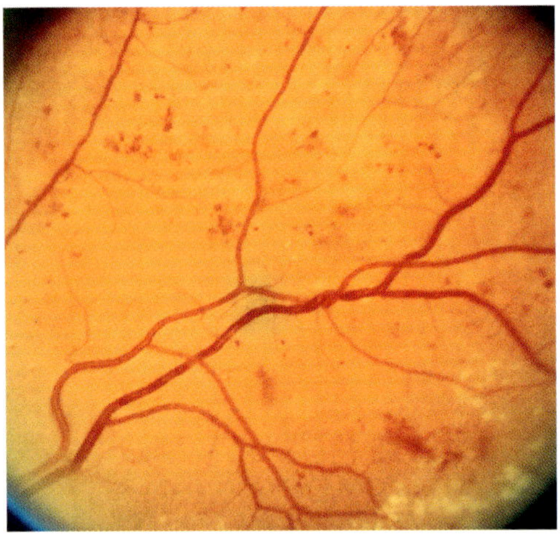
Fig. 1

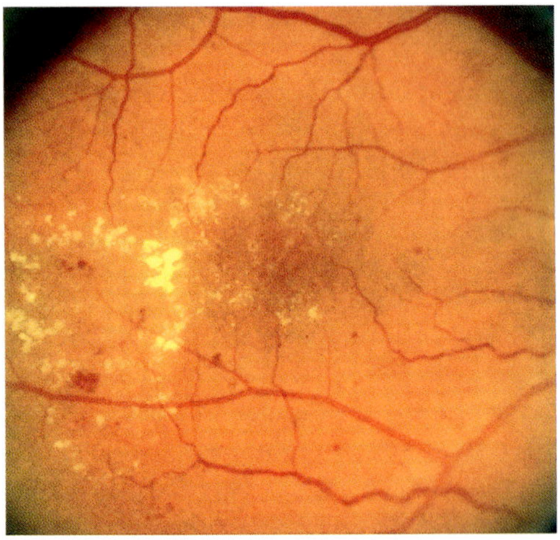
Fig. 2

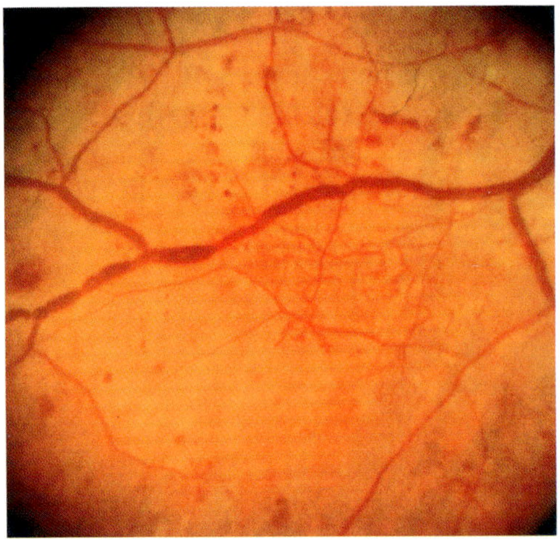
Fig. 3

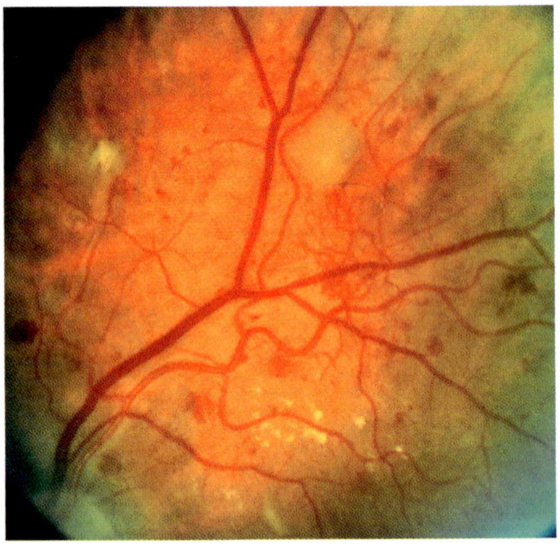
Fig. 4

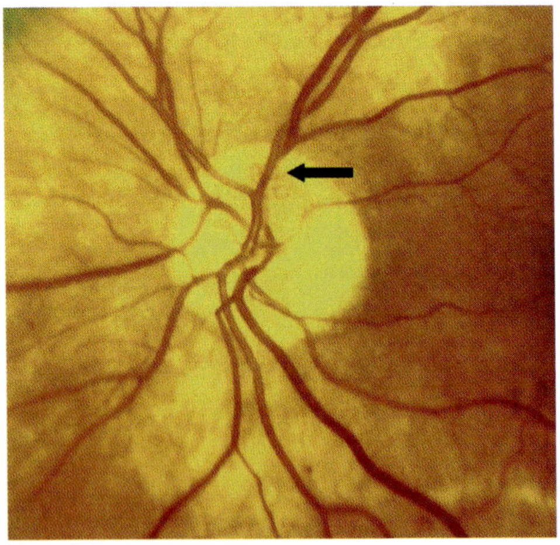
Fig. 5

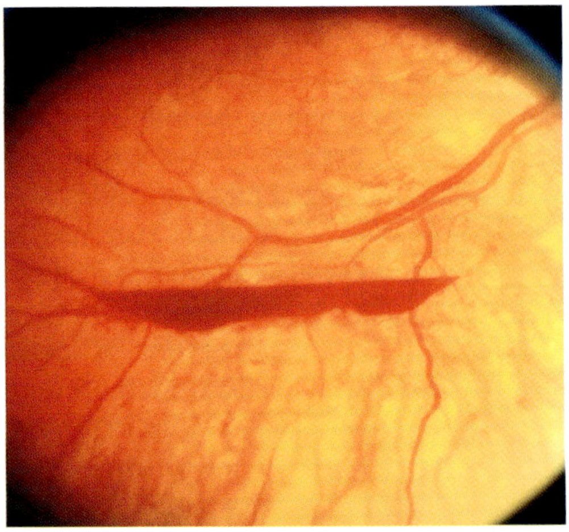
Fig. 6

Fig. 1. Standard photograph 2B demonstrating dot and blot hemorrhages and microaneurysms. (Courtesy of the Early Treatment Diabetic Retinopathy Study [ETDRS] Research Group.)

Fig. 2. Standard photograph 4 demonstrating severe hard exudates. Associated macular edema, if present, can only be appreciated either by fundus biomicroscopy or with stereophotography (Courtesy of the Early Treatment Diabetic Retinopathy Study [ETDRS] Research Group.)

Fig. 3. Standard photograph 6B demonstrating severe venous beading, IRMAs, and neovascularization elsewhere (NVE). (Courtesy of the Early Treatment Diabetic Retinopathy Study [ETDRS] Research Group.)

Fig. 4. Standard photograph 5 demonstrating hard exudates, soft exudates (cotton-wool spots), IRMAs, and NVE. (Courtesy of the Early Treatment Diabetic Retinopathy Study [ETDRS] Research Group.)

Fig. 5. Standard photograph 10A defining the lower limit of moderate neovascularization of the disk (NVD). (Courtesy of the Early Treatment Diabetic Retinopathy Study [ETDRS] Research Group.)

Fig. 6. Standard photograph 13 demonstrating preretinal hemorrhage. (Courtesy of the Early Treatment Diabetic Retinopathy Study [ETDRS] Research Group.)

This latter type of hemorrhage is also referred to as preretinal or retrohyaloid hemorrhages to emphasize its location in relation to the retina and vitreous. Unsophisticated observers may not distinguish between the types of hemorrhage, but they should be encouraged to do so because the location and configuration of hemorrhages has clinical significance.

Landmark Clinical Trials Addressing the Management of Diabetic Retinopathy

The Diabetic Retinopathy Study

Numerous anecdotal reports throughout the 1960s suggested that photocoagulation provided some benefit in patients with PDR. To determine if this was the case and to better define the indications, side effects, long-term results, and complications of photocoagulation, a clinical trial, the Diabetic Retinopathy Study (DRS), was commenced in 1971. The DRS demonstrated that scatter laser photocoagulation (panretinal photocoagulation, [PRP]) significantly reduced the risk of severe visual loss from PDR *(43)*.

The Early Treatment Diabetic Retinopathy Study

Although the DRS clearly demonstrated the beneficial effect of PRP in PDR, it did not address the questions of timing or extent of treatment nor did it clarify if photocoagulation benefited other aspects of the disease, such as macular edema. The ETDRS was designed to determine if it is preferable to perform PRP prior to the onset of neovascularization or after neovascularization had begun *(44)*. It was also designed to determine if focal laser photocoagulation for diabetic macular edema was beneficial *(13)*. Focal laser photocoagulation entails direct laser treatment to leakage sites to try to decrease leakage and improve edema. When the leakage sites were difficult to define and/or there was diffuse leakage from the vascular bed, this was referred to as diffuse diabetic macular edema and a grid of a laser was placed. The ETDRS used the term "clinically significant macular edema" or CSME to describe any one of three situations: (1) retinal thickening at or within 500 μm from the center of the macula, (2) hard exudates at or within 500 μm of the center of the macula if there is thickening of adjacent retina, or (3) an area of retinal thickening at least one disk area in size, part of which must be within one disk diameter of the center of the macula. When all eyes with diabetic macular edema were considered and irrespective of whether the edema was "clinically significant," immediate focal, or grid treatment reduced the incidence of moderate visual loss (loss of 15 or more letters on an ETDRS visual acuity chart) by approx 50% at all time-points *(13)*. On the other hand, PRP was found not to be effective in managing macular edema. In some cases, PRP may accelerate the progression of macular edema.

The ETDRS also demonstrated that early panretinal photocoagulation in eyes with severe nonproliferative diabetic retinopathy (NPDR) did not significantly alter the end point of severe visual loss (visual acuity less than 5/200 at two consecutive follow-up visits) and deferral of laser treatment until such time as high-risk PDR develops is therefore recommended, provided careful follow-up can be maintained *(44)*.

The Diabetic Retinopathy Vitrectomy Study

The Diabetic Retinopathy Vitrectomy Study (DRVS) was designed to answer the question, Is it is better to perform vitreous surgery immediately when a patient presents with a severe vitreous hemorrhage because of PDR, or should surgery be deferred to allow the hemorrhage to clear spontaneously? The results provided guidelines for the most appropriate time to perform vitrectomy surgery in type 1 and 2 diabetics with vitreous hemorrhage and in patients with severe PDR with moderate or no vitreous hemorrhage. In eyes with severe vitreous hemorrhage causing a significant reduction in vision, early vitrectomy was beneficial in type 1, but not type 2 diabetics *(45,46)*. The reason for this seems to be that type 1 diabetics with severe vitreous hemorrhage tend to have severe neovascularization, whereas most type 2 diabetics do not. In eyes with severe neovascularization and clear media, immediate vitrectomy was beneficial in both type 1 and type 2 diabetics *(47)*. Severe neovascularization carries a poor prognosis that is in part mitigated by early vitrectomy *(48)*.

Classification of Diabetic Retinopathy: Definitions and Clinical Significance

Diabetic retinopathy is classified as NPDR and PDR. Within these broad categories further subcategories or levels of retinopathy exist (*see* Table 1). These levels were defined by the ETDRS. The significance of this classification is that it allows the physician to correlate the level of retinopathy directly with the risk of progression to more severe retinopathy and, hence, the need for possible laser photocoagulation at a future date (*see* Table 1), as demonstrated by the findings of the ETDRS (*see below*). This system is therefore preferred to the older system, which broadly classified retinopathy into background and proliferative, but addressed neither the risk of progression nor the likelihood of future treatment. Accurate diagnosis of the level of retinopathy is therefore crucial because the risk of progression to PDR and, hence, any treatment depends on the specific NPDR level.

Grading of Diabetic Retinopathy and Implications for Clinical Practice

Current treatment recommendations for diabetic retinopathy are based on the results of the DRS and the ETDRS. Provided that careful follow-up can be maintained, the ETDRS recommended that patients with mild or moderate NPDR generally do not

Table 1
ETDRS Levels of Retinopathy

Mild NPDR—At least one microaneurysm, but not as severe as moderate NPDR.
The presence of mild NPDR has a 5% risk of progression to PDR within 12 mo and a 15% risk of progression to high-risk PDR within 5 yr.
Moderate NPDR—Extensive intraretinal hemorrhages and/or microaneurysms, and or cotton wool spots, venous beading, or IRMA) present, but not as extensive as severe NPDR.
There is a 12–27% risk of progression to PDR at 12 mo with the risk of progression to high-risk proliferative disease being 33% within 5 yr.
Severe NPDR—Severe intraretinal hemorrhages and microaneurysms in all four quadrants; venous beading present in two or more quadrants; or IRMA present in at least one quadrant ("4–2–1" rule).
These eyes have a 52% risk of progressing to PDR within 1 yr and a 60% risk of high-risk PDR within 5 yr.
Very severe NPDR—If any 2 of the features of severe NPDR are present, then the retinopathy is classified as been very severe NPDR.
These patients have a 75% risk of PDR within 12 mo.
Early PDR *(non-high-risk PDR)*—NVD less than a third of the disk area without preretinal or vitreous hemorrhage or NVE less that or equal to a half of the disk area without preretinal or vitreous hemorrhage.
These eyes have a 75% risk of becoming high risk within 5 yr.
High-risk PDR—NVD greater or equal to a third of the disk area, or NVD with vitreous or preretinal hemorrhage or NVE greater or equal to a half of the disk area with associated preretinal or vitreous hemorrhage.

NPDR, nonproliferative diabetic retinopathy; PDR, proliferative diabetic retinopathy; IRMA, intraretinal microvascular abnormalitites; NVD, neovascularization at the disk; NVE, neovascularization elsewhere.

require scatter laser photocoagulation and can be safely followed at 6- to 12-monthly intervals *(44)*. Intercurrent illness or pregnancy will require shorter follow-up as determined by the examining ophthalmologist. However, those patients who are approaching high-risk characteristics should be considered for laser, whereas treatment in patients with high-risk disease should not be delayed—findings that were in agreement with the DRS.

Although the ETDRS did not address the issue of timing of laser treatment of macular edema, a definite benefit was demonstrated when immediate treatment was instituted particularly when the edema was "clinically significant." Because the principal benefit of focal photocoagulation was to reduce the risk of further visual loss and not actually to improve vision, treatment of clinically significant macular edema (CSME) should be considered even when vision is 20/20. Eyes that are approaching high-risk disease and that also have CSME should undergo immediate treatment for edema in anticipation of possible future panretinal treatment if progression to high-risk disease occurs. Ideally, this should be performed 6–8 wk before the institution of scatter (panretinal) laser treatment, because of the potential deleterious effect of a panretinal laser on diabetic macular edema. On the other hand, delaying scatter treatment to treat edema in high-risk patients is not advised, because of the risk of severe visual loss. When both eyes are approaching high-risk disease, it is not unreasonable to consider initiation of scatter treatment in one eye, particularly as it may not be possible to optimize treatment if both eyes progress to high-risk disease at the same time. Finally, immediate scatter photocoagulation should be done when iris neovascularization is present, regardless of the grade of retinopathy. This is to try and prevent the potentially disastrous complication of neovascualar glaucoma.

The Role of Fluorescein Angiography in the Management of Diabetic Retinopathy

Fluorescein angiography is an important test that assists greatly in the management of diabetic retinopathy. Fluorescence occurs when blue light (wavelength of 465–490 nm) is used to excite sodium fluorescein to emit yellow–green light (520–530 nm). Fluorescein angiography is performed by injecting 25% sodium fluorescein intravenously and performing rapid sequence photography with the appropriate filters in place. Despite its low molecular weight, fluorescein does not normally diffuse out of the retinal blood vessels or across the RPE, because of the blood–retinal barrier. Because the retina is part of the central nervous system, it does not contain fenestrated capillaries like vascular beds elsewhere in the body. However, during some disease states, such as diabetic retinopathy, the blood–retinal barrier, made up of tight junctions between the retinal endothelial cells and RPE cells, can become incompetent and leak fluorescein molecules into the retina. In diabetic retinopathy, breakdown of the blood–retinal barrier can cause retinal edema that can involve the macula to cause vision loss.

Fluorescein angiography can also demonstrate other lesions of the diabetic fundus, such as capillary nonperfusion and neovascularization. Prior to treatment of CSME with laser photocoagulation, fluorescein angiography is performed to differentiate microaneurysms from small intraretinal hemorrhages and/or diffuse vascular leakage from focal leakage. Alternatively, it may demonstrate that macular edema is secondary to ischemia and, therefore, not amenable to laser treatment. Laser photocoagulation for CSME consists of "direct" treatment of microaneurysms (focal laser) or "grid" (placement of regularly spaced burns that do not target any particular lesion, but rather treat an area of diffuse leakage). In reality, almost all treatment of CSME consists of a combination of both focal and grid lasers.

Fluorescein angiography is not required to diagnose or classify PDR, but if performed, it will demonstrate leakage of fluorescein because new vessels are fenestrated. Laser treatment for retinal neovascularization consists of "scatter" or panretinal photocoagulation. The small spots of laser light are absorbed and converted to heat energy, creating small burns that are placed or "scattered" throughout the retina, except within the macular region, to prevent destruction of photoreceptors responsible for central vision. The treatment is not applied directly to the neovascularization, but regression of neovascularization often occurs because the scatter pattern of laser increases oxygenation of the retina and decreases the production of VEGF *(49)*.

OTHER CLINICALLY RELEVANT OCULAR COMPLICATIONS OF TYPE 1 DIABETES

The ravages of diabetes mellitus on the retina are long recognized by physicians and patients alike because of the effects on vision. However, all ocular structures are susceptible to the deleterious effects of the disease. Fortunately, many of these changes remain subclinical, whereas others, although not necessarily sight threatening, can have significant morbidity associated with them.

Mononeuropathies of the Extraocular Muscles

Palsies involving the third (oculomotor), fourth (superior oblique), and sixth (abducens/lateral rectus) cranial nerves occur not uncommonly in diabetes. However, despite this definite association, one must always bear in mind the potential for other pathology, including possible life-threatening disease *(50)*. Palsies of the third and sixth nerves are more commonly the result of diabetes than fourth-nerve palsies, so the latter should never be attributed to diabetes without a thorough investigation for other causes *(51,52)*. Histopathologically, diabetic mononeuropathies show occlusions of capillaries surrounding the nerves, resulting in small infarctions.

Paresis of the extraocular muscles gives rise to diplopia. However, third-nerve palsy is usually accompanied by ptosis, which is usually the presenting complaint. The ptotic lid may occlude the involved eye and prevent the symptomatic distress of diplopia. It is commonly stated that pupillary involvement in an oculomotor nerve palsy indicates aneurysm of the posterior communicating artery until proven otherwise, but pupillary involvement can occur in diabetic third-nerve palsies and although pain can also be a feature in diabetes, it is more likely to be seen in aneurysmal third-nerve palsies *(53)*.

Diabetic patients with a sixth-nerve palsy usually present with painless horizontal diplopia. However, before attributing the palsy to diabetes, other more sinister causes must be ruled out. Fourth-nerve palsies result in weakness of the superior oblique muscle, causing vertical or oblique diplopia, or sometimes a combination of both. In both fourth- and sixth-nerve palsies, patients can assume a characteristic head posture, moving their head to a position that reduces the need for the eye to move in the direction of the affected muscle.

As a general rule, in the absence of any other signs, these palsies are managed conservatively, as many will resolve entirely over 2–3 mo. However, an increase in severity of symptoms or the appearance of new symptoms should alert the physician to consider alternative diagnoses and appropriate investigations should be performed. In any event, baseline neuroimaging is reasonable, particularly when there is a third-nerve palsy.

Cataract

Age-related cataracts occur earlier, more frequently, and progress more rapidly in patients with diabetes *(54)*. Fortunately, present microsurgical techniques for cataract removal and prosthetic intraocular lens replacement are very successful and usually result in restoration of vision. However, there is some evidence that cataract surgery may be associated with acceleration of retinopathy. It is imperative that retinopathy be stable before surgery, and vigilance is warranted in the postoperative period to watch for worsening of retinopathy and instituting treatment if needed. In some instances cataracts can make examination of the retina difficult and must be removed to facilitate management of diabetic retinopathy.

Neovascular Glaucoma

Growth of NVI or rubeosis iridis occurs in less than 10% of diabetic eyes, but occurs in 40–60% of eyes with PDR *(55)*. NVI is dangerous, because the new vessels tend to grow over the trabecular meshwork, the outflow channel of the eye, resulting in intractable glaucoma. The presence of NVI, regardless of retinal status, requires prompt scatter laser photocoagulation to induce regression of these abnormal blood vessels *(56,57)*. It is postulated that scatter laser treatment decreases the release of factors from an ischemic retina that diffuse anteriorly to stimulate NVI. If intraocular pressure is already elevated, antiglaucoma medication is also commenced, but, ultimately, surgery may be required to lower intraocular pressure.

Keratopathy

Although infrequent, patients with diabetes can develop corneal problems. The diabetic cornea is known to have reduced corneal sensation *(58)*. This loss of sensation can predispose to the development of corneal abrasions or even neurotropic ulceration formation *(59)*. Those patients who develop ocular surface disorders may have delayed wound healing and this, coupled with the increased predisposition for infection in the diabetic patient, requires that they be followed closely. Because of the potential for keratopathy, diabetes is a relative contraindication for contact lens wear.

Changes in Refraction

Fluctuations in blood glucose levels can alter refraction by several diopters. Elevation of blood glucose causes osmotic swelling of the crystalline lens, which induces a myopic shift, with distant objects becoming blurred. Indeed, such fluctuations are common symptoms in recent-onset diabetes and are sometimes the presenting symptom *(60)*.

CONCLUSION

There are no cures for the ocular complications of diabetes mellitus, but provided careful and regular follow-up can be maintained by retinal specialists, most patients' retinopathy can be adequately managed with laser treatment based on guidelines derived from exemplary clinical trials. The key to successful treatment is based on the ability to grade retinopathy for which there are explicit guidelines for treatment and follow-up. When laser photocoagulation fails, vitreoretinal microsurgery offers the diabetic patient an opportunity of restoring vision in situations that previously would have inevitably led to blindness.

The deleterious effects of poor glycemic control, hypertension, hyperlipidemia, and hypercholesterolemia on the progression of diabetic retinopathy have been proven. It is imperative for ophthalmologists to work closely with internists and diabetologists to maximize glycemic control and minimize other risk factors. Effective communication between the members of a multidisciplinary health care team is the optimum way of combating the complications of diabetes.

ACKNOWLEDGMENTS

This work was supported by grants EY05951, EY12609, and P30EY1765 from the National Eye Institute, the Foundation Fighting Blindness, Lew R. Wasserman Merit Awards (PAC), Sanofi-Winthrop Foundation, The National Council for the Blind of Ireland, and unrestricted funds from Research to Prevent Blindness.

REFERENCES

1. Palmberg PF. Diabetic retinopathy. Diabetes 1977;26:703–709.
2. Klein R, Klein BEK, Moss SE, Davis MD, DeMets DL. The Wisconsin Epidemiologic Study of Diabetic Retinopathy. II Prevalence and risk of diabetic retinopathy when age at diagnosis is less than 30 years. Arch Ophthalmol 1984;102:520–526.

3. Klein R, Klein BE, Moss SE, Davis MD, DeMets DL. The Wisconsin Epidemiologic Study of Diabetic Retinopathy. III. Prevalence and risk of diabetic retinopathy when age at diagnosis is less than 30 years. Arch Ophthalmol 1984;102:527–532.
4. Engerman R, Bloodworth JMB, Nelson S. Relationship of microvascular disease in diabetes to metabolic control. Diabetes 1977;26:760–769.
5. The Diabetes Control and Complications Research Group. Progression of retinopathy with intensive versus conventional treatment in the Diabetes Control and Complications Trial. Ophthalmology 1995;102:647–661.
6. Gabbay KH. The sorbitol pathway and the complications of diabetes. N Engl J Med 1973;288:831–836
7. Brownlee M. Glycation and diabetic complications. Diabetes 1994;43:836–841
8. Lee T-S, Saltsman KA, Ohashi H, King GL. Activation of protein kinase C by elevation of glucose concentration: proposal for a mechanism in the development of diabetic complications. Proc Natl Acad Sci USA 1989;86:5141–5145
9. Barber AJ, Lieth E, Khin SA, Antonetti DA, Buchanan AG, Gardner TW. Neural apoptosis in the retina during experimental and human diabetes. Early onset and effect of insulin. J Clin Invest 1998;102: 783–791.
10. Cunha-Vaz JG, De Abreu JRF, Campos AJ, Figo GM. Early breakdown of the blood–retinal barrier in diabetes. Br J Ophthalmol 1975;59:649–656.
11. Grunwald JE, DuPont J, Riva CE. Retinal hemodynamics in patients with early diabetes mellitus. Br J Ophthalmol 1996;80:327–331.
12. The Early Treatment Diabetic Retinopathy Study Group. Fundus photographic risk factors for progression of diabetic retinopathy, ETDRS Report No. 12. Ophthalmology 1991;98:823–833.
13. The Early Treatment Diabetic Retinopathy Study Group. Photocoagulation for diabetic macular edema, ETDRS Report No. 1. Arch Ophthalmol 1985;103:1644–1652.
14. Miyamoto K, Khosrof S, Bursell S-E, Rohan R, Murata T, Clermont AC, et al. Prevention of leukostasis and vascular leakage in streptozotocin- induced diabetic retinopathy via intercellular adhesion molecule-1 inhibition. Proc Natl Acad Sci USA 1999;96:10836–10841.
15. Ozaki H, Yu A, Della N, Ozaki K, Luna JD, Yamada H, et al. Hypoxia inducible factor-1a is increased in ischemic retina: temporal and spatial correlation with VEGF expression. Invest Ophthalmol Vis Sci 1999;40:182–189.
16. Forsythe JA, Jiang B-H, Iyer NV, Agani F, Leung SW, Koos RD, et al. Activation of vascular endothelial growth factor gene transcription by hypoxia-inducible factor 1. Mol Cell Biol 1996;16:4604–4613.
17. Gerber H-P, Condorelli F, Park J, Ferrara N. Differential transcriptional regulation of the two vascular endothelial growth factor receptor genes. Flt-1, but not Flk-1/KDR, is up-regulated by hypoxia. J Biol Chem 1997;272:23,659–23,667.
18. Iyer NV, Kotch LE, Agani F, Leung SW, Laughner E, Wenger RH, et al. Cellular and developmental control of O_2 homeostasis by hypoxia-inducible factor 1alpha. Genes Dev 1998;12:149–162.
19. Campochiaro PA. Retinal and choroidal neovascularization. J Cell Physiol 2000;184:301–310.
20. The Diabetes Control and Complications Research Group. Clustering of long-term complications in families with diabetes in the diabetes control and complications trial. Diabetes 1997;46:1829–1839.
21. Kao YL, Donaghue K, Chan A, Knight J, Silink M. A novel polymorphism in the aldose reductase gene promoter region is strongly associated with diabetic retinopathy in adolescents with type 1 diabetes. Diabetes 1999;48:1338–1340.
22. Rabensteiner D, Abrahamian H, Irsigler K, Hermann KM, Kiener HP, Mayer G, et al. ACE gene polymorphism and proliferative retinopathy in type 1 diabetes: results of a case-control study. Diabetes Care 1999;22:1530–1535.
23. Kao YL, Donaghue K, Chan A, Knight J, Silink M. An aldose reductase intragenic polymorphism associated with diabetic retinopathy. Diabetes Res Clin Pract 1999;46:155–160.
24. van Ittersum FJ, de Man AM, Thijssen S, de Knijff P, Slagboom E, Smulders Y, et al. Genetic polymorphisms of the renin–angiotensin system and complications of insulin-dependent diabetes mellitus. Nephrol Dial Transplant 2000;15:1000–1007.
25. Matsubara Y, Murata M, Maruyama T, Handa M, Yamagata N, Watanabe G, et al. Association between diabetic retinopathy and genetic variations in alpha2beta1 integrin, a platelet receptor for collagen. Blood 2000;95:1560–1564.
26. Warpeha KM, Xu W, Liu L, Charles IG, Patterson CC, Ah-Fat F, et al. Genotyping and functional analysis of a polymorphic $(CCTTT)_n$ repeat of NOS2A in diabetic retinopathy. FASEB J 1999;13:1825–1832.

27. Speilman RS, Baker L, Zmijewski CM. Gene dosage and susceptibility to insulin-dependent diabetes. Ann Hum Genet 1980;4:135–150.
28. Cordell JJ, Todd JA. Multifactorial inheritance in type 1 diabetes. Trends Genet 1995;11:499–504.
29. Klein R, Klein BE, Moss SE, Davis MD, DeMets DL. Glycosylated hemoglobin predicts the incidence and progression of diabetic retinopathy. JAMA 1988;260:2864–2871.
30. Janka HU, Warram JH, Rand LI, Krolewski AS. Risk factors for progression of background retinopathy in long-standing IDDM. Diabetes 1989;38:460–464.
31. Marshall G, Garg SK, Jackson WE, Holmes DL, Chase HP. Factors influencing the onset and progression of diabetic retinopathy in subjects with insulin-dependent diabetes mellitus. Ophthalmology 1993;100:1133–1139.
32. The Diabetes Control and Complications Research Group. The effect of intensive treatment of diabetes on the development and progression of long-term complications in insulin-dependent diabetes mellitus. N Engl J Med 1993;329:977–986.
33. Group TKCS. Blood glucose control and the evolution of diabetic retinopathy and albuminuria. A preliminary multicenter trial. N Engl J Med 1984;311:365–372.
34. Group TUKPDS. Tight blood pressure control and risk of macrovascular and microvascular complications in type 2 diabetes: UKPDS 38. Br Med J 1998;317:703–713.
35. Chaturvedi N, Sjolie AK, Stephenson JM, Abrahamian H, Keipes M, Castellarin A, et al. Effect of lisinopril on progression of retinopathy in normotensive people with type 1 diabetes. The EUCLID Study Group. EURODIAB Controlled Trial of Lisinopril in Insulin-Dependent Diabetes Mellitus. Lancet 1998;351:28–31.
36. Klein BEK, Moss SE, Klein R, Surawicz TS. The Wisconsin Epidemiologic Study of Diabetic Retinopathy. XIII. Relationship of serum cholesterol to retinopathy and hard exudates. Ophthalmology 1991;98:1261–1265.
37. Chew EY, Klein ML, Ferris FLI, Remaley NA, Murphy RP, Chantry K, et al., Group ETDRS. Association of elevated serum lipid levels with retinal hard exudate in diabetic retinopathy. Arch Ophthalmol 1996;114:1079–1084.
38. Fong DS, Segal PP, Myers F, Ferris FL, Hubbard LD, Davis MD. Subretinal fibrosis in diabetic macular edema. ETDRS Report 23. Arch Ophthalmol 1997;115:873–877.
39. Davis MD, Fisher MR, Gangnon RE, Barton F, Aiello LM, Chew EY, et al. Risk factors for high-risk proliferative retinopathy and severe visual loss: Early Treatment Diabetic Retinopathy Study Report 18. Invest Ophthalmol Vis Sci 1998;39:233–252.
40. Shorb SR. Anemia and diabetic retinopathy. Am J Ophthalmol 1985;100:434–436.
41. Tesfaye S, Stevens LK, Stephenson JM, Fuller JH, Plater M, Ionescu-Tirgoviste C, et al. Prevalence of diabetic peripheral neuropathy and its relation to glycaemic control and potential risk factors: the EURODIAB IDDM complications Study. Diabetologia 1996;39:1377–1384.
42. Qiao Q, Keinanen-Kiukaanniemi S, Laara E. The relationship between hemoglobin levels and diabetic retinopathy. J Clin Epidemiol 1997;50:153–158.
43. The Diabetic Retinopathy Study Research Group. Photocoagulation treatment of proliferative diabetic retinopathy: Clinical application of Diabetic Retinopathy Study (DRS) findings, DRS Report Number 8. Ophthalmology 1981;88:583–600.
44. The Early Treatment Diabetic Retinopathy Study Group. Early photocoagulation for diabetic retinopathy, ETDRS report no. 9. Ophthalmology 1991;98(Suppl):767–785.
45. The Diabetic Retinopathy Vitrectomy Study Research Group. Early vitrectomy for severe vitreous hemorrhage in diabetic retinopathy. Two year results of a randomized trial. Diabetic Retinopathy Vitrectomy Study Report 2. Arch Ophthalmol 1985;103:1644–1652.
46. The Diabetic Retinopathy Vitrectomy Study Research Group. Early vitrectomy for severe vitreous hemorrhage in diabetic retinopathy. Four-year results of a randomized trial: Diabetic Retinopathy Vitrectomy Study Report 5. Arch Ophthalmol 1990;108:958–964.
47. The Diabetic Retinopathy Vitrectomy Study Research Group. Early vitrectomy for severe proliferative diabetic retinopathy in eyes with useful vision. Clinical application of results of a randomized trial. Diabetic Vitrectomy Study Report 4. Ophthalmology 1990;95:1321–1334.
48. The Diabetic Retinopathy Vitrectomy Study Research Group. Two-year course of visual acuity in severe proliferative diabetic retinopathy with conventional management. Diabetic Retinopathy Vitrectomy Study Report 1. Ophthalmology 1985;92:492–502.
49. Pournaras CJ, Tsacopoulos M, Strommer K, Gilodi N, Leuenberger PM. Scatter photocoagulation restores tissue hypoxia in experimental vasoproliferative microangiopathy in miniature pigs. Ophthalmology 1990;97:1329–1333.

50. Zoirrilla E, Kozak GP. Ophthalmolplegia in diabetes mellitus. Ann Intern Med 1967;67:968–976.
51. Rucker CW. Paralysis of the third, fourth, and sixth cranial nerves. Am J Ophthalmol 1958;46:787–794.
52. Rush JA, Younge BR. Paralysis of cranial nerves III, IV, and VI. Cause and prognosis in 1,000 cases. Arch Ophthalmol 1981;99:76–79.
53. Goldstein JE, Cogan DG. Diabetic opthalmoplegia with special reference to the pupil. Arch Opthalmol 1960;64:592–600.
54. Klein BE, Klein R, Moss SE. Prevalence of cataracts in a population-based study of persons with diabetes mellitus. Ophthalmology 1985;91:381–395.
55. Madsen PH. Rubeosis of the iris and haemorrhagic glaucoma in patients with proliferative diabetic retinopathy. Br J Ophthalmol 1971;55:368–371.
56. Wand M, Dueker DK, Aiello LM, Grant WM. Effects of panretinal photocoagulation on rubeosis iridis, angle neovascularization, and neovascular glaucoma. Am J Ophthalmol 1978;86:332–339.
57. Pavan PR, Folk JC, Weingeist TA, Hermsen VM, Watzle RC, Montague PR. Diabetic rubeosis and panretinal photocoagulation. Arch Ophthalmol 1983;101:882–884.
58. Ishida N, Rao GN, del Cerro M, Aquavella JV. Corneal nerve alterations in diabetes mellitus. Arch Ophthalmol 1984;102:1380–1384.
59. Hyndiuk RA, Kazarian EL, Schultz RO, Seideman S. Neurotrophic corneal ulcers in diabetes mellitus. Arch Ophthalmol 1977;95:2193–2196.
60. Waite JH, Beetham WP. The visual mechanism in diabetes mellitus: a comparitive study of 2002 diabetics and 457 non-diabetics for control. N Engl J Med 1935;212:367–379.

23 The Kidney

Diabetic Nephropathy

Abhay Vats, MD *and*
Frederick DeRubertis, MD

CONTENTS

INTRODUCTION

Diabetic nephropathy is a serious and costly microvascular complication of both type 1 and type 2 diabetes. It has been a subject of study for over two centuries. Richard Bright (1789–1858) is often credited for the observation that albuminuria reflects serious diabetic renal involvement *(1,2)*. Elliott P. Joslin (1869–1962), one of the first diabetologists stated, "the renal complications of diabetes have been unimportant in the past, but with the prolongation of life which modern treatment is bringing about they will deserve attention" *(3)*. This statement, made 5 yr before the introduction of insulin in 1917 has, unfortunately, been proven correct because more than one-third of patients entering maintenance dialysis today suffer from diabetic nephropathy. It is the most common cause of end-stage renal disease (ESRD) in the United States and the Western world. Approximately a third of type 1 diabetic patients will develop kidney disease over their lifetime and it is often associated with premature death from cardiovascular disease. Indeed, the development of albuminuria alone in diabetes significantly increases the risk of macrovascular complications and mortality *(4–7)*. The economic cost of diabetic nephropathy is, thus, substantial and exceeded $2 billion in the United States in 1991 *(8)*.

DEFINITIONS AND STAGES

Historically, diabetic nephropathy has been categorized into five stages, as shown in Table 1 *(9,10)*:

From: *Contemporary Endocrinology: Type 1 Diabetes: Etiology and Treatment*
Edited by: M. A. Sperling © Humana Press Inc., Totowa, NJ

Table 1
Stages of Diabetic Nephropathy

Stage	*UAE (μg/min)*	*GFR*	*Pathology*	*Reversible*	*Time frame*[a]
I	<20	Increased	Early renal hypertrophy	Yes	Present at diagnosis
II	<20	Increased	Increased mesangial volume	Yes	Seen after 2–3 yr
III	20–200	Increased	Increased mesangial matrix, TBM thickening, sclerosis	?	Seen after 7–10 yr
IV	>200	Normal or low	Progressive sclerosis	?	Seen after 15–18 yr
V	Variable	Renal failure	Fibrosis, sclerosis	No	Seen after 20–30 yr

Abbreviations: UAE, urinary albumin excretion; GFR, glomerular filtration rate; TBM, tubular basement membrane.

[a] Time frame indicates the typical onset of a particular stage after the diagnosis of diabetes. There can be a significant variability and overlap in the time-course.

Stage I: This is the onset of diabetic kidney disease that is characterized by renal hypertrophy and increased glomerular filtration rate (GFR > 100 mL/min per surface area). These changes are not clinically appreciable and may be reversible with good control of glycemia.

Stage II: This stage marks the beginning of the renal morphologic changes (e.g., mesangial expansion and increases in glomerular and tubular basement membrane thickness) *(10)*. In this stage, the urinary albumin excretion (UAE) remains normal, but the GFR is still elevated.

Stage III: This stage, which typically develops about 10 yr or more after the onset of diabetes, is characterized by elevated UAE. The UAE is usually in the range of 20–200 μg/min (or 30–300 mg/24 h) and is referred to as microalbuminuria (normal range: 2–8 μg/min). The dipstick for urinary protein remains negative, but systemic hypertension may be seen. Microalbuminuria may, however, decrease with angiotensin-converting enzyme (ACE) inhibitor therapy and/or improved glycemic control *(11–14)*. The UAE generally increases at a rate of approx 20% per year if there is no intervention *(15)*.

Stage IV: This is the stage of overt nephropathy. The UAE is > 200 μg/min (>300 mg/24 h) and is referred to as macroalbuminuria. The urinary dipstick tests positive for protein. The GFR in this stage may first decrease into the "normal" reference range (70–100 mL/min per surface area), because of hyperfiltration seen in early diabetic nephropathy. However, without treatment, the GFR usually falls at a rate of approx 10 mL/min/yr and this stage progresses to uremia (GFR <20 mL/min per surface area) in 5–10 yr *(16)*. Renal involvement may be irreversible at this stage.

Stage V: This is the stage of ESRD and usually develops 20–30 yr after the onset of diabetes. Uremic symptoms and minimal residual renal function usually requiring either dialysis or renal transplantation characterize this stage.

Urinary Albumin Excretion

Based on the above classification, UAE is usually the main clinically employed determinant of the stage and progression of diabetic nephropathy. As accurate serial 24-h collections of urine can be difficult to obtain, the ratio of the urinary albumin to urinary creatinine in the first morning voided specimen is also used as an index of UAE. An albumin-to-creatinine ratio (both values in milligrams) in the range

0.03–0.3 falls in the microalbuminuria range. A timed overnight urine collection can also be used instead of a 24-h collection. The reference ranges remain the same (in μg/min), as stated earlier, irrespective of the duration of collection. Although widely used, albuminuria is not a completely reliable index of renal histology in diabetic nephropathy. Thus, some diabetic patients may demonstrate significant glomerular mesangial matrix expansion, a hallmark of diabetic nephropathy, in the absence of albuminuria *(10,16,17)*. On the other hand, albuminuria may be reversibly affected by many factors, including glycemic control, hypertension, exercise, congestive heart failure, adequacy of urinary collection, and urinary tract infections *(15,16)*. Despite these caveats, UAE assessment retains a key role in the long-term evaluation of diabetic patients because microalbuminuria is a strong predictor of progression to overt nephropathy and other complications, including mortality *(6,7)*. Hence, tests for the assessment of UAE are currently recommended annually in postpubertal patients who have 5 or more years of diabetes and in all patients with onset of type 1 diabetes after 18 yr of age *(18)*.

PATHOLOGY

Pierre François-Olivier Rayer (1793–1867), a French physician known for his seminal textbook on nephrology, probably provided the first description of diabetic glomerular hypertrophy *(2)*. However, diabetic nephropathy encompasses discrete structural alterations, including renal hypertrophy, thickening of basement membranes, and progressive expansion of extracellular matrix components *(19–25)*. Morphometric studies on kidneys from patients with type 1 diabetes have shown that glomerular hypertrophy is among the earliest pathological alterations *(19–22)*. The glomerular hypertrophy is mainly consequent to the two major early lesions (i.e., increased mesangial volume and increased thickness of the glomerular basement membrane) *(20,21)*. However, these changes do not always correlate with the stages of albuminuria. Indeed, some patients with normal UAE may have the morphologic changes of diabetes, whereas some with increased UAE may have normal morphology *(16,17)*. Hence, a renal biopsy is the only definitive way to diagnose and stage diabetic nephropathy, but it is seldom used in clinical practice because of its invasive nature. Hypertrophy of renal tubular epithelium and tubular basement membrane (TBM) thickening also occur early in the course of diabetic renal involvement and are most likely the precursors of the later irreversible changes of tubular atrophy and interstitial fibrosis *(23,24)*. Advancing diabetic glomerulopathy is commonly characterized by glomerulosclerosis, which may be diffuse or exhibit a distinctive nodular form (*see* Fig. 1) as first described by Kimmelstiel and Wilson in 1936 *(25)*. These morphological changes were originally described in type 1 diabetes, but similar changes are also seen in type 2 diabetes *(26,27)*.

Pathogenesis of Diabetic Nephropathy

Diabetic nephropathy is a complex disease with multiple factors operating in concert to produce the characteristic histopathologic changes (*see* Table 2). Metabolic, hemodynamic, growth factors and genetic factors conspire in the pathogenesis of renal injury in diabetes. Some of these well-studied factors have been discussed in the chapter on molecular biology of complications. Those most pertinent to the pathogenesis of diabetic nephropathy are summarized below.

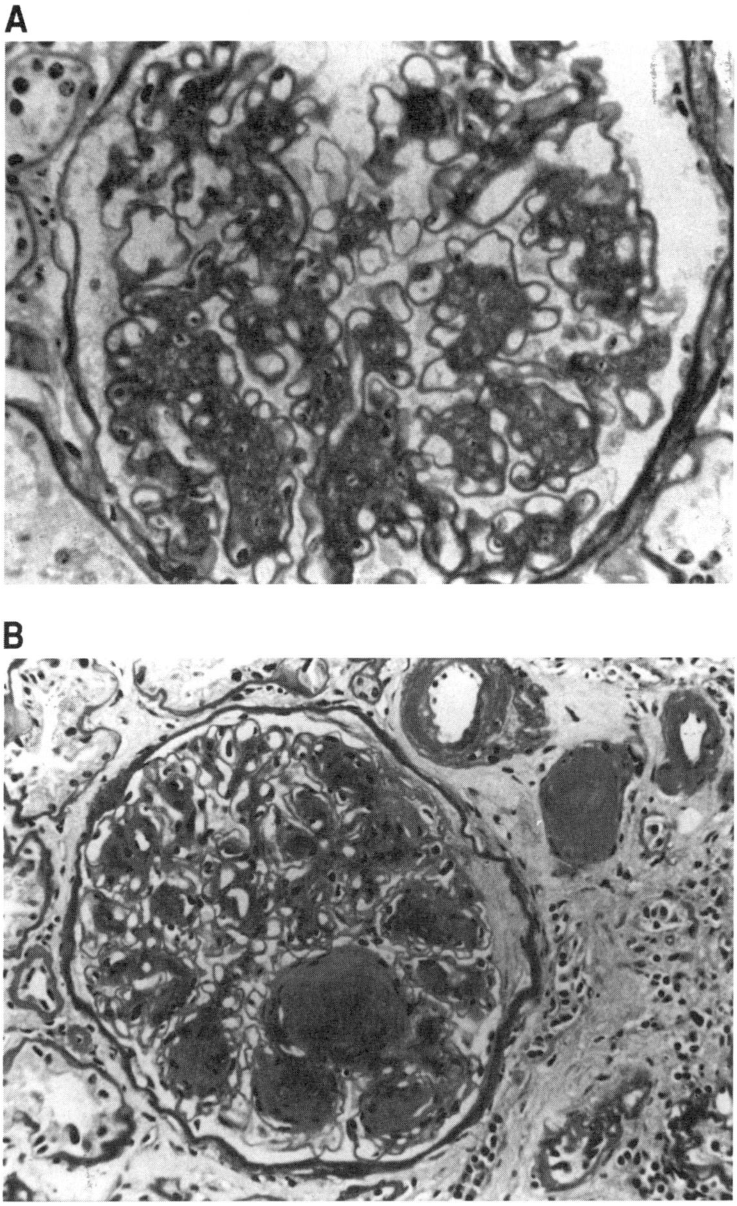

Fig. 1. Diffuse (**A**) and nodular (**B**) forms of glomerulosclerosis in patients with advanced diabetic nephropathy.

Hyperglycemia and Metabolic Factors

A central role for hyperglycemia in the pathogenesis of nephropathy and other microvascular complications has been unequivocally established in human diabetes by several well-conducted studies, including the results of the Diabetes Control and Complication Trial study (DCCT) and the United Kingdom Prospective Diabetes Study (UKPDS) *(28,29)*. In addition, normal kidneys from nondiabetic donors can develop all of the lesions of diabetic nephropathy when transplanted into diabetics *(30)*. Several

Table 2
Mechanisms Implicated in Hyperglycemia-Induced Renal Cell Injury and Mesangial Matrix Expansion

- Activation of PKC and mitogen-activated protein kinase
- Increased formation of Amadori glucose adducts
- Increased formation of glucose-derived advanced glycation end products
- Increased glucose flux through the aldose reductase pathway
- Increased glucose flux through the hexosamine pathway
- Increased production of thromboxane and other eicosanoids
- Increased oxidative and carbonyl stress
- Increased renal cell production of prosclerotic growth factors (TGF-β, PDGF-B, IGF-1, HGF), vasoactive substances (Ang II, ET-1), and chemokines (IL-8, MCP-1)

Abbreviations: PKC, protein kinase C; TGF-β, transforming growth factor-β; PDGF-B, platelet-derived growth factor-B; IGF-1, insulin-like growth factor-1; HGF, hepatocyte growth factor; Ang II, angiotensin II; ET-1, endothelin-1; IL-8, interleukin-8; MCP-1, monocyte chemotactic peptide-1.

in vitro studies have also supported direct effects of high concentrations of glucose on various renal cell lines in culture. Thus, high glucose concentrations have been shown to modulate the growth of mesangial cells and stimulate proximal tubular hypertrophy *(31,32)*. High glucose also increases the production and decreases the degradation of extracellular matrix proteins in mesangial, endothelial, and epithelial cells *(19,31–34)*. A reduction in heparan sulfate proteoglycans and alteration in the sulfation pattern is seen in glomerular mesangial and epithelial cells cultured in high glucose concentrations and may contribute to changes in charge and size permselectivity of the glomerular basement membrane in diabetes *(35,36)*. Renal cell injury seen in response to high extracellular glucose concentration is likely the result of intracellular glucose accumulation and metabolism in cells where glucose transport is largely noninsulin dependent. Thus, rat mesangial cells that overexpress one of the human glucose transporter (GLUT-1) demonstrate increased matrix protein synthesis at physiologic concentrations of extracellular glucose *(37)*. The potential metabolic mechanisms by which high glucose damages renal cells have been a focus for intense study and span a large number of interconnected pathways. The major proposed mechanisms are summarized in Table 2. These include activation of the protein kinase C (PKC) system via increased *de novo* synthesis of diacylglycerol *(38,39)*, increased activity of the polyol pathway and pentose phosphate shunt *(40)*, stimulation of cytokine *(41)* and eicosanoid production *(42–44)*, increased oxidative and carbonyl stress *(45–47)*, and increased formation of early Amadori glucose adducts *(48)* and advanced glycation end products (AGEs) *(49–51)*. The formation of AGEs and the early Amadori-glucose adducts in proteins such as serum albumin have been shown to stimulate renal expression of various growth factors, including transforming growth factor-β (TGF-β), which are important mediators of diabetic nephropathy *(52–54)*. Of note, in addition to hyperglycemia, a number of factors implicated in the pathogenesis of glomerular injury in diabetes have been shown to increase TGF-β production in cultured mesangial cell at least in part by activation of PKC (*see* Fig. 2). These include angiotensin II, thromboxane, platelet-derived growth factors, and mechanical stretch, as discussed later.

Nitric Oxide. Alterations in the production, stability, and cellular actions of nitric oxide (NO) have been implicated in the pathogenesis of diabetic nephropathy, in part

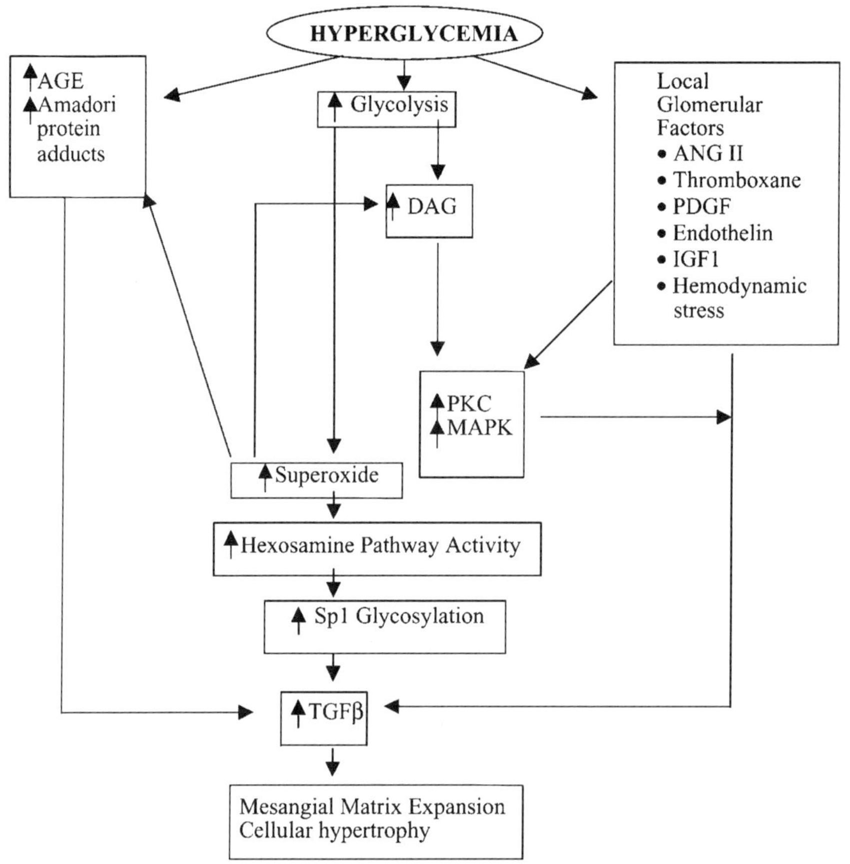

Fig. 2. Proposed metablic pathways and the central role of TGF-β in the pathogenesis of extracellular matrix expansion and renal cellular changes seen in diabetes. DAG, diacylglycerol; PDGF, platelet-derived growth factor; ANG II, angiotensin II; AGE, advanced glycation end products; PKC, protein kinase; C, MAPK, mitogen-activated protein kinase; IGF-1, insulin-like growth factor-1; TGF-β, transforming growth factor-β.

through the interaction of NO with reactive oxygen species. There is evidence that NO production may be increased early in diabetes and may contribute to the stage of glomerular hyperfiltration characteristic of this disorder *(55,56)*. However, there is also evidence for impairment of NO-mediated cellular actions in diabetes *(55)*. The latter may reflect inactivation of NO by increased production of superoxide and other reactive oxygen species in the diabetic state *(55)*. The reaction of NO with superoxide reduces NO half-life and prevents several cellular actions of NO that may protect glomeruli from injury in diabetes. In this regard, NO prevents increases in PKC activity, TGF-β production, laminin promoter activity, and matrix protein synthesis induced by culture of glomerular mesangial cells with a high concentration of glucose *(57,58)*. Antioxidants have analogous inhibitory effects on these glucose responses in mesangial cells *(59)*. Also, cyclic GMP (cGMP) responses to NO are impaired in glomeruli from diabetic rats *(60,61)*. In human diabetics, NO-dependent vasodilatory responses to cholinergic stimuli are impaired *(56)*. These responses are restored by administration of antioxidants, consistent with enhanced quenching of NO by reactive oxygen species in this disorder *(62)*. In addition to blocking cellular actions of NO, the direct reaction of NO with superoxide leads to formation of peroxynitrite, a strong oxidant with reactivity similar to the hydroxyl radical *(63)*. Peroxynitrate mediates tyrosine nitration, which can alter the function of numerous key cellular enzymes and structural proteins *(63)*. Recent studies have reported increased nitrotyrosine in placenta *(64)* and renal cortex *(65)* from diabetic rats. Thus, increased production of superoxide and other reactive oxygen species in diabetes may not only block important cellular actions of NO through quenching but also lead to formation of a strong oxidant, peroxynitrate.

Oxidant Stress. Increased mitochondrial generation of superoxide induced by high glucose in endothelial and other cells has recently been proposed as the key cellular metabolic response that fosters the formation of advanced glycation end products and also leads to activation of PKC, the polyol pathway, and the hexosamine pathway with resultant enhanced glycosylation of the transcription factor Sp1 *(66,67)*. All these metabolic responses can lead to increased cellular production of TGF-β and, thus, to mesangial matrix expansion and cellular hypertrophy (*see* Fig. 2). Overexpression of mitochondrial Mn^{2+} superoxide dismutase (SOD) in cultured vascular endothelial cells has been shown to attenuate activation of PKC, the hexosamine and polyol pathways, and the formation of advanced glycation end products in response to high glucose. In cultured mesangial cells, overexpression of either Mn^{2+}-SOD or cytoplasmic Cu^{2+}/Zn^{2+}-SOD prevents increases in collagen synthesis induced by high glucose *(68)*. Moreover, diabetic transgenic mice that overexpress Cu^{2+}/Zn^{2+}-SOD are protected from early renal injury *(68)*. These and other observations support a role for reactive oxygen species in the pathogenesis of renal cell injury in diabetes.

Pathogenetic Relevance of Metabolic Alterations. In vivo studies of experimental diabetes have supported the pathogenetic relevance of these proposed mechanisms of renal cell injury in diabetes. Thus, specific inhibition of the PKC-β isoform *(69)*, inhibitors of the formation or actions of glycation products *(51,53,54,70,71)*, administration of anti-TGF-β antibodies *(72,73)*, inhibitors of thromboxane synthesis *(42,43,74)*, or treatment with various antioxidants *(75–77)* each attenuate renal injury in experimental diabetes, possibly by interfering with the aforementioned renal cellular metabolic responses to high glucose.

Hemodynamic Changes

Early diabetic nephropathy (stages I and II) is associated with glomerular hyperfiltration, which is mediated by increased glomerular hydraulic pressure and perfusion *(78–80)*. Glomerular hypertension associated with hyperfiltration is thought to precede albuminuria and subsequent glomerulosclerosis *(80,81)*. The glomerular hemodynamic alterations and hypertrophic responses are also intricately connected *(80–82)*. Glomerular hypertrophy leads to an increase in the overall filtration surface area, and the resultant increase in the ultrafiltration coefficient furthers enhances glomerular hyperfiltration *(80,81)*. An increase in the diameter of the glomerular capillary is also seen early in the course of diabetes and it may confer a mechanical disadvantage *(82)*. According to the La Place law (tension = transmural pressure × vessel radius), increased capillary diameter increases wall tension, which may add another injurious component to the diabetic renal hypertrophy *(82)*. Several mechanisms have been proposed for glomerular hypertension-induced vascular injury. These include direct pressure injury to the mesangium and/or the endothelium and increased wall tension, leading to altered capillary wall structure and function. Also, shear stress and mechanical strain may trigger release of various growth factors *(82–84)*. For example, it has been demonstrated (*see* Fig. 2) that mechanical stimulation (stretching) of mesangial cells triggers metabolic responses that can contribute to renal injury *(83–86)*. These include activation of the PKC system and increases in TGF-β and extracellular matrix protein synthesis *(87–89)*. In addition, there is evidence that renal effects of high glucose and mechanical stretch may be additive *(82)*.

Renal Cell Growth and Prosclerotic Factors

As outlined earlier, in humans the development of irreversible renal changes of glomerulosclerosis and tubulointerstitial fibrosis in diabetes mellitus are preceded by the early hypertrophic processes in the glomerular and tubular compartments *(21–24)*. In studies of structural–functional relationships in type 1 diabetes, a close correlation was seen between mesangial expansion and other clinical parameters of progressive nephropathy (i.e., albuminuria, hypertension, and renal failure) *(90)*. Although glomerular events have been extensively studied, the importance of tubulointerstitial compartment in diabetic nephropathy and its contribution to the onset and progression of renal failure is also recognized. As the tubulointerstitium comprises the major bulk of the kidney *(91,92)*, tubular hypertrophy is probably the single largest contributor to renal hypertrophy of diabetes mellitus *(92,93)*. Various mechanisms that are operative in diabetic milieu (i.e., high glucose, nonenzymatic glycation products, and glomerular hypertension) can stimulate the synthesis and release of a number of growth factors, cytokines, chemokines, and vasoactive agents *(19,40,52,54,92)*. These factors are thought to stimulate either proliferation or hypertrophy of various renal cells, as well as increase extracellular matrix production *(92–94)*. Some of the implicated growth factors and their role in etiopathogenesis of diabetic nephropathy are discussed here (*see* Table 2)

Transforming Growth Factor-β. A large number of studies, mostly over the past decade, have identified the key role of TGF-β in the development of lesions characteristic of diabetes mellitus (*see* Fig. 2) *(95–101)*. The actions of TGF-β are mainly mediated through its effects on cellular hypertrophy and increased production of extracellular matrix proteins *(33,95–98)*. Increased renal TGF-β expression in diabetes has been demonstrated both in vitro studies and in vivo in experimental diabetes as well as humans *(95–100)*. Mesangial cells cultured in high glucose produce more TGF-β than cells grown in normal glucose *(33,102)*, an effect possibly mediated through intracellular glucosamine production *(67,103)*. Similar observations have also been made for cultured renal tubular epithelial cells grown in high-glucose medium *(32,102,104)*. In addition to the direct actions of hyperglycemia, additional mechanisms are thought to be mediated through TGF-β. The nonenzymatically generated AGEs *(52)* and the early Amadori-glucose adducts in serum albumin *(53)* can also stimulate renal expression of TGF-β *(54)*. Also, Amadori glucose adducts in albumin increases TGF-β type II receptor mRNA and protein expression in mesangial cell cultures *(54)*. As mentioned earlier, increased glomerular capillary pressure, seen in early diabetic nephropathy, can also stimulate TGF-β production *(85,87,105)*. In fact, several vasoactive factors such as angiotensin II *(106–108)*, endothelin-1 *(109)*, and thromboxane *(44,110)* may exert part of their prosclerotic effects through the secondary induction of TGF-β. Also, neutralization studies using specific anti-TGF-β antibodies, both in vivo and in vitro, have shown attenuation of renal hypertrophy and the accumulation of extracellular matrix proteins seen in diabetic nephropathy *(31,72,73)*. Thus, hyperglycemia and a number of other mechanisms associated with diabetic milieu increase the renal levels of TGF-β and also upregulate its signaling receptors, which are thought to be key events in the genesis of diabetic renal damage.

Insulin-Like Growth Factor-1. Insulin-like growth factor-1 (IGF-1) is a mitogen for cultured mesangial cells and proximal tubular cells and is also likely involved in diabetic renal hypertrophy *(111–116)*. Renal IGF-1 mRNA and protein level is elevated during the early renal hypertrophy in experimental diabetes *(114,115)*. The plasma IGF-1 and growth hormone levels are, however, not elevated *(115)*. In addition, the expression of mRNA and concentration of IGF-1 receptors kidney are both increased in experimentally induced diabetes *(116,117)*. Long-term treatment of diabetic rats with the octreotide, a somatostatin analog that antagonizes growth hormone release and lowers tissue IGF-1 levels, reduces renal hypertrophy *(118)*. IGF-1 is, thus, important in the genesis and maintenance of renal hypertrophy seen in diabetes, but it is probably not the key factor for its induction. IGF-1 most likely acts as a cofactor in modulating renal tubular growth in the diabetic proteinuric state because serum-derived IGF-1 has been shown to leak from the glomerular filtrate into the peritubular fluid *(119)*. Further studies are needed to clarify the complex role of the growth hormone, IGF-1, and IGF-1-binding proteins axis on diabetic renal hypertrophy.

Angiotensin II. The vasoactive peptide angiotensin II (Ang II) has, in addition to its hemodynamic properties, potent direct effects on several renal cell types *(106–108,120,121)*. It can stimulate cellular hypertrophy and/or proliferation as well as increase the synthesis of extracellular matrix proteins *(120–123)*. The intrarenal renin–angiotensin system has been shown to be upregulated in diabetic nephropathy and it is very likely that hyperglycemia and the locally synthesized Ang II exert additive hypertrophic and prosclerotic effects *(122–125)*. Ang II is thought to mediate its effects through TGF-β *(106)* and is involved in downregulation of proteolytic activity, thus favoring extracellular matrix accumulation *(126,127)*. Furthermore, growing cells may release vasoactive factors, which may impair blood flow to subordinate vascular beds and contribute to ischemic/fibrotic changes seen in diabetic nephropathy *(120)*. Finally, both ACE inhibitors and AT-1-receptor blockers can partially inhibit renal hypertrophy *(128,129)*. Thus, Ang II appears to be a key component and a mediator of the pathologic changes that characterize diabetic nephropathy.

Platelet-Derived Growth Factor-B. The role of platelet-derived growth factor-B (PDGF-B) as a modulator of cellular events has also been investigated in diabetic nephropathy. Increased expression of PDGF-B is associated with mesangial cell proliferation with subsequent induction of TGF-β *(130,131)*. TGF-β, in turn, has antiproliferative actions and stimulates cellular hypertrophy as well as extracellular matrix production. Upregulation of PDGF-B-chain mRNA and its receptor has also been reported in glomeruli from diabetic rats, as well as in mesangial cells cultured in high-glucose medium *(132)*. PDGF-B may, thus, mediate its actions through TGF-β synthesis in diabetic nephropathy *(131,133)*.

Hepatocyte Growth Factor Hepatocyte growth factor (HGF) is a strong mitogen of cultured renal tubular cells *(134)* and is a chief mediator of regenerative growth in both liver and kidney subsequent to injury. HGF and its tyrosine kinase receptor, which is a product of the c-met oncogene, are both upregulated in the kidneys of diabetic rats *(134)*. An increase of c-met protein in tubular cells has been shown by immunohistochemistry and high-glucose medium, in vitro, to induce HGF in cultured proximal tubular *(134)*. Thus, HGF and its receptor may also be important mediators of renal growth seen in diabetes, but their roles need to be further elucidated.

Endothelins. Analogous to Ang II, endothelin-1 is a vasoconstrictor and appears to be involved in pathogenesis of diabetic nephropathy. Glomerular expression of endothelin-1 (ET-1) mRNA is increased in streptozotocin (STZ)-diabetic rats *(109)* and urinary excretion of ET-1 is increased in diabetic Bio-Breeding (BB) rats compared to controls *(135)*. Also, plasma ET levels are higher in diabetics, especially those with retinopathy, when compared to nondiabetics *(136,137)*. Finally, the ET receptor antagonist FR139317 attenuates hyperfiltration, albuminuria, and glomerular expression of TGF-β and matrix proteins in STZ-diabetic rats *(109)*.

Thromboxane. Urinary excretion of thromboxane-B_2 (TXB) is increased in newly diagnosed type 1 diabetes *(138)* and the STZ-diabetic rat *(139)*, probably in part because of increased glomerular cell production of TX and/or that of infiltrating platelets *(140)*. In cultured mesangial cells, TX analogs activate PKC and increase TGF-β and matrix protein synthesis *(141)*. Inhibitors of TX synthesis or TX-receptor blockers attenuate albuminuria and mesangial matrix expansion in experimental diabetes *(42,43,74,75,142)*. Of note, prostaglandin E_2 (PGE_2) has effects on TGF-β and matrix protein synthesis in cultured mesangial cells opposite to those of TX, and suppresses these parameters *(42)*. Thus, the balance of vasoconstrictor vs vasodilatory eicosanoids produced in the kidney in diabetes may be one determinate of renal TGF-β and matrix protein production *(143)*.

Chemokines. Various chemokines have been implicated in the pathogenesis of glomerular hypertrophy seen in diabetes. An increased production of chemokines and infiltration of monocytes/macrophages into the glomerulus has been demonstrated in early diabetes *(41)*. The release of various growth factors and cytokines from these infiltrating cells (i.e., interleukin-8 and monocyte chemotactic peptide-1) may contribute to the histologic changes seen in diabetes *(41,144)*.

Genetic Factors in the Development of Diabetic Nephropathy

There appears to be a genetic susceptibility to the development of nephropathy in diabetes (*see* Table 3). It has been observed that some persons with diabetes progress rapidly to develop nephropathy, whereas in others, normal or near-normal renal function is maintained even after 30 or more years of diabetes. In fact, about 65% of patients with type 1 diabetes will not develop nephropathy, despite suboptimal glycemic control *(145,146)*. Hence, it appears that genetic factors are important in the genesis of diabetic nephropathy *(145–148)*. The DCCT studies showed that although a tight control of hyperglycemia can reduce the incidence of nephropathy, it did not completely eliminate this complication *(149)*. The genetic risk of developing nephropathy contrasts sharply with diabetic retinopathy, where the prevalence rates increase linearly with duration of diabetes *(150)*. There are several family-based studies that further allude to the genetic risk of nephropathy. In families with two or more type 1 diabetic siblings, the development of nephropathy in one was associated with a fourfold risk of nephropathy in the other sibling compared with a sibling of a diabetic without nephropathy *(151,152)*. This risk has been confirmed in a more recent study in which, if the proband had nephropathy, the cumulative risk of

Table 3
Genetic Factors in Diabetic Nephropathy

Population studies
• 35% Incidence of nephropathy in insulin-dependent diabetes mellitus (IDDM) irrespective of glycemic control
• Concordance with nephropathy risk in siblings
• Concordance with familial risk of hypertension and cardiovascular disease
• Discordance between retinopathy and nephropathy risk
Candidate gene studies
• Renin angiotensin system genes
Angiotensin converting enzyme (ACE)
Angiotensinogen
Angiotensin II type 1 receptor (AT-1)
• Nitric oxide synthase
• Transforming growth factor-β (TGF-β) gene
• Aldose reductase
• Heparan sulfate
• Insulin gene
• Apolipoprotein E
In vitro cell behavior
• Cellular proliferation and senescence
• Sodium–hydrogen exchanger (NHE) activity

nephropathy to diabetic siblings was 72%. This risk fell to 25%, a staggering 47% difference, when the proband did not have nephropathy *(148)*. Analysis of the DCCT data has also shown similar findings *(149)*. In several studies, there appears to be a correlation between risk of developing nephropathy and familial occurrence of hypertension and cardiovascular disease. Parents of patients with type 1 diabetes with nephropathy have been found to have higher arterial blood pressures than parents of patients without nephropathy *(153–155)*. The EURODIAB study also showed that the blood pressure is higher in the type 1 diabetes patients with parental hypertension *(156)*. Also, parents of proteinuric type 1 diabetic patients die at an earlier age, have higher arterial blood pressure, have higher incidence of cardiovascular disease, and have more hyperlipidemia and insulin resistance than parents of normoalbuminuric patients *(157,158)*. All of these observations suggest a genetic predisposition to diabetic nephropathy and, possibly, a link to hypertension. In view of the accumulating evidence that there is a genetic risk of developing nephropathy, which appears to be inherited separately from the risk of developing diabetes, a considerable effort is being made to identify such factors *(158–160)*.

There are main strategies for identifying susceptibility genes (i.e., linkage analysis and population-association [case-control] studies). Although linkage analysis has recently been used to identify a nephropathy susceptibility gene locus in type 2 diabetes, mostly association studies have been reported for genes associated with nephropathy in type 1 diabetics *(158,159)*. Such studies usually involve the comparison of allele and genotype frequencies at candidate gene loci in individuals with diabetic nephropathy and in controls. Although several studies, which have generated numerous statistically significant associations, have been published, the results many times have been inconclusive, contradictory, or require further confirmation.

Candidate Gene Studies in Diabetic Nephropathy

Early studies looked into the association of diabetic nephropathy with the major histocompatibility complex on chromosome-6-encoding human leukocyte antigens (HLA). Although HLA association has been demonstrated for microvascular disease *(160)* and twins with the DR3/4 genotype show concordance for retinopathy *(161)*, one large study (n = 675) found no association of HLA markers with diabetic nephropathy *(162)*. After the initial HLA-association studies, several candidate genes have been investigated for their association with diabetic nephropathy.

Renin–Angiotensin System Genes. The renin–angiotensin (RAS) genes are the most extensively investigated candidate genes in this regard. Elevations in prorenin, renin, angiotensin-converting enzyme (ACE), and Ang II levels have been observed in diabetic nephropathy *(163)*. Genes encoding these factors have been associated with hypertension and cardiovascular disease, both of which, as mentioned earlier, are common in patients with diabetic nephropathy and their parents. However, studies, to date, of the association of polymorphisms of ACE, angiotensinogen, and Ang II type I receptor (AT-1) genes have been inconclusive *(164–168)*. The ACE alleles may, however, have a role in the natural history of diabetic nephropathy, with ACE II genotype predicting a greater renoprotective response to ACE inhibitor therapy *(169,170)*. The patients with ACE II genotype were found to have a 51% reduction in UAE after 2 yr of lisinopril therapy compared with a 15% reduction in the *ID* group and only a 8% reduction in the *DD* group *(170)*. This altered response to the ACE inhibitor based on the genotype has also been observed in nondiabetic renal disease *(171,172)*.

Other Candidate Genes. Other major candidate genes that have been studied include nitric oxide synthase (NOS), TGF-β, aldose reductase, heparan sulfate, the insulin gene region, and apolipoprotein E. As discussed earlier, NO plays an important role in the pathogenesis of microvascular complications of diabetes. Recently, a polymorphism in one of the inducible form of human NOS gene (NOS2) promoter (CCTTT repeat polymorphism) has been associated with lowered risk of type 1 diabetic nephropathy *(173)*. Also, a polymorphism in the endothelial constitutive NOS gene (ecNOS4a allele) has been associated with increased risk of nephropathy in type 2 diabetes *(174)*. Similarly, TGF-β is a key mediator of diabetic nephropathy and its association has been reported with mutations in TGF-β gene *(175)*. Aldose reductase is an important enzyme in the polyol pathway and is thought to be a key mediator of diabetic microangiopathic complications. Polymorphism of this gene has been reported to have no association with nephropathy in type 1 diabetes, but the findings need replication *(176,177)*. Heparan sulfate is a major component of the glomerular basement membrane, in diabetic nephropathy *(35,36,178)*. An association of a heparan sulfate core protein (heparan sulfate proteoglycan 2 [HSPG2]) gene polymorphism with nephropathy has been reported *(179)*. Apolipoprotein E (ApoE) is a protein constituent of lipoproteins, and a subtle variation of ApoE can result in increased atherogenicity due to changes in lipid profile. The ApoE gene polymorphism is triallelic and the E2 allele has been associated with nephropathy *(180)*. The results on these various candidate genes require further confirmation and replication by other groups. The insulin gene region, a known susceptibility locus for diabetes (insulin-dependent diabetes mellitus [IDDM2]), has been implicated in premature atherosclerosis and has been examined as a candidate for diabetic nephropathy, but the results have been negative *(162)*.

Sodium–Hydrogen Exchanger. In addition to candidate gene studies, attempts have also been made to associate in vitro cell behavior and phenotype with the risk of diabetic nephropathy. These studies have included analysis of cellular proliferation, senescence, and various physiological mechanisms in a variety of cell types, including red blood cells, cultured skin fibrobalsts, and immortalized lymphocytes *(181–185)*. Among these various approaches, the studies on sodium–hydrogen exchanger (NHE) have been most convincing and have been replicated by different group of workers. The NHE is an integral plasma membrane protein that catalyzes the exchange of extracellular sodium for intracellular hydrogen and regulates various events such as intracellular pH, cellular proliferation, and volume *(183)*. NHE has five isoforms and NHE1 is the most widely expressed and the most studied, isoform *(183–185)*. Increased NHE activity has been demonstrated in cultured skin fibroblasts *(184)*, immortalized lymphoblasts *(185)*, and erythrocytes *(186)* of type 1 diabetic patients with nephropathy. Also, a close concordance for NHE activity was reported in cultured skin fibroblasts of type 1 diabetic siblings with similar renal involvement *(187)*. The NHE can also be activated by extracellular matrix molecules *(183)*. As the increased NHE activity persists in culture after several passages of the cells, these findings may be genetically determined and may reflect a genetic predisposition to accumulate more matrix *(182,183,188,189)*. Although the association of increased NHE activity and diabetic nephropathy has been reproduced by several workers, the measurement of NHE activity is an arduous task. Hence, more reliable and reproducible markers of genetic risk of diabetic nephropathy are needed. The recent advances in the human genome project and whole-genome approaches to identification of such markers may provide additional answers in the near future.

Diabetic nephropathy, thus, has complex and multifactorial etiology and is most likely affected by a number of environmental and genetic interactions. The search for genetic markers of diabetic nephropathy is a difficult but important task for several reasons. Identification of such genetic markers can define individuals who are predisposed to nephropathy early in the course of the diabetes who could then be very carefully followed and possibly treated with stricter glycemic control or newer options, as discussed next. Also, identification of the responsible gene(s) may provide important insights into the pathogenesis and possibly new therapeutic approaches to this disorder *(159)*.

TREATMENT AND PREVENTION OF DIABETIC NEPHROPATHY

Diabetic nephropathy is the most common cause of ESRD in the Western world and is responsible for almost a third of all the patients with ESRD in the United States. Approximately 20–30% of diabetic patients will develop kidney disease over their lifetime. However, possibly as a result of improvements in glycemic control and blood pressure therapy, the incidence of diabetic nephropathy seems to be declining *(145–147)*. Therapies to prevent or delay the progression of diabetic nephropathy are thus critical and the various strategies effective at various stages are discussed below.

Prevention of Diabetic Nephropathy: General Considerations

GLYCEMIC CONTROL

Because the causative event in diabetic nephropathy is hyperglycemia, the ideal preventive approach would be achievement of normal or near-normal glycemia. Both the DCCT and UKPDS studies clearly showed that intensive blood glucose control reduces the risk of development of nephropathy *(28,29)*. Although such results are intuitive, the intensive insulin therapy used in the DCCT *(28)* was associated with a fourfold increase in the incidence of severe hypoglycemic episodes (defined as coma or need for medical assistance) and an average gain of 4.6 kg in weight after 5 yr of intensive therapy. However, despite these concerns in the DCCT study, a 33% reduction in the development of nephropathy occurred in type 1 diabetics. Also, both the DCCT Research Group and the UKPDS concluded that there was not a minimal glycemic threshold above normal for the development of the microvascular complications of diabetes and, thus, recommended that patients attempt to achieve as tight glucose control as possible *(28,29,190)*.

Angiotensin-Converting Enzyme Inhibition and Blood Pressure Control

Hypertension plays an important role in the pathogenesis and progression of diabetic nephropathy. Hence, it is not surprising that therapies aimed at controlling blood pressure have had a positive impact on delaying progression of the disease, and ACE inhibition has been the most extensively investigated such therapy. A meta-analysis of ACE inhibitor therapy vs placebo (116 vs 119 "normotensive" patients with albuminuria) showed a 63% reduction in the progression of nephropathy (8 vs 25 patients) *(191)*. Similar results were shown in patients with type 2 diabetes *(192)*. In a prospective, double-blind multicenter study in patients with type 1 diabetes with macroalbuminuria (UAE > 500 μg/min) and a serum creatinine ≤ 2.5 mg/dL were randomized to receive either captopril ($n = 207$) or placebo ($n = 202$) *(193)*. The serum creatinine doubled in only 25 patients in the captopril group (vs 43 in the placebo group) over a median follow-up period of 3 yr ($p = 0.007$). Interestingly, captopril decreased the rate of doubling of the serum creatinine by almost 50% in patients with more advanced nephropathy (baseline serum creatinine concentration of ≥ 1.5 mg/dL) but had no significant effect on the patients with serum creatinine < 1.5 mg/dL, although it is possible that a longer follow-up might have shown an effect in this group. Also, other outcomes such as the serum creatinine and the UAE were improved in the captopril group and fewer patients had progression to dialysis or transplantation in this group compared to those in the placebo group (10% vs 15%). The continued progression of the disease in treated patients in this study, even during a relatively brief follow-up period, suggests that captopril does not completely prevent the development of renal failure, but slows the projected rate of decline of GFR in patients with macro albuminuria *(193)*. This improvement has been projected to be from the untreated rate of 10–14 mL/min per 1.73 m^2 per year to a rate of 2–5 mL/min per 1.73 m^2 per year while on ACE inhibitor therapy *(193–196)*. In addition to ACE inhibitors, AT-1 blockers also delay progression of renal disease in diabetes *(197,198)*. The renoprotective effect of ACE inhibitors and AT-1 blockers are not adequately explained by their effect on blood pressure *(197)*. The proposed mechanisms underlying these observations include a reduction of glomerular hypertension and a direct blockade of renal cellular actions of Ang II *(122–125)*. However, results of the UKPDS have confirmed earlier observations that reduction in blood pressure with agents other than ACE inhibitors (diuretics and β-blockers) also will prevent or delay renal injury in diabetes *(199)*.

Protein Restriction, Lipid Control, and Smoking Cessation

A meta-analysis of 5 small studies showed that the relative risk of progression among 108 dietary-restricted patients was reduced by almost 50% compared with those who had a more liberal protein intake in diabetic nephropathy *(200)*. More recent studies have also confirmed these observations *(201)*. Measures to correct dyslipidemia, either dietary or pharmacotherapeutic, have also been associated with improved outcome in diabetic nephropathy *(201,202)*. Smoking cessation may provide an additive protection from the risk of development of diabetic nephropathy *(203,204)*. Thus, every attempt should be made to encourage patients with diabetes to stop smoking.

Prevention of Progression at the Microalbuminuria Stage

Microalbuminuria is the most commonly used clinical marker, can be seen into stage III of diabetic nephropathy, and is usually associated with hyperfiltration (*see* Table 1). Several studies suggest that at these early stages, progression of diabetic nephropathy can be prevented. Improved glycemic control using insulin infusion pumps resulted in a decrease in the number of patients who progressed from microalbuminuria to albuminuria in the Steno studies *(205)*. In that study, the patients with high-range microalbuminuria (UAE: 100–300 mg/24 h) who were at the greatest risk for progression when treated with insulin pumps had significantly decreased progression to nephropathy over an 8-yr follow-up compared to conventional insulin treatment (of 9 patients 10 of 10 patients). However, a few studies have failed to document the protective role of tight glycemic control at this stage of disease. In the DCCT study, intensive insulin therapy in microalbuminuric patients did not significantly alter the risk of progression to macroalbuminuria over a mean follow up of 6.5 yr *(28,190)*. Also, in a study conducted in the United Kingdom, 70 type 2 diabetic patients with microalbuminuria failed to show any effect of improved glycemic control after 5 yr *(206)*. It is possible that a longer period of follow-up (≥ 10 yr) is required to see the effects of such therapy. Several studies have now demonstrated that ACE inhibitors can delay the progression from microalbuminuria to macroalbuminuria *(8,9,14)*. Whether initiation of ACE inhibitors at the microalbuminuria stage will ultimately prevent the development of ESRD is not established and would require long-term studies. Nonetheless, based on the available data, the use of ACE inhibitors in diabetic patients with microalbuminuria has now become standard and recommended treatment *(18)*.

Prevention of Progression at the Macroalbuminuria Stage

The development of macroalbuminuria (UAE: > 200 μg/min) is seen in stage IV of diabetic nephropathy. The GFR begins to decline at the rate of 5–10% per year after macroalbuminuria develops *(16)*. Patients in this stage may be very heterogenous with respect to the rate of progression of disease and compliance with therapy. The renal failure may occur in a few months in some, whereas others may have relatively normal renal function for years. Genetic factors probably play an important role in this progression. Patients with more rapid progression are also likely to have a higher incidence of smoking as well as noncompliance and these patients may represent a fundamentally different patient population than those with less advanced kidney disease. Despite the advanced state of diabetic nephropathy and variability in progression, blood pressure control is of paramount importance at this stage *(191,192)*. Some studies of intensive insulin therapy in patients with macroalbuminuria have shown no significant effect on progression to ESRD. These studies were, however, small, with relatively short-term follow-up *(207,208)*. Moreover, blood pressure control in these studies was not optimal. Recent observations have suggested that beneficial effects of improved glycemic control on the progression of overt nephropathy may become evident when combined with stricter control of hypertension (a target blood pressure of 135/80 or less) *(207)*. Similarly, in the UKPDS, attenuation of nephropathy was most pronounced in the subgroup with tight glycemic and blood pressure control *(209)*. Tight glycemic control in overt diabetic nephropathy may also benefit other microvascular complications. ACE inhibitors and/or AT-1 blockers are the agents of choice for blood pressure control in patients with diabetic nephropathy and macroalbuminuria because these agents clearly retard the progression of renal disease *(193,197)*. Dyslipidemia *(202)* and, as noted earlier, smoking may also contribute to renal injury in diabetes. Thus, despite the lack of definite evidence on the role of hyperglycemia in the progress of overt nephropathy to ESRD, current recommendations are that strict glycemic control should be part of a comprehensive regimen that includes optimal blood pressure and lipid control as well as smoking cessation in diabetics with or without overt nephropathy *(210,211)*.

Role of Early Pancreas or Islet Cell Transplantation in the Prevention or Reversal of Diabetic Nephropathy

Pancreas transplantation provides essentially euglycemic control in type 1 diabetes patients. The glycosylated hemoglobin levels usually average 5.5% with almost no hypoglycemic episodes *(212)*. Conversely, the glycosylated hemoglobin levels achieved on intensive insulin regimen in the DCCT study were only 7% and two-thirds of such patients had progression of nephropathy *(190)*. As there appears to be no minimum threshold for glycemia that prevents progression of diabetic nephropathy, the near-normal glycemic control achievable with pancreas or islet cell transplantation may be necessary to prevent or reverse diabetic nephropathy.

Indeed, pancreas transplantation has been shown to prevent or reverse the development of diabetic nephropathy *(212–214)*. It can also reverse more advanced and established diabetic nephropathy in native kidneys, although it took up to 10 yr to see such effects in one study *(214)*. In this study, eight patients with type 1 diabetes, but without uremia, who had successful pancreas transplants were followed up for 10 yr. At 5 yr, the UAE and the glomerular mesangial volume were unchanged, but after 10 yr, both the UAE and the glomerular mesangial volume had decreased substantially. However, currently, it is not clear which patients should receive a pancreas transplant to prevent or reverse diabetic nephropathy. It appears that patients with advanced renal disease but not ESRD and poor glycemic control might benefit the most with pancreas transplantation *(212)*. It is possible that kidney biopsies or clinical application of genetic markers of the nephropathy risk may be required to identify such patients. However, the benefits of pancreas transplantation must be seriously weighed against the risks of surgery and immunosuppression. Clearly, more studies are required before a role for isolated pancreas transplantation in diabetic nephropathy management is established.

Future Medical Therapies

A number of medical interventions have shown promise in experimental animals in preventing the development or attenuating the progression of diabetic nephropathy. These include aminoguanidine, an inhibitor of the formation of advanced glycation products *(54,70,71)*, anti-TGF-β antibodies *(72,73)*, thromboxane inhibitors *(42,43,74)*, antioxidants *(75,76)*, and a selective inhibitor of the PKCβ isozyme *(69)*. The efficacy of these interventions in human diabetic nephropathy remains to be established.

Treatment of Established Diabetic End-Stage Renal Disease

The development of ESRD is a major source of not only morbidity but also mortality in diabetic patients. Dialysis and renal transplantation are the only effective ways of treating established ESRD, although patients with diabetes undergoing dialysis have a lower survival rate compared with nondiabetic patients *(215)*. Kidney transplantation has been shown to improve patient survival in diabetes and is the treatment of choice for diabetic ESRD *(216)*. However, the waiting time for a cadaveric kidney transplant is continuously increasing, with more than 40,000 patients on waiting lists and only 8000 kidneys available annually in the United States *(217)*. Finally, there is increasing evidence that simultaneous pancreas kidney (SPK) transplantation may prolong patient survival more than isolated kidney transplantation in diabetic end-stage nephropathy *(212,218,219)*. In a study comparing patient survival in recipients of isolated kidney vs SPK transplantation, the 10-yr patient survival was 37% in diabetic patients with kidney transplant alone *(219)*. The 10-yr survival rate improved to 60% in SPK transplant patients with a functioning pancreas and was comparable to the rate of 72% seen in nondiabetic patients. The 10-yr survival rate was, however, only 33% in the SPK patients whose pancreas failed within the first 2 yr. These results underscore the importance of long-term euglycemia even at the late stages of this diabetic complication. With 1-yr pancreas graft survival rates of almost 90% at some centers, SPK transplantation is now increasingly accepted as the treatment of choice for patients with type 1 diabetes and kidney failure *(212,219)*. However, SPK transplantation is a technically more complex procedure (versus isolated kidney transplant) and further studies are needed to expand and establish the criteria for selecting suitable patients for this procedure.

Urinary Tract Infections in Diabetes

A twofold to fourfold higher incidence of bacteriuria has been reported in diabetic women compared to nondiabetic women, although it is not seen in men *(220–222)*. As compared with nondiabetic women, diabetic women with bacteriuria are usually asymptomatic *(223)*. However, asymptomatic bacteriuria can be a predisposing factor for overt urinary tract infections (UTIs) *(224)*. Also, diabetes predisposes patients with UTI to more severe infections of the upper urinary tract and to various complications. The upper tract is involved in up to 80% of UTIs in diabetic patients and, in contrast to nondiabetic patients, bilateral infection is more common in diabetics *(220)*.

The most common microbe in diabetics with UTI is *Escherichia coli*. However *Klebsiella* and *Proteus* sp are more frequently found in diabetic patients than in the control population *(220,221)*. Also, unusual microbes such as fungi, particularly Candida, staphylococci, and *Pasteurella multocida* may also be responsible for a small fraction of UTIs *(225–229)*. There are, possibly, multiple mechanisms underlying the reported higher frequency and severity of UTI in diabetes. Some of the proposed mechanisms include glucosuria, which favors bacterial growth, impaired bladder evacuation, increased adherence of pathogens to uroepithelial cells, and defective neutrophil function *(229,230)*.

A number of potential complications of UTI have been reported in diabetics and include pyelonephritis *(220,221)*, perinephric abscess *(231)*, emphysematous cystitis

(232–234), and renal papillary necrosis *(235,236).* Renal papillary necrosis has been one of the oldest documented and most recognized such complication *(235).* It can present with recurrent UTI, fever, renal colic, hematuria, flank, and/or abdominal pain and the diagnosis is usually established by retrograde pyelography or ultrasonography *(236).* The incidence of papillary necrosis, however, has markedly decreased in the last two decades and this condition appears to have become a rarity now. This trend of diminishing incidence is possibly related to earlier and more frequent administration of antibiotics *(237).* In addition to papillary necrosis, there is also a higher incidence of perinephric abscess in diabetics with symptomatic UTI. In one series, 36% of patients with this diagnosis had diabetes *(231). E. coli* or *Proteus* sp account for the majority (> 75%) of this complication, whereas *Staphylococcus aureus* accounts for the remainder of the cases *(220).* Symptoms include flank or abdominal, which may be present in less than 25% of cases, and persistent fever (> 4 d after the initiation of antibiotic therapy) *(231).* Ultrasonography or computed tomography are usually diagnostic. Treatment consists of hydration, surgical drainage, and parenteral antibiotics *(220,231).* Another potentially life-threatening complication of UTI in diabetics is emphysematous pyelonephritis. It most often presents as an acute medical emergency, typically in a septic diabetic patient with acute renal failure *(232–234).* The diagnosis is made radiologically, usually by plain abdominal radiography or computed tomography *(232,233).* The management of this condition has traditionally been surgical and involves nephrectomy *(234,238).* However, some recent reports have described successful treatment with medical intervention *(234).* Other potential complications of UTI in diabetic patients are the extrarenal spread of bacterial infection and generalized sepsis. These may manifest as endophthalmitis *(239),* spondylitis *(240),* and iliopsoas abscess, particularly with methicillin-resistant staphylococci *(241).* Episodes of UTI may also pose problems after renal transplantation.

Symptomatic upper urinary tract and complicated asymptomatic bacteriuria infections require systemic antibiotic therapy along with hydration and possible surgical intervention. A community-acquired symptomatic lower UTI may be managed with trimethoprim/ sulfamethoxazole, trimethoprim, or gyrase inhibitors. For nosocomially acquired UTI, sensitivity-directed antibiotic intervention is required. Certain aspects of management of UTI in diabetics, however, remain controversial. No clear benefits of prophylactic antibiotic treatment have been demonstrated for treatment in diabetic patients *(242).* The treatment of candida infection confined to the bladder is also controversial. Spontaneous resolution of funguria can occur and removal of an indwelling catheter, if one is present, is recommended as the initial intervention. Invasive candiduria can be managed with oral fluconazole or amphotericin B, by either bladder irrigation or by systemic administration *(243,244).* Systemic therapy by oral fluconazole (for 4 d) or single-dose intravenous amphotericin B has been shown to have improved cure rates compared to bladder irrigation with amphotericin B alone *(245),* although amphotericin B bladder irrigation may be also effective in some patients *(244,245).* However, currently fluconazole may be the preferred agent because of its ease of administration and relative lack of toxicity *(221).*

SUMMARY

Nephropathy is a serious complication of diabetes and considerable advances have been made over the past two decades in the understanding of its pathogenesis, especially at the cellular and molecular level. Hyperglycemia is the key requirement for the development of diabetic nephropathy, and interventions aimed at interfering with adverse metabolic actions of hyperglycemia on renal cells have shown promise in experimental diabetic nephropathy. There is also evidence that genetic factors play an important role in susceptibility, progression, and response to therapy of this serious complication. Although identification of candidate genes for diabetic nephropathy has so far been largely inconclusive or contradictory, recent advances in the human genome project and newer approaches to the study of this complex problem may shed light on the genetic factors in the near future. The treatment of early stages of nephropathy has significantly changed over the past decade with the routine use of ACE inhibitors or AT-II receptor blockers as the standard of care. However, despite improvements in medical therapy for patients with diabetic nephropathy, increasing numbers of patients with diabetes develop ESRD each year. In patients with established but not end-stage diabetic nephropathy, pancreas transplantation may be a viable choice. Recent advances in surgical techniques and immunosuppressive therapy have made kidney transplantation the therapy of choice for patients with ESRD resulting from diabetes. Simultaneous pancreas kidney transplant may, in the near future, acquire a wider role in management of this complication. Finally, in addition to diabetic nephropathy, patients with long-standing type 1 diabetes may be at a higher risk of infections of the urinary tract, which include both asymptomatic bacteruria and pyelonephritis that, at times, can lead to serious complications.

REFERENCES

1. Bright P. Dr. Richard Bright (1789–1858), The Bodley Head, London, 1983, pp. 131–142.
2. Ritz E, Zeier M, Lundin P. French and German nephrologists in the mid-19th century: the impact of Richard Bright on the continent. Am J Nephrol 1989;9:167–172.
3. Joslin EP. Treatment of Diabetes Mellitus. Lea & Febiger, Philadelphia, 1917, p. 419.
4. Borch-Johnsen K, Kreiner S. Proteinuria: value as predictor of cardiovascular mortality in insulin-dependent diabetes mellitus. Br Med J 1987;294:1651–1654.
5. Mogensen CE. Microalbuminuria predicts clinical proteinuria and early mortality in maturity onset diabetes. N Engl J Med 1984;310:356–360.
6. Marso SP, Ellis SG, Gurm HS, Lytle BW. Topol EJ. Proteinuria is a key determinant of death in patients with diabetes after isolated coronary artery bypass grafting. Am Heart J 2000;139:939–944.
7. Messent JWC, Elliott TG, Hill RD, Jarrett RJ, Keen H, Viberti GC. Prognostic significance of microalbuminuria in insulin-dependent diabetes mellitus: a twenty year follow-up study. Kidney Int 1992;41:836–839.
8. Nelson RG, Knowler WC, Pettitt DJ, Bennett PH. Kidney diseases. In: National Diabetes Group. Diabetes in America, 2nd ed. National Institutes of Health, National Institute of Diabetes and Digestive and Kidney Diseases, Bethesda, MD, 1995, pp. 349–400.
9. Bilous RW. Can we prevent or delay diabetic nephropathy? J R Coll Physicians Lond 1997;31:22–27.
10. Fioretto P, Steffes MW, Mauer M. Glomerular structure in non-proteinuric IDDM patients with various levels of albuminuria. Diabetes 1994;43:1358–1364.
11. Feldt-Rasmussen B, Mathiesen ER, Deckert T. Effect of 2 years of strict metabolic control on progression of incipient nephropathy in insulin-dependent diabetes. Lancet 1986;2:1300–1304.
12. Dahl-Jorgensen K, Hanssen KF, Kierulf P, Bjoro T, Sandvik L, Aagenaess O. Reduction of urinary albumin excretion after 4 years of continuous subcutaneous insulin infusion in insulin-dependent diabetes mellitus. Acta Endocrinol 1988;117:19–25.
13. Dahl-Jorgensen K, Bjoro T, Kierulf P, Sandvik L, Bangstad HJ, Hanssen KF. The effect of long-term strict glycemic control on kidney function in insulin-dependent diabetes mellitus: seven years result from the Oslo Study. Kidney Int 1992;41:920–923.
14. Viberti G, Mogensen CE, Groop LC, Pauls JF, European Microalbuminuria Captopril Study Group. Effect of captopril on progression to clinical proteinuria in patients with insulin-dependent diabetes mellitus and microalbuminuria. JAMA 1994;271:275–279.

15. Borch-Johnsen K, Wenzel H, Viberti GC, Mogensen CE. Is screening and intervention for microalbuminuria worthwhile in patients with insulin dependent diabetes? Br Med J 1993;306:1722–1725.
16. Viberti GC, Bilous RW, Mackintosh D, Keen H. Monitoring glomerular function in diabetic nephropathy: a prospective study. Am J Med. 1983;74:256–264.
17. Camamori MI, Fioretto P, Mauer M. The need for early predictors of diabetic nephropathy risk: is albumin excretion rate sufficient? Diabetes 2000;49:1399–1408.
18. Bennett PH, Haffner S, Kasiske BL, et al. Screening and management of microalbuminuria in patients with diabetes mellitus: recommendations to the Scientific Advisory Board of the National Kidney Foundation from an ad hoc committee of the Council on Diabetes Mellitus of the National Kidney Foundation. Am J Kidney Dis 1995;25:107–112.
19. Ziyadeh FN. The extracellular matrix in diabetic nephropathy. Am J Kidney Dis 1993;22:736–744.
20. Osterby R, Gundersen HJG. Glomerular size and structure in diabetes mellitus. I. Early abnormalities. Diabetologia 1975;11:225–229.
21. Osterby R. Morphometric studies of the peripheral glomerular basement membrane in early juvenile diabetes. I. Development of initial basement membrane thickening. Diabetologia 1972;8:84–92.
22. Mogensen CE, Andersen MJ. Increased kidney size and glomerular filtration rate in early juvenile diabetes. Diabetes 1973;22:706–712.
23. Lane PH, Steffes MW, Fioretto P, Mauer SM. Renal interstitial expansion in insulin-dependent diabetes mellitus. Kidney Int 1993;43:661–667.
24. Ziyadeh FN, Goldfarb S. The renal tubulointerstitium in diabetes mellitus. Kidney Int 1991;39:464–475.
25. Kimmelstiel P, Wilson C. Intercapillary lesions in glomeruli of the kidney. Am J Pathol 1936;12:83–97.
26. Rodby RA. Type II diabetic nephropathy: Its clinical course and therapeutic implications. Semin Nephrol 1997;17:132–147.
27. Dalla Vestra M, Saller A, Bortoloso E, Mauer M, Fioretto P. Structural involvement in type 1 and type 2 diabetic nephropathy. Diabetes Metab 2000;26(Suppl 4):8–14.
28. DCCT Research Group. The effect of intensive treatment of diabetes on the development and progression of long-term complications in insulin-dependent diabetes mellitus. N Engl J Med 1993;329:977–986.
29. United Kingdom Prospective Diabetes Study (UKPDS). Intensive blood-glucose control with sulphonylurea or insulin compared to conventional treatment and risk of complications in patients with type 2 diabetes (UKPDS 33). Lancet 1998; 1352:837–853.
30. Mauer SM, Goetz FC, McHugh CE. Long term studies of normal kidneys transplanted into patients with type I diabetes. Diabetes 1989;38:516–523.
31. Wolf G, Sharma K, Chen Y, Ericksen M, Ziyadeh FN. High glucose-induced proliferation in mesangial cells is reversed by autocrine TGF-β. Kidney Int 1992;42:647–656.
32. Ziyadeh FN, Snipes ER, Watanabe M, Alvarez RJ, Goldfarb S, Haverty TP. High glucose induces cell hypertrophy and stimulates collagen gene transcription in proximal tubule. Am J Physiol 1990;259:F704–F714.
33. Ziyadeh FN, Sharma K, Ericksen M, Wolf G. Stimulation of collagen gene expression and protein synthesis in murine mesangial cells by high glucose is mediated by activation of transforming growth factor-β. J Clin Invest 1994;93:536–542.
34. Wakisaka M, Spiro MJ, Spiro RG. Synthesis of type VI collagen in cultured glomerular cells and comparison of its regulation by glucose and other factors with that of type IV collagen. Diabetes 1994;43:95–103.
35. Van Det NF, van den Born J, Tamsa JT, et al. Effects of high glucose on the production of heparan sulfate proteoglycan by mesangial and epithelial cells. Kidney Int 1996;49:1079–1089.
36. Kasinath BS, Block JA, Singh AK, et al. Regulation of rat glomerular epithelial cell proteoglycans by high-medium glucose. Arch Biochem Biophys 1994;309:149–159.
37. Heilig CW, Concepcion LA, Riser BL, Freytag SO, Zhu M, Cortes P. Overexpression of glucose transporters in rat mesangial cells cultured in a normal glucose milieu mimics the diabetic phenotype. J Clin Invest 1994;96:149–159.
38. King GL, Ishii H, Koya D. Diabetic vascular dysfunctions: a model of excessive activation of protein kinase C. Kidney Int 1997;52:S77–S85.
39. DeRubertis FR, Craven PA. Activation of protein kinase C in glomerular cells in diabetes. Mechanisms and potential link to the pathogenesis of diabetic glomerulopathy. Diabetes 1994;43:1–8.
40. Larkins RG, Dunlop ME. The link between hyperglycaemia and diabetic nephropathy. Diabetologia 1992;35:499–504.

41. Sharma K, Ziyadeh FN. Biochemical events and cytokine interactions linking glucose metabolism to the development of diabetic nephropathy. Semin Nephrol 1997;17:80–92.
42. Ledbetter S, Copeland EJ, Noonan D, Vogeli G, Hassell JR. Altered steady-state mRNA levels of basement membrane proteins in diabetic mouse kidneys and thromboxane synthase inhibition. Diabetes 1990;39:196–203.
43. Craven PA, Melhem FT, DeRubertis FR. Thromboxane in the pathogenesis of glomerular injury in diabetes. Kidney Int 1992;42:937–946.
44. Studer RK, Negrete H, Craven PA, DeRubertis FR. Protein kinase C signals thromboxane induced increases in fibronectin synthesis and TGF-beta bioactivity in mesangial cells. Kidney Int 1995;48:422–430.
45. Baynes JW, Thorpe SR. The role of oxidative stress in diabetic complications. Curr Opin Endocrinol 1996;3:277–284.
46. Giugliano D, Ceriello A, Paolisso G. Oxidative stress and diabetic vascular complications. Diabetes Care 1996;19:257–267.
47. Santinim SA, Marra G, Giardina B, et al. Defective plasma antioxidant defenses and enhanced susceptibility to lipid peroxidation in uncomplicated IDDM. Diabetes 1997;46:1853–1858.
48. Cohen MP, Ziyadeh FN. Role of Amadori-modified nonenzymatically glycated serum proteins in the pathogenesis of diabetic nephropathy. J Am Soc Nephrol 1996;7:1–8.
49. Brownlee M. Lilly Lecture 1993. Glycation and diabetic complications. Diabetes 1994;43:836–841.
50. Makita Z, Radoff S, Rayfield EJ, et al. Advanced glycosylation end products in patients with diabetic nephropathy. N. Engl J Med 1991;325:836–842.
51. Soulis T, Cooper M, Vranes D, Bucala R, Jerums G. The effects of aminoguanidine in preventing experimental diabetic nephropathy are related to duration of treatment. Kidney Int 1996;627–634.
52. Pugliese G, Pricci F, Romeo G, et al. Upregulation of mesangial growth factor and extracellular matrix synthesis by advanced glycation end products via a receptor-mediated mechanism. Diabetes 1997;46:1881–1887.
53. Cohen MP, Masson N, Hud E, Ziyadeh F, Han DC. Clements RS. Inhibiting albumin glycation ameliorates diabetic nephropathy in the db/db mouse. Exp Nephrol 2000;8:135–143.
54. Ziyadeh FN, Han DC, Cohen J, Guo J, Cohen MP. Glycated albumin stimulates fibronectin gene expression in glomerular mesangial cells: Involvement of the TGF-[beta] system. Kidney Int 1998;53:631–638.
55. Craven PA, DeRubertis FR, Melhem MF. Nitric oxide in diabetic nephropathy. Kidney Int 1997;52(Suppl):S46–S53.
56. Keynan S, Hirshberg B, Levin-Iaina N, et al. Renal nitric oxide production during the early phase of experimental diabetes mellitus. Kidney Int 2000;58:740–747.
57. Craven PA, Studer RK, Felder J, et al. Nitric oxide inhibition of transforming growth factor-beta and collagen synthesis in mesangial cells. Diabetes 1997;46:671–681.
58. Phillips SL, DeRubertis FR, Craven PA. Regulation of the laminin C1 promoter in cultured mesangial cells. Diabetes 1999;48:2083–2089.
59. Studer RK, Craven PA, DeRubertis FR. Antioxidant inhibition of protein kinase C signalled increases in transforming growth factor-β in mesangial cells. Metabolism 1997;46:918–925.
60. Craven PA, Studer RK, DeRubertis FR. Impaired NO dependent cyclic GMP generation in glomeruli from diabetic rats: evidence for protein kinase C mediated suppression of the cholinergic response. J Clin Invest 1994;93:311–320.
61. Craven PA, Studer RK, DeRubertis FR. Impaired nitric oxide release by glomeruli from diabetic rats. Metabolism 1995;44:695–698.
62. Ting H, Timimi FK, Boles KS, et al. Vitamin C improves endothelium dependent vasodilation in patients with non insulin dependent diabetes mellitus. J Clin Invest 1996;97:22–28.
63. Beckman JS, Koppenol WH. Nitric oxide, superoxide, and peroxynitrite: the good, the bad, and the ugly. Am J Physiol 1996;271:C1424–C1437.
64. Lyall F, Gibson JL, Greer IA, et al. Increased nitrotyrosine in the diabetic placenta. Diabetes Care 1998;21:1753–1758.
65. Carmines P, Pollock JS, Ishii N, et al. Tyrosine nitration accompanies increased nitric oxide and superoxide production in renal cortex in diabetes. J Am Soc Nephrol 1999;10:393A.
66. Nishikawa T, Edelstein D, Du XL, et al. Normalizing mitochondrial superoxide production blocks three pathways of hyperglycaemic damage. Nature 2000;404:787–790.
67. Du X-L, Edelstein D, Rossetti L, et al. Hyperglycemia-induced mitochondrial superoxide overproduction activates the hexosamine pathway and induces plasminogen activator inhibitor-1 expression by increasing Sp1 glycosylation. Proc Natl Acad Sci USA 2000;97:12,222–12,226.

68. Craven PA, Melhem MF, Phillips SL, DeRubertis FR. Overexpression of Cu^{2+}/Zn^{2+} superoxide dismutase protects against early diabetic glomerular injury in transgenic mice. Diabetes 2001;50(9),2114–2115.
69. Ishii H, Jirousek MR, Koya D, et al. Amelioration of vascular dysfunctions in diabetic rats by an oral PKC β inhibitor. Science 1996;272:728–731.
70. Soulis-Liparota T, Cooper M, Papazoglou D, Clarke B, Jerums G. Retardation by aminoguanidine of development of albuminuria, mesangial expansion, and tissue fluorescence in streptozotocin-induced diabetic rat. Diabetes 1991;40:1328–1334.
71. Bucala R, Vlassara H. Advanced glycosylation end products in diabetic renal and vascular disease. Am J Kidney Dis 1995;26:875–888.
72. Sharma K, Jin Y, Guo J, Ziyadeh FN. Neutralization of TGF-β by anti-TGF-β antibody attenuates kidney hypertrophy and the enhanced extracellular matrix gene expression in STZ-induced diabetic mice. Diabetes 1996;45:522–530.
73. Ziyadeh FN, Hoffman BB, Han DC, et al. Long-term prevention of renal insufficiency, excess matrix gene expression, and glomerular mesangial matrix expansion by treatment with monoclonal anti-transforming growth factor-beta antibody in db/db diabetic mice. Proc Nat Acad Sci USA 2000;97:8015–8020.
74. Matsuo Y, Takagawa I, Koshida H, et al. Antiproteinuric effect of a thromboxane receptor antagonist, S-1452, on rat diabetic nephropathy and murine lupus nephritis. Pharmacology 1995;50:1–8.
75. Craven PA, DeRubertis FR, Kagan VE, Melhem MF, Studer RK. Effects of dietary supplementation with vitamin C or E on albuminuria, glomerular TGFβ and size in diabetes. J Am Soc Nephrol 1997;8:1405–1407.
76. Koya D, Lee IK, Ishii H, Kanoh H, King GL. Prevention of glomerular dysfunction in diabetic rats by treatment with *d*-alpha-tocopherol. J Am Soc Nephrol 1997;8:426–435.
77. Melhem MF, Craven PA, DeRubertis FR. Effects of dietary supplementation of alpha-lipoic acid on early glomerular injury in diabetes mellitus. J Am Soc Nephrol 2001;12(1):124–133.
78. Ibrahim HN, Hostetter TH. Diabetic nephropathy. J Am Soc Nephrol 1997;8:487–493.
79. Hostetter TH, Troy JL, Brenner BM. Glomerular hemodynamics in experimental diabetes mellitus. Kidney Int 1981;19:410–415.
80. O'Bryan GT, Hostetter TH. The renal hemodynamic basis of diabetic nephropathy. Semin Nephrol 1997;17:93–100.
81. Zatz R. Haemodynamically mediated glomerular injury: the end of a 15-year-old controversy? Curr Opin Nephrol Hypertens 1996;5:468–475.
82. Cortes P, Zhao X, Riser BL, Narins RG. Role of glomerular mechanical strain in the pathogenesis of diabetic nephropathy. Kidney Int 1997;51:57–68.
83. Harris RC, Haralson MA, Badr KF. Continuous stretch-relaxation in culture alters rat mesangial cell morphology, growth characteristics and metabolic activity. Lab Invest 1992;66:548–554.
84. Yasuda Kondo S, Homma T, Harris RC. Regulation of extracellular matrix by mechanical stress in rat glomerular mesangial cells. J Clin Invest 1996;98:1991–2000.
85. Riser BL, Cortes P, Zhao X, Berstein J, Dumler F, Narins RG. Intraglomerular pressure and mesangial stretching stimulate extracellular matrix formation in the rat. J Clin Invest 1992;90:1932–1943.
86. Mattana J, Singhal PC. Applied pressure modulates mesangial cell proliferation and matrix synthesis. Am J Hypertens 1995;8:1112–1120.
87. Riser BL, Cortes P, Heilig C, et al. Cyclic stretching force selectively up-regulates transforming growth factor-b isoforms in cultured rat mesangial cells. Am J Pathol 1996;148:1915–1923.
88. Homma T, Akai Y, Burns KD, Harris RC. Activation of S6 kinase by repeated cycles of stretching and relaxation in rat glomerular mesangial cells. J Biol Chem 1992;267:23,129–23,135.
89. Harris RC, Akai Y, Yasuda T, Homma T. The role of physical forces in alterations of mesangial cell function. Kidney Int 1995;45(Suppl 45):S17.
90. Mauer SM, Steffes MW, Ellis EN, Sutherland DER, Brown DM, Goetz FC. Structural–functional relationships in diabetic nephropathy. J Clin Invest 1984;74:1143–1155.
91. Nath KA. Tubulointerstitial changes as a major determinant in the progression of renal damage. Am J Kidney Dis 1992;20:1–17.
92. Schwieger J, Fine LG. Renal hypertrophy, growth factors, and nephropathy in diabetes mellitus. Semin Nephrol 1990;10:242–253.
93. Wolf G. Cellular mechanisms of tubule hypertrophy and hyperplasia in renal injury. Miner Electrolyte Metab 1995;21:303–316.
94. Abboud HE. Growth factors and diabetic nephropathy: an overview. Kidney Int 1997;52(Suppl 60):S3–S6.

95. Sharma K, Ziyadeh FN. Hyperglycemia and diabetic kidney disease: the case for transforming growth factor-[beta] as a key mediator. Diabetes 1995;44:1139–1146.
96. Border WA, Ruoslahti E. Transforming growth factor-[beta] in disease: the dark side of tissue repair. J Clin Invest 1992;90:1–7.
97. Sharma K, Ziyadeh FN, Alzahabi B, et al. Increased renal production of transforming growth factor-[beta]1 in patients with type II diabetes mellitus. Diabetes 1997;46:854–859.
98. Shankland SJ, Scholey JW. Expression of transforming growth factor-[beta]1 during diabetic renal hypertrophy. Kidney Int 1994;46:430–442.
99. Yamamoto T, Nakamura T, Noble NA, Ruoslahti E, Border WA. Expression of transforming growth factor [beta] is elevated in human and experimental diabetic nephropathy. Proc Natl Acad Sci USA 1993;90:1814–1818.
100. Sharma K, Ziyadeh FN. Renal hypertrophy is associated with upregulation of TGF-[beta]1 gene expression in diabetic BB rat and NOD mouse. Am J Physiol 1994;267:F1094–F1101.
101. Pankewycz OG, Guan JX, Bolton WK, Gomez A, Benedict JF. Renal TGF-[beta] regulation in spontaneously diabetic NOD mice with correlations in mesangial cells. Kidney Int 1994;46:748–758.
102. Mogyorosi A, Ziyadeh FN. Increased decorin mRNA in diabetic mouse kidney and in mesangial and tubular cells cultured in high glucose. Am J Physiol 1998;275(5 Pt 2):F827–F832.
103. Kolm-Litty V, Sauer U, Nerlich A, Lehmann R, Schleicher ED. High glucose-induced transforming growth factor [beta]1 production is mediated by the hexoseamine pathway in porcine glomerular mesangial cells. J Clin Invest 1998;101:160–169.
104. Rocco MV, Chen Y, Goldfarb S, Ziyadeh FN. Elevated glucose stimulates TGF-[beta] gene expression and bioactivity in proximal tubule. Kidney Int 1992;41:107–114.
105. Hirakata M, Kaname S, Chung UG, et al. Tyrosine kinase dependent expression of TGF-[beta] induced by stretch in mesangial cells. Kidney Int 1997;51:1028–1036.
106. Wolf G, Mueller E, Stahl RAK, Ziyadeh FN. Angiotensin II-induced hypertrophy of cultured murine proximal tubular cells is mediated by endogenous transforming growth factor-[beta]. J Clin Invest 1993;92:1366–1372.
107. Guh JY, Yang ML, Yang YL, Chang CC, Chuang LY. Captopril reverses high-glucose-induced growth effects on LLC-PK_1 cells partly by decreasing transforming growth factor-[beta] receptor protein expression. J Am Soc Nephrol 1996;7:1207–1215.
108. Sharma K, Eltayeb BO, McGowan TA, et al. Captopril-induced reduction of serum levels of transforming growth factor-beta1 correlates with long-term renoprotection in insulin-dependent diabetic patients. Am J Kidney Dis 1999;34:818–823.
109. Nakamura T, Ebihara I, Fukui M, Tomino Y, Koide H. Effect of a specific endothelin receptor A antagonist on mRNA levels for extracellular matrix components and growth factors in diabetic glomeruli. Diabetes 1995;44:895–899.
110. Negrete H, Studer RK, Craven PA, DeRubertis FR. Role for transforming growth factor [beta] in thromboxane-induced increases in mesangial cell fibronectin synthesis. Diabetes 1995;44:335–339.
111. Feld SM, Hirschberg R, Artishevsky A, Nast C, Adler SG. Insulin-like growth factor I induces mesangial proliferation and increases mRNA and secretion of collagen. Kidney Int 1995;48:45–51.
112. Blazer-Yost BL, Watanabe M, Haverty TP, Ziyadeh FN. Role of insulin and IGF1 receptors in proliferation of cultured renal proximal tubule cells. Biochim Biophys Acta 1992;113:329–335.
113. Hammerman MR. The growth hormone-insulin-like growth factor axis in kidney. Am J Physiol 1989;257:F503–F514.
114. Flyvbjerg A, Bornfeldt KE, Marshall SM, Arnqvist Orskov H. Kidney IGF-I mRNA in initial renal hypertrophy in experimental diabetes in rats. Diabetologia 1990;33:334–338.
115. Phillip M, Segeve Y, Zung A, et al. The accumulation of IGF-I in kidneys of streptozotocin-diabetic adult rats is not associated with elevated plasma GH or IGF-I levels. Endocrine 1995;3:689–693.
116. Werner H, Shen-Orr Z, Stannard B, Burguera B, Roberts CT, Leroith D. Experimental diabetes increases insulinlike growth factor I and II receptor concentration and gene expression in kidney. Diabetes 1990;39:1490–1497.
117. Sugimoto H, Shikata K, Makino H, Ota K, Ota Z. Increased gene expression of insulin-like growth factor-I receptor in experimental diabetic rat glomeruli. Nephron 1996;72:648–653.
118. Flyvbjerg A, Marshall SM, Frystyk J, Hansen KW, Harris AG, Orskov H. Octreotide administration in diabetic rats: effects on renal hypertrophy and urinary albumin excretion. Kidney Int 1992;41:805–812.
119. Hirschberg R. Bioactivity of glomerular ultrafiltrate during heavy proteinuria may contribute to renal tubulo-interstitial lesions: evidence for a role of insulin-like growth factor I. J Clin Invest 1996;98:116–124.

120. Wolf G. Molecular mechanisms of angiotensin II in the kidney: emerging role in the progression of renal disease beyond haemodynamics. Nephrol Dial Transplant 1998;13:1131–1142.
121. Wolf G. Vasoactive substances as regulators of renal growth. Exp Nephrol 1993;1:141–151.
122. Wolf G, Ziyadeh FN. The role of angiotensin II in diabetic nephropathy: emphasis on nonhemodynamic mechanisms. Am J Kidney Dis 1997;29:153–163.
123. Kennefick TM, Anderson S. Role of angiotensin II in diabetic nephropathy. Semin Nephrol 1997;17:441–447.
124. Wolf G, Neilson EG, Goldfarb S, Ziyadeh FN. The influence of glucose concentration on angiotensin II-induced hypertrophy of proximal tubular cells in culture. Biochem Biophys Res Commun 1991;176:902–909.
125. Wolf G, Neilson EG. Angiotensin II induces cellular hypertrophy in cultured murine proximal tubular cells. Am J Physiol 1990;259:F768–F777.
126. Wolf G, Neilson EG. Angiotensin II as a renal growth factor. J Am Soc Nephrol 1993;3:1531–1540.
127. Ling H, Vamvakas S, Schaefer L, Schnittler HJ, Schaefer RM, Heidland A. Angiotensin II-induced cellular hypertrophy: Potential role of impaired proteolytic activity in cultured LLC-PK_1 cells. Nephrol Dial Transplant 1995;10:1305–1312.
128. Haijinazarian M, Cosio FG, Nahman NS, Mahan JD. Angiotensin-converting enzyme inhibition partially prevents diabetic organomegaly. Am J Kidney Dis 1994;23:105–117.
129. Sassy-Prigent C, Heudes D, Jouquey S, et al. Morphometric detection of incipient glomerular lesions in diabetic nephropathy in rats: protective effects of ACE inhibition. Lab Invest 1995;73:64–71.
130. Young BA, Johnson RJ, Alpers CA, et al. Cellular events in the evolution of experimental diabetic nephropathy. Kidney Int 1995;47:935–944.
131. Throckmorton DC, Brodgen AP, Min B, Rasmussen H, Kashgarian M. PDGF and TGF-[beta] mediate collagen production by mesangial cells exposed to advanced glycosylation end products. Kidney Int 1995;48:111–117.
132. Nakamura T, Fukui M, Ebihara I, et al. mRNA expression of growth factors in glomeruli from diabetic rats. Diabetes 1993;42:450–456.
133. Inaba T, Ishibashi S, Gotoda T, et al. Enhanced expression of platelet-derived growth factor-[beta] receptor by high glucose. Involvement of platelet-derived growth factor in diabetic angiopathy. Diabetes 1996;45:507–512.
134. Ishibashi K, Sasaki S, Sakamoto H, et al. Hepatocyte growth factor is a paracrine factor for renal epithelial cells: stimulation of DNA synthesis and Na,K-ATPase activity. Biochim Biophys Res Commun 1992;182:960–965.
135. Morabito E, Corsico N, Arrigoni Martelli E. Endothelins urinary excretion in spontaneously diabetic db/db rats. Life Sci 1995;56:13–18.
136. Takahashi K, Ghatei MA, Lam H-C, O'Halloran, OJ, Bloom SR. Elevated plasma endothelin in patients with diabetes mellitus. Diabetologia 1990;33:306–310.
137. Ferri C, Laurenti O, Bellini C, et al. Circulating endothelin-1 levels in lean non-insulin-dependent diabetic patients. Am J Hypertens 1995;8:40–47.
138. Craven PA, Caines MA, DeRubertis FR. Sequential alterations in glomerular prostaglandin and thromboxane synthesis in diabetic rats: relationship to the hyperfiltration of early diabetes. Metabolism 1987;36:95–103.
139. Gambardella S, Andreani D, Cancelli A, et al. Renal hemodynamics and urinary excretion of 6-keto prostaglandin F 1a, and thromboxane B2 in newly diagnosed type I diabetic patients. Diabetes 1988;37:1044–1048.
140. DeRubertis FR, Craven PA. Contribution of platelet thromboxane production to enhanced urinary excretion and glomerular production of thromboxane and to the pathogenesis of albuminuria in the streptozotocin-diabetic rat. Metabolism 1992;41:90–96.
141. Bruggeman LA, Horigan EA, Horikoshi S, Ray PE, Klotman PE. Thormboxane stimulates synthesis of extracellular matrix proteins in vitro. Am J Physiol 1991;261:F488–F494.
142. Craven PA, Patterson M, DeRubertis FR. Role of enhanced arachidonate availability through the phospholipase A_2 pathway in the mediation of increased prostaglandin synthesis by glomeruli from diabetic rats. Diabetes 1988;37:429–435.
143. Pricci E, Pugliese G, Mene P, et al. Regulatory role of eicosanoids in extracellular matrix overproduction induced by long-term exposure to high glucose in cultured rat mesangial cells. Diabetologia 1996;39:1055–1062.
144. Banba N, Nakamura T, Matsumura M, Kuroda H, Hattori Y, Kasai K. Possible relationship of monocyte chemoattractant protein-1 with diabetic nephropathy. Kidney Int 2000;58:684–690.

145. Anderson AR, Christiansen IS, Anderson JK, Kreiner S, Deckert T. Diabetic nephropathy in type 1 (insulin-dependent) diabetes: an epidemiological study. Diabetologia 1983;25:496–501.
146. Krolewski AS, Warram JH, Christlieb AR, Busick EJ, Kahn CR. The changing natural history of nephropathy in type 1 diabetes. Am J Med 1985;78:785–793.
147. Parving HH, Hommel E. Prognosis in diabetic nephropathy. Br Med J 1989;299:230–233.
148. Quinn M, Angelico MC, Warram JH, Krolewski AS. Familial factors determine the development of diabetic nephropathy in patients with IDDM. Diabetologia 1996;39:940–945.
149. DCCT. Clustering of long term complications in families with diabetes in the Diabetes Control and Complications Trials. Diabetes 1997;46:1829–1839.
150. Klein R, Klein BEK, Moss SE. The Wisconsin Epidemiologic study of Diabetic Retinopathy: II. Prevalence and risk of diabetic retinopathy when age at diagnosis is less than 30 years. Arch Ophthalmol 1984;102:527–532.
151. Seaquist ER, Goetz FC, Rich S, Barbosa J. Familial clustering of diabetic kidney disease. Evidence for genetic susceptibility to diabetic nephropathy. N Engl J Med 1989;320:1161–1165.
152. Borch-Johnsen K, Norgaard K, Hommel E, et al. Is diabetic nephropathy an inherited complication? Kidney Int 1992;41:719–722.
153. Viberti GC, Keen H, Wiseman MJ. Raised arterial pressure in parents of proteinuric insulin-dependent diabetics. Br Med J 1987;295:515–518.
154. Krolewski AS, Canessa H, Warram JH, et al. Predisposition to hypertension and susceptibility to renal disease in insulin-dependent diabetes mellitus. N Engl J Med 1988;318:140–145.
155. Barzilay J, Warram JH, Bak M, Laffel LM, Canessa M, Krolewski AS. Predisposition to hypertension: risk factor for nephropathy and hypertension in IDDM. Kidney Int 1992;41:723–730.
156. Roglic G, Colhoun HM, Stevens LK, Lemkes HH, Manes C, Fuller JH. Parental history of hypertension and parental history of diabetes and microvascular complications in insulin dependent diabetes mellitus: the EURODIAB IDDM complications study. Diabet Med 1998;15:418–426.
157. Viberti G. Why do we invoke genetic susceptibility for diabetic nephropathy. Kidney Int 1999;55:2526–2527.
158. Vardarli I, Baier LJ, Hanson RL, et al. Gene for susceptibility to diabetic nephropathy in type 2 diabetes maps to 18q22.3–33. Kidney Int 2002;62:2176–2183.
159. Bain S, Chowdhury T. Genetics of diabetic nephropathy and microalbuminuria. J Royal Soc Med 2000;93:62–66.
160. Barbosa J, Saner B. Do genetics factors play a role in the pathogenesis of diabetic microangiopathy? Diabetologia 1984;27:487–492.
161. Pyke D, Tattersall R. Diabetic retinopathy in identical twins. Diabetes 1973;22:613–618.
162. Chowdhury TA, Dyer PH, Mijovic CH, Dunger D, Barnett AH, Bain SC. HLA and insulin genes in diabetic nephropathy. Diabetologia 1999;42:1017–1020.
163. Hallab M, Bled F, Ebran JM. Elevated serum angiotensin converting enzyme activity in type 1, insulin dependent diabetic subjects with persistent microalbuminuria. Acta Diabetol 1992;29:82–85.
164. Schmidt S, Schone N, Ritz E. Association of ACE gene polymorphism and diabetic nephropathy? The Diabetic Nephropathy Study Group. Kidney Int 1995;47:1176–1181.
165. van Ittersum FJ, de Man AM, Thijssen S, et al. Genetic polymorphisms of the renin–angiotensin system and complications of insulin-dependent diabetes mellitus. Nephrol Dial Transplant 2000;15:1000–1007.
166. Tarnow L, Cambien F, Rossing P, et al. Lack of relationship between an insertion/deletion polymorphism in the angiotensin I-converting enzyme gene and diabetic nephropathy and proliferative retinopathy in IDDM patients. Diabetes 1995;44:489–494.
167. Doria A, Warram JH, Krolewski AS. Genetic predisposition to diabetic nephropathy. Evidence for a role of the angiotensin I-converting enzyme gene. Diabetes 1994;43:690–695.
168. Tarnow L, Cambien F, Rossing P, et al. Angiotensin-II type 1 receptor gene polymorphism and diabetic microangiopathy. Nephrol Dial Transplant 1996;11:1019–1023.
169. Chowdhury TA, Dyer PH, Kumar S, et al. Lack of association of angiotensin II type 1 receptor gene polymorphism with diabetic nephropathy in insulin-dependent diabetes mellitus. Diabet Med 1997;14:837–840.
170. Parving HH, Jacobsen P, Tarnow L, et al. Effect of deletion polymorphism of angiotensin converting enzyme gene on progression of diabetic nephropathy during inhibition of angiotensin converting enzyme: observational follow up study. Br Med J 1996;313:591–594.
171. Penno G, Chaturvedi N, Talmud PJ, et al. Effect of angiotensin-converting enzyme (ACE) gene polymorphism on progression of renal disease and the influence of ACE inhibition in IDDM patients. Diabetes 1998;47:1507–1511.

172. van Essen GG, Rensma PL, de Zeeuw D, et al. Association between angiotensin-converting-enzyme gene polymorphism and failure of renoprotective therapy. Lancet 1996;347:94–95.
173. Johannesen J, Tarnow L, Parving HH, Nerup J, Pociot F. CCTTT-Repeat polymorphism in the human NOS2-promoter confers low risk of diabetic nephropathy in type 1 diabetic patients. Diabetes Care 2000;23:560–562.
174. Neuberger S, Baba T, Watanabe T. Association of nitric oxide synthase gene polymorphism with an increased risk for progression to diabetic nephropathy in type 2 diabetes. Diabetes 2000;49:500–503.
175. Pociot F, Hansen PM, Karlsen AE, Langdahl BL, Johannesen J, Nerup J. TGF-[beta]1 gene mutations in insulin-dependent diabetes mellitus and diabetic nephropathy. J Am Soc Nephrol 1998;9:2302–2307.
176. Heesom AE, Hibberd ML, Millward A, Demaine AG. Polymorphism in the 5′-end of the aldose reductase gene is strongly associated with the development of diabetic nephropathy in type I diabetes. Diabetes 1997;46:287–291.
177. Dyer PH, Chowdhury TA, Dronsfield MJ, Dunger D, Barnett AH, Bain SC. The 5′-end polymorphism of the aldose reductase gene is not associated with diabetic nephropathy in Caucasian type I diabetic patients. Diabetologia 1999;42:1030.
178. Deckert T, Feldt Rasmussen B, Borch-Johnsen K, Jensen T, Kofoed-Enevoldsen A. Albuminuria reflects widespread vascular damage. The Steno Hypothesis. Diabetologia 1989;32:219–226.
179. Hansen PM, Chowdhury TA, Deckert T, Hellgren A, Bain SC, Pociot F. Genetic variation of the heparan sulphate proteogylcan gene (perlecan gene). Association with albumin excretion in IDDM patients. Diabetes 1997;46:1658–1659.
180. Chowdhury TA, Dyer PH, Kumar S, et al. Association of apolipoprotein e2 allele with diabetic nephropathy in subjects with insulin dependent diabetes mellitus. Diabetes 1998;47:278–281.
181. Hardman TC, Dubrey SW, Leslie DG, Hafiz M, Noble MI, Lant AF. Erythrocyte sodium–lithium countertransport and blood pressure in identical twin pairs discordant for insulin dependent diabetes. Br Med J 1992;305:215–219.
182. Ng LL, Quinn PA, Baker F, Carr SJ. Red cell Na^+/Li^+ countertransport and Na^+/H^+ exchanger isoforms in human proximal tubules. Kidney Int 2000;58:229–235.
183. Trevisan R, Viberti GC. Sodium–hydrogen antiporter: its possible role in the genesis of diabetic nephropathy. Nephrol Dial Transplant 1997;12:643–645.
184. Trevisan R, Li LK, Messent J, et al. Na^+/H^+ antiport activity and cell growth in cultured skin fibroblasts of IDDM patients with nephropathy. Diabetes 1992;41:1239–1246.
185. Ng LL, Davies JE, Siczkowski M, et al. Abnormal sodium–lithium antiporter phenotype and turnover of immortalized lymphoblasts from type 1 diabetic patients with nephropathy. J Clin Invest 1994;93:2750–2757.
186. Koren W, Koldanov R, Pronin VS, et al. Enhanced erythrocyte Na^+/H^+ exchange predicts diabetic nephropathy in patients with IDDM. Diabetologia 1998;41:201–205.
187. Trevisan R, Fioretto P, Barbosa J, Mauer M. Insulin-dependent diabetic sibling pairs are concordant for sodium–hydrogen antiport activity. Kidney Int 1999;55:2383–2389.
188. Fioretto P, Steffes MW, Barbosa J, Rich SS, Miller ME, Mauer M. Is diabetic nephropathy inherited? Studies on glomerular structure in type 1 diabetic sibling pairs. Diabetes 1999;48:865–869.
189. Krolewski AS, Canessa M, Warram JH, et al. Predisposition to hypertension and susceptibility to renal disease in insulin-dependent diabetes mellitus. N Engl J Med 1988;318:140–145.
190. DCCT Collaborative Group. The absence of a glycemic threshold for the development of long-term complications: the perspective of the Diabetes Control and Complications Trial. Diabetes 1996;45:1289–1298.
191. Kasiske BL, Kalil RS, Ma JZ, Liao M, Keane WF. Effect of antihypertensive therapy on the kidney in patients with diabetes: a meta-regression analysis. Ann Intern Med 1993;118:129–138.
192. Ravid M, Lang R, Rachmani R, Lishner M. Long-term renoprotective effect of angiotensin-converting enzyme inhibition in non-insulin-dependent diabetes mellitus: a 7-year follow-up study. Arch Intern Med 1996;156:286–289.
193. Lewis EJ, Hunsicker LG, Bain RP, Rohde RD, Collaborative Study Group. The effect of angiotensin-converting-enzyme inhibition on diabetic nephropathy. N Engl J Med 1993;329:1456–1462.
194. Parving HH, Rossing P, Hommel E, Smidt UM. Angiotensin-converting enzyme inhibition in diabetic nephropathy: ten years' experience. Am J Kidney Dis 1995;26:99–107.
195. Mulec H, Johnsen SA, Bjorck S. Long-term enalapril treatment in diabetic nephropathy. Kidney Int 1994;45(Suppl):S141–S144.

196. Laffel LMB, McGill JB, Gans DJ, North American Microalbuminuria Study Group. The beneficial effect of angiotensin-converting enzyme inhibition with captopril on diabetic nephropathy in normotensive IDDM patients with microalbuminuria. Am J Med 1995;99:497–504.
197. Brenner BM, Cooper ME, de Zeeuw D, et al. Effects of losartan on renal and cardiovascular outcomes in patients with type 2 diabetes and nephropathy. N Eng J Med 2001;345:861–869.
198. Parvirg HH, Lehnert H, Brochner-Mortensen J, et al. The effect of irbesartan on the development of diabetic nephropathy in patients with type 2 diabetes. N Engl J Med 2001;345:870–878.
199. UK Prospective Diabetes Study Group. Efficacy of atenolol and captopril in reducing the risk of macrovascular complications in type 2 diabetes (UKPDS 39) Br Med J 1998;317:713–720.
200. Pedrini MT, Levey AS, Lau J, Chalmers TC, Wang PH. The effect of dietary protein restriction on the progression of diabetic and nondiabetic renal diseases: a meta-analysis. Ann Intern Med 1996;124:627–632.
201. Gin H, Rigalleau V, Aparicio M. Lipids, protein intake, and diabetic nephropathy. Diabetes Metab 2000;26(Suppl 4):45–53.
202. Tonolo G, Ciccarese M, Brizzi P, et al. Reduction of albumin excretion rate in normotensive microalbuminuric type 2 diabetic patients during long-term simvastatin treatment. Diabetes Care 1997;20:1891–1895.
203. Chase HP, Garg SK, Marshall G, et al. Cigarette smoking increases the risk of albuminuria among subjects with type I diabetes. JAMA 1991;265:614–617.
204. Ritz E, Ogata H, Orth SR. Smoking: a factor promoting onset and progression of diabetic nephropathy. Diabetes Metab 2000;26(Suppl 4):54–63.
205. Feldt-Rasmussen B, Mathiesen ER, Jensen T, Lauritzen T, Deckert T. Effect of improved metabolic control on loss of kidney function in type 1 (insulin-dependent) diabetic patients: an update of the Steno studies. Diabetologia 1991;34:164–170.
206. Microalbuminuria Collaborative Study Group, United Kingdom. Intensive therapy and progression to clinical albuminuria in patients with insulin dependent diabetes mellitus and microalbuminuria. Br Med J 1995;311:973–977.
207. Alaveras AEG, Thomas SM, Sagriotos A, Viberti GC. Promoters of progression of diabetic nephropathy: the relative roles of blood glucose and blood pressure control. Nephrol Dial Transplant 1997;12(Suppl 2):71–74.
208. Bos H, Andersen S, Rossing P, et al. Role of patient factors in therapy resistance to antiproteinuric intervention in nondiabetic and diabetic nephropathy. Kidney Int 2000;57(Suppl 75):32–37.
209. ADA Position Statement: Implications of the UKPDS. Diabetes Care 1991;22(Suppl 1):S27–S31.
210. ADA Position Statement: Standards of Care for Patients with Diabetes Mellitus. Diabetes Care 1999;22(Suppl 1):S32–S41.
211. Best JD. O'Neal DN. Diabetic dyslipidaemia: current treatment recommendations. Drugs 2000;59:1101–1111.
212. Stegall MD, Larson TS, Kudva YC, et al. Pancreas transplantation for the prevention of diabetic nephropathy. Mayo Clin Proc 2000;75:49–56.
213. Bohman SO, Tyden G, Wilczek H, et al. Prevention of kidney graft diabetic nephropathy by pancreas transplantation in man. Diabetes 1985;34:306–308.
214. Fioretto P, Steffes MW, Sutherland DER, Goetz FC, Mauer M. Reversal of lesions of diabetic nephropathy after pancreas transplantation. N Engl J Med 1998;339:69–75.
215. Port FK, Wolfe RA, Mauger EA, Berling DP, Jiang K. Comparison of survival probabilities for dialysis patients vs cadaveric renal transplant recipients. JAMA 1993;270:1339–1343.
216. Basadonna G, Matas AJ, Gillingham K, et al. Kidney transplantation in patients with type I diabetes: 26-year experience at the University of Minnesota. Clin Transpl 1992;227–235.
217. Tilney NL. A crisis in transplantation: too much demand for too few organs. Transplant Rev 1998;12:112–120.
218. Gruessner AC, Sutherland DER. Pancreas transplants for United States (US) and non-US cases as reported to the International Pancreas Transplant Registry (IPTR) and to the United Network for Organ Sharing (UNOS). Clin Transpl 1997;45–59.
219. Tyden G, Tollemar J, Bolinder J. Combined pancreas and kidney transplantation improves survival in patients with end-stage diabetic nephropathy. Clin Transplant 2000;14:505–508.
220. Joshi N, Caputo GM, Weitekamp MR, Karchmer AW. Primary care: infections in patients with diabetes mellitus. N Engl J Med 1999;341(25):1906–1912.
221. Ronald A, Ludwig E. Urinary tract infections in adults with diabetes. Int J Antimicrob Agents 2001;17:287–292

222. Patterson JE, Andriole VT. Bacterial urinary tract infections in diabetes. Infect Dis Clin North Am 1995;9:25–51.
223. Geerlings SE, Stolk RP, Camps MJ, et al. Asymptomatic bacteriuria may be considered a complication in women with diabetes. Diabetes Mellitus Women Asymptomatic Bacteriuria Utrecht Study Group. Diabetes Care 2000;23:744–749.
224. Geerlings SE, Stolk RP, Camps MJ, Netten PM, Collet TJ, Hoepelman AI. Risk factors for symptomatic urinary tract infection in women with diabetes. Diabetes Care 2000;23:1737–1741.
225. Lye WC, Chan RKT, Lee EJC, et al. Urinary tract infections in patients with diabetes mellitus. J Infect 1992;24:169–174.
226. Kobayashi T, Ieiri T, Asada M, et al. A case of *Pasteurella multocida* urinary tract infection in non-insulin-dependent diabetes mellitus. J Jpn Diabetes Soc 1997;40:341–346.
227. Jacobs LG, Skidmore EA, Cardoso LA, et al. Bladder irrigation with amphotericin B for treatment of fungal urinary tract infections. Clin Infect Dis 1994;18:313–318.
238. Frye KR, Donovan JM, Drach GW. Torulopsis glabrata urinary infections: a review. J Urol 1988;139:1245–1249.
229. Hoepelmann IM. Urinary tract infection in patients with diabetes mellitus. Int J Antimicrob Agents 1994;4:113–116.
230. Barkai L, Szabo L. Urinary bladder dysfunction in diabetic children with and without subclinical cardiovascular autonomic neuropathy. Eur J Pediatr 1993;152:190–192.
231. Edelstein H, McCabe RE. Perinephric abscess: modern diagnosis and treatment in 47 cases. Medicine 1988;67:118–131.
232. Tahir H, Thomas G, Sheerin N, Bettington H, Pattison JM, Goldsmith DJ. Successful medical treatment of acute bilateral emphysematous pyelonephritis. Am J Kidney Dis 2000;36:1267–1270.
233. Egawa S, Utsunomiya T, Uchida T, et al. Emphysematous pyelonephritis, ureteritis, and cystitis in a diabetic patient. Urol Int 1994;52:178.
234. Sailesh S, Randeva HS, Hillhouse EW, Patel V. Fatal emphysematous pyelonephritis with gas in the spinal extradural space in a patient with diabetes. Diabet Med 2001;18:68–71.
235. Turner FC. Necrosis of the pyramids of one kidney. Trans Pathol Soc London 1939;159:1887–1888.
236. Eknoyan G. Renal papillary necrosis in diabetic patients. In: Mogensen CE, ed. The Kidney and Hypertension in Diabetes Mellitus. Kluwer Academic, Boston, 1996, pp. 461–468.
237. Smitherman KO, Peacock JE Jr. Infectious emergencies in patients with diabetes mellitus. Med Clin North Am 1995;79:53–77.
238. Waldherr R, Ilkenhans C, Ritz E. How frequent is glomerulonephritis in diabetes mellitus type II? Clin Nephrol 1992;37:271–273.
239. Walmsley RS, David DB, Allan RN, et al. Bilateral endogenous *Escherichia coli* endophthalmitis: a devastating complication in an insulin-dependent diabetic. Postgrad Med J 1996;72:361–363.
240. Ogata M, Sato A, Takahashi Y, et al. A case of pyogenic spondylitis associated with diabetes mellitus. J Tokyo Wom Med Coll 1991;61:645–650.
241. Suzuki H, Miyake T. A case of diabetes mellitus associated with iliopsoas abscess caused by MRSA. J Jpn Diabetes Soc 1995;38:965–969.
242. Gluckman SJ, Dinubile MJ. Controversial issues in the management of urinary tract infections. Curr Opin Infect Dis 1992;5:50–56.
243. Wong-Beringer A, Jacobs RA, Guglielmo J. Treatment of funguria. JAMA 1992;20:2780–2785.
244. Leu HS, Huang CT. Clearance of funguria with short-course antifungal regimens: a prospective, randomized, controlled study. Clin Infect Dis 1995;20:1152–1157.
245. Jacobs LG, Skidmore EA, Freeman K, Lipschultz D, Fox N. Oral fluconazole compared with bladder irrigation with amphotericin B for treatment of fungal urinary tract infections in elderly patients. Clin Infect Dis 1996;22:30–35.

24 Diabetic Peripheral and Autonomic Neuropathy

Eva L. Feldman, MD, PhD,
Martin J. Stevens, MD,
and James W. Russell, MD, MS

CONTENTS

INTRODUCTION

Several distinct syndromes affecting the peripheral nervous system occur in diabetic patients. Diabetes affects sensory and motor nerves in a distal to proximal pattern producing diabetic polyneuropathy (DPN). DPN is a common complication of type 1 diabetes and represents the most frequently diagnosed DPN in the Western world *(1–3)*. Diabetes also affects the autonomic nervous system, leading to diabetic autonomic neuropathy (DAN) *(4–6)*. Nerve roots and the lumbosacral plexus are targets of diabetes-mediated injury leading to diabetic polyradiculopathy, also known as diabetic amyotrophy *(5)*. Diabetes can also impair cranial nerve function, especially cranial nerves III and IV, as well as multiple individual peripheral nerves, leading to the syndrome of diabetic mononeuritis multiplex *(5)*. These various forms of DPN are presented in Table 1 and are discussed in more detail in a recent review *(5)*. This chapter will focus on the two most common neuropathic complications, DPN and DAN, with a short discussion of polyradiculopathy and mononeuropathies. The pathogenesis, diagnosis, epidemiology, and treatment of DPN and DAN will be addressed with an emphasis, when possible, on type 1 diabetic patients.

From: *Contemporary Endocrinology: Type 1 Diabetes: Etiology and Treatment*
Edited by: M. A. Sperling © Humana Press Inc., Totowa, NJ

Table 1
Diabetes Mellitus: Potential Peripheral Nervous System Complications

A. Mononeuropathy or mononeuritis multiplex
  1. Isolated cranial or peripheral nerve involvement (e.g., CN III, ulnar, median, femoral, or peroneal)
  2. If confluent, may resemble polyneuropathy
B. Radiculopathy, polyradiculopathy, or plexopathy
  1. Thoracic
  2. Lumbosacral
  3. Diabetic amyotrophy
  4. Lumbosacral plexopathy
C. Autonomic neuropathy
D. Polyneuropathy
  1. Diffuse sensorimotor
  2. Painful sensory

Source: Adapted from Greene DA, Feldman EL, Stevens MJ, Sima AAF, Albers JW, Pfeifer MA. Diabetic neuropathy. In: Porte D Jr, Sherwin RS, Rifkin H, eds. Ellenberg and Rifkin's Diabetes Mellitus, 5th ed. Appleton & Lange, Stamford, CT, 1997, pp. 1009–1076.

PATHOGENESIS OF DPN AND DAN

Although the exact etiology of DPN and DAN is unknown, the Diabetes Control and Complications Trial (DCCT) confirmed the long-held concept that DPN and DAN are the result of sustained hyperglycemia in type 1 patients and not insulin deficiency and/or autoimmunity alone *(7)*. The mechanisms underlying the metabolic and vascular changes that occur in complication-prone tissues in the presence of acute and chronic hyperglycemia are an active area of research. Multiple etiologies have been proposed to underlie the development of DPN and DAN. These include altered polyol metabolism, abnormal lipid or amino acid metabolism, protein glycation (i.e., formation of advanced glycation end productions [AGE]), blunted nitric oxide production, altered neurotrophism, and autoimmune mechanisms *(8)*. More recently, the idea has emerged that these alterations in cellular metabolism occur in concert and as a consequence of glucose-mediated oxidative stress *(8)*.

Early after the induction of diabetes, high glucose leads to cellular oxidative stress and accumulation of reactive oxygen species (ROS). In healthy cells, free-radical scavengers detoxify superoxide ($O_2\cdot^-$) and hydroxyl (·OH) radicals, preventing mitochondrial and cellular injury and maintaining normal cellular function. Superoxide dismutase is a key enzyme in cellular detoxification. Superoxide dismutase detoxifies superoxide ($O_2\cdot^-$) into hydrogen peroxide, which is reduced in the mitochondria by glutathionine. Reduction (detoxification) of hydrogen peroxide generates an oxidized glutathione disulfide. To regenerate glutathione, glutathione disulfide is reduced by NADPH. In diabetes, conversion of glucose to sorbitol is linked to the oxidation of NADPH to $NADP^+$. This leads to *depletion of the NADPH* needed for regenerating glutathione. Thus, early after the induction of diabetes, metabolic defects lead to loss of NADPH that limits the nerve's ability to scavenge ROS, leading to a vicious cycle of oxidative stress, mitochondrial dysfunction, nerve ischemia, and damage. Collectively, these insults allow ROS to injure complication-prone tissues such as nerve. Unchecked, ROS produce (1) lipid, DNA, and protein peroxidation *(9–12)*, (2) ischemia and reduced nerve blood flow *(13–16)*, and (3) cellular apoptosis *(17,18)*.

These alterations in cellular metabolism result in peripheral nervous system damage and the signs and symptoms of DPN. In the diabetic rat, measures of oxidative stress and reduced levels of circulating antioxidants parallel DPN, and blocking oxidative stress in the diabetic animal prevents the development of DPN. Antioxidants restore normal blood flow and sciatic and saphenous nerve conduction velocities in streptozotocin (STZ) diabetic rats *(9,11–14,16)*. Treatment with insulin decreases ROS activity in diabetes and prevents DPN *(10–12)*. Antioxidant therapy may ameliorate DPN and DAN in man. Lipid peroxidation measured as increased serum lipid peroxides is a marker of oxidative stress and is well documented in diabetic patients with microvascular complications *(19)*.

Recent interest has emerged about the role of autoimmunity in the development of DAN complicating type 1 diabetes. Risk factors for the development of DAN include age, glycemic control, duration of diabetes, and the presence of microvascular and macrovascular complications. Interestingly, a correlation has been found to hypoglycemia *(20)*, hyperinsulinemia, and hyperlipidema *(21)*. Mechanistically, many of the pathologic pathways implicated in DPN are thought to be important in the development of DAN *(22)*. A weak correlation has been found between the presence of autoantibodies against the sympathetic nervous system and scintigraphically detected deficits of cardiac sympathetic innervation in type 1 diabetic subjects *(23)*. Complement-fixing autoantibodies to the vagus, sympathetic ganglia, and adrenal medulla have been identified in up to 30% of type 1 diabetic subjects *(24)*. Others have found that antibodies against autonomic nervous system antigens are inconsistently found in diabetes and may be associated with coincidental autoimmunity against other organs *(25)*. In a study of 64 newly diagnosed, and 142 long-duration type 1 diabetic subjects, and 57 nondiabetic neuropathic subjects, sympathetic and parasympathetic ganglia autoantibodies were found much more frequently in diabetic compared to nondiabetic neuropathic subjects. There was, however, only a trend toward an increased number of sympathetic ganglia antibodies in long-duration DAN subjects. These data confirm that autonomic ganglia autoantibodies are common in type 1 diabetes, but their role in the pathogenesis of DAN remains uncertain *(26)*.

EPIDEMIOLOGY OF DPN

Approximately half of all patients with diabetes will develop DPN during their lifetime, with a clinical course and severity that correlates with the length of their diabetes and their level of glycemic control *(2,27–33)*. Although the exact estimates of the frequency of DPN differ among the various studies, this is more likely the result of diagnostic criteria and terminology rather than marked differences in the prevalence of DPN. Although multiple clinical tools are used to diagnose and stage DPN, the specific required clinical criteria remain a source of investigation *(22,34–36)*. Some studies may employ symptoms, whereas another study may use strict changes in nerve physiology. Despite these differences in study design, there are several recurring themes that emerge from the available data; specifically, DPN occurs in both types 1 and 2 diabetes, with an average prevalence of 50% and is strongly associated with diabetes duration and level of glycemic control *(4)*.

Pirart reported a 12% prevalence rate of DPN in a cohort of 4400 newly diagnosed diabetic outpatients *(37)*. After 25 yr of longitudinal care, over 50% of these patients had DPN *(37)*. A cross-sectional multicenter study in the United Kingdom of 6487 type

1 and 2 diabetic patients reported a low prevalence of DPN in young adults (5% in patients 20–29 yr of age), whereas 44% of older patients, 70–79 yr of age, had neuropathy. This study defined DPN with a nine-point symptom score and a simple clinical assessment of sensory function in the foot and ankle reflexes *(30)*. A recent study from Spain reported similar rates of DPN prevalence and severity *(38)*. A screening tool that assessed pinprick and vibration in the great toe and ankle reflexes *(39)* was applied to 8757 types 1 and 2 diabetic patients and 32.3% of patients had scores reflective of diabetic DPN *(27)*. The extent of DPN was then further quantified in the 2033 affected patients using a quantitative neurological examination and nerve conduction studies. The severity of DPN correlated with duration of diabetes and age, with half of the patients having mild to moderate DPN *(27)*. The Rochester Diabetic Neuropathy Study, now over 15 yr old, has reported that 54% of insulin-dependent and 45% of non-insulin-dependent diabetic patients had DPN *(29)*.

There are several studies that report the presence of DPN in either type 1 or type 2 patients, rather than combining the two study populations. At the onset of the DCCT, 39% of 278 healthy type 1 diabetic patients had DPN defined by either an abnormal examination and/or abnormal nerve electrophysiology *(40)*. In the Pittsburgh Epidemiology of Diabetes Complications Study, 18% of type 1 patients aged 18–29 yr had DPN. This prevalence sharply increased 58% in the >30 yr-old group *(41)*. The EURODIAB complications study confirmed the findings that age, duration of diabetes, and glycemic control are strongly associated with DPN. In this study, 28% of the 3250 type 1 patients from 16 European countries had confirmed DPN *(31,42)*. The estimates of DPN in young children with type 1 diabetes vary widely *(43)*, in part the result of the diagnostic criteria employed in individual studies *(44,45)*. Using abnormal nerve conduction studies to define subclinical DPN, individual studies report 29% *(46)*, 57% *(47)*, and 68% *(48)* of type 1 diabetic children were neuropathic, with the majority of abnormalities in the lower limbs *(47)*. The Danish Study Group of Diabetes in Childhood found that 62% of 339 type 1 diabetic patients had DPN, defined by quantitative loss of vibratory sensation. These patients had a median age of 21 yr and a 13-yr median duration of diabetes *(49)*. Similar statistics emerge from three prospective studies of type 2 patients with the reported prevalence of DPN being 22% after 4 yr of diabetes *(50)* and 42% and 49% after 10 *(28)* and 12 yr *(51)*, of diabetes respectively.

Diabetic polyneuropathy is associated with significant patient morbidity and is the leading cause of foot infections, ulcers, and nontraumatic limb amputations *(52–54)*. The national annual direct cost in the United States of diabetic foot ulcers is estimated to be $5 billion, with a loss of patient productivity contributing an additional indirect cost of $400 million *(55)*. Between 1995 and 1996, the average Medicare expenditure for a nondiabetic patient was $5226. In contrast, the cost for a diabetic patient was $15,309 and 25% of this amount was spent on the treatment of foot ulcers *(55)*. On average, one out of every six to seven diabetic patients will require an amputation secondary to DPN *(52)*. Thus, DPN is generally conceded to be an extraordinarily common complication of diabetes, causing significant morbidity and financial burden.

EPIDEMIOLOGY OF DAN

Like DPN, DAN is a common complication of diabetes. DAN may be categorized as subclinical or clinical, dependent on whether the clinical manifestations of autonomic denervation are present. Subclinical autonomic neuropathy does not often occur in isolation and is usually found in association with DPN. It may only be detected by using cardiovascular reflex tests, which assess the integrity of complex reflex arcs or by more direct tests of peripheral sympathetic function.

The prevalence of DAN, however, depends on the diagnostic criteria used together with the reference population to which it is being compared. If, for example, a single abnormality in one autonomic reflex test (i.e., beat-to-beat heart rate variability) is used as the sole criteria, then deficits can be found in many diabetic subjects. If the definition of DAN is defined by an additional abnormality in a different reflex arc, then, clearly, the prevalence will be lower. In general, significant abnormalities of cardiovascular reflex testing can be identified in approx 16–20% of diabetic subjects *(56–62)*. For example, in the EURODIAB complications study and an earlier report *(57)*, abnormalities of heart rate variability (HRV) were detected in approx 19% and 25%, respectively, of subjects. Other studies have estimated the prevalence of abnormalities of both HRV and the Valsalva ratio to be approx 17% *(63)*. In the DCCT, in the primary prevention cohort, the young healthy type 1 diabetics were found to have deficits in beat-to-beat HRV in less than 2% and in the Valsalva ratio of 6%. In subjects with baseline complications, this prevalence was increased to approx 6% for both defects *(64,65)*.

However, symptoms of autonomic dysfunction are distinctly rarer *(60–62)*. There is considerable uncertainty as to whether the development of DAN is more frequent in the patient with type 1 diabetes. Indeed, young women with type 1 diabetes appear to be particularly susceptible to the development of aggressive, early-onset autonomic failure, which may develop in the absence of other chronic complications. This risk appears to be particularly great if there is an associated history of an eating disorder. There does not appear to be an equivalent syndrome in patients with type 2 diabetes.

Standardized tests of autonomic function may demonstrate early abnormalities in parasympathetic cardiac denervation without associated deficits in sympathetic innervation *(66)*. However, conventional reflex measures utilize indirect methods that typically detect early abnormalities in parasympathetic integrity, but are relatively insensitive to sympathetic deficits. In type 2 diabetes, for example, the frequency of parasympathetic DAN has been reported to be 20% at 5 yr and 65% at 10 yr *(67)* and sympathetic DAN 7% at 5 yr and 24% at 10 yr. The prevalence of sympathetic deficits has been re-evaluated with the recent introduction of radiolabeled analogs of norepinephrine, which are actively taken up by the sympathetic nerve terminals of the heart *(68–78)*. These radiolabeled tracers are not substrates for monoamine oxidase in the cytosol and achieve rapid equilibrium across both the neuronal axoplasm and vesicular membranes and, therefore, mark the position of functioning sympathetic nerve terminals. Retention of these tracers within the sympathetic neuron will be abnormal if several different components of neuronal function have been perturbed by diabetes. For example, alterations of neuronal type 1 amine uptake or vesicular storage, as well as complete neuronal loss, may both lead to impaired tracer retention. Quantitative scintigraphic assessment of the pattern of sympathetic innervation of the human heart is possible with either [^{131}I] metaiodobenzylguanidine (MIBG) or [^{11}C] hydroxyephedrine (HED). In cross-sectional studies, deficits of LV [^{123}I] MIBG and [^{11}C] HED retention have been identified in type 1 *(23,79–81)* (plus HED) and type 2 *(82–86)* diabetic subjects with HED *(87–90)* and without *(70,72,73,75,91,92)* abnormalities on cardiovascular reflex testing and have been reported even in newly diagnosed diabetes *(74)*. In type 1 diabetic subjects, abnormalities of [^{11}C] HED retention affecting between 4% and 8% of the left ventricle have been identified in 40% of otherwise healthy subjects without deficits on cardiovascular reflex testing. In the mild DAN subjects, defects were observed only in the distal inferior wall of the left ventricle, whereas in the severe DAN subjects, defects extended to involve the distal and proximal anterolateral and inferior walls. The presence of an abnormal Valsalva ratio or the presence of symptomatic orthostasis *(72,75)* predicted a deficit of left ventricular tracer retention of greater than 40%. The ability of the currently available reflex tests of autonomic function to correctly classify subjects free of DAN (specificity) was 0.86 and their ability to correctly classify those with DAN (sensitivity) was 0.67 *(75)*. Deficits of autonomic innervation have been more widely characterized using MIBG-single photon emission computed tomography (SPECT). This technique has demonstrated widespread abnormalities of myocardial tracer retention, and, indeed, deficits have been reported in metabolically compromised newly diagnosed IDDM subjects that are at least partially correctable by intensive insulin therapy *(88)*. Therefore, these deficits most likely reflect hyperglycemia-induced neuronal dysfunction, which is sensitive to rapidly improved metabolic control and not more advanced neuronal loss. Unfortunately, a clinically useful tracer for the quantitative direct assessment of parasympathetic integrity has not yet been developed and so, currently, the evaluation of this component of autonomic integrity remains dependent upon HRV assessments.

CLINICAL PRESENTATION OF DPN

Diabetic polyneuropathy can be staged as subclinical (class I) and clinical (class II) (*see* Table 2) *(93)*. Patients with subclinical DPN lack clinical signs or symptoms but have peripheral nerve dysfunction measured by nerve conduction studies and/or quantitative sensory testing. Clinical DPN is present in patients with signs and/or symptoms and abnormal nerve conduction studies and/or quantitative sensory testing (*see* Table 2). DPN is not a single entity; it encompasses several distinct syndromes. Each syndrome has an individual pattern, but as they frequently coexist in the same patient, it can be difficult to distinguish distinct syndromes.

The most common subtype of DPN is distal symmetric sensorimotor polyneuropathy, a clinical syndrome with sensory deficits and symptoms that far surpass motor involvement *(36,94)*. In this chapter, the term DPN is synonymous with this form of diabetic neuropathy. Sensory loss begins in the most distal portions of the feet and progresses proximally. Once loss reaches approximately mid-calf, the patient begins to experience sensory loss in the fingertips. This constitutes the classic "stocking-glove" distribution of DPN. In the most advanced cases of this type of DPN, vertical bands of sensory loss occur on the chest as the truncal nerves become affected *(4,95)*.

The specific signs and symptoms a patient experiences depend on the affected classes of nerve fibers. When large-diameter myelinated sensory nerve fibers are lost, a patient experiences loss of vibratory and position sense in a distal to proximal gradient. In severe cases, large myelinated motor fibers are affected, producing a pattern of distal weakness. Frequently, large-fiber loss is asymptomatic and is detected by a health caregiver during a foot exam. The depressed vibratory sensation and position sense is accompanied by diminished or absent Achilles tendon reflexes. In contrast, loss of small thinly or unmyelinated sensory fibers leads to a loss of pain and thermal sensation. When this class of fibers is predominantly involved, a patient often experiences neuropathic pain, dysesthesias, and/or paresthesias *(4,15,96)*. There are patients who experience a loss of both large and small sensory and motor function and who remain

Table 2
Classification and Staging of Diabetic Neuropathy

Class I: Subclinical Neuropathy[a]
- A. Abnormal Electrodiagnostic Tests (EDX)
  - 1. Decreased nerve conduction velocity
  - 2. Decreased amplitude of evoked muscle or nerve action potential
- B. Abnormal Quantitative Sensory Testing (QST)
  - 1. Vibratory/tactile
  - 2. Thermal warming/cooling
  - 3. Other
- C. Abnormal Autonomic Function Tests (AFT)
  - 1. Diminished sinus arrhythmia (beat-to-beat heart rate variation)
  - 2. Diminished sudomotor function
  - 3. Increased pupillary latency

Class II: Clinical Neuropathy
- A. Diffuse Neuropathy
  - 1. Distal symmetric sensorimotor polyneuropathy
    - a. Primarily small-fiber neuropathy
    - b. Primarily large-fiber neuropathy
    - c. Mixed
  - 2. Autonomic neuropathy
    - a. Abnormal pupillary function
    - b. Sudomotor dysfunction
    - c. Genitourinary autonomic neuropathy
      - (1) Bladder dysfunction
      - (2) Sexual dysfunction
    - d. Gastrointestinal autonomic neuropathy
      - (1) Gastric atony
      - (2) Gallbladder atony
      - (3) Diabetic diarrhea
      - (4) Hypoglycemia unawareness (adrenal medullary neuropathy)
    - e. Cardiovascular autonomic neuropathy
    - f. Hypoglycemic unawareness
- B. Focal Neuropathy
  - 1. Mononeuropathy
  - 2. Mononeuropathy multiplex
  - 3. Plexopathy
  - 4. Radiculopathy
  - 5. Cranial neuropathy

[a] Neurological function tests are abnormal, but no neurological symptoms or clinically detectable neurological deficits indicative of a diffuse or focal neuropathy are present. Class I "Subclinical Neuropathy" is further subdivided into Class Ia if an AFT or QST abnormality is present, Class Ib if EDX or AFT and QST abnormalities are present, and Class Ic if an EDX and either AFT or QST abnormalities or both are present.

Source: Adapted from American Diabetes Association. Report and recommendations of the San Antonio conference on diabetic neuropathy. Consensus statement. Diabetes 1988;37:1000–1004.

relatively asymptomatic. These individuals may present with late complications such as ulceration or neuroarthropathy ("Charcot's joints") of the foot *(97)*. The other diffuse form of clinical diabetic neuropathy is DAN, which is discussed in detail in this chapter, because of its high occurrence in type 1 patients. DAN often, but not always, accompanies DPN and can impair virtually any sympathetic or parasympathetic autonomic function *(5,98)*.

There are focal forms of diabetic neuropathy that correspond to dysfunction in the distribution of single or multiple peripheral nerves ("mononeuropathy" and "mononeuropathy multiplex"), cranial nerves, regions of the brachial or lumbosacral plexuses ("plexopathy"), or the nerve roots ("radiculopathy"). Diabetic mononeuropathy multiplex, plexopathy, and radiculopathy are primarily disorders of type 2 diabetes and are rarely seen in type 1 patients. Even in type 2 patients, these focal forms of nerve dysfunction are rare. When they occur, signs and symptoms happen abruptly and are frequently self-limiting *(5)*. "Femoral neuropathy," which actually represents a lumbar polyradiculopathy, is a disorder of older type 2 patients. Patients present with unilateral thigh pain followed by motor weakness and sensory loss at the level of the lumbar plexus or lumbar roots as well as the femoral nerve *(99)*. Thoracic radiculopathies are also a disorder of older type 2 diabetic patients and present as severe bandlike thoracic or abdominal pain. These individuals are often initially thought to have an acute abdomen.

Mononeuropathies are common in both types 1 and 2 diabetes, especially isolated nerve entrapment at the wrist (median mononeuropathy), at the elbow (ulnar mononeuropathy), and at the fibular head (peroneal mononeuropathy) *(100)*. These are similar to the mononeuropathies that occur in nondiabetic patients. Among cranial nerve mononeuropathies, the third cranial nerve is most frequently involved. Patients experience unilateral pain, diplopia, and ptosis, whereas pupillary function remains intact in a syndrome termed "diabetic ophthalmoplegia." Diabetic ophthalmoplegia can occur in the absence of DPN; there are reports of bilateral as well as recurrent diabetic ophthalmoplegia *(101)*.

In summary, distal symmetric polyneuropathy and autonomic neuropathy (DAN) are common, diffuse, and generally progressive disorders, whereas the focal neuropathies are rare, sudden in onset, often self-limited, and occur primarily in older patients with diabetes.

CLINICAL PRESENTATION OF DAN

The symptoms of DAN are often very subtle and insidious in onset and may be unrecognized. Alternatively, because the symptoms of DAN can be so diverse and reproduce the appearance of many other disease processes, the patient may be subjected to extensive diagnostic evaluation without reward. In common with other forms of diabetic neuropathy, DAN is essentially a diagnosis of exclusion. The most prominent clinical signs and symptoms of autonomic involvement complicating diabetes include the gastrointestinal tract system, cardiovascular system, bladder, sex organs, ocular pupil, sweat glands, and adrenal medullary system. The clinical presentations of this multiple-organ involvement are discussed in the following sections.

Gastrointestinal Autonomic Neuropathy

The most common presenting symptom of gastrointestinal autonomic neuropathy is constipation *(102)*. Other gastrointestinal tract problems that may present include gastric atony, gallbladder atony, and "diabetic diarrhea" or incontinence *(102)*. DAN may also present as esophageal motility disorders such as dysphagia, retrosternal pain, and "heartburn." Diabetic diarrhea is characterized by severe nocturnal exacerbations and may be secondary to intestinal motility abnormalities, sphincter malfunction, bacterial overgrowth, pancreatic exocrine insufficiency, and/or bile salt malabsorption. It is characterized by up to 20 bowel movements per day, with stool volumes greater than 300 g/d. Fluid losses from diabetic diarrhea, which may accompany gastric atony, may result in severe dehydration requiring parenteral fluid therapy. Autonomic neuropathy of the gallbladder results in a stasis of bile salts that may "spill over" into the intestines at inappropriate times. Additionally, stasis and cholestrol elevation may predispose to the development of cholelithiasis.

Delayed gastric emptying rate should be considered in type 1 subjects with unusual variability in postprandial blood glucose levels that cannot be explained by variable diet/exercise patterns or insulin dosing. Symptoms may be exacerbated by the use of rapid-acting insulin analogs, which may result in profound early hypoglycemia. These insulins may need to be administered 30–45 min after eating to avoid hypoglycemia. Solid-phase radionuclide gastric emptying studies may be helpful in confirming a diagnosis of delayed gastric emptying, but may be normal in the presence of symptoms *(103)* and, conversely, abnormal in the absence of symptoms. Diagnosis of delayed solid-phase gastric emptying requires assessment of the gastric emptying time by nuclear medicine studies. This involves the ingestion of radiolabeled solid food and determining the time for 50% of this meal to empty from the stomach. This is the most sensitive and specific way to diagnose delayed gastric emptying. Nuclear studies can also measure liquid-phase gastric emptying. An abnormal upper gastrointestinal (GI) series can also be performed (which measures liquid-phase gastric emptying) and usually indicates the existence of abnormal solid-phase gastric emptying. However, a normal liquid-phase gastric emptying does not exclude abnormal solid-phase emptying. More recently, the [^{13}C]octanoic acid breath test has been shown to be an accurate measure of delayed gastric emptying in diabetic subjects, which correlates with the presence of symptoms and DAN and appears not to be affected by the degree of hyperglycemia. Magnetic resonance imaging has been used as a means of diagnosing delayed gastric emptying, which has a high specificity but lower sensitivity compared to standardized radio-opaque marker techniques *(104)*.

Unfortunately, a close correlation between symptoms and objective assessments of abnormal gastric emptying does not always occur. For example, only 60% of patients with symptoms suggestive of delayed gastric emptying have been reported to have diagnostic solid-phase gastric emptying studies *(103)*. The majority of subjects with widely fluctuating blood glucose values have abnormal solid-phase gastric emptying studies but are often free of symptoms of gastric atony. Therefore, symptoms indicative of gastric atony are insensitive and unreliable predictors of prolonged gastric emptying. Patients with symptoms consistent with gastroparesis and unstable diabetes should undergo solid-phase gastric emptying studies.

Genitourinary Autonomic Neuropathy

Involvement of the genitourinary system in DAN may result in syndromes including cystopathy, retrograde ejaculation, erectile impotence and vaginal atrophy, and dyspareunia *(105)*.

Diabetic cystopathy occurs early in the natural history of DAN and often has an insidious onset and progression with few symptoms. The most common findings are inability to sense when the bladder is full, increased postvoid residual volume, decreased contractility of the detrusor that may progress to detrusor areflexia, and decreased urinary flow. There is loss of autonomic afferent innervation that results in infrequent urination. Efferent bladder deficits result in incomplete emptying. These abnormalities typically result in frequent urinary tract infections and overflow incontinence, with dribbling and poor urinary stream. More than two bladder infections per year (especially in men) should alert the physician to possible bladder neuropathy and elicit appropriate diagnostic procedures. A postvoiding residual of greater than 150 cm^3 is consistent with the diagnosis of diabetic cystopathy and should be confirmed by a urological consultation and a cystometrogram. Coexistent urologic conditions (such as bladder outlet obstruction) may be present and should be excluded.

It has been reported that 50% of diabetic men and 30% of diabetic women have some degree of sexual dysfunction *(106,107)*. Retrograde ejaculation reflects loss of coordinated internal sphincter closure with external vesicle sphincter relaxation during ejaculation and may become apparent as cloudy urine postcoitally, reflecting the presence of sperm. Diagnosis of retrograde ejaculation entails documentation of a low sperm count in the ejaculate. Impotence is commonly reported in DAN patients and usually occurs in the presence of other systemic manifestations of either somatic or autonomic neuropathy, but an attempt should be made to exclude other causes, including psychogenic, endocrine, vascular, iatrogenic (secondary to drugs, including antihypertensives, anticholinergics, antidepressants, and narcotics). Hormonal abnormalities should be screened by serum testosterone and prolactin levels. Nocturnal penile tumescence monitoring may be necessary to differentiate organic from psychogenic impotence. A penile/brachial blood pressure index below normal (<0.70) should initiate an angiogram.

In women, decreased vaginal lubrication may result in vaginal wall atrophy and dyspareunia. Diagnosis of female sexual dysfunction requires a directed questioning in order to elicit a history of dyspareunia, the use of vaginal lubricants, or a combination of both.

Abnormal Pupillary Function

Diabetes can result in altered balance of the pupillary parasympathetic and sympathetic tone, with relative sparing of the parasympathetic limb, which results in a smaller than normal pupil at rest *(108–111)*. This tends to make dark adaptation difficult. No specific therapy is required, but patients should be warned to allow more time when entering poorly illuminated areas and take extra caution with night driving.

Peripheral Autonomic Denervation

Peripheral autonomic denervation can have many clinical manifestations and contributes to changes to the skin texture, edema, venous prominence, callus formation, loss of nails, and sweating abnormalities of the feet. Diabetic subjects with neuropathic foot ulceration have been shown to have greater impairment of power spectral analysis of heart-rate variation than subjects with neuropathy without a history of foot ulcers, despite no differences being found for nerve conduction velocities *(112)*. Diabetic autonomic sudomotor dysfunction is commonly manifested by asymptomatic distal anhidrosis of the lower extremities that decreases thermal-regulatory capacity *(113)*. This may produce a symptomatic compensatory increase in truncal and facial sweating. Gustatory sweating *(113)* is an abnormal profuse sweating that accompanies the ingestion of certain foods, particularly cheeses. This abnormality of sudomotor function can be quite irritating and will often be volunteered by the patient. It is highly specific for DAN.

Other clinical manifestations of peripheral autonomic denervation include prominent veins in the lower extremities secondary to arteriovenous shunting *(114,115)*. High peripheral blood flow may play an important role in the development of Charcot arthropathy (neuroarthropathy) by weakening bones in the foot, thereby predisposing to fractures. Peripheral edema is also common in patients with DAN and can become severe and disabling and lead to skin breakdown and sepsis.

Defective Glucose Counterregulation

The autonomic nervous system mediates the counterregulatory response to hypoglycemia in the type 1 diabetic patient. This counterregulatory response to hypoglycemia is comprised of an increase in hepatic glucose production and decreased peripheral glucose uptake. Patients with long-standing diabetes with or without autonomic neuropathy may not have typical autonomic warning signs of hypoglycemia, such as sweating and tachycardia. However, recent studies have not confirmed an etiologic association between DAN and hypoglyemia unawareness. Hypoglycemic unawareness should not be used as a criterion to make the diagnosis of autonomic neuropathy and it may occur in diabetes as a result of improved glycemic control, or recurrent hypoglycemia. The normal glucagon response to hypoglycemia deteriorates within 1–5 yr after the diagnosis of type 1 diabetes. The epinephrine response to hypoglycemia from the adrenal medulla is delayed *(116)*, a defect that tends to worsen with increasing duration of type 1 diabetes. It is greatly diminished or totally lost with diabetes of 14–31 yr duration. Therefore, absent glucagon together with abnormal epinephrine responses to hypoglycemia greatly diminish glucose counterregulation. In subjects with type 1 diabetes, perhaps the major risk associated with severe DAN is severe hypoglycemia *(117)*. This may play a major role in the pathogenesis of sudden cardiac death associated with DAN. In the EURODIAB IDDM Complications Study, compared to subjects who had not experienced a severe hypoglycemic episode in the previous year, subjects who had experienced an episode were older, had a longer duration of diabetes, had better glycemic control, and had abnormal HRV and postual orthostasis with an odds ratio of 1.7 after controlling for other factors. Thus, the risk of severe hypoglycemia appears to be modestly increased in DAN subjects *(118)*. Interestingly, pancreas transplantation improves epinephrine response and normalizes hypoglycemia symptom recognition in subjects with DAN *(119)*, implicating a reversible component in some subjects. Therefore, particular care should be taken in patients with type 1 diabetes complicated by DAN to avoid hypoglycemia, which may result in the rather unsatisfying compromise of less strict metabolic control.

Cardiovascular Autonomic Neuropathy

In general, cardiovascular autonomic neuropathy (CAN) can be divided into three main syndromes: abnormal exercise-induced cardiovascular performance, orthostatic hypotension, and cardiac denervation syndrome.

Abnormal Cardiovascular Exercise Performance

Advanced CAN may result in reduced cardiovascular performance during exercise, which may or may not be noticed by the patient. The cardiovascular response to exercise is impaired in CAN subjects *(120)* in the absence of coronary artery disease or cardiomyopathy. The exercise-induced rise in cardiac output is proportional to the resting vagal tone as measured by resting beat-to-beat HRV. The DAN subject typically has a resting tachycardia and increased cardiac perfusion with impaired maximal vasodilatory response *(75)*. Decreased exercise capacity needs to be considered when prescribing exercise regimens.

Postural Hypotension

Postural hypotension produces weakness, dizziness, visual impairment, and syncope that are at times difficult to distinguish from hypoglycemia or vertigo. Orthostasis results from a combination of both central and peripheral cardiovascular sympathetic denervation and is defined as a fall in systolic blood pressure in excess of 30 mm Hg. It results in part from a failure of vasoconstriction in both splanchnic and peripheral vascular beds. There is a loss of diurnal variation of blood pressure in patients with DAN, with nocturnal supine hypertension, which may also be evident to a lesser degree in healthy diabetic patients *(121)*. Patients with a profound disability resulting from postural hypotension are, fortunately, rare. There can be a great day-to-day variability of orthostatic symptoms, which may be aggravated by insulin therapy *(122)* and food *(123)*. The mechanism of postprandial hypotension in DAN is unclear, but vasodilatory gut peptides have been implicated. A hematocrit should also be checked because anemia can result from erythropoetin (EPO) deficiency secondary to renal denervation, which may greatly exacerbate orthostatic symptoms.

Cardiac Denervation Syndrome

Cardiac denervation at its most extreme results in a fixed heart rate (usually 80–90 beats per minute) that is unresponsive to exercise, stress, or sleep. As mentioned earlier, both parasympathetic and sympathetic activity to the heart declines soon after the development of diabetes. Perhaps there is an initial imbalance in the rate of decline, with a rapid development of reduced parasympathetic tone and a relative increase in sympathetic tone, giving rise to an increase in resting heart rate (at this time, the resting heart rate may be 110–120 beats per minute). With progression of sympathetic deficits, the heart rate progressively slows. Eventually, with advanced involvement of both parasympathetic and sympathetic innervation, a cardiac denervation syndrome exists. Potential consequences of advanced cardiac denervation include abnormal myocardial blood flow regulation, cardiovascular instability during anesthesia, and increased susceptibility to cardiac arrhythmias and sudden death. Afferent autonomic pathways are also involved in the cardiovascular denervation syndrome, which increases the risk for painless ischemic heart disease.

Regional cardiac sympathetic hyperactivity is associated with the development of malignant ventricular arrhythmias, particularly when accompanied by reduced protective parasympathetic tone and myocardial ischemia *(124)*. The highest mortality rates are usually observed in subjects with advanced deficits of cardiovascular sympathetic innervation *(58)*. A recent meta-analysis of diabetic patients concluded that the mortality of DAN-free subjects over 5.5 yr was approx 5%, and this increased to 27% with the development of abnormal cardiovascular reflex tests *(125)*. Other studies agree that 5-yr mortality in subjects with advanced CAN approaches 30% *(59)*. Diabetic patients have increased mortality after myocardial infarction, which is thought to reflect increased susceptibility to arrythmogenic triggers such as CAN. Compared to nondiabetic subjects, patients with type 1 diabetes have a lower incidence of myocardial infarction events in the morning, with an increase observed in the evening. This may reflect decreased morning sympathetic activation in diabetic subjects and impaired evening parasympathetic and fibrinolytic activity *(126,127)*. Considerable interest has centered upon the role of abnormal myocardial electrical activity in arrythmogenesis, including, for example, QT prolongation and altered ventricular repolarization *(128)*. In the EURODIAB Type 1 Complications Study, the prevalence of QT prolongation was 16% overall [11% in men, 21% in women *(129)*]. The potential mechanisms whereby cardiac denervation increases the risks of myocardial instability have begun to be addressed using scintigraphic techniques. The radiotracer [^{123}I]-MIBG has been extensively utilized to explore the contribution of the sympathetic nervous system to enhanced cardiac risk. Decreased inferior and posterior left-ventricular (LV) [^{123}I]-MIBG retention occurs in subjects with silent *(130,131)* or symptomatic *(131)* myocardial ischemia. Abnormal myocardial [^{123}I]-MIBG uptake correlates with altered LV diastolic filling *(79,132)* and electrophysiological defects involving the QT interval *(81)* and QT dispersion *(133)*. Impaired retention of LV [^{123}I]-MIBG in diabetic subjects is also predictive of sudden death *(134)*.

Studies using the sympathetic tracer C-11 HED have shown that abnormalities of left-ventricular sympathetic innervation begin distally in the LV, spread circumferentially and proximally involving anterior, inferior, and lateral ventricular walls, reflecting a proximal–distal progression in the severity of neuropathy *(72)*. Interestingly, despite extensive cardiac denervation, "islands" of proximal myocardial persist that demonstrate a 30% increase of [^{11}C]-HED retention above the same regions in the CAN-free subjects *(88)*. Despite this increase of tracer retention, no appreciable washout of tracer is observed in the proximal segments, consistent with normal regional tone but regional sympathetic hyperinnervation. Distally, [^{11}C]-HED retention is decreased in severe CAN by ~approx 30%, and, thus, dramatic gradient of sympathetic innervation is observed in advanced CAN that may enhance electrical and chemical instability *(75)*. Positron-emission tomography (PET) has been used to explore myocardial blood flow/innervation relationships in type 1 diabetic subjects. Maximal impairment in vasodilatory capacity is found in the "hyperinnervated" proximal myocardial segments *(68)*. Other reports have confirmed that DAN is associated with impaired vasodilation of coronary resistance vessels to sympathetic stimulation that is related to the severity of the sympathetic nerve dysfunction *(135)*. These regions also demonstrate paradoxical reductions of myocardial perfusion on sympathetic stimulation *(136)*, suggesting that this region of the heart may be the focus of instability particularly during exercise, hypoglycemia, or acute myocardial ischemia.

TREATMENT OF DPN

As part of our treatment approach of DPN, we first carefully establish that the neuropathy is the result of diabetes. Table 3 lists the differential diagnoses of sensorimotor polyneuropathies. Importantly, DPN is a symmetric, sensory greater than motor, slowly progressive disorder. Generalized neuropathies that present in an asymmetric pattern with more motor involvement or with an acute course need to be thoroughly investigated by a neurologist.

Once the diagnosis is established, there are three general therapeutic approaches to the treatment of DPN. Preventive management strategies (e.g., education and hygiene) are designed to deal with potential risk. Palliative management strategies are designed to alleviate specific symptoms of DPN (e.g., pain, foot deformities, or ulcers)

Table 3
Differential Diagnosis of Diabetic Neuropathy

I. Distal Symmetric Polyneuropathy
- A. Metabolic
  1. Diabetes mellitus
  2. Uremia
  3. Folic acid/cyanocobalamin deficiency
  4. Hypothyroidism
  5. Acute intermittent porphyria
- B. Toxic
  1. Alcohol
  2. Heavy metals (lead, mercury, arsenic)
  3. Industrial hydrocarbons
  4. Various drugs
- C. Infectious or Inflammatory
  1. Sarcoidosis
  2. Leprosy
  3. Periarteritis nodosa
  4. Other connective-tissue diseases (e.g., systemic lupus erythematosus)
- D. Other
  1. Dysproteinemias and paraproteinemias
  2. Paraneoplastic syndrome
  3. Leukemias and lymphomas
  4. Amyloidosis
  5. Hereditary neuropathies

II. Pains and Paresthesias Without Neurological Deficit
- A. Early small-fiber sensory neuropathy
- B. Psychophysiologic disorder (e.g., severe depression, hysteria)

III. Autonomic Neuropathy Without Somatic Component
- A. Shy–Drager syndrome (progressive autonomic failure)
- B. Diabetic neuropathy with mild somatic involvement
- C. Riley–Day syndrome
- D. Idiopathic orthostatic hypotension

IV. Diffuse Motor Neuropathy Without Sensory Deficit
- A. Guillain–Barré syndrome
- B. Primary myopathies
- C. Myasthenia gravis
- D. Heavy-metal toxicity

V. Femoral Neuropathy (sacral plexopathy)
- A. Degenerative spinal-disk disease (e.g., Paget's disease of the spine)
- B. Intrinsic spinal-cord-mass lesion
- C. Equina cauda lesions
- D. Coagulopathies

VI. Cranial Neuropathy
- A. Carotid aneurysm
- B. Intracranial mass
- C. Elevated intracranial pressure

(continued)

Table 3 *(continued)*

VII. Mononeuropathy Multiplex
  A. Vasculidites
  B. Amyloidosis
  C. Hypothyroidism
  D. Acromegaly
  E. Coagulopathies

Source: Adapted from Greene DA, Feldman EL, Stevens MJ, Sima AAF, Albers JW, Pfeifer MA. Diabetic neuropathy. In: Porte D Jr, Sherwin RS, Rifkin H, eds. Ellenberg and Rifkin's Diabetes Mellitus, 5th ed., 1997, pp. 1009–1076.

Table 4
Drugs Used in the Treatment of Painful Diabetic Neuropathy

1. Nonsteroidal Drugs
   Ibuprofen 600 mg qid
   Sulindac 200 mg bid
2. Antidepressant Drugs
   Amitriptyline 50–150 mg at night
   Nortriptyline 50–150 mg at night
   Imipramine 100 mg qd
   Paroxetine 40 mg qd
   Trazadone 50–150 mg tid
3. Antiepileptic Drugs
   Gabapentin 600–1200 mg tid
   Carbamazipine 200 mg qid
4. Others
   Ultram 50–100 mg bid
   Mexiletine 150–450 mg/qd
   Capsacin 0.075% qid
   Transcutaneous nerve stimulation

Source: Adapted from Greene DA, Feldman EL, Stevens MJ, Sima AAF, Albers JW, Pfeifer MA. Diabetic neuropathy. In: Porte D Jr, Sherwin RS, Rifkin H, eds. Ellenberg and Rifkin's Diabetes Mellitus, 5th ed., 1997, pp. 1009–1076.

(137,138). Definitive therapeutic strategies are targeted against specific pathogenetic components of DPN *(138–140)*. Currently, glycemic control is the only effective definitive therapy *(141)*. The development of future adjunct therapies to prevent and potentially reverse the neurological damage that underlies the clinical manifestations of DPN awaits clearer understanding of the responsible pathogenetic mechanisms *(142)*.

Approximately 20% of patients experience painful DPN. We have recently reviewed our approach to treatment of painful DPN *(143)*. Table 4 lists the agents most commonly used to ameliorate symptoms in painful DPN. Each agent in Table 4 has been tested in a double-blind placebo-controlled trial for its efficacy in the treatment of painful DPN. Our approach is stepwise. If burning and dysesthesias are the prominent complaints, either an antidepressant such as amitriptyline or an antiepileptic, in particular, gabapentin, is begun and slowly titrated to maximum tolerated doses. If pain persists, a second agent is added;

for example, if the patient is on an antidepressant, then an antiepileptic is added. Careful monitoring of side effects, especially excessive drowsiness, is mandatory. If maximal combination therapy is reached, a third agent is added for those patients still incapacitated by pain. The choice of this agent depends on the patient's age; younger patients tolerate the addition of Ultram, whereas older patients may experience intolerable side effects. A pain clinic is needed by a small percentage of patients when this stepwise approach fails.

TREATMENT OF DAN

Intensification of metabolic control, which can retard the development or slow the progression of DAN, should significantly improve the overall prognosis for diabetes. Improved metabolic control has been reported to slow the progression of HRV deficits in type 1 diabetic patients in some studies *(144–146)* but not in others *(147,148)*. As described earlier, in the DCCT, intensive therapy was able to slow the progression and development of abnormal autonomic tests *(65)*. More recent studies have confirmed that strict glycemic control can reverse early deficits of autonomic function in subjects with type 1 diabetes *(78,149)*. More advanced deficits are more resistant. The variability of the reported beneficial effects of good glycemic control on the development or progression of DAN could reflect a number of factors, including inadequacy of glycemic control, insufficient study duration, too advanced DAN, or the insensitivity of the cardiovascular autonomic function tests utilized.

Gastrointestinal Autonomic Neuropathy

Treatment of Gastric Atony

After the diagnosis of gastric atony has been made (usually using a solid-phase gastric emptying study), therapy is directed toward addressing the imbalance of opposing metabolic influences on the stomach, including defective cholinergic and predominant dopaminergic tone. The initial approach comprises intensifying diabetes control, which will facilitate neurogenic stimulation of gastric emptying. The presence of hyperglycemia by itself has been shown to delay gastric emptying of liquids and solids in both diabetic and healthy individuals *(150)*. In general, high-fiber diet should be avoided in these patients because it can delay gastric emptying. Initial pharmacological approaches include the use of the dopamine antagonist metoclopramide (10 mg 1–2 h before meals). This is usually well tolerated but can result in a distressing acute extrapyramidal reaction or, more chronically, can precipitate hyperprolactinemia and galactorrhea. Formerly, myenteric acetylcholine release could be potentiated using cisapride, but this is now only available for intractable gastroparesis under carefully controlled "research" purposes, because of concerns about precipitating arrythmias secondary to QTc prolongation in patients with DAN. The dopamine antagonist domeridone (20 mg qid, 30 min before meals) is also highly effective and is often useful in subjects in whom metoclopramide has failed. However, doperidone is not yet available in the United States and has to be obtained from Canada *(151)*. Erythromycin is also used in the therapy of gastroparesis. It can promote gastric emptying in patients with gastroparesis secondary to autonomic neuropathy *(152)* via stimulation of motilin receptors. In general, oral erythromycin (250 mg qid) tends to be rather disappointing, and it seems to be most effective when used intravenously (3 mg/kg every 8 h) for the control of acute exacerbations. Bethanechol, a parasympathetic agonist (10–30 mg 1–2 h before meals) has also been used infrequently. Again, caution should be used because these drugs in combination may produce extrapyramidal symptoms. Small, frequent, high-caloric liquid-rich meals may also be used in extreme cases. In patients with intractable episodes of vomiting necessitating recurrent hospital admissions, which is often accompanied by considerable weight loss, nourishment may need to be provided by gastrostomy. Bypass surgery has been used as a last resort and can lead to a dramatic remission of symptoms in carefully selected patients.

Diabetic Diarrhea

Diabetic diarrhea more commonly complicates type 1 than type 2 diabetes *(153)*. The therapeutic approach to the management of diabetic diarrhea first involves the exclusion of other etiologies, such as functional bowel syndrome or sprue. A positive hydrogen breath test may indicate bacterial overgrowth secondary to intestinal hypomotility. A coarse of broad-spectrum antibiotics such as tetracycline, ampicillin, or metronidazole may be successful in about half the cases if given at the onset of the attack. If no improvement is observed, then bile salt binders (e.g., cholestyramine) may be tried. Clonidine has also proved to be useful in some cases. Severe, intractable diarrhea may respond to octreotide (100 μg tid, sc), but care must be taken because the associated instability of diabetes control and randomized clinical trials have not yet been performed. When diarrhea is secondary to aberrant hypermotility, loperamide up to 16 mg/d can be helpful *(154)*.

Genitourinary Autonomic Neuropathy

The management of a neurogenic bladder includes regular urinations, with patients instructed to empty the bladder every 4 h even in the absence of the sensation of fullness, which may be coupled with the Crude maneuver. Other maneuvers to increase the force of bladder contraction include the parasympathetic agonist bethanechol (10–30 mg three times a day). An α_1-blocker, such as doxazosin, can help sphincter. Self-catheterization may also be required. In more severe or refractory cases, an internal sphincter resection can enhance bladder emptying. Finally, severe sympathetic efferent neuropathy may require suprapubic catheterization to prevent urinary retention.

Erectile dysfunction (ED) has many potential etiologies (including concurrent medical therapy) and so a careful initial evaluation is important in order to provide a targeted therapeutic approach. The presence of ED should alert the physician to perform a search for other modifiable cardiovascular risk factors, as cardiovascular events are reported to be increased in these subjects *(155)*. Patients with psychogenic impotence should initially receive appropriate counseling before any other therapeutic maneuvers are undertaken *(156)*. Testosterone supplementation should be provided if free-testosterone levels are inadequate. Atherosclerosis with resulting low penile blood flow may require a vascular surgery consultation. In males, therapy can include 50 mg or 100 mg sildenafil *(157)*, a selective inhibitor of cyclic guanosine monophosphate-specific phosphodiesterase type 5 that is effective in about 50–60% of subjects [and must not be given with organic nitrates because hypotension and fatal cardiovascular events can occur *(158)*]. The dose may need to be reduced in patients with renal failure and hepatic dysfunction. The duration of the drug effect is approx 4 h. Other alternatives include the alprostadil urethral suppository MUSE (125–1000 μg), yohimbine, an α_2-adrenergic blocker (5.4 mg tid), use of a suction apparatus, and various prosthetic devices such as semirigid, malleable, inflatable, and self-contained. Thirty milligrams of papaverine plus 1 mg of phentolamine or prostaglandin E (alprostadil, 20 μg) will result in an increase of blood flow into the penis, resulting in tumescence and rigidity. A constricting band must then be applied to the base of the penis, which must be immediately removed after intercourse. Sustained erections in excess of 2 h may require immediate medical therapy with epinephrine to avoid priapism. Retrograde ejaculation, a cause of infertility, has been successfully treated with an antihistamine *(159)*. Treatment for female sexual dysfunction involves recognition, vaginal lubricants, and estrogen creams *(160)*.

Gustatory Sweating

Gustatory sweating can occasionally be the patient's most disabling symptom and a cause of a great deal of social embarrassment. The most effective therapeutic approach is 0.1 mg bid clonidine. Other treatments such as oxybutynin at 5 mg qd may be an alternative, but is probably less successful. Other anticholinergic drugs have been used successfully, but may be less well tolerated than the condition itself.

Orthostatic Hypotension

The first step in the management of orthostatic hypotension is the discontinuation, where possible, of long-acting hypotensive agents that may be contributing to the problem. Occasionally, the patient can be switched to a shorter-acting agent (captopril, e.g.) and the timing of the dose altered in order to minimize daytime orthostatic changes. Other non-neuropathic etiologies such as volume depletion, adrenal insufficiency, anemia, and hypothyroidism should be addressed. Typical initial approaches to the problem include elevating the head of the bed by 30° during the night, instructing the patient to make changes in posture slowly—"stand-in-stages"— and use of body stockings (which have to be at least waist high). The latter often do not meet with much success, however, because of the fact that much of the fluid pooling is not in the lower extremities, but in the splanchnic circulation. Plasma volume expanders such as a high-salt diet or fludrocortisone (up to 0.4 mg/d), which also increases catecholamine sensitivity *(161)*, can be used. The sympathomimetic agent midodrine is useful in the treatment of orthostatic hypotension in nondiabetic patients in doses up to 40 mg/d *(162)*. However, midodrine may be less effective in subjects with severe neuropathy. Care has to be taken, because of the risk of increasing nocturnal supine hypertension. Atrial tachypacing has also been advocated in severe cases, but, in our experience, it may not be helpful. Erythropoetin (5000 U/wk) has been shown to improve orthostasis *(163)* and improve quality of life, particularly in patients who exhibit anemia of autonomic failure, and may work, in part, by directly modulating small-nerve-fiber function in addition to ameliorating the anemia.

Cardiorespiratory Arrest

Type 1 patients with DAN may be particularly susceptible to abnormal ventilatory responses to hypoxia and hypercapnea and obstructive sleep apnea *(164,165)*. This may increase the risk of nocturnal hypoxia and respiratory arrests. Nocturnal sleep studies are important in these subjects, as is a trial of continuous positive airway pressure *(166)*.

SUMMARY

In summary, DPN and DAN represent common, disabling complications of types 1 and 2 diabetes. This chapter has discussed the basic pathogenesis, signs, and symptoms of DPN and DAN, along with known symptomatic treatment. An increased understanding of pathogenesis will lead to improved therapies in the future.

ACKNOWLEDGMENTS

The authors would like to thank Judith Boldt for expert secretarial assistance. This work was supported by the Juvenile Diabetes Research Foundation Center for the Study of Complications in Diabetes (ELF, MJS, JWR) and the National Institutes of Health (RO1 NS38849) (ELF).

REFERENCES

1. Currie CJ, Morgan CL, Peters JR. The epidemiology and cost of inpatient care for peripheral vascular disease, infection, neuropathy, and ulceration in diabetes. Diabetes Care 1998;21:42–48.
2. Morgan CL, Currie CJ, Stott NC, Smithers M, Butler CC, Peters JR. The prevalence of multiple diabetes-related complications. Diabet Med 2000;17:146–151.
3. Martyn CN, Hughes RA. Epidemiology of peripheral neuropathy. J Neurol Neurosurg Psychiatry 1997;62:310–318.
4. Feldman EL, Stevens MJ, Greene DA. Diabetic neuropathy. In: Turtle JR, Kaneko T, Osato S, eds. Diabetes in the New Millennium. The Endocrinology and Diabetes Research Founation of the University of Sydney, Sydney, 1999, pp. 387–402.
5. Windebank AJ, Feldman EL. Diabetes and the nervous system. In: Aminoff MJ, ed. Neurology and General Medicine, 3rd ed. Churchill Livingstone, New York, 2001, pp. 341–364.
6. Feldman EL, Stevens MJ, Russell JW, Greene DA. Diabetic neuropathy. In: Becker KL, ed. Principles and Practice of Endocrinology and Metabolism, 3rd ed. Lippincott Williams & Wilkins, Philadelphia, 2001, pp. 1391–1399.
7. Stevens MJ, Feldman EL, Thomas T, Greene DA. Pathogenesis of diabetic neuropathy. In: Veves A, ed. Clinical Management of Diabetic Neuropathy. Humana, Totowa, NJ, 1998, pp. 13–48.
8. Feldman EL, Windebank AJ. Growth factors and peripheral neuropathy. In: Dyck PJ, Thomas PK, eds. Diabetic Neuropathy, 2nd ed. WB Saunders, Philadelphia, 1998, pp. 377–386.
9. van Dam PS, Bravenboer B. Oxidative stress and antioxidant treatment in diabetic neuropathy. Neurosci Res Commun 1997;21:41–48.
10. Feldman EL, Stevens MJ, Greene DA. Pathogenesis of diabetic neuropathy. Clin Neurosci 1997;4:365–370.
11. Greene DA, Obrosova I, Stevens MJ, Feldman EL. Pathways of glucose-mediated oxidative stress in diabetic neuropathy. In: Packer L, Rosen P, Tritschler HJ, King GL, Azzi A, eds. Antioxidants in Diabetes Management. Marcel Dekker, New York, 2000, pp. 111–119.
12. Greene DA, Stevens MJ, Obrosova I, Feldman EL. Glucose-induced oxidative stress and programmed cell death in diabetic neuropathy. Eur J Pharmacol 1999;375:217–223.
13. Low PA, Nickander KK, Tritschler HJ. The roles of oxidative stress and antioxidant treatment in experimental diabetic neuropathy. Diabetes 1997;46(Suppl 2):S38–S42.
14. Tomlinson DR. Future prevention and treatment of diabetic neuropathy. Diabetes Metab 1998;24(Suppl 3):79–83.
15. Zochodne DW. Diabetic neuropathies: features and mechanisms. Brain Pathol 1999;9:369–391.
16. Cameron NE, Cotter MA. Metabolic and vascular factors in the pathogenesis of diabetic neuropathy. Diabetes 1997;46(Supp 2):S31–S37.
17. Russell JW, Sullivan KA, Windebank AJ, Herrmann DN, Feldman EL. Neurons undergo apoptosis in animal and cell culture models of diabetes. Neurobiol Dis 1999;6:347–363.
18. Anderson KM, Seed T, Ou D, Harris JE. Free radicals and reactive oxygen species in programmed cell death. Med Hypotheses 1999;52:451–463.
19. Androne L, Gavan NA, Veresiu IA, Orasan R. In vivo effect of lipoic acid on lipid peroxidation in patients with diabetic neuropathy. In Vivo 2000;14:327–330.
20. Cohen JA, Jeffers BW, Faldut D, Marcoux M, Schrier RW. Risks for sensorimotor peripheral neuropathy and autonomic neuropathy in non-insulin-dependent diabetes mellitus (NIDDM). Muscle Nerve 1998;21:72–80.

21. Gottsater A, Ahmed M, Fernlund P, Sundkvist G. Autonomic neuropathy in type 2 diabetic patients is associated with hyperinsulinaemia and hypertriglyceridaemia. Diabet Med 1999;16:49–54.
22. Vinik AI, Park TS, Stansberry KB, Pittenger GL. Diabetic neuropathies. Diabetologia 2000;43:957–973.
23. Schnell O, Muhr D, Dresel S, et al. Autoantibodies against sympathetic ganglia and evidence of cardiac sympathetic dysinnervation in newly diagnosed and long-term IDDM patients. Diabetologia 1996;39:970–975.
24. Ejskjaer N, Arif S, Dodds W, et al. Prevalence of autoantibodies to autonomic nervous tissue structures in type 1 diabetes mellitus. Diabet Med 1999;16:544–549.
25. Stroud CR, Heller SR, Ward JD, Hardisty CA, Weetman AP. Analysis of antibodies against components of the autonomic nervous system in diabetes mellitus. Q J Med 1997;90:577–585.
26. Muhr-Becker D, Ziegler AG, Druschky A, et al. Evidence for specific autoimmunity against sympathetic and parasympathetic nervous tissues in type 1 diabetes mellitus and the relation to cardiac autonomic dysfunction. Diabet Med 1998;15:467–472.
27. Fedele D, Comi G, Coscelli C, et al. A multicenter study on the prevalence of diabetic neuropathy in Italy. Diabetes Care 1997;20:836–843.
28. Partanen J, Niskanen L, Lehtinen J, Mervaala E, Siitonen O, Uusitupa M. Natural history of peripheral neuropathy in patients with non-insulin-dependent diabetes mellitus. N Engl J Med 1995;333:89–94.
29. Dyck PJ, Kratz KM, Karnes JL, et al. The prevalence by staged severity of various types of diabetic neuropathy, retinopathy, and nephropathy in a population-based cohort: the Rochester Diabetic Neuropathy Study. Neurology 1993;43:817–824.
30. Young MJ, Boulton AJM, Macleod AF, Williams DRR, Sonksen PH. A multicentre study of the prevalence of diabetic peripheral neuropathy in the United Kingdom hospital clinic population. Diabetologia 1993;36:150–154.
31. Tesfaye S, Stevens LK, Stephenson JM, et al. Prevalence of diabetic peripheral neuropathy and its relation to glycaemic control and potential risk factors: the EURODIAB IDDM Complications Study. Diabetologia 1996;39:1377–1384.
32. Molyneaux LM, Constantino MI, McGill M, Zilkens R, Yue DK. Better glycaemic control and risk reduction of diabetic complications in type 2 diabetes: comparison with the DCCT. Diabetes Res Clin Pract 1998;42:77–83.
33. Klein R, Klein BE, Moss SE. Relation of glycemic control to diabetic microvascular complications in diabetes mellitus. Ann Intern Med 1996;124:90–96.
34. Dyck PJ, O'Brien PC. Quantitative sensation testing in epidemiological and therapeutic studies of peripheral neuropathy. Muscle Nerve 1999;22:659–662.
35. Dyck PJ, Davies JL, Litchy WJ, O'Brien PC. Longitudinal assessment of diabetic polyneuropathy using a composite score in the Rochester Diabetic Neuropathy Study cohort. Neurology 1997;49:229–239.
36. Feldman EL, Stevens MJ, Russell JW, Greene DA. Diabetic neuropathy. In: Taylor S, ed. Current Review of Diabetes. Current Medicine, Inc., Philadelphia, PA,1999, pp. 71–83.
37. Pirart J. Diabetes mellitus and its degenerative complications; a prospective study of 4,400 patients observed between 1947 and 1973. Diabetes Care 1978;1:168–188.
38. Cabezas-Cerrato J. The prevalence of clinical diabetic polyneuropathy in Spain: a study in primary care and hospital clinic groups. Neuropathy Spanish Study Group of the Spanish Diabetes Society (SDS). Diabetologia 1998;41:1263–1269.
39. Feldman EL, Stevens MJ, Thomas PK, Brown MB, Canal N, Greene DA. A practical two-step quantitative clinical and electrophysiological assessment for the diagnosis and staging of diabetic neuropathy. Diabetes Care 1994;17:1281–1289.
40. The DCCT Research Group. Factors in the development of diabetic neuropathy: baseline analysis of neuropathy in the feasibility phase of the Diabetes Control and Complications Trial (DCCT). Diabetes 1988;37:476–481.
41. Maser RE, Steenkiste AR, Dorman JS, et al. Epidemiological correlates of diabetic neuropathy. Report from Pittsburgh Epidemiology of Diabetes Complications Study. Diabetes 1989;38:1456–1461.
42. Toeller M, Buyken AE, Heitkamp G, Berg G, Scherbaum WA. Prevalence of chronic complications, metabolic control and nutritional intake in type 1 diabetes: comparison between different European regions. EURODIAB Complications Study group. Horm Metab Res 1999;31:680–685.
43. Donaghue KC, Silink M. Diabetic neuropathy in childhood. Diabetes Nutr Metab 1999;12:154–160.
44. Torigoe K, Numata O, Yazaki S, et al. Sympathetic skin response in diabetic children: do diabetic children have diabetic neuropathy? Pediatr Int 1999;41:631–636.

45. Karavanaki K, Baum JD. Prevalence of microvascular and neurologic abnormalities in a population of diabetic children. J Pediatr Endocrinol Metab 1999;12:411–422.
46. el Bahri-Ben Mrad F, Gouider R, Fredj M, Ben Becher S, Mrad-Mazigh S, Mrabet A. Childhood diabetic neuropathy: a clinical and electrophysiological study. Funct Neurol 2000;15:35–40.
47. Meh D, Denislic M. Subclinical neuropathy in type I diabetic children. Electroencephalogr Clin Neurophysiol 1998;109:274–280.
48. Bao XH, Wong V, Wang Q, Low LC. Prevalence of peripheral neuropathy with insulin-dependent diabetes mellitus. Pediatr Neurol 1999;20:204–209.
49. Olsen BS, Johannesen J, Sjolie AK, et al. Metabolic control and prevalence of microvascular complications in young Danish patients with type 1 diabetes mellitus. Danish Study Group of Diabetes in Childhood. Diabet Med 1999;16:79–85.
50. Sands ML, Shetterly SM, Franklin GM, Hamman RF. Incidence of distal symmetric (sensory) neuropathy in NIDDM. The San Luis Valley Diabetes Study. Diabetes Care 1997;20:322–329.
51. de Wytt CN, Jackson RV, Hockings GI, Joyner JM, Strakosch CR. Polyneuropathy in Australian outpatients with type II diabetes mellitus. J Diabetes Complic 1999;13:74–78.
52. Frykberg RG. Epidemiology of the diabetic foot: ulcerations and amputations. Adv Wound Care 1999;12:139–141.
53. Resnick HE, Valsania P, Phillips CL. Diabetes mellitus and nontraumatic lower extremity amputation in black and white Americans: the National Health and Nutrition Examination Survey Epidemiologic Follow-up Study, 1971–1992. Arch Intern Med 1999;159:2470–2475.
54. Thomas PK. Diabetic peripheral neuropathies: their cost to patient and society and the value of knowledge of risk factors for development of interventions. Eur Neurol 1999;41(Suppl 1):35–43.
55. Bloomgarden ZT. American Diabetes Association Annual Meeting, 1999: nephropathy and neuropathy. Diabetes Care 2000;23:549–556.
56. Hilsted J, Jeensen SB. A simple test for autonomic neuropathy in juvenile diabetics. Acta Med Scand 1979;205:385–387.
57. Dryberg T, Benn J, Christiansen J, Hilsted J, Nerup J. Prevalence of diabetic autonomic neuropathy measured by simple bedside tests. Diabetologia 1981;20:190–194.
58. Ewing DJ, Martyn CN, Young RJ, Clarke BF. The value of cardiovascular autonomic function tests: 10 years experience in diabetes. Diabetes Care 1985;8:491–498.
59. Kennedy WR, Navarro X, Sakuta M, Mandell H, Knox CK, Sutherland DE. Physiological and clinical correlates of cardiorespiratory reflexes in diabetes mellitus. Diabetes Care 1989;12:399–408.
60. Canal N, Comi G, Saibene V, Musch B, Pozza G. The relationship between peripheral and autonomic neuropathy in insulin-dependent diabetes: a clinical and instrumental evaluation. In: Canal N, Pozza G, eds. Peripheral Neuropathies. Elsevier, Amsterdam, 1978, pp. 247–255.
61. Ewing DJ, Campbell IW, Clarke BF. Assessment of cardiovascular effects in diabetic autonomic neuropathy and prognostic implications. Ann Intern Med 1980;92:308–311.
62. Young RJ, Ewing DJ, Clarke BF. Nerve function and metabolic control in teenage diabetics. Diabetes 1983;32:142–147.
63. Neil HA, Thompson AV, John S, McCarthy ST, Mann JI. Diabetic autonomic neuropathy: the prevalence of impaired heart rate variability in a geographically defined population. Diabet Med 1989;6:20–24.
64. The Diabetes Control and Complications Trial Research Group. The effect of intensive diabetes therapy on the development and progression of neuropathy. Ann Intern Med 1995;122:561–568.
65. The Diabetes Control and Complications Trial Research Group. The effect of intensive diabetes therapy on measures of autonomic nervous system function in the Diabetes Control and Complications Trial (DCCT). Diabetologia 1998;41:416–423.
66. Wieling W, Borst C, van Dongen T, et al. Relationship between impaired parasympathetic and sympathetic cardiovascular control in diabetes mellitus. Diabetologia 1983;24:422–427.
67. Toyry JP, Niskanen LK, Mantysaari MJ, Lansimies EA, Uusitupa MIJ. Occurrence, predictors and clinical significance of autonomic neuropathy in NIDDM. Diabetes 1996;45:308–315.
68. Stevens MJ, Dayanikli F, Raffel DM, et al. Scintigraphic assessment of regionalized defects in myocardial sympathetic innervation and blood flow regulation in diabetic patients with autonomic neuropathy. J Am Coll Cardiol 1998;31:1575–1584.
69. Mantysaari M, Kuikka J, Mustonen J, et al. Noninvasive detection of cardiac sympathetic nervous dysfunction in diabetic patients using [^{123}I] metaiodobenzylguanidine. Diabetes 1992;41:1069–1075.
70. Kreiner G, Woltzt M, Fasching P. Myocardial *m*-[^{123}I] iodobenzylguanidine scintigraphy for the assessment of adrenergic cardiac innervation in patients with IDDM. Diabetes 1995;44:543–549.

71. Langer A, Freeman ME, Josse RG, Armstrong PW. Metaiodobenzylguanidine imaging in diabetes mellitus: assessment of cardiac sympathetic denervation and its relation to autonomic dysfunction and silent myocardial ischemia. J Am Coll Cardiol 1995;25:610–618.
72. Allman KC, Stevens MJ, Wieland DM, et al. Noninvasive assessment of cardiac diabetic neuropathy by carbon-11 hydroxyephedrine and positron emission tomography. J Am Coll Cardiol 1993;22:1425–1432.
73. Schnell O, Kirsch C-M, Stemplinger J. Scintigraphic evidence for cardiac sympathetic dysinnervation in long-term IDDM patients with and without ECG-based autonomic neuropathy. Diabetologia 1995;38:1345–1352.
74. Schnell O, Muhr D, Weiss M, Dresel S, Haslbeck M, Standl E. Reduced myocardial 123I-metaiodobenzylguanidine uptake in newly diagnosed IDDM patients. Diabetes 1996;45:801–805.
75. Stevens MJ, Raffel DM, Allman KC, et al. Cardiac sympathetic dysinnervation in diabetes: implications for enhanced cardiovascular risk. Circulation 1998;98:961–968.
76. Ziegler D, Weise F, Langen KJ, et al. Effect of glycaemic control on myocardial sympathetic innervation assessed by [123I]metaiodobenzylguanidine scintigraphy: a 4-year prospective study in IDDM patients. Diabetologia 1998;41:443–451.
77. Schnell O, Muhr D, Dresel S, Weiss M, Haslbeck M, Standl E. Partial restoration of scintigraphically assessed cardiac sympathetic denervation in newly diagnosed patients with insulin-dependent (type 1) diabetes mellitus at one-year follow-up. Diabet Med 1997;14:57–62.
78. Stevens MJ, Raffel DM, Allman KC, Schwaiger M, Wieland DM. Regression and progression of cardiac sympathetic dysinnervation in diabetic patients with autonomic neuropathy. Metabolism 1999;48:92–101.
79. Kreiner G, Wolzt M, Fasching P, et al. Myocardial *m*-[123I]iodobenzylguanidine scintigraphy for the assessment of adrenergic cardiac innervation in patients with IDDM. Comparison with cardiovascular reflex tests and relationship to left ventricular function. Diabetes 1995;44:543–549.
80. Schnell O, Kirsch CM, Stemplinger J, Haslbeck M, Standl E. Scintigraphic evidence for cardiac sympathetic dysinnervation in long-term IDDM patients with and without ECG-based autonomic neuropathy. Diabetologia 1995;38:1345–1352.
81. Langen KJ, Ziegler D, Weise F, et al. Evaluation of QT interval length, QT dispersion and myocardial *m*-iodobenzylguanidine uptake in insulin-dependent diabetic patients with and without autonomic neuropathy. Clin Sci (Colch) 1997;93:325–333.
82. Hattori N, Tamaki N, Hayashi T, et al. Regional abnormality of iodine-123-MIBG in diabetic hearts. J Nucl Med 1996;37:1985–1990.
83. Turpeinen AK, Vanninen E, Kuikka JT, Uusitupa MI. Demonstration of regional sympathetic denervation of the heart in diabetes. Comparison between patients with NIDDM and IDDM. Diabetes Care 1996;19:1083–1090.
84. Shimabukuro M, Chibana T, Yoshida H, Nagamine F, Komiya I, Takasu N. Increased QT dispersion and cardiac adrenergic dysinnervation in diabetic patients with autonomic neuropathy. Am J Cardiol 1996;78:1057–1059.
85. Murata K, Sumida Y, Murashima S, et al. A novel method for the assessment of autonomic neuropathy in type 2 diabetic patients: a comparative evaluation of 123I-MIBG myocardial scintigraphy and power spectral analysis of heart rate variability. Diabet Med 1996;13:266–272.
86. Freeman MR, Newman D, Dorian P, Barr A, Langer A. Relation of direct assessment of cardiac autonomic function with metaiodobenzylguanidine imaging to heart rate variability in diabetes mellitus. Am J Cardiol 1997;80:247–250.
87. Mantysaari M, Kuikka J, Mustonen J, et al. Noninvasive detection of cardiac sympathetic nervous dysfunction in diabetic patients using [123I]metaiodobenzylguanidine. Diabetes 1992;41:1069–1075.
88. Mantysaari M, Kuikka J, Mustonen J, et al. Measurement of myocardial accumulation of 123I-metaiodobenzylguanidine for studying cardiac autonomic neuropathy in diabetes mellitus. Clin Auton Res 1996;6:163–169.
89. Langer A, Freeman MR, Josse RG, Armstrong PW. Metaiodobenzylguanidine imaging in diabetes mellitus: assessment of cardiac sympathetic denervation and its relation to autonomic dysfunction and silent myocardial ischemia. J Am Coll Cardiol 1995;25:610–618.
90. Wei K, Dorian P, Newman D, Langer A. Association between QT dispersion and autonomic dysfunction in patients with diabetes mellitus. J Am Coll Cardiol 1995;26:859–863.
91. Kim SJ, Lee JD, Ryu YH, et al. Evaluation of cardiac sympathetic neuronal integrity in diabetic patients using iodine-123 metaiodobenzylguanidine. Eur J Nucl Med 1996;23:401–406.

92. Claus D, Feistel H, Brunholzl C, Platsch G, Neundorfer B, Wolf F. Investigation of parasympathetic and sympathetic cardiac innervation in diabetic neuropathy: heart rate variation versus meta-iodo-benzylguanidine measured by single photon emission computed tomography. Clin Auton Res 1994;4:117–123.
93. Greene DA, Feldman EL, Stevens MJ, Sima AAF, Albers JW, Pfeifer MA. Diabetic Neuropathy. In: Porte Jr D, Sherwin R, eds. Diabetes Mellitus, 5th ed. Appleton & Lange, East Norwalk, CT, 1997, pp. 1009–1076.
94. Boulton AJ, Malik RA. Diabetic neuropathy. Med Clin North Am 1998;82:909–929.
95. Dyck PJB, Dyck PJ. Diabetic polyneuropathy. In: Dyck PJ, Thomas PK, eds. Diabetic Neuropathy, 2nd ed. WB Saunders, Philadelphia, 1999, pp. 255–278.
96. Russell J, Karnes J, Dyck P. Sural nerve myelinated fiber density differences associated with meaningful changes in clinical and electrophysiological measurements. J Neurol Sci 1996;135:114–117.
97. Fabrin J, Larsen K, Holstein PE. Long-term follow-up in diabetic Charcot feet with spontaneous onset. Diabetes Care 2000;23:796–800.
98. Freeman R. Diabetic autonomic neuropathy: an overview. In: Veves A, ed. Clinical Management of Diabetic Neuropathy. Humana, Totowa, NJ 1998, pp. 181–208.
99. Said G, Thomas PK. Proximal diabetic neuropathy. In: Dyck PJ, Thomas PK, eds. Diabetic Neuropathy, 2nd ed. WB Saunders, Philadelphia, 1999, pp. 474–480.
100. Wilbourn AJ. Diabetic entrapment and compression neuropathies. In: Dyck PJ, Thomas PK, eds. Diabetic Neuropathy, 2nd ed. WB Saunders, Philadelphia, 1999, pp. 481–508.
101. Smith BE. Cranial neuropathy in diabetes mellitus. In: Dyck PJ, Thomas PK, eds. Diabetic Neuropathy, 2nd ed. WB Saunders, Philadelphia, 1999, pp. 457–467.
102. Feldman M, Schiller LR. Disorders of gastrointestinal motility associated with diabetes mellitus. Ann Intern Med 1983;98:378–384.
103. Pfeifer MA. Diabetic neuropathy can affect the physician's ability to treat the diabetic patient. J KY Med Assoc 1986;84:101–103.
104. Lehmann R, Borovicka J, Kunz P, et al. Evaluation of delayed gastric emptying in diabetic patients with autonomic neuropathy by a new magnetic resonance imaging technique and radio-opaque markers. Diabetes Care 1996;19:1075–1082.
105. Kaplan SA, Blaivas JG. Diabetic cystopathy. J Diabet Complic 1988;2:133–139.
106. Ellenberg M. Sexual function in diabetic patients. Ann Intern Med 1980;92:331–333.
107. Schiavi RC, Hogan B. Sexual problems in diabetes mellitus: psychological aspects. Diabetes Care 1979;2:9–17.
108. Smith SE, Smith SA, Brown PM, Fox C, Sonksen PH. Pupillary signs in diabetic autonomic neuropathy. Br Med J 1978;2:924–927.
109. Hreidarsson AB. Pupil motility in long-term diabetes. Diabetologia 1979;17:145–150.
110. Pfeifer MA, Cook D, Brodsky J, et al. Quantitative evaluation of sympathetic and parasympathetic control of iris function. Diabetes Care 1982;5:518–528.
111. Pfeifer MA, Weinberg CR, Cook DL, et al. Autonomic neural dysfunction in recently diagnosed diabetic subjects. Diabetes Care 1984;7:447–453.
112. Aso Y, Fujiwara Y, Inukai T, Takemura Y. Power spectral analysis of heart rate variation in diabetic patients with neuropathic foot ulceration. Diabetes Care 1998;21:1173–1177.
113. Thomas PK, Eliasson S. Peripheral Neuropathy. WB Saunders, Philadelphia, 1975.
114. Edmonds ME, Archer AG, Watkins PJ. Ephedrine: a new treatment for diabetic neuropathic oedema. Lancet 1983;1:548–551.
115. Edmonds ME, Roberts VC, Watkins PJ. Blood flow in the diabetic neuropathic foot. Diabetologia 1982;22:9–15.
116. Amiel SA, Tamborlane WV, Simonson DC, Sherwin RS. Defective glucose counterregulation after strict glycemic control of insulin-dependent diabetes mellitus. N Engl J Med 1987;316:1376–1383.
117. Meyer C, Grossmann R, Mitrakou A, et al. Effects of autonomic neuropathy on counterregulation and awareness of hypoglycemia in type 1 diabetic patients. Diabetes Care 1998;21:1960–1966.
118. Stephenson JM, Kempler P, Perin PC, Fuller JH. Is autonomic neuropathy a risk factor for severe hypoglycaemia? The EURODIAB IDDM Complications Study. Diabetologia 1996;39:1372–1376.
119. Kendall DM, Rooney DP, Smets YF, Salazar BL, Robertson RP. Pancreas transplantation restores epinephrine response and symptom recognition during hypoglycemia in patients with long-standing type I diabetes and autonomic neuropathy. Diabetes 1997;46:249–257.
120. Hilsted J. Pathophysiology in diabetic autonomic neuropathy: cardiovascular, hormonal, and metabolic studies. Diabetes 1982;31:730–737.

121. Hornung RS, Mahler RF, Raftery EB. Ambulatory blood pressure and heart rate in diabetic patients: an assessment of autonomic function. Diabet Med 1989;6:579–585.
122. Page MM, Watkins PJ. Provocation of postural hypotension by insulin in diabetic autonomic neuropathy. Diabetes 1976;25:90–95.
123. Stevens MJ, Edmonds ME, Foster AVM, Watkins PJ. Selective neuropathy and preserved vascular responses in the diabetic Charcot foot. Diabetologia 1992;35:148–154.
124. Willich SN, Maclure M, Mittleman M, Arntz HR, Muller JE. Sudden cardiac death. Support for a role of triggering in causation. Circulation 1993;87:1442–1450.
125. Ziegler D. Cardiovascular autonomic neuropathy: clinical manifestations and measurement. Diabetes Rev 1999;7:342–357.
126. ISIS-2 (Second International Study of Infarct Survival) Collaborative Group. Morning peak in the incidence of myocardial infarction: experience in the ISIS-2 trial. Eur Heart J 1992;13:594–598.
127. Aronson D, Weinrauch LA, D'Elia JA, Tofler GH, Burger AJ. Circadian patterns of heart rate variability, fibrinolytic activity, and hemostatic factors in type I diabetes mellitus with cardiac autonomic neuropathy. Am J Cardiol 1999;84:449–453.
128. Sawicki PT, Kiwitt S, Bender R, Berger M. The value of QT interval dispersion for identification of total mortality risk in non-insulin-dependent diabetes mellitus. J Intern Med 1998;243:49–56.
129. Veglio M, Borra M, Stevens LK, Fuller JH, Perin PC. The relation between QTc interval prolongation and diabetic complications. The EURODIAB IDDM Complication Study Group. Diabetologia 1999;42:68–75.
130. Matsuo S, Takahashi M, Nakamura Y, Kinoshita M. Evaluation of cardiac sympathetic innervation with iodine-123-metaiodobenzylguanidine imaging in silent myocardial ischemia. J Nucl Med 1996;37:712–717.
131. Koistinen MJ, Airaksinen KE, Huikuri HV, et al. No difference in cardiac innervation of diabetic patients with painful and asymptomatic coronary artery disease. Diabetes Care 1996;19:231–233.
132. Mustonen J, Mantysaari M, Kuikka J, et al. Decreased myocardial ^{123}I-metaiodobenzylguanidine uptake is associated with disturbed left ventricular diastolic filling in diabetes. Am Heart J 1992;123:804–805.
133. Shimabukuro M, Chibana T, Yoshida H, Nagamine F, Komiya I, Takasu N. Increased QT dispersion and cardiac adrenergic dysinnervation in diabetic patients with autonomic neuropathy. Am J Cardiol 1996;78:1057–1059.
134. Kahn JK, Sisson JC, Vinik AI. Prediction of sudden cardiac death in diabetic autonomic neuropathy. J Nucl Med 1988;29:1605–1606.
135. Di Carli MF, Bianco-Batlles D, Landa ME, et al. Effects of autonomic neuropathy on coronary blood flow in patients with diabetes mellitus. Circulation 1999;100:813–819.
136. Stevens MJ. New imaging techniques for cardiovascular autonomic neuropathy: a window on the heart. Diabetes Technol Ther 2001;3:9–22.
137. Levin ME. Foot lesions in patients with diabetes mellitus. Endocrinol Metab Clin North Am 1996;25:447–462.
138. Benotmane A, Mohammedi F, Ayad F, Kadi K, Azzouz A. Diabetic foot lesions: etiologic and prognostic factors. Diabetes Metab 2000;26:113–117.
139. Litzelman DK, Marriott DJ, Vinicor F. Independent physiological predictors of foot lesions in patients with NIDDM. Diabetes Care 1997;20:1273–1278.
140. Dyck PJ, Davies JL, Wilson DM, Service FJ, Melton LJ, O'Brien PC. Risk factors for severity of diabetic polyneuropathy: intensive longitudinal assessment of the Rochester Diabetic Neuropathy Study cohort. Diabetes Care 1999;22:1479–1486.
141. Greene DA, Stevens MJ, Feldman EL. Glycemic control. In: Dyck PJ, Thomas PK, eds. Diabetic Neuropathy, 2nd ed. WB Saunders, Philadelphia, 1998, pp. 297–315.
142. Greene DA, Stevens MJ, Feldman EL. Diabetic neuropathy: scope of the syndrome. Am J Med 1999;107(2B):2S–8S.
143. Simmons Z, Feldman EL. The pharmacologic treatment of painful diabetic neuropathy. Clin Diabetes 2000;18:116–118.
144. The Diabetes Control and Complications Trial Research Group. The effect of intensive treatment of diabetes on the development and progression of long-term complications in insulin-dependent diabetes mellitus. N Engl J Med 1993;329:977–986.
145. Diabetes Control and Complications Trial (DCCT) Research Group. Effect of intensive diabetes treatment on nerve conduction in the diabetes control and complications trial. Ann Neurol 1995;38:869–880.

146. Jakobsen J, Christiansen JS, Kristoffersen I, et al. Autonomic and somatosensory nerve function after 2 years of continuous subcutaneous insulin infusion in type I diabetes. Diabetes 1988;37:452–455.
147. Lauritzen T, Frost-Larsen K, Larsen HW, Deckert T. Two-year experience with continuous subcutaneous insulin infusion in relation to retinopathy and neuropathy. Diabetes 1985;34(Suppl 3):74–79.
148. Ziegler D, Dannehl K, Wiefels K, Gries FA. Differential effects of near-normoglycaemia for 4 years on somatic nerve dysfunction and heart rate variation in type I diabetic patients. Diabet Med 1992;9:622–629.
149. Burger AJ, Weinrauch LA, D'Elia JA, Aronson D. Effect of glycemic control on heart rate variability in type I diabetic patients with cardiac autonomic neuropathy. Am J Cardiol 1999;84:687–691.
150. Rayner CK, Samsom M, Jones KL, Horowitz M. Relationships of upper gastrointestinal motor and sensory function with glycemic control. Diabetes Care 2001;24:371–381.
151. McLeod JG, Tuck RR. Disorders of the autonomic nervous system: Part 2. Investigation and treatment. Ann Neurol 1987;21:519–529.
152. Janssens J, Peeters TL, Vantrappen G. Improvement of gastric emptying in diabetic gastroparesis by erythromycin. N Engl J Med 1990;322:1028–1031.
153. Lysy J, Israeli E, Goldin E. The prevalence of chronic diarrhea among diabetic patients. Am J Gastroenterol 1999;94:2165–2170.
154. Nakabayashi H, Fujii S, Miwa U, Seta T, Takeda R. Marked improvement of diabetic diarrhea with the somatostatin analogue octreotide. Arch Intern Med 1994;154:1863–1867.
155. Vinik A, Erbas T, Stansberry K. Gastrointestinal, genitourinary, and neurovascular disturbances in diabetes. Diabetes Rev 1999;7:358–378.
156. Schiavi RC. Psychological treatment of erectile disorders in diabetic patients. Ann Intern Med 1980;92:337–339.
157. Sildenafil Study Group. Oral sildenafil in the treatment of erectile dysfunction. N Engl J Med 1998;338:1397–1404.
158. Rendell MS, Rajfer J, Wicker PA, Smith MD. Sildenafil for treatment of erectile dysfunction in men with diabetes: a randomized controlled trial. Sildenafil Diabetes Study Group. JAMA 1999;281:421–426.
159. Andaloro VAJ, Dube A. Treatment of retrograde ejaculation with brompheniramine. Urology 1975;5:520–522.
160. Enzlin P, Mathieu C, Vanderschueren D, Demyttenaere K. Diabetes mellitus and female sexuality: a review of 25 years' research. Diabet Med 1998;15:809–815.
161. Chobanian AV, Volicer L, Tifft CP, Gavras H, Liang CS, Faxon D. Mineralocorticoid-induced hypertension in patients with orthostatic hypotension. N Engl J Med 1979;301:68–73.
162. Kaufmann H, Brannan T, Krakoff L, Yahr MD, Mandeli J. Treatment of orthostatic hypotension with a peripheral alpha adrenergic agonist (midodrine). Neurology 1988;38:951–956.
163. Hoeldtke RD, Streeten DH. Treatment of orthostatic hypotension with erythropoietin. N Engl J Med 1993;329:611–615.
164. Sobotka PA, Liss HP, Vinik AI. Impaired hypoxic ventilatory drive in diabetic patients with autonomic neuropathy. J Clin Endocrinol Metab 1986;62:658–663.
165. Ficker JH, Dertinger SH, Siegfried W, et al. Obstructive sleep apnoea and diabetes mellitus: the role of cardiovascular autonomic neuropathy. Eur Respir J 1998;11:14–19.
166. Veale D, Chailleux E, Hoorelbeke-Ramon A, et al. Mortality of sleep apnoea patients treated by nasal continuous positive airway pressure registered in the ANTADIR observatory. Association Nationale pour le Traitement A Domicile de l'Insuffisance Respiratoire chronique. Eur Respir J 2000;15:326–331.

the muscles of the lower leg. Normally, innervation of the small intrinsic muscles of the foot keep the bones and tendons in proper alignment. Without the correct alignment, the toes are pulled up and do not touch the ground when walking. This is known as a claw deformity. The change in the position of the toes shifts the metatarsal heads toward the plantar surface. This is a common site of ulceration in diabetic patients, especially the areas beneath the first and fifth metatarsal heads. As the disease progresses, there is collapse of the midfoot with loss of the plantar arch. This, in turn, results in further deformity of the foot, and, ultimately, a rocker-bottom deformity. The sensory neuropathy causes the foot to be insensate with loss of protective sensory function.

A foot ulcer commonly begins as a minor wound, usually traumatic in origin. The abnormal shape of the foot leads to the development of pressure points that cannot be felt by the patient. The patient continues to walk on his/her foot until an ulcer occurs. Improperly fitting shoes are a common cause of foot ulcer. Wounds also occur from trauma and foreign bodies from walking barefoot, improper nail trimming, and burns from hot bath water. The autonomic neuropathy results in decreased sweating with cracking of the skin. The cracks become portals of entry for bacteria, resulting in infection. The autonomic neuropathy also leads to opening of arteriovenous shunts, which redirect blood flow away from the nutrient capillaries of the skin *(7)*.

Diabetic patients also develop foot wounds because of peripheral vascular disease. The accepted risk factors for atherosclerosis include diabetes, smoking, hyperlipidemia, and hypertension. Diabetes is a risk factor for atherosclerosis; however, the atherosclerotic process is the same in patients whether or not they have diabetes *(8)*. There are some differences, however. Diabetic patients develop atherosclerosis at a younger age and the disease progresses more rapidly in diabetic patients. The pattern of occlusion is also different.

The atherosclerosis in these patients is commonly in the tibial arteries. Patients often have a palpable popliteal pulse but none in the foot. It was once thought that diabetic patients had so-called "small-vessel disease," with occlusion of very small arteries, but that is not true. Minor trauma leads to wounds that do not heal. These wounds commonly become infected. When treated with antibiotics, the treatment may be ineffective, as there is inadequate blood supply to carry the antibiotics to the foot to the site of infection. Uncontrolled infection and gangrene then necessitate amputation. Obviously, it is better to prevent wounds with good foot care (*see* Table 1).

Most wounds of the foot in patients with diabetes occur in the forefoot. Wounds on the plantar surface commonly are caused by inadequate protection while walking. On the other hand, wounds on the dorsum of the foot commonly occur from rubbing on an improperly fitting shoe. It is of interest to note that the distribution of forefoot ulcers is equal on the dorsal and plantar surface of the foot. Because ulcers on the dorsum of the foot almost always occur because of rubbing from a poorly fitting shoe in a patient with sensory neuropathy, half of forefoot ulcers could be prevented by properly fitting footwear.

There are a number of other factors associated with ulceration. These patients have limited joint mobility. Limited motion in the metatarsal phalyngeal joint is associated with ulceration. Increased pressure is placed on the toe of a patient while walking if he/she has reduced range of motion in dorsiflexion at the metatarsal phalyngeal joint. Excessive callus over bony prominences is associated with elevated plantar pressure. The increased pressure may then serve to stimulate further callus formation. Removal of the callus may then reduce the likelihood of ulceration.

Table 1
Good Foot Care

1. Inspect foot daily for cuts, blisters, and abrasions.
2. Bathe feet carefully and dry between toes. Do not use extremely hot water.
3. Do not soak feet.
4. Use antifungal powder on feet as needed.
5. Use moisturizing cream on dry skin.
6. Have nails trimmed properly.
7. Wear properly fitting shoes. Patients often need custom shoes with fitted inserts.
8. Do not walk barefoot.
9. Seek professional help for all wounds.
10. Do not use a heating pad or hot water bottle if feet are cold.

Table 2
Risk Factors Associated with Amputation

1. Age
2. Gender
3. Race
4. Duration of diabetes
5. Poor glycemic control
6. Atherosclerosis of lower extremities
7. Neuropathy with loss of protective sensation and foot deformity
8. Limited joint mobility
9. Smoking

The combination of neuropathy, atherosclerotic arterial occlusive disease, and infection can lead to gangrene and necessitate amputation. Three independent predictors of foot ulceration have been identified. These include absence of the Achilles' tendon reflex, inability to sense the 5.07 (10 g) Semmes–Weinstein monofilment, and a transcutaneous oxygen tension (TcPO2) of less than 30 mm Hg *(6)*. In many cases, ulceration leads to amputation. The risk factors associated with amputation include age, duration of diabetes, race, poor glycemic control, poor foot care, and inadequate patient education (Table 2).

ASSESSMENT

Treatment of a diabetic foot ulcer begins with assessment of neuropathy and arterial occlusive disease by history and physical examination. There may be a history suggesting generalized atherosclerosis. These patients often have coronary artery disease and cerebrovascular disease, as well as peripheral vascular disease. Many patients have a history of claudication *(9)*. Some have had a prior amputation. A detailed evaluation of pulses will determine the degree and location of atherosclerotic occlusion. An easily palpable pulse is, in general, good evidence of adequate arterial circulation. If pulses are not easily palpated, the patient should be evaluated in the noninvasive peripheral vascular laboratory *(10)*. Ankle pressure should be measured using a hand-held Doppler device. A ratio of pressure at the ankle to pressure in the arm in the brachial

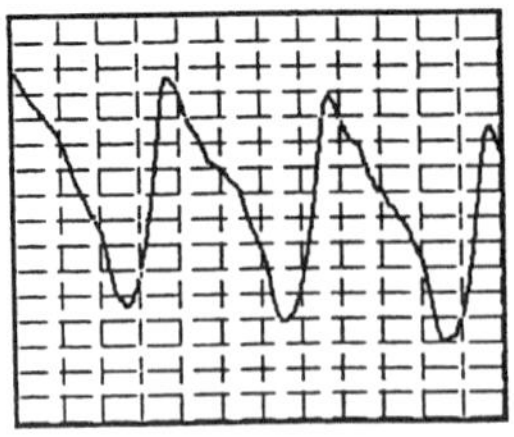

Normal Triphasic Arterial Waveform

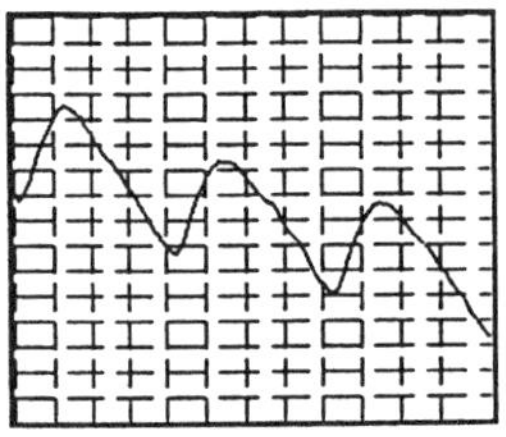

Biphasic Waveform Indicating Hemodynamically Significant Obstruction

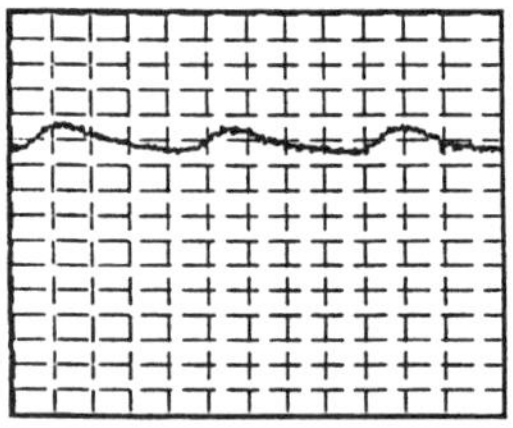

Monophasic Waveform with Severe Arterial Stenosis or Occlusion

Fig. 1. Three waveforms from the vascular lab.

artery allows calculation of an ankle/brachial index (ABI). A normal ABI is 0.9–1.1. Patients with claudication commonly have an ABI of less than 0.7. Rest pain from inadequate arterial blood supply is found in patients with an ABI of less than 0.4. Tissue loss occurs most commonly when the ABI is less than 0.3.

One may be mislead, however, when calculating the ABI in a patient with diabetes. Diabetic patients commonly have very calcified and, thus, hardened arteries. When inflating a blood pressure cuff to measure the pressure needed to occlude arterial flow, some of the squeeze of the cuff is used to overcome the stiffness of the arterial wall, thus suggesting an arterial blood pressure that is falsely elevated. If one relies only on ABI to determine the adequacy of arterial blood pressure, he/she may not recognize ischemia. Of course, a low pressure is strong evidence of arterial occlusive disease. If the pressure is high, then arterial waveforms derived by Doppler or pulse-volume recording may still suggest arterial occlusion. A normal waveform is triphasic (*see* Fig. 1). With hemodynamically significant narrowing, it becomes biphasic, then monophasic with severe occlusive disease. A normal or elevated ABI with a dampened waveform is good evidence of calcified arteries, falsely elevated pressures, and ischemia. Toe pressures may be measured as well. The digital arteries are less likely to be calcified; thus, toe pressures may be a better indicator of arterial disease. However, many laboratories are not equipped with cuffs small enough to measure toe pressures *(11)*.

TcPO2 measurements in the noninvasive peripheral vascular laboratory may be quite helpful. TcPO2 is a measurement of skin perfusion. TcPO2 is measured with an electrode placed on the skin. The skin is then heated to 44°C to allow maximum vasodilitation. The TcPO2 is about 80% of an arterial pO_2 determined by direct arterial sampling. A normal TcPO2 is defined as 55 mm Hg or greater. It has been determined that a TcPO2 of 30 mm Hg or greater is needed for wound healing. Even if the patient has arterial occlusive disease, collateral arterial blood flow with a TcPO2 of 30 mm Hg or greater may be adequate for healing. There are no risks or complications from TcPO2 measurement. A low TcPO2 suggests inadequate oxygenation of the tissues and further evaluation with angiography may be warranted. Although this test is not reimbursed by third-party payers in some states, it may be cost-effective to measure TcPO2, as it may direct the management of the patient.

Patients with ulcers secondary to ischemia will heal only with improved arterial inflow *(12)*. Although angioplasty has low risk, it is often not appropriate in these patients, as most patients with ischemic ulceration have severe disease, too extensive for angioplasty. Most have tandem lesions. The atherosclerotic occlusive disease is most severe in the tibial arteries. Bypass to the foot using the saphenous vein has proven to be successful and durable with patency rates of 80% or greater at 3 yr. Hyberbaric oxygen therapy (HBO) does not appear to play a significant role in the management of these patients.

Infection plays a major role in this disease. In general, the signs of inflammation including erythema, induration, warmth, tenderness, and pain with motion are present, if there is infection. Although these patients have an insensate foot, they may have pain when infection is present. An X-ray of the foot may be helpful in determining if osteomyelitis is present. It must be remembered, however, that changes of osteomyelitis on X-ray do not occur until it has been present for 3 wk. It is helpful to probe the wound with a sterile cotton-tipped applicator. If one can probe to the bone, osteomyelitis may be present in as many as 85% of cases. If one probes to the bone, debridement of the wound is indicated, with the surgeon prepared to resect the infected bone, if found.

TREATMENT

Proper debridement is an important component in the treatment of diabetic foot ulcers. Debridement has been shown to improve the healing of diabetic foot ulcers *(13)*. Wounds debrided aggressively appear to heal better. The initial debridement should include callus, necrotic tissue, pale granulation tissue, and infected bone. These should also be removed at any follow-up visit. Debridement allows an accurate assessment of the extent and depth of the ulcer and whether there is infection in the bone. It provides complete drainage of pus and removes the tissues with the highest bacterial counts per gram. Debridement also helps to determine if there is involvement of a tendon or joint. Sharp debridement with a knife is the most effective method to remove necrotic tissue. It can often be performed in an office setting, as these patients commonly have sensory neuropathy. There may be pain, bleeding, and transient bacteremia.

Debridement can be performed in other ways. Erymatic debriding agents will remove necrotic tissue; however, they must be applied daily over a period of time to remove all necrotic tissue. Also, bacterial counts increase in the devitalized tissue, increasing the risk of infection. It is difficult to remove large amounts of necrotic debris using these agents. Saline-moistened gauze placed on a wound and allowed to dry will mechanically debride a wound, but this may be associated with pain and bleeding. There is also the possibility that some newly formed epithelium will be damaged by this technique. Occlusive dressings placed on uninfected wounds will provide some measure of autolytic debridement.

Debridement is quite important in the management of diabetic foot wounds, in that undrained pockets of pus may be recognized during debridement. Fibroblasts, the fundamental cell of wound healing, become senescent in the chronic wound. Removal of these cells at the time of debridement with replacement by young fibroblasts may stimulate the healing process. The bleeding caused by debridement attracts platelets into the wound to control hemorrhage. These same platelets release growth factors from their α granules to trigger the healing cascade. Debridement also allows tissue sampling for culture. All diabetic foot ulcers contain bacteria. The wounds are in "bacterial balance." Infected wounds have greater than 10^5 bacteria per gram of tissue and will not heal unless the bacterial count is reduced. Debridement mechanically removes the tissues most heavily laden with bacteria. Routine swabbing of dry surface wounds is of very limited benefit in determining the bacteria responsible for infection with cellulitis. Culture of organisms on the surface of a wound does not correlate with cultures of pus or tissue taken from the deepest level of debridement.

In general, patients with diabetes have multiple flora in their wounds. Wounds present for less than 1 mo have Gram-positive micro-organisms. Wounds present for more than 1 mo have Gram-negative enteric organisms. Twenty-five percent of diabetic wounds have anaerobic bacteria.

The choice of proper antibiotics for infected diabetic ulcers depends on an understanding of the bacteria likely to be present in the wounds *(14)*. In new wounds with Gram-positive bacteria, the micro-organisms are most commonly staphylococcus or streptococcus. Appropriate antibiotics include cephalexin, amoxicillin/clavulanate, or clindamycin. In older wounds with Gram-negative organisms and anaerobic bacteria, broad-spectrum antibiotics may be more appropriate. Milder infections can be treated with a lactam/lactamase inhibitor combination such as ampicillin/sulbactam, orpiperi-cillin/tazobactam, or clindamycin with a fluoroquinolone. Severe infections may require imipenem/cilastatin or the combination of vancomycin, azetreonam, and metronidazole. Antibiotic therapy should be adjusted based on culture and sensitivity of the micro-organisms identified.

Therapeutic shoes are critical in preventing ulceration in patients with diabetic neuropathy or peripheral vascular disease. Once a patient has healed an ulcer, diabetic footwear can lower the chance of recurrent ulceration. The abnormal shape of the foot leads to areas of high pressure on the plantar surface. A molded shoe with a custom molded insert will reduce areas of high pressure on the plantar surface as well as the lateral aspects of the foot. For those patients with a claw toe deformity, an extra depth shoe may prevent ulceration on the dorsum of the foot. Custom fit shoes prevent ulceration and may also decrease callus development.

A patient with an ulcer can reduce weight-bearing by using crutches, a walker, or wheelchair. If the ulcer is on the forefoot, the patient can also use a half-shoe designed to avoid bearing weight only on the heel. Excessive callus formation, undermining of the epithelial margins of the ulcer, and clefts within the granulation tissue are signs that the patient is walking on his/her foot without adequate protection.

If there is lower extremity edema, one should elevate his/her leg, at least to the level of the heart. There is probably no benefit to leg elevation if no edema is present. Patients with arterial occlusive disease may complain of pain with leg elevation. These patients need the benefit of gravity to perfuse their lower extremity. They often sleep in a chair or recliner or keep their leg off the side of the bed. This is often a clue to the presence of ischemia.

Ulcer Care

Despite the fact that diabetic ulcers are quite common, there are still no universally accepted standards of care. There is no consensus on wound care, creams and salves, or dressings. Most experts in wound care will, however, agree on some issues. The foot, including the wound, should be washed with mild soap and water. Harsh agents such as undiluted alcohol, peroxide, iodine solutions, vinegar, or bleach probably play no role in wound care. Washing with soap and water will remove bacteria and necrotic debris. Soaking has no benefit. It can cause maceration of the tissues and lead to worsening infection. The sensory neuropathy can allow a burn to occur if the water is too hot or harsh chemicals are used. Whirlpool therapy is probably also of limited benefit. It will only provide superficial debridement and, when prolonged, also leads to maceration. Whirlpool therapy does not stimulate development of circulation. A whirlpool can be contaminated with bacteria, especially Pseudomonas.

A dressing serves to keep the wound moist while healing occurs. Saline-moistened gauze is an acceptable dressing but must be changed twice a day. Hydrogels have an osmolarity similar to saline but are less likely to dry out and need to be changed only every other day. Topical antibiotic salves keep the wound moist while keeping the bacterial colony count low. They do not penetrate a wound to a significant degree and thus cannot be used as the sole treatment of an infected wound.

Total contact casting (TCC) has been used to treat diabetic neurotrophic foot ulcers *(15)*. TCC promotes healing of these wounds by reducing pressure and shear stress on the foot. By using TCC, pressure over an ulcer is reduced by spreading the force on the foot over a large area, thus lowering pressure per unit area *(16)*. Peak plantar pressures can be reduced 40–80% using TCC. TCC increases the percentage of ulcers which heal and shortens the time to complete healing.

Total contact casting is most appropriate in treating partial or full thickness ulcers secondary to sensory neuropathy. It should not be used in the face of infection or gangrene. There are risks to using TCC. Rubbing by the cast may cause new ulcers to form. This is especially true in patients who also have peripheral arterial occlusive disease. Therefore, a lowered ABI of less than 0.4 and perhaps less than 0.7 is considered to be a contraindication to TCC. It cannot be used in patients with significant edema, as the cast will not fit properly once the swelling has resolved. Patients may remain ambulatory while in a cast, once the cast has dried. The cast protects the foot from further trauma. The cast does impair patient mobility and may not be appropriate for a patient who is at increased risk for falling. The cast needs to be changed every 1–2 wk, thus eliminating the need for daily dressing changes.

The cast must be applied by a technician trained in this procedure. A small thin dressing is placed over the ulcer. Antifungal powder is placed between the toes. The toes and bony prominances are protected with felt and foam padding. The foot is placed in the neutral position with a 90° angle at the ankle. A layer of plaster is applied first and molded to the foot. This is reinforced with a second stronger acrylic layer. The patient must be monitored carefully for signs of infection, and if found, the cast must be removed.

Total contact casting is now considered by some to be the gold standard for healing diabetic neurotrophic foot ulcers. Although it is less costly than some other forms of therapy, there are still a limited number of health care providers trained in the use of this technique.

Most wounds heal with good care. If the wound does not heal by 50% in area within a month or so of treatment, one should look for underlying infection, unrecognized ischemia, or inadequate off-loading. If none of these are present, then newer therapeutic modalities should be considered. Modern wound healing involves manipulation of the cellular environment. For example, it is recognized that fibroblasts in a chronic wound have less ability to replicate or produce proteins than fibroblasts from the same patient found elsewhere in the body. The replacement of senescent fibroblasts may be one of the benefits of debriding a chronic wound.

The cellular environment is under the control of growth factors. These are polypeptides that control the growth, differentiation, and function of cells *(17)*. They are present in most tissues of the body. They are found in the platelets and released by the platelets as they come into the wound to control hemorrhage. Within 48 h, they are released by the macrophage and continue to influence the wound environment until healing has occurred. Growth factors have been harvested from platelets, a product known as a "platelet releasate" *(18)*. At this time, there is not universal agreement on the benefit of a topically applied platelet releasate in wound healing. There is no approved platelet releasate. Isolated growth factors have also been used to heal diabetic ulcers. Platelet-derived growth factor (PDGF) has been shown to be of benefit in treating diabetic neurotrophic foot ulcers in several randomized prospective blinded trials *(19–21)*. Known as REGRANEX, it is currently approved for healing refractory diabetic foot ulcers.

There has been great interest in living-skin equivalents. These are living cells, cultured from human donors. Epidermal cells have been grown over a dermis of bovine collagen and dermal fibroblasts. Fibroblasts have also been grown over a bioabsorbable mesh. These skin equivalents may help wounds to heal by producing cytokines and matrix proteins. These growth factors and other proteins then influence wound healing. The cells of the living-skin equivalent probably do not survive long term, but stimulate healing by the patient's own cells. It may be that these skin equivalents may be of benefit in healing diabetic foot ulcers. It is hoped that these living cells can be transfected with human genes known to promote wound healing. Their exact role in wound healing remains yet to be defined.

In summary, foot problems in diabetic patients are a leading cause of amputation. This is a huge economic burden on the health care system. Although there are newer therapies to heal leg ulcers, it is much better to prevent these wounds with good foot care. This should be emphasized in diabetic patients with peripheral neuropathy and peripheral vascular disease. If a wound does develop, it is likely to heal if the blood supply is adequate, there is no infection, the glucose is under good control, pressure-relief footwear is used, and the wound is kept moist.

REFERENCES

1. Reiber G, Lipsky B, Gibbons G. The burden of diabetic foot ulcers. Am J Surg 1998;176:55–105.
2. Borssen B, Bergenheim T, Lithner F. The epidemiology of foot lesions in diabetic patients aged 15–50 years. Diabet Med 1990;7:438–444.
3. Moss S, Klein R, Klein B. The prevalence and incidence of lower extremity amputation in a diabetic population. Arch Intern Med 1992;152:610–616.
4. Rith-Najarian S, Stolusky T, Gohdes D. Identifying diabetic patients at high risk for lower extremity amputation in a primary care setting. Diabetes Care 1992;15:1386–1389.
5. Reiber G, Boyko E, Smith D. Lower extremity foot ulcers and amputations in diabetes. In: National Diabetes Data Group, ed. Diabetes in America, 2nd ed. Department of Health and Human Services (DHHS), Washington, DC, 1995.
6. McNeely M, Boyko E, Ahroni J, et al. The independent contributions of diabetic neuropathy and vasculopathy in foot ulceration: how great are the risks? Diabetes Care 1995;18:216–219.
7. Boulton A, Scarpello J, Ward J. Venous oxygenation in the diabetic neuropathic foot: evidence of arterial venous shunting. Diabetologia 1981;22:6–10.
8. Weitz J, Byrne J, Clagett G. Diagnosis and treatment of chronic arterial insufficiency of the lower extremities: a critical reviews. Circulation 1996;94:3026–3049.
9. Bowers B, Valentine R, Myers S. The natural history of patients with claudication with toe pressures of 40 mm Hg or less. J Vasc Surg 1993;18:506–511.
10. Jaff M, Dorros G. The vascular laboratory: a critical component required for successful management of peripheral arterial occlusive disease. J Endovasc Surg 1998;5:146–158.
11. Holstein P. The distal blood pressure predicts healing of amputations on the feet. Acta Orthop Scand 1984;55:227–233.
12. LoGerfo F, Gibbons G, Pomposelli F. Trends in the care of the diabetic foot: expanded role of arterial reconstruction. Arch Surg 1992;127:617–621.
13. Steed D, Donahoe D, Webster M, Lindsley L. The Diabetic Ulcer Study Group. Effect of extensive debridement and treatment on the healing of diabeticfoot ulcers. J Am Coll Surg 1996;183:61–64.
14. Foot Care. American Diabetes Association Consensus Conference Report. Diabetes Care, 1999;22.
15. Helm P, Walker S, Pullium G. Total contact casting in diabetic patients with neuropathic foot ulcerations. Arch Phys Med Rehabil 1984;65:691–693.
16. Conti S, Martin R, Chaytor E, et al. Plantar pressure measurements during ambulation in weight bearing conventional short leg casts and total contact casts. Foot Ankle Int 1996;17:464–469.
17. Hunt TK, LaVan EB. Enhancement of wound healing by growth factors. N Engl J Med 1989;321:111–112.
18. Steed D. Diabetic Ulcer Study Group. Clinical evaluation of recombinant human platelet-derived growth factor for the treatment of lower extremity diabetic ulcers. J Vasc Surg 1995;21:71–81.
19. Steed D, Goslen J, Holloway A. CT-102 activated platelet supernatant topical versus placebo: a randomized prospective double blind trial in healing of chronic diabetic foot ulcers. Diabetes Care 1992;15:1598–1604.
20. Wieman J, Smiel J, Steed D. Efficacy and safety of recombinant human platelet derived growth factor-BB (becaplermin) in patients with nonhealing lower extremity diabetic ulcers: A phase III randomized double blind study.
21. Lynch SE, Nixon JC. Role of platelet-derived growth factor in wound healing: synergistic effects with growth factors. Proc Natl Acad Sci USA 1987;84:7696–7697.

26 Atherosclerosis in Type 1 Diabetes

Wael Emad Eid, MD, *Siripoom McKay*, MD,
Finnbogi Karlsson, MD,
and Alan J. Garber, MD, PhD

CONTENTS

INTRODUCTION

Since the discovery and commercialization of insulin, heart and kidney diseases have replaced ketotic coma as the major cause of death in type 1 diabetes. In this chapter, we will review the epidemiology, the biochemical mechanisms, and the prevention of atherosclerosis in type 1 diabetes.

There are few published data examining the etiology of macrovascular disease in type 1 diabetes. Krolewski et al. *(1)* examined the risk of coronary heart disease in three cohorts of type 1 diabetic subjects: (1) those diagnosed in 1939 ($n = 65$), (2) those diagnosed in 1949 ($n = 84$), and (3) those diagnosed in 1959 ($n = 143$). The study correlated mortality from heart disease in these patients with regard to age, age of onset of diabetes, and presence of nephropathy. Mortality rates in diabetic subjects were compared to rates in matched cohorts drawn from the Framingham database *(2)*. By January 1981, 80 patients from the original cohort had died, 204 were alive, and 8 were untraceable. Thirty-five percent ($n = 28$) of the deaths were attributable to coronary artery disease (CAD) and 11% ($n = 9$) were sudden deaths not clearly attributable to CAD. As shown in Fig. 1, the risk of CAD increased with patient age. In the same figure, there is a striking difference between the subjects with type 1 diabetes *(3)* and the Framingham cohort. In both cohorts, there are no CAD deaths prior to the age of 30. However, by age 55, about one-third of the men and women in the Joslin cohort had died of CAD, compared with 8% of men and 4% of women in the Framingham cohort.

From: *Contemporary Endocrinology: Type 1 Diabetes: Etiology and Treatment*
Edited by: M. A. Sperling © Humana Press Inc., Totowa, NJ

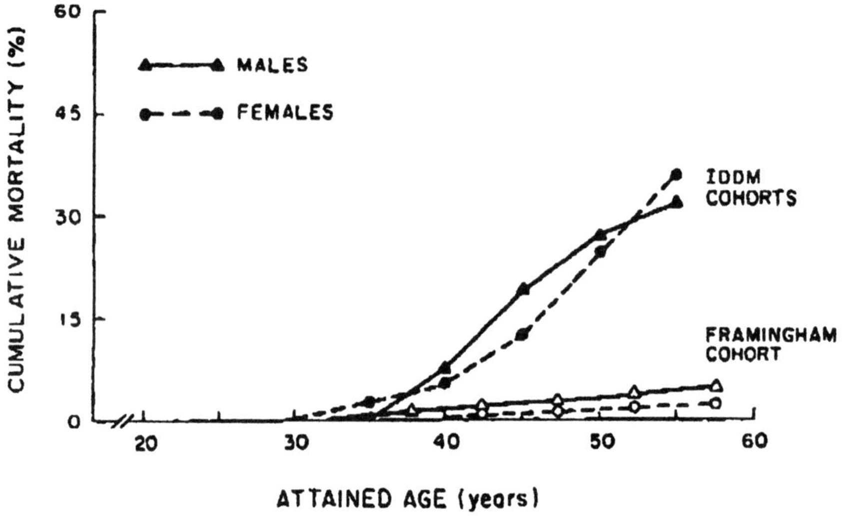

Fig. 1. Cumulative mortality resulting from coronary artery disease up to age 55 yr in patients with insulin-dependent diabetes mellitus (IDDM) and in the population of the Framingham Heart Study *(14,20)*. Unpublished data courtesy of Adrienne Cupples, PhD. Krolewski AS, Kosinki EJ, Warren JH, et al. Magnitude and determinants of coronary artery disease in juvenile-onset, insulin-dependent diabetes mellitus. Am J Cardiol 1987; 59:750–755.

This amounts to a 4.2-fold increase in CAD mortality in men and an 8.4 increase in women. It is noteworthy that the presence of type 1 diabetes completely eliminated the gender difference in the risk of CAD between men and women, so that the protective effect of being a premenopausal female was not evident in type 1 diabetic patients.

Krolewski also showed clearly that CAD mortality was not related to age of onset of diabetes. Subjects diagnosed with diabetes prior to the age of 10 yr had CAD mortality rates similar to those diagnosed at age 15–20 yr. This suggests that type 1 diabetes clearly accelerates the progression of atherosclerotic disease. Although there appears to be no increase in CAD associated with the prepubertal duration of diabetes, there is markedly increased CAD risk associated with nephropathy, which, in turn, is strongly associated with the duration of diabetes. In a follow-up period of 20–40 yr, patients with overt nephropathy had 15 times the risk of fatal CAD compared to those without nephropathy.

Tuomilehto et al. *(4,5)* compiled similar data from the Finnish registry of subjects with type 1 diabetes. They were able to capture not only deaths but also all hospitalizations for CAD and stroke using International Classification of Diseases (ICD) codes. Their patient population was younger than the Joslin population. Subjects were diagnosed with type 1 diabetes before the age of 18 and were newly diagnosed between January 1965 and December 1979. As in the Joslin data, they found an increase in the prevalence of CAD with increasing age. Diabetic subjects with nephropathy had a 10.3 risk ratio (RR) of CAD compared to those without. It is of note that although both studies show that type 1 diabetic subjects without nephropathy had a lower risk of CAD than those with nephropathy, the risk in the type 1 diabetic without nephropathy is still significantly higher than that of the general population. Compared to the general Finnish population, patients with type 1 diabetes without nephropathy had a 3.8-fold (female) to 4.5-fold (male) increase in cardiovascular risk, including stroke and CAD.

Other large epidemiological studies, although not exclusively focused on diabetes, have also yielded interesting data. For example, the Nurses Health Survey studied 226 nurses with type 1 diabetes *(6)*. They had nearly twice the incidence of atherosclerosis than the 1483 nurses with type 2 diabetes and 12.2-fold greater CAD risk than the nondiabetic population.

ANGIOGRAPHIC AND AUTOPSY DATA

Angiographic and autopsy evidence shows that compared to nondiabetic controls, subjects with type 1 diabetes have more diffuse coronary lesions and more severe stenosis *(7)*. Valsania *(8)* compared the coronary angiograms from 32 type 1 diabetic subjects to those of 31 age-, gender-, and symptom-matched nondiabetics. Subjects were presumed to have type 1 diabetes based on age of onset prior to 30 yr of age. Severe (>70% narrowing of lumen) multivessel disease was more common in the diabetic than the control subjects. Moreover, diabetic subjects tended to have multiple lesions within a given vessel. In those with left coronary lesions, 37% of the diabetic subjects had proximal, as well as distal, stenosis of >70% compared to only 10% of control subjects. For the right coronary artery, proximal and distal narrowing was found in 44% of diabetic and 33% of control subjects. This study did not match for hypertension and hypercholesterolemia in the two groups, but based on a multiple logistic regression analysis that took these factors into account, the relative odds of >70% stenosis in two or more vessels was 26.2 times greater in the diabetic than the control subjects. In contrast, hypercholesterolemia, hypertension, and smoking increased the risk of >70% stenosis, far less than type 1 diabetes *per se*.

PATHOGENESIS AND TREATMENT OF THE MACROVASCULAR COMPLICATIONS OF TYPE 1 DIABETES

Because hyperglycemia is the obvious biochemical hallmark and diagnostic criterion for type 1 diabetes, it is often assumed that hyperglycemia plays a primary causal role in the macrovascular complications of diabetes. Although epidemiological studies such as the Wisconsin Epidemiologic Study of Diabetic Retinopathy (WESDR) *(9)* of Klein and colleagues clearly implicate the duration and severity of hyperglycemia as associated with CAD risk, causation has not been clearly established thus far in any interventional trial with type 1 or even type 2 diabetes. The Diabetes Control and Complications Trial (DCCT) *(10)* studied 1441 type 1 patients with diabetes randomized to an intensive treatment vs a conventional treatment program. Intensive treatment reduced HbA1c levels to a mean on treatment value of 7.2% over the 6-yr trial. Conventional therapy resulted in an HbA1c of 9.1%. Although this treatment benefit reduced microvascular complications by 50–60%, no significant benefit was seen for macrovascular events. Similar disparities were seen in other interventional trials performed in patients with type 2 diabetes. Both the United Kingdom Prospective Diabetes Study (UKPDS) *(11)* and the Kumamoto trials *(12)* showed substantial reductions in microvascular complications with intensive treatment. In general, eye and kidney complications were reduced 30–35% per 1% reduction of HbA1c. However, there were no significant treatment benefits seen with macrovascular complications. It is, therefore, clear that we must look beyond glycemic control alone if we are to impact favorably the excess atherosclerosis of patients with type 1, as well as type 2 diabetes.

Unlike patients with type 2 diabetes who have, if anything, a superabundance of CAD risk factors, patients with type 1 diabetes have a scarcity of traditional CAD risk factors. Lipid profiles are generally normal or even quite good with high levels of high-density lipoprotein (HDL) cholesterol when glucose is well controlled. Triglycerides and low-density lipoprotein (LDL) cholesterol are rarely elevated unless the diabetes is poorly controlled *(13)*. Alterations of LDL particle size distribution are common in type 2 diabetes, in which small dense phenotype B LDL particles of increased atherogenic potential predominate as the consequence of insulin resistance *(14)*. This shift in LDL particle size is rarely seen in type 1 diabetes. However, as in type 2 diabetes, glycation of apolipoproteins with an increased potential for lipid oxidation is noted in type 1 diabetes. This undoubtedly contributes in part to the excess atherosclerosis of poorly controlled type 1 diabetes *(15)*. Oxidized LDL is, therefore, a prime candidate for therapeutic intervention. In type 2 diabetes, bulk LDL reduction with HMG-CoA-reductase inhibitors reduced coronary events 23–54% in three different secondary prevention trials (Scandinavian Simvastin Survival Study [4S]; Cholesterol and Current Events [CARE]; the Long-term Intervention with Pravastatin in Ischemic Disease [LIPID] Study Group) *(16–18)*. Although uninvestigated in type 1 diabetes, the presumption is very strong that aggressive LDL reduction to levels below 100 mg/dL should be beneficial in type 1 diabetes as well as type 2 diabetes and, therefore, should be an important focus for therapeutic intervention, if necessary. In context of these considerations, HMG-CoA-reductase inhibitor therapy is often indicated in patients with type 1 diabetes. On the other hand, fibric acid derivatives are rarely indicated, because disorders of triglyceride-rich lipoproteins and HDL cholesterol metabolism are generally well managed by intensification of diabetes control. Hypertriglyceridemia and/or low HLD cholesterol levels result from poorly controlled diabetes and not from an underlying insulin-resistant state. Improved glycemic control, reduced carbohydrate intake, and reduction or elimination of alcohol should eliminate such a dyslipidemia. Secondary causes such as overt nephropathy and hypothyroidism also must be excluded *(19)*.

THE ROLE OF ADVANCED GLYCOSYLATION END PRODUCTS

Despite the absence of a clear, convincing demonstration of a causal relationship between hyperglycemia and atherosclerosis, as would be provided by a successful interventional trial, there are much epidemiological data and in vitro experimentation to suggest such a linkage. Protein glycation is a clear mechanism by which hyperglycemia may give rise to diabetic complications *(20)*.

Accumulation of lipids and lipoproteins in the arterial wall leading to the formation of fatty streaks is an important step in the formation of advanced atherosclerotic lesions. It has been widely speculated that oxidative modification of LDL in vivo results in a reduced affinity for the LDL receptors and enhanced uptake of the modified lipoprotein by scavenger receptors on macrophages and vascular smooth muscle cells *(21)*. Glycation of LDL is a physiologically relevant modification *(22)*. Vascular endothelium expresses receptors for advanced glycation end products (AGEs) and it is likely that AGE LDL can be transcytosed by the endothelium and can lead directly to the accumulation of AGEs in the vessel wall. In addition, it has been shown that intracellular accumulation of AGEs may promote phenotypic conversion of smooth muscle cells and foam-cell formation within the atherosclerotic plaque *(21,23)*. AGE adducts residing in vessel walls are known to interfere with endothelial nitric oxide synthase

(NOS) and the vasodilatory action of (NO). AGEs react chemically directly with NO to inactivate it and block NO-mediated vasodilatation. AGE-infused nondiabetic animals show diabeticlike disruption of vasorelaxation or vasodilation processes. Accumulation of AGEs on collagen causes stiffening of the collagen fibers as the result of AGE crosslinking, thereby affecting arterial and cardiac mechanical properties even without clinical CAD *(24)*.

Endothelial dysfunction leading to enhanced procoagulant activity may result from exposure of endothelial cells to AGEs in vitro. Furthermore, vascular endothelial cells react to AGEs by causing downregulation of the anticoagulant thrombomodulin and promotion of transendothelial migration by monocytes *(25)*. Vlassara et al.*(26)* reported an accelerated atherogenic potential in AGE-infused rabbits, characterized by a significant increase in expression of vascular cell adhesion molecule-1 (VCAM-1) and intracellular adhesion molecule-1 (ICAM-1) on the endothelial surface of the rabbit aorta. These AGE-induced changes were markedly accelerated in animals placed on a cholesterol-rich diet.

Taken together, it is apparent that AGEs can cause significant dysfunctional changes to the macrovascular endothelium in ways that can potentiate vessel wall atherogenesis, hypertension, or prothrombotic events *(27)*. For these reasons, scrupulous glycemic control is important in type 1 diabetes. Clearly, elimination of hyperglycemia will minimize the microvascular complications of type 1 diabetes and may possible improve the risk of macrovascular complications. It should also be noted that albuminuria is quantitatively the greatest single risk factor for atherosclerosis in type 1 diabetes. Whether this reflects a causal relationship or a linkage to other factors such as hypertension, which is an independent risk factor for both microvascular and macrovascular disease, is unknown *(28)*.

ENDOTHELIAL DYSFUNCTION

Endothelial dysfunction is present in both type 1 and type 2 diabetes with normal urinary albumin excretion, suggesting that such dysfunction is a feature of the diabetic state *per se (29)*. Endothelial dysfunction is generalized in microalbuminuric type 1 diabetes patients, in that it affects many aspects of endothelial function such as the regulation of vascular resistance, vascular permeability, coagulation, and fibrinolysis *(30,31)*. Recent studies have suggested a primary disturbance of endothelium-dependent vascular dilation as a causative mechanism of early atherogenesis in type 1 diabetes *(32,33)*. This may reflect a possible deficit in the bioactivity of endothelium-derived relaxing factor (EDRF) or NO. Such dysfunction may evolve over time and reflect both the duration and severity of the diabetic state. However, several findings are in conflict with this hypothesis. Early in uncomplicated type 1 diabetes, there is near-normal microvascular dilation and an increase in microvascular blood flow, both in human and animal models *(34)*. Studies in humans using the response to intra-arterial infusion of cholinergic agents as an estimate of NO-mediated endothelial-dependent vasodilation and the response to nitroprusside as a measure of endothelial-independent vasodilation have produced conflicting results in diabetes. These studies are limited by the small number of subjects investigated and have generally failed to exclude microalbuminuric patients as well as patients with new type 1 disease *(32,33,35)*. These studies investigated endothelial-dependent vasodilation in resistance vessels but not in conduit vessels, which are the type of vessel most prone to develop atherosclerotic lesions; endothelial dysfunction in the brachial artery parallels that seen in the coronary artery *(36)*.

Arterial compliance is an important property of the vascular system that provides the smooth, continuous flow of blood to the periphery while maintaining optimal systolic blood pressure. Reduced arterial compliance, reflecting functional or structural alterations in the vascular wall, is associated with increased systolic and decreased diastolic blood pressure *(36)*. It is a major determinant of an increased pulsatile pressure, which has implications for cardiovascular disease that are distinct from those of an elevated mean arterial pressure *(36)*. Specifically, vascular stiffening may result in systolic hypertension, ventricular hypertrophy, diastolic dysfunction, and secondary coronary artery disease. Increased pulse pressure may modulate the sensitivity of the endothelial cells to shear stress, which, in turn, accelerates atherosclerosis. These conditions are common in the advanced stages of type 1 diabetes *(37)*.

Berry et al. *(38)* compared 25 individuals with uncomplicated type 1 diabetes (mean age of 22 ± 4 yr and mean duration of disease 8 ± 4.6 yr) with 30 healthy controls matched for age, sex, body mass index (BMI), lipid, and blood pressure variables. He found arterial compliance to be reduced by 29% in type 1 diabetic patients ($p < 0.05$). Giannattasio et al. *(39)*. also showed arterial compliance to be reduced in young patients with type 1 diabetes ($p < 0.01$) before the development of overt microvascular or macrovascular disease. Lambert et al. *(40)* investigated 24-h ambulatory blood pressure profiles and arterial distensibility in 32 normoalbuminuric type 1 diabetic patients (diabetes duration ≤ 7 yr) and 32 healthy control subjects on diets containing 50 mmol and 200 mmol sodium per day. They noted increases in daytime diastolic blood pressure on the high-sodium diets; these were significantly higher in the diabetic patients than in control subjects ($p < 0.05$). On a high-sodium regimen, femoral artery distensibility was significantly decreased in the diabetic patients compared with the control subjects ($p < 0.05$). Intervention with angiotensin-converting enzyme inhibition in the diabetic patients on high sodium diets decreased daytime diastolic blood pressure and increased femoral artery distensibility mostly because of decreasing blood pressure.

The increased sodium sensitivity of the blood pressure in uncomplicated type 1 diabetes is supported by several observations. First, proximal tubular reabsorption of sodium, total-body exchangeable sodium, and extracellular fluid volume are increased in type 1 diabetes *(41–43)*. Type 1 patients are usually hyperinsulinemic. Second, in animal studies, sodium sensitivity has been shown to play a major role in the response of the blood pressure to insulin *(44)*. A blunted nocturnal decline in arterial blood pressure has been demonstrated in type 1 diabetes *(45–47)*. Such findings are associated with left-ventricular hypertrophy, enhanced cardiovascular and renal complications, and retinopathy *(48)*. Poor glycemic control has been shown to be associated with lack of physiological decline in nocturnal blood pressure in adolescents and young adults with type 1 diabetes *(49)*. On the other hand, glycemic improvement even over a short period of time (days) may improve the nocturnal blood pressure variation close to normal. This may be the result of, at least in part, to an attenuated insulin stimulation of sympathetic activity *(50)*.

THE ROLE OF THE SYMPATHETIC NERVOUS SYSTEM

Insulin, in addition to its metabolic effects, exerts potent effects on vascular tone *(51)*. It can also increase the sympathetic nervous system activity, which, by virtue of vasoconstriction, could reduce vascular compliance. Autonomic neuropathy may also contribute to the increased sudden death and excess cardiovascular mortality in type 1

Table 1
Chemoprevention of Atherosclerosis in Type 1 Diabetes

Reverse endothelial dysfunction with ACE inhibition
Normalize blood pressure if necessary
Reduce the prothrombotic state with ASA and ADP receptor antagonist if necessary
Normalize glycemic control
Treat residual hyperlipidemia

ACE, angiotensin-converting enzyme; ASA, acetyl salicylic acid; ADP, adenosine diphosphate.

diabetes. Its presence is associated with silent ischemia, QT-interval lengthening *(52)* and dispersion (difference between the maximum and minimum value of the QTc interval in different leads of the electrocardiogram [ECG] recording), cardiorespiratory arrest, poor outcome of myocardial infarction and increased mortality *(53)*. Heart-rate variability (HRV) correlates significantly with long-term metabolic control and arterial stiffness (carotid artery) *(54,55)*. Strict glycemic control slows and may partially reverse diabetic cardiac autonomic neuropathy *(56)*.

Cardiac sympathetic dysinnervation (CSD) is the result of chronic hyperglycemia and perhaps irreversible neuronal abnormalities *(57,58)*. Substantial metabolic improvement, however, partially restores cardiac sympathetic innervation, indicating the presence of a reversible component of CSD in these patients *(59,60)*. Aronson et al. have shown a loss of the nocturnal predominance of parasympathetic activity in type 1 diabetics *(61)*. This may also predispose to the development of diastolic dysfunction, hypertension, increased aortic stiffness, and increased risk of sudden cardiac death in type 1 diabetes *(62,63)*. In addition to the burden of autonomic nervous dysfunction (AND) on the heart, coronary heart disease remains the most common cause of premature death in type 1 diabetics. There is also evidence of existence of specific heart disease of diabetes in type 1 diabetes *(64)*. Di Bello et al. did find altered behavior in myocardial tissue reflectivity to ultrasound in type 1 diabetics. This pattern may be used as a very early index of a diabetic cardiomyopathy *(65)*.

Endothelial dysfunction can be improved by angiotensin-converting enzyme (ACE) inhibitor therapy, particularly with agents impacting tissue ACE activity. Thus, in the Heart Outcomes Prevention Evaluation (HOPE) study with predominantly type 2 diabetes patients, ramipril reduced CAD recurrence and CAD mortality *(66)*. Such therapy should be considered for all type 1 diabetic patients, even without evidence of microalbuminuria. In particular, small increases in systolic or diastolic pressures (5–10 mm Hg) should be treated aggressively even if pressure is still within the generally accepted normal range. In all cases, blood pressure should be reduced below 130/80 mm Hg *(67,68)*. If albuminuria is present to any extent, treatment with ACE inhibitors and secondary agents should aim to normalize albumin excretion regardless of attained blood pressure. Even mild orthostasis should be tolerated in an effort to eliminate microalbuminuria.

Endothelial dysfunction is also associated with a prothrombotic state resulting from increased plasminogen activator inhibitor 1 (PAI-1) secretion and a shift in the prostaglandin/prostacyclin balance toward thrombosis. Abnormal platelet aggregation and shortened platelet survival is also well known in type 1 diabetes. Patients with diabetes have increased intravascular thrombosis and a twofold increase in sudden death

(69). Aspirin therapy in the predominantly type 1 diabetic patients of the Early Treatment of Diabetic Retinopathy Study (ETDRS) reduced fatal and nonfatal myocardial infarction by approx 20% *(70)*. Confirmation of this observation was seen by the Antiplatelet Trialists Collaboration *(71)*. Thus, in the absence of contraindications, aspirin therapy (81–325 mg/d) is a mainstay of a successful coronary prevention program in patients with type 1 diabetes. The appearance of a vascular event despite aspirin chemoprevention is an indication for more intense antiplatelet treatments such as the addition (not substitution) of the ADP receptor antagonist clopidegrel *(72)*.

As we have seen, there is yet no known single mechanism accounting for the increased atherosclerosis of type 1 diabetes. No single treatment has been shown to eliminate this complication. However, it is abundantly clear that aggressive treatment of all traditional risk factors for atherosclerosis such as hypertension, hyperlipidemia, endothelial dysfunction, and the prothrombotic state may go far toward reducing the atherosclerotic burden on the diabetic patient.

REFERENCES

1. Krolewski AS, Kosinski EJ, Warram JH, Leland OS, Busick EJ, Asmal AC, et al. Magnitude and determinants of coronary artery disease in juvenile-onset, insulin-dependent diabetes mellitus. Am J Cardiol 1987;59(8):750–755.
2. Dawber TR, Kannel WB. The Framingham study. An epidemiological approach to coronary heart disease. Circulation 1966;34(4):553–555.
3. Marble A. Late complications of diabetes. A continuing challenge. The Elliott P. Joslin Memorial Lecture of the German Diabetes Federation. Diabetologia 1976;12(3):193–199.
4. Miettinen H, Lehto S, Salomaa V, Mahonen M, Niemela M, Haffner SM, et al. Impact of diabetes on mortality after the first myocardial infarction. The FINMONICA Myocardial Infarction Register Study Group. Diabetes Care 1998;21(1):69–75.
5. Tuomilehto J, Borch-Johnsen K, Molarius A, Forsen T, Rastenyte D, Sarti C, et al. Incidence of cardiovascular disease in type 1 (insulin-dependent) diabetic subjects with and without diabetic nephropathy in Finland. Diabetologia 1998;41(7):784–790.
6. Colditz GA, Manson JE, Hankinson SE. The Nurses Health Study: 20-year contribution to the understanding of health among women. J Wom Health 1997;6(1):49–62.
7. Crall FV Jr, Roberts WC. The extramural and intramural coronary arteries in juvenile diabetes mellitus: analysis of nine necropsy patients aged 19 to 38 years with onset of diabetes before age 15 years. J Med 1978;64(2):221–230.
8. Valsania P, Zarich SW, Kowalchuk GJ, Kosinski E, Warram JH, Krolewski AS. Severity of coronary artery disease in young patients with insulin-dependent diabetes mellitus. Am Heart J 1991;122(3 Pt 1):695–700.
9. Moss SE, Klein R, Klein BE. Cause-specific mortality in a population-based study of diabetes. Am J Public Health 1991;81:1158–1162.
10. The Diabetes Control and Complications Trial Research Group. The effect of intensive treatment of diabetes on the development and progression of long-term complications in insulin-dependent diabetes mellitus. N Engl J Med 1993;329(14):977–986.
11. UK Prospective Diabetes Study (UKPDS) Group. Intensive blood-glucose control with sulphonylureas or insulin compared with conventional treatment and risk of complications in patients with type 2 diabetes (UKPDS 33). Lancet 1998;352(9131):837–853.
12. Ohkubo Y, Kishikawa H, Araki E, Miyata T, Isami S, Motoyoshi S, et al. Intensive insulin therapy prevents the progression of diabetic microvascular complications in Japanese patients with non-insulin-dependent diabetes mellitus: a randomized prospective 6-year study. Diabetes Res Clin Pract 1995;28(2):103–117.
13. Sosenko JM, Breslow JL, Miettinen OS, Gabbay KH. Hyperglycemia and plasma lipid levels: a prospective study of young insulin-dependent diabetic patients. N Engl J Med 1980;302:650–654.
14. Stewart MW, Laker MF, Dyer RG, Game F, Mitcheson J, Winocour PH, et al. Lipoprotein compositional abnormalities and insulin resistance in type II diabetic patients with mild hyperlipidemia. Arteriosclerosis Thromb 1993;13:1046–1052.

15. Lyons TJ, Jenkins AJ. Glycation, oxidation, and lipoxidation in the development of the complications of diabetes: a carbonyl stress hypothesis. Diabetes Rev 1997;5:365–391.
16. Scandinavian Simvastatin Survival Study Group. Randomized trial of cholesterol lowering in 4444 patients with coronary disease: Scandinavian Simvastatin Survival Study (4S). Lancet 1994;344: 1383–1389.
17. Sacks FM, Pfeffer MA, Moye LA, et al. The effect of pravastatin on coronary events after myocardial infarction in patients with average cholesterol levels. N Engl J Med 1996;335:1001–1009.
18. The Long Term Intervention with Pravastatin in Ischemic Disease (LIPID) Study Group. Prevention of cardiovascular events and death with pravastatin in patients with coronary heart disease and a broad range of initial cholesterol levels. N Engl J Med 1998;339:1349–1357.
19. American Diabetes Association. Management of dyslipidemia in adults with diabetes. Position Statement. Diabetes Care 2001;24(Suppl 1):s58–s61.
20. Bucala R. Lipid and lipoprotein modification by advanced glycosylation end-products: role in atherosclerosis. Exp Physiol 1997;82(2):327–337.
21. Stitt AW, Vlassara H. Advanced glycation end-products: impact on diabetic complications. In: Betteridge JD, ed. Diabetes: Current Perspectives. Blackwell Science, Malden, MA, 2000, pp. 67–92.
22. Bucala R, Makita Z, Koschinsky T, Cerami A, Vlassara H. Lipid advanced glycosylation: pathway for lipid oxidation in vivo. Proc Natl Acad Sci USA 1993;90(14):6434–6438.
23. Horiuchi S, Sano H, Higashi T, Ikeda K, Jinnouchi Y, Nagai R, et al. Extra- and intracellular localization of advanced glycation end-products in human atherosclerotic lesions. Nephrol Dial Transplant 1996;11(Suppl 5):81–86.
24. Chappey O, Dosquet C, Wautier MP, Wautier JL. Advanced glycation end products, oxidant stress and vascular lesions. Eur J Clin Invest 1997;27(2):97–108.
25. Bloomgarden ZT. American Diabetes Association Annual Meeting, 1999: dyslipidemia, endothelial dysfunction, and glycosylation. Diabetes Care 2000;23(5):690–698.
26. Vlassara H, Fuh H, Donnelly T, Cybulsky M. Advanced glycation endproducts promote adhesion molecule (VCAM-1, ICAM-1) expression and atheroma formation in normal rabbits. Mol Med 1995;1(4):447–452.
27. Vlassara H, Bucala R. Recent progress in advanced glycation and diabetic vascular disease: role of advanced glycation end product receptors. Diabetes 1996;45 (Suppl 3):S65–S66.
28. Vlassara H. Intervening in atherogenesis: lessons from diabetes. Hosp Pract (Off Ed) 2000;35(11):25–39.
29. Lambert J, Aarsen M, Donker AJ, Stehouwer CD. Endothelium-dependent and -independent vasodilation of large arteries in normoalbuminuric insulin-dependent diabetes mellitus. Arteriosclerosis Thromb Vasc Biol 1996;16(5):705–711.
30. Elliott TG, Cockcroft JR, Groop PH, Viberti GC, Ritter JM. Inhibition of nitric oxide synthesis in forearm vasculature of insulin-dependent diabetic patients: blunted vasoconstriction in patients with microalbuminuria. Clin Sci (Colch) 1993;85(6):687–693.
31. Messent JW, Elliot TG, Hill RD, Jarrett RJ, Keen H, Viberti GC. Prognostic significance of microalbuminuria in insulin-dependent diabetes mellitus: a twenty-three year follow-up study. Kidney Int 1992;41(4):836–839.
32. Johnstone MT, Creager SJ, Scales KM, Cusco JA, Lee BK, Creager MA. Impaired endothelium-dependent vasodilation in patients with insulin-dependent diabetes mellitus. Circulation 1993;88(6):2510–2516.
33. Steinberg HO, Baron AD. Insulin-dependent diabetes mellitus and nitrovasodilation. Important and complex interactions. Circulation 1997;95(3):560–561.
34. Cleland SJ, Petrie JR, Ueda S, Elliott HL, Connell JM. Insulin as a vascular hormone: implications for the pathophysiology of cardiovascular disease. Clin Exp Pharmacol Physiol 1998;25(3–4):175–184.
35. Smits P, Kapma JA, Jacobs MC, Lutterman J, Thien T. Endothelium-dependent vascular relaxation in patients with type I diabetes. Diabetes 1993;42:148–153.
36. Mikhail N, Tuck ML, Insulin and the vasculature. Curr Hypertens Rep 2000;2(2):148–153.
37. Contreras F, Rivera M, Vasquez J, De la Parte MA, Velasco M. Diabetes and hypertension physiopathology and therapeutics. J Hum Hypertens 2000;14(Suppl 1):S26–S31.
38. Berry KL, Skyrme-Jones RA, Cameron JD, O'Brien RC, Meredith IT. Systemic arterial compliance is reduced in young patients with IDDM. Am J Physiol 1999;276(6 Pt 2):H1839–H1845.
39. Giannattasio C, Failla M, Piperno A, Grappiolo A, Gamba P, Paleari F, et al. Early impairment of large artery structure and function in type I diabetes mellitus. Diabetologia 1999;42(8):987–994.
40. Lambert J, Pijpers R, van Ittersum FJ, Comans EF, Aarsen M, Pieper EJ, et al. Sodium, blood pressure, and arterial distensibility in insulin-dependent diabetes mellitus. Hypertension 1997;30(5):1162–1168.
41. Feldt-Rasmussen B, Mathiesen ER, Deckert T, Giese J, Christensen NJ, Bent-Hansen L, et al. Central role for sodium in the pathogenesis of blood pressure changes independent of angiotensin,

aldosterone and catecholamines in type 1 (insulin-dependent) diabetes mellitus. Diabetologia 1987;30(8):610–617.
42. Strojek K, Grzeszczak W, Lacka B, Gorska J, Keller CK, Ritz E. Increased prevalence of salt sensitivity of blood pressure in IDDM with and without microalbuminuria. Diabetologia 1995;38(12):1443–1448.
43. Wedler B, Brier ME, Wiersbitzky M, Gruska S, Wolf E, Kallwellis R, et al. Sodium kinetics in salt-sensitive and salt-resistant normotensive and hypertensive subjects. J Hypertens 1992;10(7):663–669.
44. Brands MW, Hildebrandt DA, Mizelle HL, Hall JE. Hypertension during chronic hyperinsulinemia in rats is not salt-sensitive. Hypertension 1992;19(1 Suppl):I83–I89.
45. Azar ST Birbari A. Nocturnal blood pressure elevation in patients with type 1 diabetes receiving intensive insulin therapy compared with that in patients receiving conventional insulin therapy. J Clin Endocrinol Metab 1998;89(9):3190–3193.
46. van Ittersum FJ, Spek JJ, Praet IJ, Lambert J, IJzerman RG, Fischer HR, et al. Ambulatory blood pressures and autonomic nervous function in normoalbuminuric type I diabetic patients. Nephrol Dial Transplant 1998;13(2):326–332.
47. Verdecchia P, Porcellati C, Schillaci G, Borgioni C, Ciucci A, Battistelli M, et al. Ambulatory blood pressure. An independent predictor of prognosis in essential hypertension. Hypertension 1994;24(6):793–801.
48. Palatini P, Penzo M, Racioppa A, Zugno E, Guzzardi G, Anaclerio M, et al. Clinical relevance of night-time blood pressure and of daytime blood pressure variability. Arch Intern Med 1992;152(9):1855–1860.
49. Young LA, Kimball TR, Daniels SR, Standiford DA, Khoury PR, Eichelberger SM, et al. Nocturnal blood pressure in young patients with insulin-dependent diabetes mellitus: correlation with cardiac function. J Pediatr 1998;133(1):46–50.
50. Ferreira SR, Cesarini PR, Vivolo MA, Zanella MT. Abnormal nocturnal blood pressure fall in normotensive adolescents with insulin-dependent diabetes is ameliorated following glycemic improvement. Braz J Med Biol Res 1998;31(4):523–528.
51. Cleland SJ, Petrie JR, Ueda S, Elliott HL, Connell JM. Insulin as a vascular hormone: implications for the pathophysiology of cardiovascular disease. Clin Exp Pharmacol Physiol 1998;25(3–4):175–184.
52. Galetta F. Franzoni F, Prattichizzo F, Tintori G, Cinotti F, Taccola D, et al. QT dispersion in insulin-dependent diabetics. G Ital Cardiol 1999;29:675–678.
53. Valensi P, Sachs RN, Harfouche B, Lormeau B, Paries J, Cosson E, et al. Predictive value of cardiac autonomic neuropathy in diabetic patients with or without silent myocardial ischemia. Diabetes Care 2001;24(2):339–343.
54. Burger AJ. Short- and long-term reproducibility of heart rate variability in patients with long-standing type I diabetes mellitus. Am J Cardiol 1997;80:1198–1202.
55. Jensen-Urstad K. Decreased heart rate variability in patients with type 1 diabetes mellitus is related to arterial wall stiffness. J Intern Med 1999;245:57–61.
56. Burger AJ, Weinrauch LA, D'Elia JA, Aronson D. Effect of glycemic control on heart rate variability in type I diabetic patients with cardiac autonomic neuropathy. Am J Cardiol 1999;84(6):687–691.
57. Ziegler D. Effect of glycaemic control on myocardial sympathetic innervation assessed by [^{123}I]metaiodobenzyguanidine scintigraphy: a 4-year prospective study in IDDM patients. Diabetologia 1998;41:443–451.
58. Schnell O. Three-year follow-up on scintigraphically assesed cardiac sympathetic denervation in patients with long-term insulin-dependent (type I) diabetes mellitus. J Diabetes Complic 1997;11:307–313.
59. Muhr-Becker D. Scintigraphically assessed cardiac sympathetic dysinnervation in poorly controlled type 1 diabetes mellitus: one-year follow-up with improved metabolic control. Exp Clin Endocrinol Diabetes 1999;107:306–312.
60. Schnell O. Partial restoration of scintigraphically assessed cardiac sympathetic denervation in newly diagnosed patients with insulin-dependent (type 1) diabetes mellitus at one-year follow-up Diabet Med 1997;14:57–62.
61. Aronson D. Circadian patterns of heart rate variability, fibrinolytic activity, and hemostatic factors in type I diabetes mellitus with cardiac autonomic neuropathy. Am J Cardiol 1999;84:449–453.
62. Ahlgren AR. Increased aortic stiffness in women with type 1 diabetes mellitus is associated with diabetes duration and autonomic nerve function. Diabet Med 1999;16:291–297.
63. Weston PJ, James MA, Panerai RB, McNally PG, Potter JF, Thurston H. Evidence of defective cardiovascular regulation in insulin-dependent diabetic patients without clinical autonomic dysfunction. Diabetes Res Clin Pract 1998;42(3):141–148.

64. Galderisi M, Anderson KM, Wilson PW, Levy D. Echocardiographic evidence for the existence of a distinct diabetic cardiomyopathy (the Framingham Heart Study). Am J Cardiol 1991;68(1):85–89.
65. Di Bello V, Giampietro O, Matteucci E, Giorgi D, Bertini A, Piazza F, et al. Ultrasonic tissue characterization analysis in type 1 diabetes: a very early index of diabetic cardiomyopathy? G Ital Cardiol 1998;28(10):1128–1137.
66. Yusuf S, Sleight P, Pogue J, Bosch J, Davies R, Dagenais G. Effects of an angiotensin-converting-enzyme inhibitor, ramipril, on cardiovascular events in high-risk patients. The Heart Outcomes Prevention Evaluation Study Investigators. N Engl J Med 2000;342(3):145–153.
67. Birkenhager WH, Staessen JA, Gasowski J, de Leeuw PW. Effects of antihypertensive treatment on endpoints in the diabetic patients randomized in the Systolic Hypertension in Europe (Syst-Eur) trial. J Nephrol 2000;13(3):232–237.
68. Birkenhager WH, Staessen JA. Treatment of diabetic patients with hypertension. Curr Hypertens Rep 1999;1(3):225–231.
69. Jokl R, Colwell JA. Arterial thrombosis and atherosclerosis in diabetes. Diabetes Rev 1997;5:316–330.
70. ETDRS Investigators. Aspirin effects on mortality and morbidity in patients with diabetes mellitus. Early Treatment Diabetic Retinopathy Study Report 14. JAMA 1992;268(10):1292–1300.
71. Collins R, Baigent C, Sandercock P, Peto R. Antiplatelet therapy for thromboprophylaxis: the need for careful consideration of the evidence from randomised trials. Antiplatelet Trialists' Collaboration. Br Med J 1994;309(6963):1215–1217.
72. Jarvis B, Simpson K. Clopidogrel: a review of its use in the prevention of atherothrombosis. Drugs 2000;60(2):347–377.

27 Cutaneous Complications of Type 1 Diabetes

Jean L. Bolognia, MD *and*
Irwin M. Braverman, MD

CONTENTS

INTRODUCTION

In this chapter on the cutaneous complications of diabetes mellitus, we include a broad range of clinical entities. Several of the disorders such as acanthosis nigricans (AN) and candidal infections are more familiar to nondermatologists, whereas others are rarely discussed except in dermatologic texts. Examples of the latter include disseminated granuloma annulare and bullous diabeticorum. Our goal is to provide descriptions of these disease entities that are sufficiently practical so as to lead to their clinical recognition and appropriate management. Several of the entities may be more common in patients with type 2 diabetes mellitus, but also may occur in patients with type 1 diabetes.

SCLEREDEMA

Although patients with this disorder develop induration (hardening) of the skin, *scleredema* should not be confused with the distinctly different disease, *scleroderma.* The

From: *Contemporary Endocrinology: Type 1 Diabetes: Etiology and Treatment*
Edited by: M. A. Sperling © Humana Press Inc., Totowa, NJ

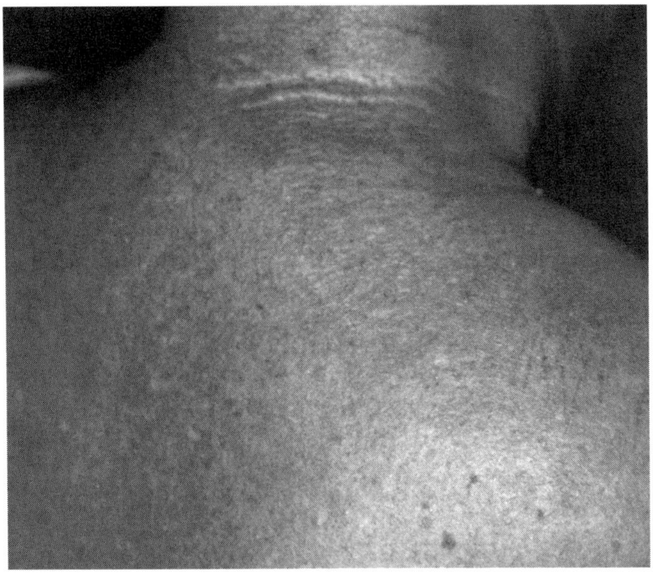

Fig. 1. Peau d'orange appearance of the upper back in a patient with scleroderma. The areas of involvement are firm to palpation.

basic abnormality in scleredema is an increased deposition of glycosaminoglycans (mucin)—in particular, hyaluronic acid—within the dermis. The upper back is the most common site of involvement, followed by the neck, upper arms, and upper chest. Occasionally, there is facial involvement and, rarely, cardiac or esophageal involvement. Given the often subtle changes in the appearance of the skin, the diagnosis may be missed unless the skin is palpated. Then, the induration of the skin becomes obvious.

Visual clues to the diagnosis include prominent openings of the hair follicles and diffuse erythema. The former can give the skin an appearance that resembles the peel of an orange, hence the term *peau d'orange* (*see* Fig. 1). The diffuse erythema is most commonly observed on the upper back and, on occasion, it is misdiagnosed as treatment-resistant cellulitis. Although patients may notice a tightening of the skin, more frequently they comment on decreased mobility of the neck. The onset, however, is usually insidious. By physical examination, there is decreased range of motion, especially dorsal extension of the neck.

The diagnosis of scleredema is based on the above-outlined clinical features as well as the histologic finding of increased deposits of mucin within the dermis. The disorder is then further subdivided based on the presence or absence of diabetes mellitus. In 1 study of 33 patients with scleredema, those with diabetes usually had the late-onset, but insulin-requiring, form and were difficult to control *(1)*. Of the group of patients without diabetes, some will be found to have a monoclonal gammopathy *(2)* or a preceding streptococcal infection.

An improvement of scleredema has been reported following better diabetic control via insulin, intravenous administration of prostaglandin E_1, high-dose penicillin, psoralens plus ultraviolet A (PUVA), electron beam therapy, intralesional corticosteroids, and oral tocopherol acetate plus hyaluronidase *(3–5)*. However, these therapeutic interventions are based primarily on case reports and small series of patients enrolled in open clinical trials. Based on personal experience, our initial therapeutic intervention in symptomatic patients

Table 1
Prevalence of Limited Joint Mobility (LJM) in Children 7–18 yr Old with Type 1 Diabetes and Percent of Those Children with Mild or Moderate/Severe LJM

	Prevalence of LJM			*Severity of LJM*		
Year	*No LJM*	*LJM*	*p-Value*[a]	*Mild*	*Moderate/severe*	*p-Value*[a]
1976–1978 ($n = 515$)	357 (69%)	158 (31%)		103 (65%)	55 (35%)	
1998 ($n = 312$)	290 (93%)	22 (7%)	<0.001	20 (91%)	2 (9%)	0.0253

[a] Exact χ^2.
Source: ref. *9,* with permission of the publisher.

is a 12-wk course of PUVA therapy. More specific treatments for scleredema should emerge once the underlying pathophysiology of the disease is better understood.

WAXY SKIN AND STIFF JOINTS (CHEIROARTHROPATHY)

In the dermatologic literature, the descriptive term "waxy skin and stiff joints" appears more commonly than the term "cheiroarthropathy." The most common site of cutaneous involvement is the hands and, like scleredema, it can sometimes be confused with scleroderma. Clinically, the skin on the dorsal surface of the hands is waxy in appearance and somewhat taut *(6)*. A simple screening test is to ask the patient to bring his or her hands together with the palmar surfaces apposed as if one were about to pray. Patients with cheiroarthropathy will be unable to extend their fingers to the degree required for the interphalangeal joints to approximate one another *(7)*. In other words, there will be a gap between the palmar surfaces of the fingers; this is sometimes referred to as the "prayer sign." However, a more precise assessment of joint involvement can be accomplished via passive extension *(8)*.

In a study of 309 patients (ages 1–28 yr) with insulin-dependent diabetes, 30% were found to have limited mobility of small and large joints *(7)*. Thickened waxy skin that could not be tented was noted on the dorsae of the hands in one-third of the patients with limited joint mobility, but only in those whose joint involvement was judged to be either moderate or severe. Of note, a life-table analysis demonstrated that after 16 yr of diabetes, there was an 83% risk of developing microvascular complications if joint involvement were present, but only a 25% risk if it were absent. Presumably, the cheiroarthropathy is a reflection of more widespread abnormalities in connective tissue metabolism including an increase in the glycosylation or crosslinking of collagen *(6)*. Thus, this complication mirrors overall metabolic control and is associated with high values of HbA_{1c}. Although cheiroarthropathy may be seen in poorly controlled adolescents, its incidence in this age group has declined as methods of metabolic control have improved (*see* Table 1) *(9)*.

In biopsy specimens from the wrist of three diabetic patients with waxy skin, a marked increase in the thickness of the dermis was noted, as was an accumulation of connective tissue in the lower dermis *(7)*. By high-resolution ultrasonography, an increase in the thickness of the skin of the hands was confirmed in patients with clinically waxy skin *(10)*. In one brief report, three of four patients were noted to have undergone a reduction in skin thickness over a period of 3 mo following the initiation of insulin therapy via a portable-pump infusion *(11)*. Given the correlation between the incidence of cheiroarthropathy and diabetic control, the primary therapy remains attention to metabolic control in order to prevent its occurrence, although genetic predisposition may contribute.

DIABETIC DERMOPATHY

Diabetic dermopathy is characterized by hyperpigmented macules (<1 cm) and patches (>1 cm) on the extensor surfaces of the distal lower extremities (i.e., the shins). Less commonly, similar lesions are found on the lateral foot and distal thigh *(12)*. Secondary findings include superficial white scale as well as atrophy; in some patients, there may be preceding erythema. Additional names for this disorder include "shin spots" *(13)* and "pigmented pretibial patches" *(14)*.

Although the exact cause of diabetic dermopathy is not known, a leading theory is that it is an abnormal reaction to trauma. In 1 study, 16 of 19 patients with diabetes and dermopathy developed atrophic circumscribed skin lesions at the sites of experimentally induced thermal trauma whereas none of the 25 controls and only 1 of the 16 diabetic patients without dermopathy developed similar lesions *(15)*. The possibility has been raised that this abnormal response to trauma is a reflection of an underlying microangiopathy. For example, an increased frequency of retinopathy (39.1%) was observed in a series of 23 patients with diabetic dermopathy when compared to a group of 77 diabetics without dermopathy (incidence of retinopathy = 6.9%) *(16)*. In a more recent study of 173 patients with diabetes, 69 of whom had dermopathy, an increased incidence of retinopathy, nephropathy, and neuropathy was observed in those with diabetic dermopathy *(17)*.

Diabetic dermopathy is observed in up to 50% of patients with diabetes, both insulin dependent and non-insulin dependent *(13,16)*, with a M : F ratio of 2 : 1. As a result, these hyperpigmented macules are the most common cutaneous finding in diabetes. With such a high incidence, it should come as no surprise that diabetic dermopathy is not as specific a clinical finding as entities such as waxy skin and stiff joints. To date, the only treatment for diabetic dermopathy is avoidance of trauma.

ULCERATIONS OF THE LOWER EXTREMITIES

In the general population, the most common cause of lower extremity ulcers is venous hypertension, and patients with diabetes, especially as they age, certainly can develop venous hypertension. Venous ulcers are often located above the medial or lateral malleolus and are usually painless. Clues to the diagnosis are frequently found in the surrounding skin and include edema, varicosities, stasis dermatitis, a yellow-brown discoloration due to hemosiderin, and induration of the skin as a result of lipodermatosclerosis. However, in comparison to the general population, individuals with diabetes are more prone to the development of ulcers resulting from atherosclerosis and microangiopathy, peripheral neuropathy (mal perforans), necrobiosis lipoidica diabeticorum (NLD), calciphylaxis, and soft tissue infections.

In comparison to venous ulcers, arterial ulcers involve the toes and distal foot more frequently; they also favor the anterior tibial surface. Arterial ulcers are usually painful, especially at night, are often accompanied by claudication, and tend to have a "dry" base. Clues to the diagnosis are found in the surrounding skin and include pallor, dry skin (xerosis), brittle nails, a decrease in the density of hair, and a shiny appearance to the skin *(18)*. An examination for pallor with elevation and hyperemia with dependency can be performed, but an actual assessment of blood flow is essential. Following palpation of peripheral pulses, the ankle/brachial pressure index can be measured by Doppler, both at rest and following exercise. Radiographic studies are then performed to confirm the presence of surgically correctable disease. Therapeutic interventions include cessation of smoking, angioplasty, endarterectomy, and revascularization via bypass surgery.

Cholesterol emboli also can give rise to lower extremity ulcerations and represent yet another consequence of atherosclerosis. The resulting ischemia of the skin is reflected in angulated areas of blue to violet gray discoloration. Ulcerations as a result of calciphylaxis have a similar clinical appearance, and livedo reticularis (a blue to violet netlike pattern due to sluggish blood flow within the superficial venous plexus) often accompanies both entities. In patients with diabetes, the most common cause of calciphylaxis is secondary hyperparathyroidism in the setting of chronic renal failure.

The plantar surface of the foot is a very unusual location for an ulcer, and as a result, the possibility of a cutaneous malignancy such as a squamous cell carcinoma (e.g., epithelioma cuniculatum) or amelanotic melanoma is often entertained. However, in the presence of a peripheral neuropathy, the most likely diagnosis is a neuropathic ulcer or mal perforans. These ulcers are usually at the sites of greatest pressure and shearing forces (e.g., the metatarsal heads and heels). Clinically, there is often a thick keratotic rim surrounding the ulcer, and in order to heal a neuropathic ulcer, there must be a reduction in pressure via the use of orthotics, debridement, and exclusion of underlying osteomyelitis. Topical application of platelet-derived growth factor can also be added to the therapeutic regimen.

NECROBIOSIS LIPOIDICA DIABETICORUM

NLD is a reflection of the degenerative changes observed in the dermis histologically and the yellow color of mature lesions (presumably caused by the granulomatous inflammation in the dermis allowing the visualization of subcutaneous fat). An estimated 0.3% of patients with diabetes develop NLD and the lesions most commonly (approx 85%) appear on the extensor surfaces of the distal lower extremities (i.e., the shins) *(12)* (*see* Fig. 2). Additional locations include the distal upper extremities and the face and scalp. Initially, the lesions are red–brown in color and then over time acquire a yellow color centrally. In mature lesions, there is associated epidermal atrophy and deep dermal/subcutaneous blood vessels are easily visualized.

There is some disagreement as to the proportion of patients with NLD who have frank diabetes. The range that is usually cited is 40–65%, based primarily on clinical series from the 1950s and 1960s *(19)*. In a more recent retrospective study of consecutive patients seen over a period of 25 yr, only 7 (11%) of 65 patients with classic biopsy-proven NLD had diabetes mellitus at presentation *(20)*. However, the lesions are not pathognomic, as the diagnosis of NLD can predate the onset of diabetes and additional patients with NLD have equivocal glucose tolerance tests as well as family histories of diabetes. In patients with type 1 and 2 diabetes, the presumed underlying

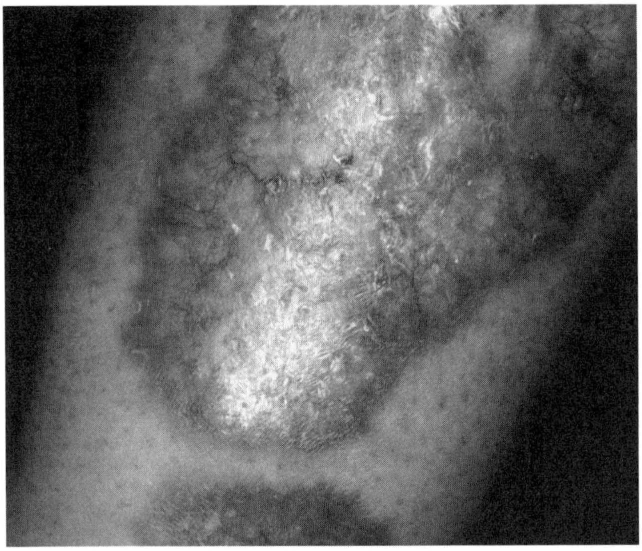

Fig. 2. Plaque of necrobiosis lipoidica diabeticorum on the shin; note the atrophy and easily visualized superficial blood vessels.

etiology, as in the case of diabetic dermopathy, is microangiopathy. A higher incidence of both diabetic nephropathy and retinopathy was observed in children and adolescents with NLD in comparison to those without NLD, suggesting an association with poor metabolic control *(21)*. Histologically, granulomatous inflammation surrounds degenerated collagen and elastin (necrobiosis).

Clinical improvement of NLD lesions has been reported following the use of topical corticosteroids (including class I) with or without occlusion, intralesional corticosteroids, oral clofazamine, oral pentoxifylline, and oral acetylsalicylic acid (ASA) plus dipyridamole *(22–26)*. The reported therapeutic success of topical and intralesional corticosteroids as well as clofazamine and pentoxifylline is based on case reports and small series of patients. Clinical trials involving antithrombotic agents were based in part on the presence of microangiopathy and the observation that platelets in diabetics may have an increased tendency to aggregate. However, a double-blind, placebo-controlled trial of ASA plus dipyridamole in 14 patients with NLD failed to demonstrate any differences between the treatment and control groups *(27)*. Similar negative findings were observed in a randomized, double-blind 6-mo trial of low-dose ASA *(28)*.

Up to one-third of patients with NLD of the lower extremities can develop ulcerations within the lesions. In addition to the above-outlined therapies, single or small series of patients with ulcerative NLD have been treated with topical granulocyte–macrophage colony-stimulating factor (GM-CSF), tretinoin or collagen, hyperbaric oxygen, oral nicotinamide, oral corticosteroids, and oral cyclosporine (29–35). Treatment of the ulcers also includes local care and elevation of the legs *(24)*. Glucose levels in patients receiving nicotinamide should be monitored because the dosage of insulin may need to be adjusted. The use of potent immunosuppressives is reserved for those individuals with significant morbidity.

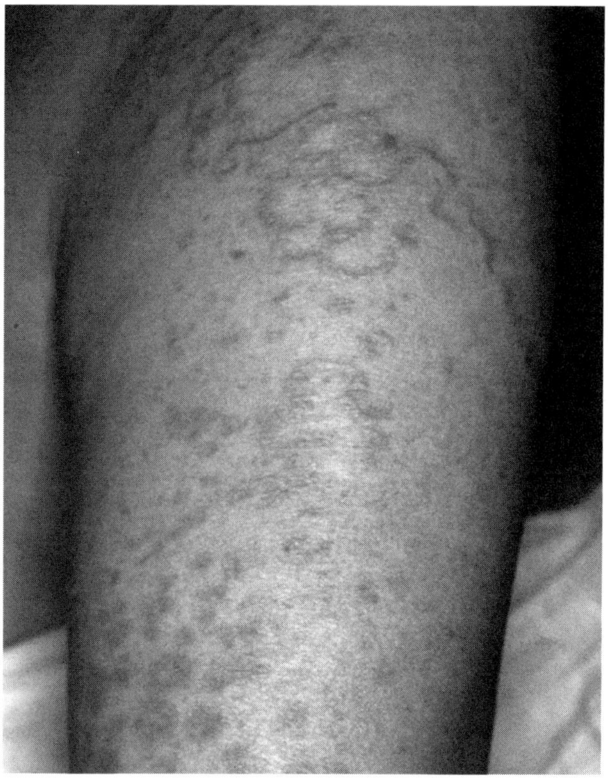

Fig. 3. Generalized granuloma annulare with multiple annular and arciform lesions composed of coalescent papules.

DISSEMINATED GRANULOMA ANNULARE

Granuloma annulare (GA) is an idiopathic disorder that occurs in both children and adults. The individual lesions are pink to skin-colored papules and they often coalesce to form rings and arcs, hence the term *annulare.* In the classic form of the disease, lesions are found predominantly on the distal extremities. One theory advanced to explain the distribution of GA is that it represents an unusual granulomatous reaction to trauma or arthropod bites. Occasionally, a patient will have generalized or widespread lesions of GA (*see* Fig. 3) and this is the form of GA associated with diabetes mellitus. In 1 series of 100 patients with generalized GA, 21% were shown to have diabetes *(36).*

Treatment of GA overlaps significantly with that of NLD (as outlined earlier). For example, initial therapy, especially for localized disease, consists of topical corticosteroids (including class I) with or without occlusion and intralesional corticosteroids *(24).* For the generalized form of GA, systemic therapies are often required, as topical agents and intralesional injections can prove impractical. When the lesions are inflammatory, high-dose oral niacinamide (500 mg tid) is usually our initial treatment of choice *(37).* If this medication fails and the patient is still concerned about the appearance of the cutaneous eruption, oral PUVA can be prescribed *(38).* There are also scattered reports of the use of oral retinoids, dapsone, clofazamine, antimalarials, pentoxifylline, and cyclosporine for the treatment of widespread GA *(23,24).*

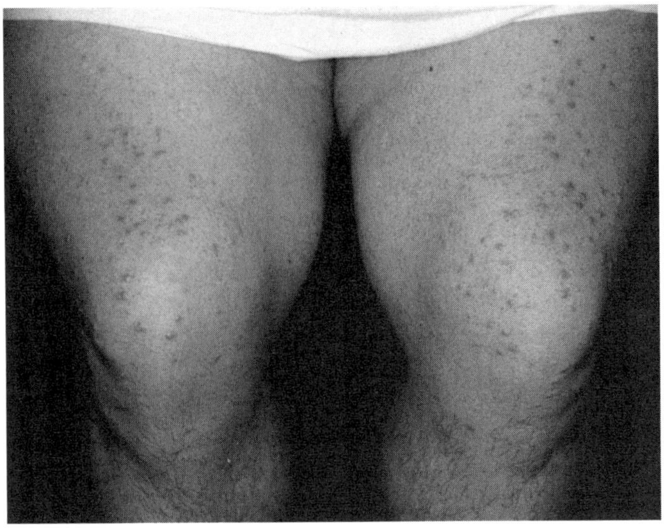

Fig. 4. Eruptive xanthomas on the lower thighs and knees in a patient with poorly controlled diabetes and hypertriglyceridemia. The papules are discrete and firm to palpation.

XANTHOMAS

Of the major forms of cutaneous xanthomas—planar, tendinous, tuberous, and eruptive—it is the latter one that serves as a cutaneous manifestation of the hypertriglyceridemia that can complicate poorly controlled diabetes mellitus. Eruptive xanthomas are usually 3–7 mm in diameter and have a central yellow hue and a peripheral erythematous rim (*see* Fig. 4). The most common locations for eruptive xanthomas are the extensor surfaces of the extremities, in particular, the elbows and the knees, and the buttocks. The yellow color is a reflection of the accumulation of lipids with macrophages in the dermis, and if the clinical diagnosis is in question, a biopsy specimen can be obtained. Rapid resolution of eruptive xanthomas follows the return of metabolic control, as the hypertriglyceridemia is the result of the effect of hypoinsulinemia on lipid metabolism, especially the activity of lipoprotein lipase.

ACANTHOSIS NIGRICANS

Clinical descriptions of acanthosis nigricans (AN) usually emphasize its velvety texture and relative hyperpigmentation. However, these characteristic findings are not the result of increased melanin production or thickening (acanthosis) of the epidermis, as is sometimes assumed. Rather, they are a reflection of an increased folding of the superficial layers of the skin leading to an accordionlike configuration that is best appreciated by gently stretching the skin. Recognition of this phenomenon aids in the identification of AN in unusual locations and provides some insight into suggested treatment options.

The most common locations for AN are the flexural surfaces of the body—in particular, the neck and axillae (*see* Fig. 5). However, AN can involve extensor surfaces, especially the skin overlying the elbows, knees, and the small joints of the hands and feet. Although the diagnosis of AN always prompts a mental review of associated systemic diseases or syndromes, the most common underlying disease is obesity, with its associ-

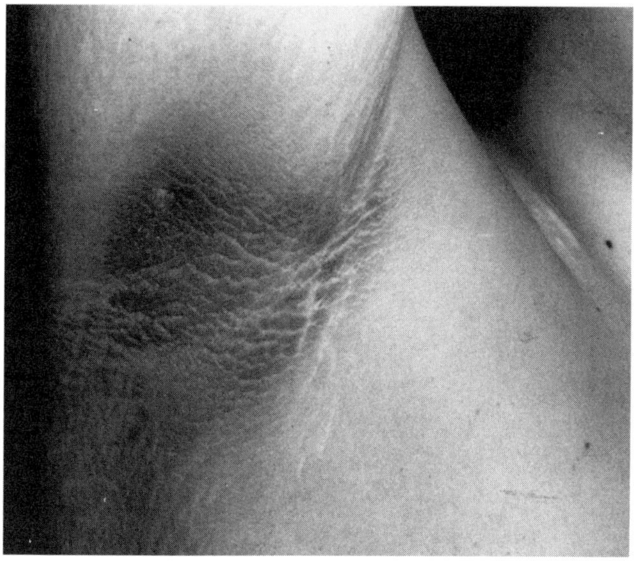

Fig. 5. Velvety hyperpigmentation in the axilla of a patient with acanthosis nigricans.

ated insulin resistance and hyperinsulinemia. Some dermatologists prefer to refer to the form of AN associated with obesity as "pseudo-AN," but given the overlap in underlying pathophysiology between this form of the disease and AN associated with diabetes, use of the term "pseudo" may be unnecessary. Although AN is a hallmark of insulin resistance with hyperinsulinemia and, hence, is typically seen in type 2 diabetes, it may occur in the obese patient with type 1 diabetes or atypical diabetes mellitus.

Insulin resistance with AN is characteristic of Kahn's type A syndrome, which is the result of defects in the insulin receptor or downstream targets and Kahn's type B syndrome, which is the result of circulating anti-insulin receptor antibodies *(39)*. In the type B syndrome, cutaneous manifestations of other autoimmune disorders such as lupus erythematosus and Sjogren's syndrome may be present. Clinical signs of hyperandrogenemia (e.g., hirsutism, acne vulgaris, and androgenetic alopecia) can be seen in prepubertal and postpubertal women with insulin resistance, explained in part by insulin–ovary interactions and often referred to as the HAIR-AN syndrome (HyperAndrogenism; Insulin Resistance; Acanthosis Nigricans).

One explanation proposed for the epidermal hyperplasia seen in AN is binding of excess amounts of circulating insulin to insulinlike growth factor receptors on keratinocytes and fibroblasts *(40)*. Therapies for AN include weight loss and topical agents such as urea, tretinoin, and α-glycolic acids *(24,41)*. For widespread and severe cases of AN, there are scattered case reports of the use of oral retinoids *(42)*. However, the side effects of oral retinoids, which include hypertriglyceridemia and fetal abnormalities, must be balanced against their use, especially in light of the observation that AN reappears soon after discontinuation of the medication.

BULLOUS DIABETICORUM

Bland bullae that lack a traumatic, inflammatory, or infectious etiology can arise spontaneously in the skin of patients with diabetes mellitus *(43)*. The most common location for these bullae is the distal lower extremity, although they have been described on the hands and forearms *(44);* the lesions can be up to 8 cm in diameter and are subepidermal or intraepidermal in location. The majority, but not all, of the patients have evidence of peripheral neuropathy *(44)*. In contrast to the water-like contents of friction bullae, the fluid within diabetic bullae is said to be more viscous and "stringy."

To decrease symptoms resulting from pressure and stretching of the skin, the contents of the bulla can be drained. However, it is important to avoid the temptation to remove the blister roof; the detached epidermis should be left in place to serve as a natural barrier or "bandaid." Topical antibiotics such as mupirocin can be applied and the surrounding skin should be observed for signs of soft tissue infection. Otherwise, there are no specific treatments.

ACQUIRED PERFORATING DERMATOSIS

The perforating disorders are a group of cutaneous diseases that share a common phenomenon—the outward elimination of dermal contents via "claws" formed by downgrowths of the epidermis. Clinically, actual plugs of degenerated collagen and elastin (admixed with keratin) are seen perforating through the epidermis to the surface of the skin. The primary systemic disease associated with perforating disorders is chronic renal failure (CRF)—in particular, CRF resulting from diabetes mellitus. Occasionally, patients will have just diabetes in the absence of renal failure. In individuals with no underlying illness, specific names such as perforating folliculitis, Kyrle's disease, and reactive perforating collagenosis are usually applied *(45)*. Because there is often clinical overlap, especially in diabetics with CRF, the term "acquired perforating dermatosis" is commonly used *(46)*.

At least 10% of patients with diabetic nephropathy on maintenance hemodialysis will have evidence of acquired perforating dermatosis *(47)*. The lower extremity is the most common site of involvement, and individual lesions are red–brown to skin-colored, dome-shaped papules and nodules with central keratotic cores (*see* Fig. 6). Sometimes, the patient will have manually removed these plugs and a history of such activity can serve as clue to the diagnosis. A common complaint in patients with renal failure-associated perforating disease is pruritus, and vigorous scratching has been proposed as an inciting event in the formation of lesions. The differential diagnosis includes prurigo simplex and prurigo nodularis, entities that reflect simple picking and rubbing, but, centrally, one sees a hemorrhagic crust in these lesions and not a keratotic plug. Often, histologic examination of a representative lesion is necessary to confirm the diagnosis.

In the treatment of acquired perforating dermatosis, an attempt is always made to reduce pruritus through the use of topical antipruritics (e.g., pramoxine, corticosteroid lotions) and oral antihistamines. However, this is not a particularly easy task. Individual lesions can be injected with triamcinolone or they can be destroyed via curettage or cryosurgery. There have been case reports where a reduction in the number of lesions was observed following the use of keratolytics *(45)*, topical tretinoin *(48)*, or ultraviolet B (UVB) phototherapy *(49)*, and, more recently, transcutaneous electrical nerve stimulation was advocated as effective in reducing the associated pruritus *(50)*. However, the vast array of treatment modalities is merely a reflection of the lack of a consistently effective therapy.

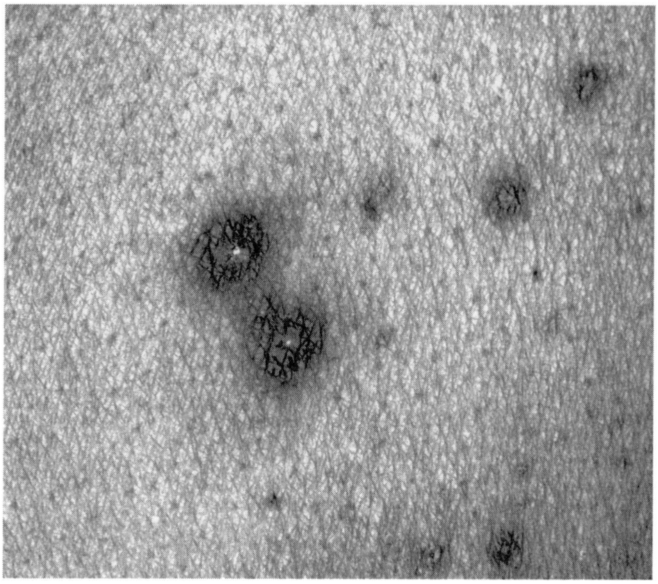

Fig. 6. Dome-shaped papules with central keratotic cores in a patient with acquired perforating dermatosis and diabetic nephropathy.

INFECTIONS

Patients with diabetes mellitus tend to have more extensive or serious bacterial infections of the skin and soft tissues, in particular infections resulting from *Staphylococcus aureus, Streptococcus* spp., and Gram-negative bacilli. Recurrent furunculosis or folliculitis as a result of *S. aureus* should prompt a search for nasal carriage either in the patient or a family member. A 1-wk course of intranasal mupirocin can be used to treat the nasal carriers. In addition to Gram-negative cellulitis *(51)* and malignant otitis externa secondary to *Pseudomonas aeruginosa,* patients with diabetes are at risk for the development of necrotizing fasciitis *(52,53)*. Early diagnosis of necrotizing fasciitis does require a high index of suspicion.

Although textbooks often emphasize the more dramatic association of diabetes with mucormycosis of the face and sinuses *(54),* the most common fungal infection is cutaneous candidiasis (*see* Fig. 7). Clinically, candidal infections can present as perleche, thrush, intertrigo, balanitis, vulvovaginitis, and chronic paronychia with nail plate involvement.

DRUG REACTIONS TO INSULIN

Rarely, injections of insulin result in generalized systemic reactions such as urticaria, angioedema, and serum sickness-like illnesses. More commonly, reactions to insulin are localized to the sites of injection. The risk of a systemic reaction to insulin is related to the source and purification of the insulin, with bovine insulin having the highest incidence, and human insulin the lowest *(55)*. In addition, the systemic reaction may be caused by another component of the insulin preparation, such as protamine. Treatment options for individuals receiving human insulin include desensitization and use of the insulin analog lispro.

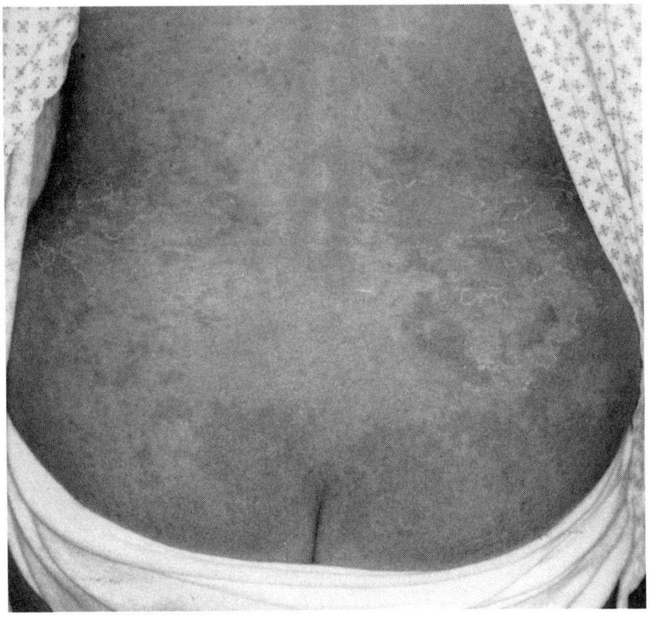

Fig. 7. Widespread cutaneous candidiasis in a patient with diabetes mellitus who had recently completed a course of broad-spectrum antibiotics.

There are two major types of localized reactions to subcutaneous injections of insulin: allergic and lipodystrophic. The latter group is then subdivided into either lipohypertrophy or lipoatrophy *(16)*. Localized allergic reactions are characterized by pruritus in addition to erythema and induration; less often, the skin changes are those of dermatitis. These reactions may be immediate or delayed. As with systemic reactions, the "allergen" may be a component of the insulin preparation (e.g., zinc, protamine, or diluent) rather than the insulin itself. An even more elusive cause of allergic reactions is the presence of small quantities of natural latex rubber antigens in insulin injection materials *(56,57)*. Finally, sterile abscesses can occur at the sites of injections.

Localized areas of lipoatrophy as a result of subcutaneous injections of insulin are fairly easy to recognize. The frequency of this side effect has decreased as the use of monocomponent and human insulin has increased. In fact, treatment of localized lipoatrophy consists of switching to human insulin, injection of human insulin into the sites of lipoatrophy (beginning at the periphery and progressing toward the center), and rotation of sites over a 30-d cycle *(24)*. In patients already receiving human insulin, the use of a jet injector may prove beneficial *(58)*.

In contrast to lipoatrophy, lipohypertrophy results in an elevation or thickening of the skin (*see* Fig. 8) rather than an indentation due to loss of subcutaneous tissue. The clinical appearance is not the only problem, for the presence of lipohypertrophy can lead to delayed absorption of insulin. Unfortunately, the incidence of this side effect has not been decreasing. Other than rotation of injection sites, treatment options are rather limited. Recently, however, there have been reports of clinical improvement following liposuction *(59)* and use of the insulin analog lispro *(60)*. Finally, continuous subcutaneous insulin infusions are associated with the reactions just outlined as well as a second set of cutaneous side effects ranging from bacterial infections at the injection

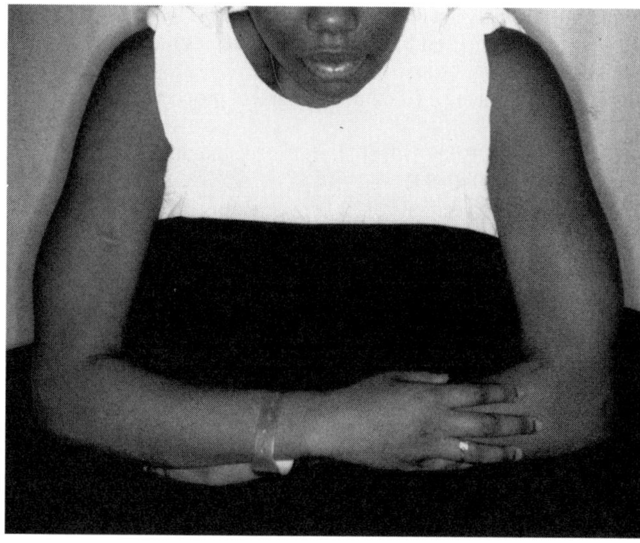

Fig. 8. Lipohypertrophy of the midportions of both upper extremities at the sites of insulin injections.

site to contact dermatitis from components of the infusion system (e.g., components of the glue used in the infusion pump sets) *(61)*.

CONCLUDING REMARKS

There is a wide spectrum of cutaneous manifestations of diabetes mellitus, from NLD to insulin-induced lipohypertrophy. Some of these diseases are reflections of hyperglycemia (e.g., cheiroarthropathy); others are related to the long-term consequences of microangiopathy, macroangiopathy and neuropathy (e.g., ischemic ulcers and neuropathic ulcers). Improvements in metabolic control as well as the purity of insulin and its delivery have resulted in a significant reduction in the frequency of a few of these dermatologic complications, but much remains to be learned about genetic susceptibility, underlying pathophysiology, and more specific treatments.

REFERENCES

1. Venencie PY, Powell FC, Su WP, Perry HO. Scleredema: a review of thirty-three cases. J Am Acad Dermatol 1984;11:128–134.
2. Grudeva-Popova J, Dobrev H. Biomechanical measurement of skin distensibility in scleredema of Buschke associated with multiple myeloma. Clin Exp Dermatol 2000;25:247–249.
3. Ikeda Y, Suehiro T, Abe T, et al. Severe diabetic scleredema with extension to the extremities and effective treatment using prostaglandin E1. Intern Med 1998;37:861–864.
4. Hager CM, Sobhi HA, Hunzelmann N, et al. Bath–PUVA therapy in three patients with scleredema adultorum. J Am Acad Dermatol 1998;38:240–242.
5. Rho YW, Suhr KB, Lee JH, Park JK. A clinical observation of scleredema adultorum and its relationship to diabetes. J Dermatol 1998;25:103–107.
6. Burton JL. Thick skin and stiff joints in insulin-dependent diabetes mellitus. Br J Dermatol 1982;106:369–371.
7. Rosenbloom AL, Silverstein JH, Lezotte DC, et al. Limited joint mobility in childhood diabetes mellitus indicates increased risk for microvascular disease. N Engl J Med 1981;305:191–194.
8. Rosenbloom AL. Limited joint mobility in insulin dependent childhood diabetes. Eur J Pediatr 1990;149:380–388.

9. Infante JR, Rosenbloom AL, Silverstein JH, Garzarella L, Pollock BH. Changes in frequency and severity of limited joint mobility in children with type 1 diabetes mellitus between 1976–78 and 1998. J Pediatr 2001;138:33–37.
10. Nikkels-Tassoudji N, Henry F, Letawe C, et al. Mechanical properties of the diabetic waxy skin. Dermatology 1996;192:19–22.
11. Lieberman LS, Rosenbloom AL, Riley WJ, et al. Reduced skin thickness with pump administration of insulin. N Engl J Med 1980;303:940–941.
12. Huntley AC. The cutaneous manifestations of diabetes mellitus. J Am Acad Dermatol 1982;7:427–455.
13. Danowski TS, Sabeh G, Sarver ME, et al. Shin spots and diabetes mellitus. Am J Med Sci 1966;251:570–575.
14. Bauer MJ, Levan NE, Frankel A, Bach J. Pigmented pretibial patches. Arch Dermatol 1966;93:282–286.
15. Lithner F. Cutaneous reactions of the extremities of diabetics to local thermal trauma. Acta Med Scand 1975;198:319–325.
16. Vijayasingam SM, Thai AC, Chan HL. Non-infective skin associations of diabetes mellitus. Ann Acad Med Singapore 1988;17:526–535.
17. Shemer A, Bergman R, Linn S, et al. Diabetic dermopathy and internal complications in diabetes mellitus. Int J Dermatol 1998;37:113–115.
18. Ryan TJ, Burnand K. Diseases of the veins and arteries—leg ulcers. In: Champion RH, Burton JL, Ebling FJG, eds. Rook/Wilkinson/Ebling Textbook of Dermtaology, 5th ed. Blackwell Scientific, London, 1992, pp. 1963–2013.
19. Muller SA, Winkelmann RK. Necrobiosis lipoidica diabeticorum. A clinical and pathological investigation of 171 cases. Arch Dermatol 1966;93:272–281.
20. O'Toole E, Kennedy U, Nolan JJ, et al. Necrobiosis lipoidica: only a minority of patients have diabetes mellitus. Br J Dermatol 1999;140:283–286.
21. Verrotti A, Chiarelli F, Amerio P, Morgese G. Necrobiosis lipoidica diabeticorum in children and adolescents: a clue for underlying renal and retinal disease. Pediatr Dermatol 1995;12:220–223.
22. Goette DK. Resolution of necrobiosis lipoidica with exclusive clobetasol propionate treatment. J Am Acad Dermatol 1990;22:855–856.
23. Juhlin L. Treatment of psoriasis and other dermatoses with a single application of a corticosteroid left under a hydrocolloid occlusive dressing for one week. Acta Derm Venereol 1989;69:355–357.
24. Bolognia JL, Braverman I. Skin and subcutaneous tissues. In: DeFonzo RA, ed. Current Therapy of Diabetes Mellitus. Mosby, St. Louis, MO, 1998, pp. 210–217.
25. Mensing H. Clofazimine—therapeutische alternative bei necrobiosis lipoidica and granuloma annulare. Hautarzt 1989;40:99–103.
26. Littler CM, Tschen EH. Pentoxifylline for necrobiosis lipoidica diabeticorum. J Am Acad Dermatol 1987;17:314–316.
27. Statham B, Finlay AY, Marks R. A randomized double blind comparison of an aspirin dipyridamole combination versus a placebo in the treatment of necrobiosis lipoidica. Acta Derm Venereol 1981;61:270–271.
28. Beck H-I, Bjerring P, Rasmussen I, et al. Treatment of necrobiosis lipoidica with low-dose acetylsalicylic acid. Acta Derm Venerol 1985;65:230–234.
29. Remes K, Ronnemaa T. Healing of chronic leg ulcers in diabetic necrobiosis lipoidica with local granulocyte–macrophage colony stimulating factor treatment. J Diabetes Complic 1999;13:115–118.
30. Heymann WR. Necrobiosis lipoidica treated with topical tretinoin. Cutis 1996;58:53–54.
31. Spenceri EA, Nahass GT. Topically applied bovine collagen in the treatment of ulcerative necrobiosis lipoidica diabeticorum. Arch Dermatol 1997;133:817–818.
32. Weisz G, Ramon Y, Waisman D, Melamed Y. Treatment of necrobiosis lipoidica diabeticorum by hyperbaric oxygen. Acta Dermato-Venereol 1993;73:447–448.
33. Handfield-Jones S, Jones S, Peachey R. High dose nicotinamide in the treatment of necrobiosis lipoidica. Br J Dermatol 1988;118:693–696.
34. Dwyer CM, Dick D. Ulceration in necrobiosis lipoidica—a case report and study. Clin Exp Dermatol 1993;18:366–369.
35. Darvay A, Acland KM, Russell-Jones R. Persistent ulcerated necrobiosis lipoidica responding to treatment with cyclosporin. Br J Dermatol 1999;141:725–727.
36. Dabski K, Winkelmann RK. Generalized granuloma annulare: clinical and laboratory findings in 100 patients. J Am Acad Dermatol 1989;20:39–47.
37. Ma A, Medenica M. Response of generalized granuloma annulare to high-dose niacinamide. Arch Dermatol 1983;119:836–839.

38. Kerker BJ, Huang CP, Morison WL. Photochemotherapy of generalized granuloma annulare. Arch Dermatol 1990;126:359–361.
39. Hogan PA. Cutaneous manifestations of endocrine disease. In: Harper J, Oranje A, Prose N. eds. Textbook of Pediatric Dermatology. Blackwell Science, Oxford, 2000, pp. 1623–1650.
40. Cruz PD Jr, Hud JA Jr. Excess insulin binding to insulin-like growth factor receptors: proposed mechanism for acanthosis nigricans. J Invest Dermatol 1992;98:82S–85S.
41. Darmstadt GL, Yokel BK, Horn TD. Treatment of acanthosis nigricans with tretinoin. Arch Dermatol 1991;127:1139–1140.
42. Katz RA. Treatment of acanthosis nigricans with oral isotretinoin. Arch Dermatol 1980;116:110–111.
43. Cantwell AR, Martz W. Idiopathic bullae in diabetics. Bullosis diabeticorum. Arch Dermatol 1967;96:42–44.
44. Toonstra J. Bullosis diabeticorum. Report of a case and review of the literature. J Am Acad Dermatol 1985;13:799–805.
45. Patterson JW. The perforating disorders. J Am Acad Dermatol 1984;10:561–581.
46. Rapini RP, Herbert AA, Drucker CR. Acquired perforating dermatosis. Evidence for combined transepidermal elimination of both collagen and elastic fibers. Arch Dermatol 1989;125:1074–1078.
47. Hurwitz RM, Melton ME, Creech FT 3rd, et al. Perforating folliculitis in association with hemodialysis. Am J Dermatopathol 1982;4:101–108.
48. Berger RS. Reactive perforating collagenosis of renal failure/diabetes responsive to topical retinoic acid. Cutis 1989;43:540–542.
49. Hurwitz RM. The evolution of perforating folliculitis in patients with chronic renal failure. Am J Dermatopathol 1985;7:231–239.
50. Chan LY, Tang WY, Lo KK. Treatment of pruritus of reactive perforating collagenosis using transcutaneous electrical nerve stimulation. Eur J Dermatol 2000;10:59–61.
51. Brook I, Frazier EH. Clinical features and aerobic and anaerobic microbiological characteristics of cellulitis. Arch Surg 1995;130:786–792.
52. Gonzalez MH. Necrotizing fasciitis and gangrene of the upper extremity. Hand Clin 1998;14:635–645.
53. Eke N. Fournier's gangrene: a review of 1726 cases. Br J Surg 2000;87:718–728.
54. Tierney MR, Baker AS. Infections of the head and neck in diabetes mellitus. Infect Dis Clin North Am 1995;9:195–216.
55. Zürcher K, Krebs A. Cutaneous Drug Reactions, 2nd ed. Karger, Basel, 1992, pp. 236–241.
56. MacCracken J, Stenger P, Jackson T. Latex allergy in diabetic patients: a call for latex-free insulin tops. Diabetes Care 1996;19:184.
57. Towse A, O'Brien M, Twarog FJ, et al. Local reaction secondary to insulin injection. A potential role for latex antigens in insulin vials and syringes. Diabetes Care 1995;18:1195–1197.
58. Logwin S, Conget I, Jansa M, et al. Human insulin-induced lipoatrophy. Successful treatment using a jet-injection device. Diabetes Care 1996;19:255–256.
59. Barak A., Har-Shai Y, Ullmann Y, et al. Insulin-induced lipohypertrophy treated by liposuction. Ann Plastic Surg 1996;37:415–417.
60. Roper NA, Bilous RW. Resolution of lipohypertrophy following change of short-acting insulin to insulin lispro (Humalog). Diabet Med 1998;15:1063–1064.
61. Busschots AM, Meuleman V, Poesen N, et al. Contact allergy to components of glue in insulin pump infusion sets. Contact Derm 1995;33:205–206.

28 Infection and Diabetes

Nirmal Joshi, MD, FACP

CONTENTS

INTRODUCTION

An increased propensity to infections in patients with diabetes has been well known. However, contrary to common belief, this association is not supported by strong evidence. A critical re-evaluation of this association has received somewhat increased attention lately. Some infections clearly occur uniquely and, indeed, almost exclusively in the diabetic population. Others are more common, and still others have a different and more aggressive clinical course in the diabetic host. There is well-established data that improved glycemic control decreases morbidity and mortality associated with several infections in patients with diabetes. However, some studies have failed to prove a clearly causal relationship between hyperglycemia and infections *(1)*.

MECHANISMS OF IMMUNITY IN DIABETES

Several factors affecting the immune system may increase the susceptibility to infections in patients with diabetes mellitus. White blood cell abnormalities have been demonstrated in the form of impaired adherence, chemotaxis, phagocytosis, and microbicidal function *(2,3)*. The intracellular killing of organisms by leukocytes is mediated by release of toxic free radicals, superoxides, and hydrogen peroxide. This phenomenon is referred to as the "respiratory burst" and is defective in patients with diabetes mellitus *(4)*. Polymorphonuclear function is further affected by a state of persistent low-level activation by advanced glycation end products (AGEs). This hyperexcited

From: *Contemporary Endocrinology: Type 1 Diabetes: Etiology and Treatment*
Edited by: M. A. Sperling © Humana Press Inc., Totowa, NJ

Table 1
Infections in Diabetes: Predisposing Factors

Primary Factors
- Phagocytic dysfunction
- Myeloperoxidase deficiency
- Complement pathway defects
- Cytokine (IL-1, TNF) mediated

Secondary Factors
- Use of intravascular access lines
- Indwelling urinary catheters
- Antibiotic misuse/resistance
- Frequent hospitalization
- Neuropathy
- Gastroparesis, reflux, and aspiration
- Total parenteral nutrition

Table 2
Classification of Infections in Diabetes

A. Common Infections with Increased Incidence in Diabetic Patients
   1. Urinary tract infections
   2. Respiratory tract infections
   3. Soft tissue infections

B. Infections Predominantly Occurring in Diabetic Patients
   1. Malignant otitis externa
   2. Rhinocerebral mucormycosis
   3. Necrotizing fasciitis
   4. Fournier's gangrene
   5. Emphysematous infections
      - Emphysematous cholecystitis
      - Emphysematous pyelonephritis, pyelitis, and cystitis
   6. Infections in diabetic foot

C. Micro-organisims Strongly Associated with Infections in Patients with Diabetes
   1. *Candida* species
   2. Group B streptococcus
   3. *Klebsiella* species
   4. Hepatitis C

D. Infections Resulting from Iatrogenic Causes
   1. Insulin injection
   2. Penile implants
   3. Dialysis

state leads to spontaneous activation of the respiratory burst and release of myeloperoxidase, elastase, and other neutrophil granule components that (1) may lead to a "burnt-out" or tolerant polymorphonuclear cell that responds less vigorously when stimulated by an infectious pathogen and (2) may initiate pathologic processes leading to vascular injury *(5)*. Studies have demonstrated an improvement in phagocytic function with enhanced glycemic control *(6)*. Complement-mediated functions may also be affected by hyperglycemia *(7)*. Stress-related hyperglycemia also causes release of cytokines that affect carbohydrate metabolism *(8)*. However, humoral immunity and response to vaccines appears to be normal.

Other than the primary mechanisms described, secondary causes predisposing diabetic patients to infections include frequent hospitalization, delayed wound healing, and loss of skin integrity as a result of ischemia and chronic renal failure (*see* Table 1).

A clinically helpful classification of infections in patients with diabetes is presented in Table 2. Table 3 summarizes clinical features and diagnosis of selected infections in patients with diabetes.

COMMON INFECTIONS OCCURRING IN PATIENTS WITH DIABETES

These infections, although occurring commonly in the normal host, are more severe and associated with an increased complication rate in patients with diabetes.

Urinary Tract Infection

Urinary tract infection (UTI) is commonly encountered in patients with diabetes *(9)*. However, studies have failed to demonstrate significant differences in epidemiological, clinical, and microbiological features of UTI in patients with or without diabetes except for a relative difficulty in eradicating infection in the former group *(10)*. Asymptomatic bacteruria occurs with a higher frequency; one study demonstrated a 26% incidence in diabetic women compared to 6% in controls *(11)*. Whether this increase is the result of an increased use of urinary catheters in these women or to diabetes itself has been debated *(12)*. Other possible reasons for the increased incidence includes the presence of diabetic neuropathy, which affects the sympathetic and parasympathetic afferent fibers, causing decreased reflex detrusor activity. Impaired bladder sensations result in bladder distension, increased residual urine volume, vesicoureteral reflux, and recurrent upper UTI *(1,13)*. Coexisting vaginitis, cystocoele, and rectocoele may also predispose to UTI.

Escherichia coli is the most common etiologic bacterial pathogen, other organisms being *Klebsiella pneumoniae* and *Proteus mirabilis*. *Pseudomonas aeruginosa* should be suspected if there is history of recent instrumentation or hospitalization. Candiduria is not uncommonly encountered and may signify contamination of the urine specimen, benign saprophytic colonization of the catheter, and lower UTI, or may be indicative of true invasive infection of the upper and/or lower urinary tract *(14)*.

Uncomplicated UTI may be asymptomatic. Lower-tract infection presents as dysuria, frequency, or urgency. UTI involvement maybe up to fivefold more frequent in diabetic than in nondiabetic patients. Further, bilateral kidney involvement is more frequent *(15)*. Clinical features are otherwise similar to those in nondiabetic patients, ranging from mild flank pain to fever with chills, vomiting, and costo-vertebral angle tenderness. Prominent systemic features and a palpable renal mass should raise suspicion of perinephric abscess. A poor response to antibiotics may be caused by complications, which may include papillary necrosis or perinephric abscess. Symptoms of papillary necrosis include flank and abdominal pain accompanied by fever. In one published series of patients with perinephric abscess, 36% had underlying diabetes *(16)*. Although localized clinical findings such as flank or abdominal mass are highly suggestive, they are present in only one-fourth of cases. One study noted that fever persisting for more than 4 d after initiating antibiotic therapy was the most useful factor in differentiating perinephric abscess from uncomplicated pyelonephritis *(17)*.

Table 3
Clinical Features and Diagnosis of Selected Infections in Patients with Diabetes

Infection	*Clinical features*	*Diagnostic procedure*	*Organisms*
Urinary tract			
Acute bacterial cystitis	Increased urinary frequency, dysuria, suprapubic pain	Urine culture	*E. coli,* proteus species
Acute pyelonephritis	Fever, flank pain	Urine culture	*E. coli,* proteus species
Emphysematous pyelonephritis	Fever, flank pain, poor response to antibiotics	Radiography or CT scan	*E. coli,* other Gram-negative bacilli
Perinephric abscess	Fever, flank pain, poor response to antibiotics	Ultrasonography or CT scanning	*E. coli,* other Gram-negative bacilli
Respiratory tract			
Community-acquired pneumonia	Cough, fever	Chest radiography	*S. pneumoniae, S. aureus, H. influenzae,* atypical pathogens, Gram-negative bacilli
Invasive otitis externa	Ear pain, otorrhea, hearing loss, cellulitis	Clinical examination, MRI	*P. aeruginosa*
Rhinocerebral mucormycosis	Facial or ocular pain, fever or lethargy, black nasal eschar	Clinical examination, MRI, pathological findings	*Mucor* and *Rhizopus* species
Necrotizing fasciitis	Local pain, redness, crepitus, bullous skin lesions	Radiography, CT scan	Gram-negative bacilli, anaerobes, and group A streptococci
Emphysematous cholecystitis	Fever, right-upper-quadrant pain	Radiography	Gram-negative bacilli, anaerobes
Foot infections	Ulcers, cellulitis, ischemia, osteomyelitis	Plain radiograph, cultures, probe to bone test	Gram-positive cocci, anaerobes, and Gram-negative bacilli

Urine culture should be done before initiation and after completion of antimicrobial therapy to document infection and bacteriologic cure. Blood culture is indicated in a toxic patient. Leukocytosis and pyuria are usually present. Plain abdominal radiograph is useful to rule out obstructive uropathy and emphysematous infection. Ultrasonography is a more sensitive, safe, and inexpensive technique for initial screening. Ultrasound or computed tomography (CT) scan confirm the diagnosis of renal abscess, mass, presence of air in the urinary tract, and extent of perinephric spread of infection. The diagnosis of papillary necrosis is made by retrograde pyelography.

Uncomplicated UTI may be treated with fluoroquinolones, doxycycline trimethoprim-sulfamethoxazole, nitrofurantoin, ampicillin, or amoxycillin. Trimethoprim-sulfamethoxazole potentiates the hypoglycemic effect of oral antihyperglycemic agents and must be used with caution. Complicated infections require hospitalization and therapy with parenteral antibiotics. Intravenous therapy is continued until fever resolves followed by oral antibiotics to complete at least 2 wk of treatment. Bacteriologic cure needs to be confirmed by culture. Whereas fungal infection of the upper tract clearly requires systemic antifungal therapy with amphotericin B or fluconazole, the appropriate treatment of candida infection confined to the bladder remains controversial *(18)*. Distinguishing such infection from colonization is clinically difficult. The presence of symptoms or pyuria suggests infection. Funguria resolves in many cases without therapy. Removal of an indwelling catheter, if present, is recommended as initial intervention. Treatment options include bladder irrigation with amphotericin *(19)*, a single intravenous dose of amphotericin *(20)*, or oral fluconazole *(21)*. Fluconazole is preferred because of its ease of administration and relative safety

Respiratory Tract Infections

Whether diabetes constitutes an independent risk factor for an increased incidence or severity of common upper or lower respiratory tract infections is not clear. The overall incidence of community-acquired pneumonia may not be higher in patients with diabetes than in the normal host *(22)*. The odds ratio for death associated with diabetes was only 1.3 (95% confidence interval, 1.1–1.5) in one large meta-analysis of community-acquired pneumonia *(23)*. However, the incidence of bacteremia, delayed resolution, and recurrence may, indeed, be higher. Further, infection caused by certain specific micro-organisms clearly occurs with an increased frequency in diabetes. These include *St. aureus,* Gram-negative bacteria, *Mycobacterium tuberculosis,* and *Mucor.* Another group of infections, although not necessarily occurring more frequently, are associated with increased morbidity and mortality in patients with diabetes. These include infections caused by streptococci, legionella and influenza *(24)*.

Patients with diabetes who develop pneumococcal pneumonia are at an increased risk of bacteremia as well as a higher mortality *(25,26)*. Pneumococcal vaccine response rates are similar to nondiabetic hosts. During epidemics of influenza, there is an increased mortality and an increased incidence of bacterial pneumonia and ketoacidosis in patients with diabetes. The increased incidence of nasal colonization with *St. aureus* in diabetics combined with reduced pulmonary ciliary clearance in patients with influenza leads to an increased incidence of staphylococcal pneumonia. *Influenza and pneumococcal vaccines are therefore recommended for all diabetic patients.*

Up to 30% of diabetic patients are nasal carriers of *St. aureus* compared to 11% of healthy individuals *(27)* and this is a major pathogen in both community-acquired and nosocomial pneumonias. Gram-negative bacteria are acquired by aspiration, hematogenous spread, or contaminated equipment. The concomitant use of histamine (H2) blockers increases the potential for colonization in hospitalized individuals. Individuals with diabetes have an increased incidence of tuberculosis and more advanced disease at the time of diagnosis. This is especially true among patients on chronic hemodialysis. *Aspergillus* species, *Coccidioides immitis,* and *Cryptococcus neoformans* can cause primary pneumonia in the diabetic host.

Cough and fever are the usual initial complaints in diabetic patients with pneumonia. Diabetic ketoacidosis may be the initial manifestation. Complications of pneumonia include pleural effusion, empyema, lung necrosis, metastatic infections, and bacteremia.

Investigations include complete hemogram, blood glucose, serum electrolytes, renal function tests, and arterial blood gas analysis to assess the acid–base status. Sputum should be Gram-stained, cultured, and checked for acid-fast bacilli and fungi. A routine chest radiograph may be normal initially or may show segmental, lobar, or bilateral pulmonary infiltrates. Pulmonary tuberculosis may have an atypical radiographic presentation with higher incidence of lower-lobe disease, cavitation, pleural effusion, and multilobe involvement.

Table 4
Treatment of Selected Infections in Patients with Diabetes

Infection	*Preferred drugs*[a]	*Alternative drugs*[a]	*Other treatment*
Urinary tract—acute bacterial cystitis	Trimethoprim-sulfamethoxazole, double strength, 1 pill twice daily	Fluoroquinolones (e.g., Ciprofloxacin 250 mg, twice daily, or ofloxacin 200 mg, twice daily	
Fungal cystitis	Fluconazole, 200 mg, orally on d 1, then 100 mg/d for 4 d	Amphotericin B bladder irrigation (50 mg/L of sterile water at 40 mL/h for 24–48 h), or single dose of amphotericin B, 0.3 mg/kg	Removal of urinary catheter
Acute pyelonephritis	Fluoroquinolones (e.g., ciprofloxacin 400 mg, intravenously every 12 h, or ofloxacin 400 mg, every 12 h)	Ampicillin, 2 g intravenously every 6 h, plus gentamycin 5 mg/kg every 24 h, or ceftriaxone, 2 g, intravenously per day, or piperacillin, 3 g intravenously every 6 h	Early surgical intervention if emphysematous pyelonephritis
Perinephric abscess (associated with staphylococcal bacteremia)	Nafcillin, 2 g intravenously every 4 h	Cefazolin, 2 g, intravenously every 8 h, or vancomycin, 15 mg/kg intravenously every 6 h	Surgical drainage
Community-acquired pneumonia (outpatient management)	Macrolide (e.g., erythromycin, 500 mg, orally every 6 h, or azithromycin, 500 mg, orally on d 1, then 250 mg/d on d 2–5)	Doxycycline, 100 mg, twice daily	
Community-acquired pneumonia (hospitalized patient)	Cefuroxime, 0.75 g, intravenously every 6 h, or ceftriaxone, 1–2 g, intravenously per day; consider adding erythromycin, 0.5–1.0 g, intravenously every 6 h (or azithromycin, 500 mg, intravenously per day, or doxycycline, 100 mg, intravenously every 12 h)	Levofloxacin, 500 mg, intravenously every 24 h, or doxycycline, 100 mg, intravenously every 12 h	
Invasive otitis externa	Ciprofloxacin, 400 mg, intravenously every 12 h, and topical antipseudomonal or acetic acid drops	Ceftazidime, 2 g, intravenously every 8 h, or imipenem, 500 mg, intravenously every 6 h	Surgical debridement
Rhinocerebral mucormycosis	Amphotericin B, target dose, 1.0–1.5 mg/kg/d; total dose, 2.5–3.0 g		Surgical debridement; aggressive management of ketoacidosis (if present)

(continued)

Table 4 *(continued)*

Infection	*Preferred drugs*[a]	*Alternative drugs*[a]	*Other treatment*
Necrotizing fasciitis	Penicillin G, 24 million U intravenously per day, plus clindamycin, 900 mg, intravenously every 8 h, and gentamycin, 5 mg/kg, intravenously per day	Ceftriaxone, 2 g, intravenously every 24 h, plus clindamycin, 900 mg, intravenously every 8 h	Prompt surgical debridement
Emphysematous cholecystitis	Ampicillin-sulbactam, 3 g intravenously every 6 h	Ampicillin, 2 g, intravenously every 6 h, plus gentamycin, 5 mg/kg every 24 h, plus clindamycin, 900 mg, intravenously every 8 h (or metronidazole, loading dose of 15 mg/kg, intravenously, followed by 7.5 mg/kg, intravenously every 6 h), or ceftriaxone, 2 g intravenously every 24 h plus clindamycin (or metronidazole)	Emergency cholecystectomy required

[a] All doses are for normal renal and hepatic function.

Empiric antimicrobial agents for community-acquired pneumonia include macrolides, β-lactam agents, and newer quinilones (*see* Table 4). Aminoglycosides are used with caution in view of renal dysfunction in diabetic patients and the potential for ototoxicity. Antimicrobial drug regimens for the treatment of tuberculosis are similar to those used in nondiabetic patients; pyridoxine is an important adjunct to reduce the frequency of isoniazid induced neuropathy.

Soft Tissue Infections

It is well recognized that both bacterial and fungal deep soft tissue infections occur with increased frequency in the diabetic population. Pyomyositis refers to infection of muscle without infection of contiguous tissue. This infection by *St. aureus* occurs in muscles that have recently undergone trauma, often a minor strain or light blunt injury leading to hematoma formation. Pyogenic organisms reach the site hematogenously and lead to abscess formation. Clinical features include fever, pain, and swelling with pockets of pus formation. Computed tomography (CT) scan or magnetic resonance imaging (MRI) define the location and extent of disease involvement. Empiric antibiotic therapy directed toward *St. aureus* and CT-guided or open incision and drainage is required.

Cutaneous mucormycosis caused by organisms of the Mucoraceae family incuding *Rhizopus, Mucor,* and *Absidia* genera leads to infection that may be mild or result in gangrene. Biopsy shows invasion of skin by hyphal elements. Treatment involves surgical debridement and intravenous amphotericin B.

Specific soft tissue infections are discussed later in the chapter.

INFECTIONS OCCURRING PREDOMINANTLY IN PATIENTS WITH DIABETES

Malignant Otitis External/Invasive Otitis Externa

This potentially life-threatening condition occurs in elderly diabetic patients and involves the external auditory canal and skull. *Pseudomonas aeruginosa* is the most common etiologic agent. However, it has also been described secondary to colonization of the external ear canal by *Aspergillus* species *(28)*.

Presenting clinical features include ear discharge, severe pain, and hearing impairment, often in the absence of fever. Examination of the auditory canal shows edema, intense cellulitis, and polypoid granulation tissue. Cranial osteomyelitis and intracranial spread of infection may occur *(29)*. There may be involvement of the facial nerve.

Gram's stain, culture, and biopsy of debrided necrotic tissue distinguishes this condition from uncomplicated noninvasive otitis externa. MRI is useful in defining soft tissue and bone involvement. Some studies have reported utility of gallium-67 single-photon emission tomography in the clinical management and follow up of malignant otitis externa *(30)*.

Early referral to an otolaryngologist can be life-saving. Treatment involves repeated surgical debridement of necrotic tissue. Systemic therapy consists of antipseudomonal antibiotics, including quinolones, imipenem, or cephalosporins with antipseudomonal coverage. Adjunctive topical therapy includes antibiotics or acetic acid drops. Duration of therapy is often 4–6 wk or longer. Failure to respond to above therapy should raise suspicion of colonization with *Aspergillus* species.

Rhinocerebral Mucormycosis

Almost 50% of cases of rhinocerebral mucormycosis occur in patients with diabetes *(31)*. Fungi of the *Rhizopus* and *Mucor* species are the most common etiologic agents of this clinical entity. These fungi are ubiquitous saprophytic organisms, not uncommonly infecting the immunocompromised host *(32)*. Ketoacidosis temporarily disrupts host defense mechanisms, thereby permitting growth of *Rhizopus oryzae*. Such growth is inhibited by correcting acidosis *(33)*. These fungi have a predilection to invade blood vessels, causing infarction and necrosis.

Five clinical forms of mucormycosis are described: rhinocerebral, pulmonary, gastrointestinal, primary cutaneous, and disseminated, of which rhinocerebral has the highest frequency and mortality *(32)*. Disease onset may be with nasal stuffiness, epistaxis, and facial or ocular pain. A unique physical finding is a characteristic black necrotic eschar on the nasal turbinates or palate *(34)*. Later, proptosis and chemosis may occur. This may be accompanied by fever and varying degrees of obtundation. Ophthalmoplegia may be present. Complications include cavernous sinus thrombosis with multiple cranial nerve palsies, visual loss, brain abscesses, and carotid artery or jugular vein thrombosis with associated neurological deficits.

Swab cultures from the eschar site are usually inadequate for diagnosis, as the organism is invasive and not often superficial *(35)*. Punch biopsy of the lesion followed by fungal stains and culture confirm the diagnosis. Histologic examination reveals broad, nonseptate, haphazardly branching hyphae invading tissue. Blood culture has a low yield. CT or MRI scans of the head reveal air-fluid levels in the sinuses as well as involvement of the deep tissues of the nose, cavernous sinus, and central nervous system.

Aggressive surgical debridement and drainage of infected sinuses along with systemic amphotericin B and tight glycemic control is crucial *(14)*. Liposomal amphotericin B has been used *(36,37)*.

Necrotizing Fasciitis (Meleney's Synergistic Gangrene, Acute Dermal Gangrene, Necrotizing Erysipelas)

This is an uncommon soft tissue infection that spreads along fascial planes with relative initial sparing of skin and underlying muscle. As the infection progresses, necrosis of the overlying skin occurs as a result of thrombosis of cutaneous vessels.

Bacteriologically, two types of infection are described. Type I infection is caused by a combination of at least one anaerobe and one or more facultative anaerobes such as streptococci or enterobacteriaceae. Type II infection is caused by group A β-hemolytic streptococci alone or in combination with staphylococci *(38)*. Recently, Howard et al. have described necrotizing fasciitis on exposure of nonintact skin to salt-water-borne halophilic marine *vibrios (39)*. Tissue damage and systemic toxicity are as a result of release of endogenous cytokines and bacterial toxins.

The most common sites for infection include the abdominal wall, perineum, and extremities. Visceral metastatic abscesses may form in various viscera. The source of introduction of the pathogen may be unknown or may follow surgery *(40)*, minor trauma, or hematogenous spread from a distant site. Most cases involving the vulva occur in obese diabetic patients and often begin as Bartholin's gland duct abscess or a vulvar abscess *(41,42)*.

Severe local pain with relative paucity of local signs of inflammation characterize early disease *(43)*. Fever and systemic toxicity may be marked. An erythematous, swollen, tender, hot area of cellulitis spreads along unseen fascial planes to involve contiguous areas away from the original site of involvement.

Thrombosis leads to serous and subsequently hemorrhagic bullae, gangrene, ulceration, and "dishwater pus" because of liquefactive necrosis. Lymphadenitis and lymphangitis are rare. Crepitance is palpable in approximately half of the cases. Destruction of subcutaneous nerves leads to anesthesia.

Early diagnosis is aided by a high index of suspicion and the ability to pass a probe unimpeded along normally adherent fascial planes *(44)*. The necrotic center of the lesion is preferred for obtaining both aerobic and anaerobic cultures and Gram's stain in contrast to the leading edge of the lesion in cellulitis. Plain radiographs, ultrasonography, CT scan, and MRI may aid the diagnosis by detecting soft tissue gas and define extent of disease.

Surgical intervention forms the cornerstone of therapy. Early and adequate surgical debridement and fasciotomy play a key role in reducing mortality. Antibiotics are very important adjunctive therapy. The choice of antibiotics include penicillin or cephalosporins in combination with an aminoglycoside and anaerobic coverage with either clindamycin or metronidazole. Following initial empiric therapy, continued antibiotic therapy can be tailored according to culture and susceptibility results.

Fournier's Gangrene

This is a syndrome of synergistic, polymicrobial, necrotizing fasciitis of the perineum, scrotum, and penis. The prevalence of coexisting diabetes ranges from 32% to 60% *(45,46)*. Other predisposing factors include alcoholism, steroid use, cancer chemotherapy, and acquired imnunodeficiency syndrome (AIDS) *(47)*.

Various aerobic and anaerobic bacteria causing coinfection include *E. coli, Bacteroides,* staphylococci, *Proteus* species, streptococci, *Pseudomonas* species, and enterococci. *Clostridium perfringens* is present in more than 90% of cases with myonecrosis *(48).*

Clinically, this condition begins with a prodromal phase of malaise and scrotal discomfort that progresses to frank scrotal pain and clinical toxicity. Cutaneous manifestations include blistering, induration, bronzing, necrosis, and ulceration. In later stages, scrotal swelling, foul-smelling discharge, and crepitance develop. Pain may decrease with the onset of gangrene *(49).* Rarely, Fournier's gangrene may be the initial clinical presentation of diabetes *(50).*

Diagnosis is mainly clinical. Plain films of the abdomen may reveal subcutaneous gas prior to crepitance being appreciated. Proctoscopy may show the source of infection as well as the extent of anal and rectal involvement. A retrograde urethrogram will define the necessity for suprapubic diversion in the case of massive urinary extravasation. Ultrasound findings may include normal testes, a thickened scrotal wall, and subcutaneous gas. Specialized techniques like CT and MRI can identify the underlying treatable cause and extent of involvement.

Fournier's gangrene is a surgical emergency. Extensive unroofing is necessary. Urinary or fecal diversion and laparotomy may be required. Typically, the bladder, rectum, and testes will be spared from necrosis because of their separate, nonperineal blood supply. Rarely, orchiectomy may be necessary *(50).* The choice of antibiotics is similar to that for necrotizing fasciitis. Supportive care includes volume expanders, blood, clotting factors, and sufficient supplemental calories. Hemodialysis may be required in a few cases *(49).* Although controversial, hyperbaric oxygen therapy has given excellent results in some cases *(46,51).*

Mortality rates for Fournier's gangrene are high. Advanced age, extensive disease, deranged renal functions, sepsis, and shock are factors that predict a poor clinical outcome.

Emphysematous Cholecystitis

Emphysematous cholecystitis is a rare variant of acute cholecystitis caused by ischemia of the gallbladder wall and infection with gas-producing organisms. Approximately 35–55% of cases have underlying diabetes mellitus *(52–54).* It is thought to result from acalculous cystic duct obstruction, with inflammatory edema eventually causing cystic artery occlusion. Colonization by gas-forming organisms causes coagulative necrosis of the mucosa, venous congestion, gangrene, and eventually, gallbladder perforation. Gallstones are present in only 50% of patients with emphysematous cholecystitis. Bacteria most frequently cultured include anaerobes, such as *Clostridium* species, and aerobes, such as *E. coli.*

Although clinically similar to acute cholecystitis, some differences are notable. This condition has a male predominance, gangrene of the gallbladder and perforation are more frequent, and the overall mortality is substantially higher (15% vs less than 4%) than in patients with acute cholecystitis. The clinical manifestations may be otherwise indistinguishable from acute cholecystitis. Patients may present with biliary colic, anorexia, nausea, vomiting, and fever with chills. Toxicity is marked and jaundice may develop in the late stages because of obstruction of bile ducts. The gallbladder may be palpable in one-quarter to one-half of patients. Murphy's sign (characteristic tenderness on palpation of the right upper quadrant) may be absent in some cases because of underlying diabetic neuropathy. Crepitus on palpation is an omnious sign. Gangrene, localized perforation sealed by the omentum, abscess formation, or generalized peritonitis are dreaded complications.

Plain X-ray is diagnostic. Gas appears 1–2 d after onset of symptoms in the lumen or within the gallbladder wall as a distinctive gaseous ring. CT scan is more sensitive and shows similar findings. Ultrasound reveals high-level echoes outlining the gallbladder wall.

Initiation of appropriate antibiotics and early cholecystectomy is crucial. Laparoscopic cholecystectomy has been described as safe and feasible *(55)*.

Emphysematous Pyelonephritis and Cystitis

Emphysematous pyelonephritis is a rare necrotizing infection of the renal parenchyma and perirenal tissue that is characterized by gas formation in the intrarenal and perirenal spaces. The most common causative bacterial pathogen causing this infection is *E. coli.* Hyperglycemia and ishemic necrosis of renal parenchyma as a result of microangiopathy produce an ideal substrate for growth of microrganisms. *Escherichia coli, Proteus mirabilis,* and *Klebsiella pneumoniae* ferment glucose, lactate, and products from necrotic tissue to carbon dioxide, hydrogen, nitrogen and unknown gases, resulting in the accumulation of gas in tissue *(56,57)*. Over 90% of cases occur in diabetic patients *(58)* and may accompany ureteral obstruction. Papillary necrosis can complicate it in about 21% of cases *(59)*.

The symptoms are suggestive of acute pyelonephritis and include chills and fever, flank pain, nausea and vomiting, dysuria, lethargy, and altered sensorium. Spread of infection to perirenal space produces a crepitus *(60,61)*. Contralateral flank pain may occur. This reflects an atypical "mirror pain" secondary to a renal or ureteric calculus *(62)*. Bilateral involvement may occur infrequently.

The failure of fever to resolve after 3–4 d of treatment of UTI should raise the possibility of this infection. Laboratory investigations reveal leucocytosis, hyperglycemia, azotemia, and pyuria. Screening abdominal films demonstrate air in the renal parenchyma in 85% of cases *(63)*. Ultrasound reveals similar findings. Intravenous programs may show obstruction but can be hazardous in view of deranged renal function. CT scanning is the diagnostic test of choice. Type I emphysematous pyelonephritis refers to renal necrosis with a total absence of fluid content on CT scan or the presence of a mottled, streaky gas pattern on radiograph, or CT scan with lung window display. This has a poor prognosis. Type II emphysematous pyelonephritis is characterized by the presence of renal or perirenal fluid and a bubbly, loculated gas pattern, or the presence of gas in the collecting system and has a better outcome. Other poor prognostic factors include a serum creatinine of greater than 1.4 mg/dL and thrombocytopenia *(64)*.

Initial treatment, in addition to actively controlling hyperglycemia, consists of appropriate intravenous antibiotics and vigorous hydration. Nephrectomy has been considered standard surgical treatment. However, a more conservative approach with antibiotics, insulin, and drainage of the affected kidney has been described *(65)*.

Other Emphysematous Infections

Emphysematous pyelitis is distinguished from emphysematous pyelonephritis in that gas is localized to the renal collecting system, X-ray reveals gas following the outline of the renal pelvis, intravenous antibiotics and relieving obstruction are sufficient therapy, and overall mortality is lower *(66)*.

Emphysematous cystitis is a rare disease. Characteristic features include pneumaturia or hematuria. It is associated with vesicocolic or vesicovaginal fistula. X-Ray abdomen shows air in the bladder wall, intramural air bubbles, or air-fluid level in the lumen. Antibiotics and relief of bladder outlet obstruction are therapeutic.

Renal Papillary Necrosis

Necrosis and sloughing of the renal papillae is five times more prevalent in diabetic than nondiabetic patients and can lead to acute or slowly progressive renal failure. The patient has fever and persistent flank pain despite being on antibiotics. Other noninfectious causes like analgesic abuse, obstruction, and sickle cell disease have to be ruled out. Voided medullary tissue may be present on urinalysis. Although ultrasound or CT scan may be done, retrograde pyelogram is diagnostic. A "ring sign" is present when a separated papilla is surrounded by contrast medium *(67)*. This may show characteristic calcification *(68)*. Parenteral antibiotics, drainage to relieve obstruction, and dialysis support, if required, are the mainstay of treatment.

MICRO-ORGANISMS STRONGLY ASSOCIATED WITH INFECTIONS IN PATIENTS WITH DIABETES

Patients with diabetes sem to be at a disproportionately high risk for infections with certain micro-organisms. The prevalence of diabetes was reported to be 27.5% in one study of nonpreganant adults with group B streptococcal bacteremia *(69)*. Several series report an incidence of underlying diabetes of up to 30–60% in patients with a variety of *Klebsiella* infections such as bacteremia, liver abscess, thyroid abscess, and endophthalmitis *(70–73)*. Among enteric pathogens, *Campylobacter* and *Salmonella enteritidis* have been reported with increased frequency in patients with diabetes *(74,75)*. There is a strong association of diabetes with chronic hepatitis C virus (HCV) *(76)*. Additionally, patients with HCV-related cirrhosis have an increased incidence of diabetes compared to patients with cirrhosis resulting from other causes *(77,78)*. Although an increased incidence of staphylococcal infections has been noted in diabetic patients, a careful recent review did not confirm this association *(79)*.

The association of candidal infection and diabetes has been well known. Candidiasis in patients with diabetes is generally localized. Intertrigenous candidiasis involves moist skin folds of inframammary, axillary, inguinal and intergluteal areas, and webs of fingers and toes in obese individuals. It produces characteristic beefy red plaques surrounded by satellite pustules or papules. Candida vulvovaginitis is common in women with diabetes *(14)*. Oropharyngeal candidiasis is a well-documented complication of uncontrolled diabetes mellitus.

Although the overall incidence of AIDS in patients with diabetes may not be higher than in the general population, metabolic adverse effects of drug therapy in AIDS may result in hyperglycemia. Pentamidine therapy in the treatment of *Pneumocystis carinii* pneumonia affects glucose homeostasis and may result in hypoglycemia or hyperglycemia with clinical diabetes. Use of protease inhibitors (PIs) for supression of HIV-1 replication has been associated with hyperglycemia, insulin resistance, and new-onset diabetes *(80,81)*.

INFECTIONS RESULTING FROM IATROGENIC CAUSES

Infection occurring from self-injection of insulin is quite uncommon. In one study, no injection site infection was demonstrated despite a lack of "traditional practices," such as cleaning the vial and skin or even washing hands before injection *(82)*. More recently, it has been demonstrated that it is therapeutically effective to administer insulin through clothing. Further, such practice is not associated with an increased incidence of infection However, it is not uncommon to develop needle-site abscesses in patients on subcutaneous insulin infusion (SII) *(83)*.

Diabetic patients constitute a significant minority of individuals undergoing penile implants. Several studies have failed to demonstrate an increase in rate of infection is noted in the diabetic host *(84)*. Similarly, although underlying diabetes is a common problem in patients with end-stage renal disease on dialysis therapy, infection rates in patients on continuous ambulatory peritoneal dialysis (CAPD) are comparable to nondiabetic subjects *(85)*. This is also true for patients receiving chronic intermittent peritoneal dialysis *(86)*.

OTHER ISSUES RELATING TO INFECTION AND DIABETES

Current guidelines from the Centers for Diseases Control (CDC) recommend that all diabetic patients receive influenza and pneumococcal vaccination. Despite these recommendations, a recent review by the CDC and the Council of State and Territorial Epidemiologists (CSTE) suggested that only 52% of diabetic patients reported receiving the influenza vaccination in the past 12 mo and only 33.2% recalled receiving pneumococcal vaccination at all. When prescribing antibiotics in the diabetic patient, particular caution is warranted to avoid nephrotoxicity as well as the potential for eye toxicity. Also, when administering oral antibiotics, the effects of gastropathy on oral absorption should be considered. Maintenance of good hygiene, particularly in the context of foot care, is crucial in patients with diabetes.

REFERENCES

1. Wheat LJ. Infection and diabetes mellitus. Diabetes Care 1980;3:187–197.
2. Delamaire M, Maugendre D, Moreno M, et al. Impaired leucocyte function in diabetic patients. Diabet Med 1997;14:29–34.
3. Gallacher SJ, Thomson G, Fraser WD, et al. Neutrophil bactericidal function in diabetes mellitus: evidence for association with blood glucose control. Diabet Med 1995;12:916–920.
4. Marhoffer W, Stein M, Maeser E, Federlin K. Impairment of polymorphonuclear leucocyte function and metabolic control of diabetes. Diabetes Care 1992;15:256–260.
5. Calvet HM, Yoshikawa TT. Infections in diabetes. Infect Dis Clin North Am 2001;15:407–421.
6. MacRury SM, Gemmell CG, Paterson KR, et al. Changes in phagocytic function with glycemic control in diabetic patients. J Clin Pathol 1989;42:1143–1157.
7. Hostetter MK. Handicaps to host defences: effects of hyperglycemia on C3 and *Candida albicans.* Diabetes 1990;39:271–175.
8. Ling P, Bistrian B, Mendez B, et al. Effects of systemic infusion of endotoxin, tumour necrosis factor, and interleukin-1 on glucose metabolism in the rat: relationship to endogenous glucose metabolism and peripheral tissue glucose uptake. Metabolism 1994;43:279–284.
9. Sobel JD. Pathogenesis of urinary tract infection-role of host defences. Infect Dis Clin North Am 1997;11(3):531–549.
10. Bonadio M, Meini M, Gigli C, et al. Urinary tract infection in diabetic patients. Urol Int 1999;63(4):215–219.
11. Geerlings SE. Asymptomatic bacteruria may be considered a complication in women with diabetes. Diabetes Mellitus Women ASB Utrecht Study Group. Diabetes Care 2000;23:744–749.
12. Geerlings SE, Stolk RP, Camps MJL, et al. Risk factors for symptomatic urinary tract infection in women with diabetes. Diabetes Care 2000;23:1737–1741.
13. Frimodt-Moller C. Diabetic cystopathy I–IV. Dan Med Bull 1976;23:267–294.
14. Vasquez JA, Sobel JD. Fungal infections in diabetes. Infect Dis Clin North Am 1995;9:97–116.
15. Ellenbogen PH, Talner LB. Uroradiology of diabetes mellitus. Urology 1976;8:413–419.

16. Edelstein H, Mc Cabe RE. Perinephric abcess: modern diagnosis and treatment in 47 cases. Medicine (Balt) 1988;67:118–131.
17. Thorley JD, Jones SR, Sanford JP. Perinephric abcess. Medicine (Balt) 1974;53:441–451.
18. Wong-Beriger A, Jacobs RA, Guglielmo J. Treatment of funguria. JAMA 1992;20:2780–2785.
19. Wise GJ, Kozinn PJ, Goldberg P. Amphotericin B as a urologic irrigant in the management of noninvasive candiduria. J Urol 1982;128:82–84.
20. Fisher JF, Hicks BC, Dipiro JT, Venable J, Fincher RM. Efficacy of a single intravenous dose of amphotericin B in urinary tract infections caused by Candida. J Infect Dis 1987;156:685–687.
21. Leu HS, Huang CT. Clearance of funguria with short-course antifungal regimens: a prospective, randomized, controlled study. Clin Infect Dis 1995;20:1152–1157.
22. Woodhead MA, Macfarlane JT, McCracken JS, et al. Prospective study of the etiology and outcome of pneumonia in the community. Lancet 1987;1:671–674.
23. Fine MJ, Smith MA, Crason CA, et al. Prognosis and outcomes of patients with community-acquired pneumonia: a meta-analysis. JAMA 1996;257:134–141.
24. Koziel H, Koziel MJ. Pulmonary complications of diabetes mellitus:pneumonia. Infect Dis Clin North Am 1995;9:65–96.
25. Marrie TJ. Bacteraemic pneumococcal pneumonia: a continuously evolving disease. J Infect 1992;24:247–255.
26. Bouter KP, Diepersloot RJ, van Romunde LK, et al. Effect of epidemic influenza on ketoacidosis, pneumonia and death in diabetes mellitus: a hospital register survey of 1976–1979 in the Netherlands. Diabetes Res Clin Pract 1991;12:61–68.
27. Lipsky BA, Pecoraro RE, Chen MS, et al. Factors affecting staphylococcal colonization among NIDDM outpatients. Diabetes Care 1987;10:483.
28. Phillips P, Bryce G, Shepherd J, et al. Invasive external otitis caused by Aspergillus. Rev Infect Dis 1990;12:277–281.
29. Slattery WH III, Brackmann DE. Skull base osteomyelitis: malignant external otitis. Otolaryngol Clin North Am 1996;29:795–806.
30. Stokkel MP, Takes RP, van Eck-Smit BL, Baatenburg de Jong RJ. The value of quantitative gallium-67 single-photon emission tomography in the clinical management of malignant external otitis. Eur J Nucl Med 1997;24:1429–1432.
31. Joshi N, Caputo GM, Weitekamp MR, et al. Primary care: infections in patients with diabetes mellitus. N Engl J Med 1999;341:1906–1912.
32. Rinaldi MG. Zygomycosis. Infect Dis Clin North Am 1989;3:19–41.
33. Artis WM, Fountain JA, Delcher HK, Jones HE. A mechanism of susceptibility to mucormycosis in diabetic ketoacidosis: transferrin and iron availability. Diabetes 1982;31(12):1109–1114.
34. Smith HW, Kirchner JA. Cerebral mucormycosis: a report of three cases. Arch Otolaryngol 1958;68:715–726.
35. Cunha BA. Infections in non leukopenic compromised hosts (diabetes mellitus, SLE, steroids, and asplenia) in critical care. Crit Care Clin 1998;14(2):263–282.
36. Raj P, Vella EJ, Bickerton RC. Successful treatment of rhinocerebral mucormycosis by a combination of aggressive surgical debridement and the use of systemic liposomal amphotericin B and local therapy with nebulized amphotericin—a case report. J Laryngol Otol 1998;112:367–370.
37. Saltoglu N, Tasova Y, Zorludemir S, et al. Rhinocerebral zygomycosis treated with liposomal amphotericin B and surgery. Mycoses 1998;41:45–49.
38. Giuliano A, Lewis F, Hadley K, et al. Bacteriology of Necrotizing fasciitis. Am J Surg 1977;134:52–57.
39. Howard RJ, Bennett NT. Infections caused by halophilic marine *Vibrio* bacteria. Ann Surg 1993;217:525–531.
40. McHenry CR, Piotrowskii JJ, Petrinic D, et al. Determinants of mortality for necrotizing soft-tissue infections. Ann Surg 1995;221:558–565.
41. Farley DE, Katz VL, Dotters DJ. Toxic shock syndrome associated with vulvar necrotizing fasciitis. Obstet Gynecol 1993;82:660–662.
42. Jayatunga AP, Kaplan S, Paes TRF. Survival after retroperitoneal nacrotizing fasciitis. Br J Surg 1993;80:981.
43. Ward RG, Walsh MS. Necrotizing fasciitis: 10 years' experience in a district general hospital. Br J Surg 1991;78:488–489.
44. Chelsom J, Halstenen A, Haga T, et al. Necrotizing fasciitis due to group A streptococci in western Norway: incidence and clinical features. Lancet 1994;344:1111–1115.

45. Clayton MD, Fowler JE Jr, Sharifi R, et al. Causes, presentation and survival of 57 patients with necrotizing fasciitis of the male genitalia. Surg Gynaecol Obstet 1990;170:49–55.
46. Smith GL, Bunker CB, Dinneen MD. Fournier's gangrene. Br J Urol 1998;81:347–355.
47. Elem B, Ranjan P. Impact of immunodeficiency virus (HIV) on Fournier's gangrene: Observations in Zambia. Ann R Coll Surg Engl 1995;77:283–286.
48. Paty R, Smith AD. Gangrene and Fournier's gangrene. Urol Clin North Am 1992;19:149–162.
49. Vick R, Carson CC. Fournier's disease. Urol Clin North Am 1999;26:841–849.
50. Cheng TJ. Fournier's gangrene as the initial clinical manifestation of diabetes mellitus. J Formos Med Assoc 1996;95(2):184–186.
51. Pizzorno R, Bonini F, Donelli F, et al. Hyperbaric oxygen therapy in the treatment of Fournier's disease in 11 male patients. J Urol 1997;158:837–840.
52. Abengowe CU, McManamon PJM. Acute emphysematous cholecystitis. Can Med Assoc J 1974;111:1112–1114.
53. Mentzer RM, Golden GT, Chandler JG, Horsley JS. A comparative appraisal of emphysematous cholecystitis. Am J Surg 1975;129:10–15.
54. Tellez LG, Rodriguez-Montes JA, de Lis SF, Marten LG. Acute emphysematous cholecystitis: report of twenty cases. Hepatogastroenterology 1999;46:2144–2148.
55. Banwell PE, Hill AD, Menzies-Gow N, Darzi A. Laparoscopic cholecystectomy: safe and feasible in emphysematous cholecystitis. Surg Laporos Endosc 1994;4:189–191.
56. Huang J, Chen K. Ruann M. Mixed acid fermentation of glucose as a mechanism of emphysematous urinary tract infection. J Urol 1991;146:148–151.
57. Yang W, Shen N. Gas-forming infection of the urinary tract: an investigation of fermentation as a mechanism. J Urol 1990;143:960–964.
58. Smitherman KO, Peacock JE Jr. Infectious emergencies in patients with diabetes mellitus. Med Clin North Am 1995;79:53–77.
59. Michaeli J, Mogle P, Perlberg S, Heiman S, Caine M. Emphysematous pyelonephritis. J Urol 1984;131:203–208.
60. Ahlering TC, Boyd SD, Hamilton CL, et al. Emphysematous pyelonephritis: a five year experience with 13 patients. J Urol 1985;134:1086–1088.
61. Pappas S, Peppas TA, Sotiropoulas A, et al. Emphysematous pyelonephritis: a case report and review of literature. Diabet Med 1993;10:574–576.
62. Clark AJ, Norman RW. "Mirror pain" as an unusual presentation of renal colic. Urology 1998;51:116–118.
63. Evanoff GV, Thompson CS, Foley R, et al. Spectrum of gas within the kidney: emphysematous pyelonephritis and pyelitis. Am J Med 1987;83:149–154.
64. McGorry DM, Kroser, J. Teekel-Taylor L, et al. Emphysematous pyelonephritis presenting as an acute abdomen. Infect Urol 1999;23:162–165.
65. George J, Chakravarthy S, John GT, et al. Bilateral emphysematous pyelonephritis responding to non surgical management. Am J Nephrol 1995;15:172–174.
66. Patterson JE, Andriole VT. Bacterial urinary tact infections in diabetes. Infect Dis Clin North Am 1997;11:735–750.
67. Ellenbogen PH, Talner LB. Uroradiology of diabetes mellitus. Urology 1976;8:413–419.
68. Rodriguez-de- Velasquez A, Yoder IC, Velasquez PA, et al. Imaging the effects of diabetes in the genitourinary system. Radiographics 1995;15:1051.
69. Farley MM, Harvey RC, Stull T, et al. A population based assessment of invasive disease due to group B streptococcus in nonpregnent adults. N Engl J Med 1993;328:1807–1811.
70. Leibovici L, Samra Z, Konisberger H, Kalter-Leibovici O, Pitlik SD, Drucker M, Bacteremia in adult diabetic patients. Diabetes Care 1991;14:89–94.
71. Wang JH, Liu YC, Lee SS, et al. Primary liver abcess due to Klebsiella pneumoniae in Taiwan. Clin Infect Dis 1998;26:1434–1438.
72. Chee SP, Ang CL. Endogenous *Klebsiella* endophthalmitis – a case series. Ann Acad Med Singapore 1995;24:473–478.
73. Li CC, Wang CH, Tsan KW. Graves' disease and diabetes mellitus associated with acute suppurative thyroiditis: a case report. Chung Hua I Hsueh Tsa Chih (Taipei) 1997;59:59–64.
74. Neal K, Slack R. Diabetes mellitus, antisecretory drugs and other risk factors for *Campylobacter* gastro-enteritis in adults: a case control study. Epidemiol Infect 1997;119:307–311.
75. Telzak EE, Greenberg MSZ, Budnick LD, et al. Diabetes mellitus—a newly described risk factor for infection with *Salmonella enteritidis*. J Infect Dis 1991;164:538–541.

76. Fraser GM, Harman I, Meller N, et al. Diabetes mellitus is associated with chronic hepatitis C but not chronic hepatitis B infection. Israel J Med Sci 1996;32:526.
77. Allison M, Wreghitt T, Palmer C, et al. Evidence for a link between hepatitis C virus and infection and diabetes mellitus in a cirrhotic population. J Hepatol 1994;21:1135.
78. Farell FJ, Keeffe EB. Diabetes and the hepatobiliary system. Clin Liver Dis 1998;2:119–131.
79. Breen JD, Karchmer AW. *Staphylococcus aureus* infections in diabetic patients. Infect Dis Clin North Am 1995;9:11–24.
80. Tsiodras S, Mantzoros C, Hammer S, Samore M. Effects of protease inhibitors on hyperglycemia, hyperlipidemia, and lipodystrophy—a five year cohort study. Arch Intern Med 2000;160:2050–2056.
81. Carr A, Samaras K, Thorisdottir A, Kaufmann GR, et al. Diagnosis, prediction, and natural course of HIV-1 protease inhibitor-associated lipodystrophy, hyperlipidaemia, and diabetes mellitus: a cohort study. Lancet 1999;353:2093–2099.
82. Borders LM, Bingham PR, Riddle MC. Traditional insulin-use practices and incidence of bacterial contamination and infection. Diabetes Care 1984;7:121–127.
83. Brink SJ, Stewart C. Insulin pump treatment in insulin dependent diabetic children, adolescents and young adults. JAMA 1986;255:617–621.
84. Montague DK. Periprosthetic infections. J Urol 1987;138:68–69.
85. Amair P, Khanna R, Leibel B, et al. Continuous ambulatory peritoneal dialysis in diabetics with end-stage renal disease. N Engl J Med 1982;306:625–630.
86. Kraus ES, Spector DA. Characteristics and sequelae of peritonitis in diabetics and nondiabetics receiving chronic intermittent peritoneal dialysis. Medicine (Balt) 1983;62:52–57.

29 Pancreas Transplantation

R. Paul Robertson, MD

CONTENTS

INTRODUCTION

Pancreas transplantation is viewed by many as a last resort for diabetic patients undergoing great difficulty controlling their glucose levels despite intensive medical management, which usually involves a trial of continuous subcutaneous insulin infusion through a portable pump. Relegation of pancreas transplantation to the position of last resort arguably results in its not being considered as often as it should be. Even in the 21st century, when we know the success rate for pancreas transplantation is comparable to those for other organs, this procedure is not considered as often as is transplantation of the liver, kidney, lung, and heart. The reason that is usually given is that diabetes mellitus is not as life threatening as diseases that culminate in transplantation of the other organs. This therapeutic formulation is a debatable one, given the severity of secondary complications that diabetic patients encounter.

The purpose of this chapter is to examine the benefits of pancreas transplantation in the context of the challenge to tightly control glycemia in all diabetic patients. The chapter will recapitulate the history of pancreas transplantation, consider problems with the immunosuppressive drugs required to maintain the allograft, examine graft and the patient survival rates, consider the beneficial effects on glycemic control and chronic complications, and assess the overall risks of this procedure.

From: *Contemporary Endocrinology: Type 1 Diabetes: Etiology and Treatment*
Edited by: M. A. Sperling © Humana Press Inc., Totowa, NJ

THE NEED TO TIGHTLY CONTROL GLYCEMIA

Until 1993, the need to intensively control glucose levels in patients with diabetes mellitus was frequently debated. In that year, however, publication of the results of the Diabetes Control and Complications Trial (DCCT) settled the argument *(1)*: 1441 patients with insulin-dependent diabetes mellitus were randomly assigned to intensive therapy, administered either with an external insulin pump or by multiple daily insulin injections, or to conventional therapy. The amount of insulin given in the intensively managed group was determined by frequent blood glucose monitoring. The patients assigned to conventional therapy were treated with one or two daily insulin injections. Patients were followed for an average of 7 yr with close attention to the appearance and progression of secondary complications. Intensive therapy reduced the adjusted mean risk for the development of retinopathy by 76% compared to conventional therapy. Intensive therapy also slowed the progression of existing retinopathy by 54%. Intensive therapy reduced the occurrence of microalbuminuria by 39%, albuminuria by 54%, and clinical neuropathy by 60%. The chief adverse affect associated with intensive therapy was an increase in severe hypoglycemia. Thus, this trial put to rest any doubts that tight control of glucose levels in type 1 diabetic patients would result in a lessening of the secondary complications of the disease.

The most difficult issue surrounding intensive therapy is the danger of unanticipated hypoglycemia. As with hyperglycemia and secondary complications, hypoglycemia and symptom unawareness are also associated with increased morbidity and mortality. Consequently, the insulin-treated patient is often faced with a difficult choice of less meticulous maintenance of glycemia and hemoglobin A1c levels in order to diminish the incidence of hypoglycemic reactions.

The normal defense mechanisms against hypoglycemia consist primarily of glucagon release from α-cells of the pancreatic islet followed shortly afterward by epinephrine release from the adrenal medulla *(2)*. Cortisol and growth hormone secretion serve more chronic, long-term protective roles. Glucagon released into the portal circulation travels quickly to hepatocytes to induce glycogenolysis, which releases glucose into the systemic circulation via the hepatic vein. Glucagon is normally secreted when circulating glucose levels reach 50–60 mg/dL. Soon thereafter, epinephrine is secreted and also stimulates glycogenolysis. In the early stages of diabetes mellitus, patients retain the ability to release glucagon and epinephrine during hypoglycemia. However, within several years, the glucagon response begins to diminish and is then lost in most patients *(3)*. Eventually, the epinephrine response is also compromised although not usually not totally absent *(4)*. The most serious aspect of this clinical scenario is that patients with recurrent hypoglycemia lose their ability to fully sense low circulating glucose levels in the 50- to 60-mg/dL range (*see* Chapter 7). The normal complement of symptoms include warmth, palpitations, hunger, and sweating. If severe, hypoglycemia can cause visual blurring, sleepiness, obtundation, confusion, and even death. Early in the disease, the diabetic patient quickly learns to depend on these signals to take corrective action to restore the glucose level to normal. With time, however, recurrent hypoglycemia gradually reduces the threshold for symptoms so they do not begin until the patient encounters glucose levels much lower than 50–60 mg/dL. Consequently, diabetic patients often encounter seriously low glucose levels—often as low as 25–35 mg/dL—without experiencing any symptoms.

It is now appreciated that avoidance of recurrent hypoglycemia relieves the diabetic patient of many of these problems *(5–7)*. Careful loosening of insulin-based management and avoidance of hypoglycemia allows a return of full symptom awareness and thereby lessens the risk for serious hypoglycemic episodes. However, this is frustrating for the diabetic patient who, by loosening glycemic control, is placed at a higher risk for the complications of chronic hyperglycemia. Hence, the ideal regimen would avoid both hyperglycemia and hypoglycemia.

HISTORY OF PANCREAS TRANSPLANTATION

The first pancreas transplantations in patients with type 1 diabetes were reported in 1966 *(8)*. Two patients with long-standing diabetes and end-stage renal disease underwent simultaneous pancreas and kidney transplantation. One patient had an extended period of insulin independence, but the other did not. Over the next decade, other pancreas transplantations were attempted, but these were met with limited success. Less than 10% of early transplant patients achieved and maintained insulin independence and normal glycemia. Only a small fraction were insulin independent 1 yr after transplantation.

Significant improvements in surgical technique, treatment of acute rejection, and management of immunosuppression and infection began in the late 1970s. More experience was gained in this procedure and success rates improved. This history has led to the current American Diabetes Association recommendations that (1) pancreas transplantation should be considered in patients scheduled to have a kidney transplantation because of end-stage diabetic renal disease and (2) pancreas transplantation alone should be considered without kidney transplantation if patients encounter frequent acute and severe metabolic complications, such as hypoglycemia, that require medical attention, despite rigorous attempts at insulin-based management to control glucose levels *(9)*.

PANCREAS TRANSPLANTATION: THE OPERATIVE PROCEDURE AND THE NEED FOR IMMUNOSUPPRESSIVE DRUGS

The usual source of a transplanted pancreas is a patient who has recently died (i.e., a cadaveric organ donation). Uncommonly, a segment (usually the distal half) of a pancreas that is donated by a living family member is used. The whole or segment of pancreas is transplanted into the pelvis of the recipient and iliac vessels of the recipient are used for arterial supply and venous drainage. However, this causes hyperinsulinemia because these vessels deliver insulin from the allograft directly into the systemic circulation, thereby bypassing the normal first-pass hepatic metabolism of the hormone before it reaches the systemic circulation *(10)*. More recently, attempts are being made to surgically construct portal venous drainage for pancreas grafts because of concerns about adverse consequences of hyperinsulinemia on blood pressure and atherosclerosis.

Usually, the transplanted pancreas is still attached to a small portion of the donor duodenum that contains the exit of the pancreatic duct. In one variation of the procedure, the duodenal segment and pancreatic duct outlet is oversewn onto the urinary bladder. An alternative approach is to use a portion of the small bowel rather than the bladder for drainage of the duodenal segment. Either approach allows the exocrine enzymes, such as amylase and lipase, to be safely excreted outside the body. Advantages of bladder drainage include the use of urinary amylase to monitor for rejection and the avoidance of small-bowel complications such as obstruction and infection. Advantages of enteric drainage include the avoidance of urinary infections, acidosis (resulting from loss of bicarbonate), hematuria, and reflex pancreatitis. In all variations, the native pancreas is left untouched so that it continues to deliver normal exocrine secretions for the recipient's small intestine.

Since the advent of pancreas transplantation, multiple immunosuppression regimens have been designed. Currently, the most conventional approach includes antibody induction with either a monoclonal or a polyclonal agent directed against T-cells. Long-term maintenance is provided by triple-drug therapy with a calcineurin inhibitor (cyclosporine or tacrolimus), an antimetabolite (usually mycophenolate mofetil), and corticosteroids. Most recently, attempts are being made to eliminate corticosteroids from chronic immunosuppressive maintenance because of their adverse effects on bone metabolism, susceptibility to infections, and cosmesis.

SURVIVAL OF GRAFTS AND PATIENTS

When the procedure of pancreas transplantation was originally devised, the organ and patient survival rates were very poor. The poor patient survival rates may have been more a reflection of the severity of diabetes in the patients in whom transplantation was attempted than the operative procedure itself. Since 1966, however, organ survival rate has improved dramatically. Between the years 1994 and 1997, the patient survival rate was greater than 93% at 1 and 3 yr posttransplant (*see* Fig. 1) whether the pancreas was transplanted alone (PTA), simultaneously with a kidney (SPK), or after a kidney has been transplanted previously (PAK) *(11)*. The majority of deaths was the result of cardiovascular disease and usually occurred more than 3 mo after discharge from the hospital. By comparison, the mortality rate 1 yr after the much less invasive procedure of pancreatic islet transplantation was 5% *(12)*. Consequently, it seems likely that the mortality rate associated with pancreas transplantation is more related to cardiovascular complications of chronic diabetes than to the operative procedure of transplantation itself.

Organ survival rates vary with the type of procedure. Between 1994 and 1997, these rates were 82% for SPK, 71% for PAK, and 62% for PTA (*see* Fig. 1) 1 yr after pancreas transplantation *(11)*. Three years after transplantation, these rates were 79%, 64%, and 52%, respectively. The lower survival for PTA is thought to be related to the fact that detection of pancreas rejection is made easier when the procedure is SPK or PAK because the serum creatinine increments during kidney rejection serve as sentinels for pancreas rejection. When a pancreas alone is transplanted with urinary bladder drainage of exocrine secretions, the less sensitive indices of decreasing urinary amylase, increasing serum amylase, and increasing blood glucose levels are felt to be late signals for rejections. If enteric rather than urinary bladder drainage has been used for PTA, only the sign of rising blood glucose is available. Rejection episodes occur commonly within days of, or years after, successful transplantation. Threatened rejection is treated by hospitalizing the patient and intensively accelerating immunosuppression. Usually, threatened rejection is treated successfully so that the patient maintains the graft. When rejection is suspected, cystoscopic transduodenal (in the case of urinary bladder drainage of the graft) or transcutaneous biopsy with ultrasound guidance is used to confirm the diagnosis or the rejection. Although the possibility of recurrent autoimmune attack is

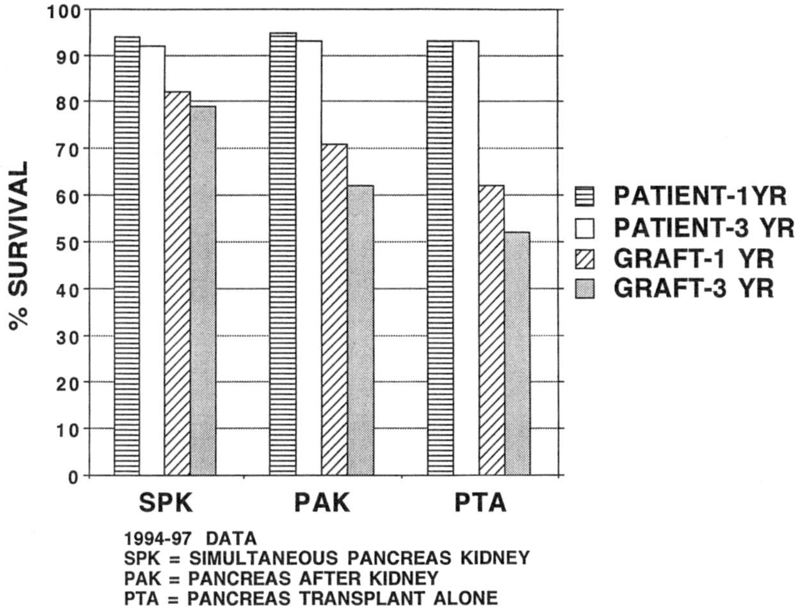

Fig. 1. Patient and pancreas graft survival 1 and 3 yr posttransplantation. (International Pancreas Transplant Registry; data from ref. *11*.)

considered, that seems unlikely to be a cause of recurrent diabetes because the patient receives immunosuppressive drugs that are known to suppress primary autoimmune function and because the transplanted organ is from a non-self source.

BENEFICIAL EFFECTS ON GLYCEMIC CONTROL

As opposed to exogenous insulin-based therapy, successful pancreas transplantation reliably restores endogenous insulin secretion and uniquely maintains glucose levels in the normal range without significant hypoglycemia for many years. Many investigators have detailed the beneficial effects of pancreas transplantation on insulin secretion and carbohydrate metabolism. In a study of 96 pancreas-transplanted patients, fasting plasma glucose, hemoglobin A1c, glucose-induced insulin secretion, and arginine-induced glucagon secretion were maintained at normal levels for up to 5 yr *(13)*. The degree of normalization of hemoglobin A1c levels is better with pancreas transplantation than with the intensive insulin-based management used in the DCCT (*see* Fig. 2). In a more recent study of 16 patients who had successfully undergone a pancreas transplant 10–18 yr earlier, all recipients had normal levels of fasting blood glucose, intravenous glucose tolerance, and hemoglobin A1c level *(14)*. Fifteen of the 16 patients stated that their quality of life had improved after transplantation. This study established that concerns over long-term deterioration, as distinct from rejection, of pancreatic grafts should not be a major obstacle when deciding whether or not to recommend pancreas transplantation. These positive clinical outcomes of transplanted pancreases are impressive in their own right, but all the more so considering that the recipients are treated with immunosuppressive drugs that by themselves diminish β-cell function. Steroid treatment is a well-known cause of peripheral insulin resistance, which, in turn, places more secretory

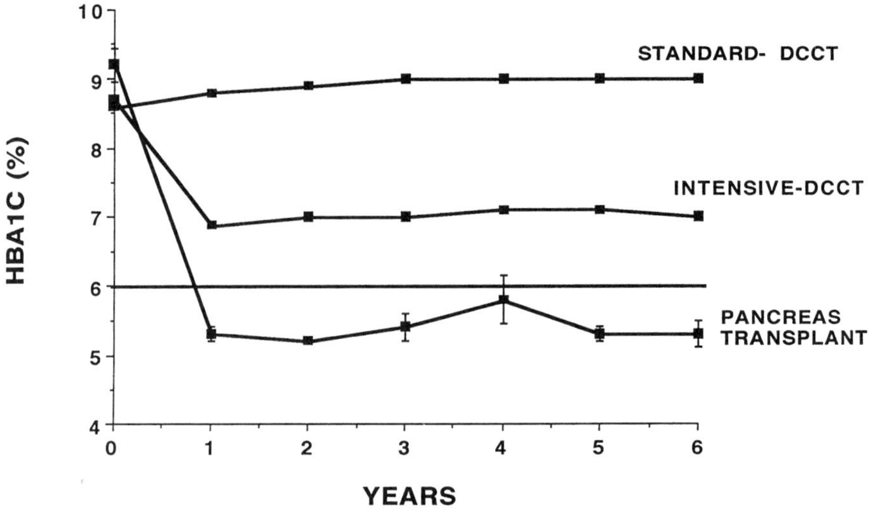

Fig. 2. Comparison of hemoglobin A1c levels following successful pancreas transplantation to hemoglobin A1c levels obtained during standard and intensive therapy in the Diabetes Control and Complications Trial (DCCT). Solid line at 6% represents upper limit of normal. (Data from refs. *1* and *13*.)

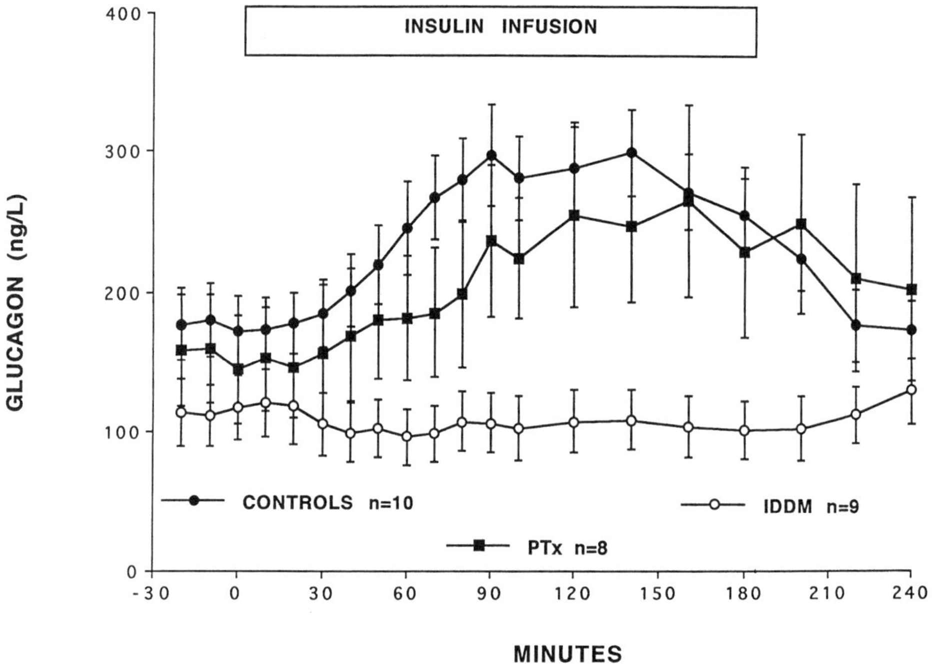

Fig. 3. Glucagon responses during hypoglycemia induced by an insulin infusion (stepped hypoglycemic clamp). Glucagon responses in type 1 diabetic patients are absent, whereas after successful pancreas transplantation (PTx), glucagon responses are normal. (Data from ref. *23*.)

demands on the islet. In addition, glucocorticoids, calcineurin inhibitors, and mycophenolate mofetil also directly inhibit insulin secretion *(15–22)*.

As mentioned earlier, patients who have had type 1 diabetes for many years typically have sluggish to absent counterregulatory hormonal responses and glucose recovery during

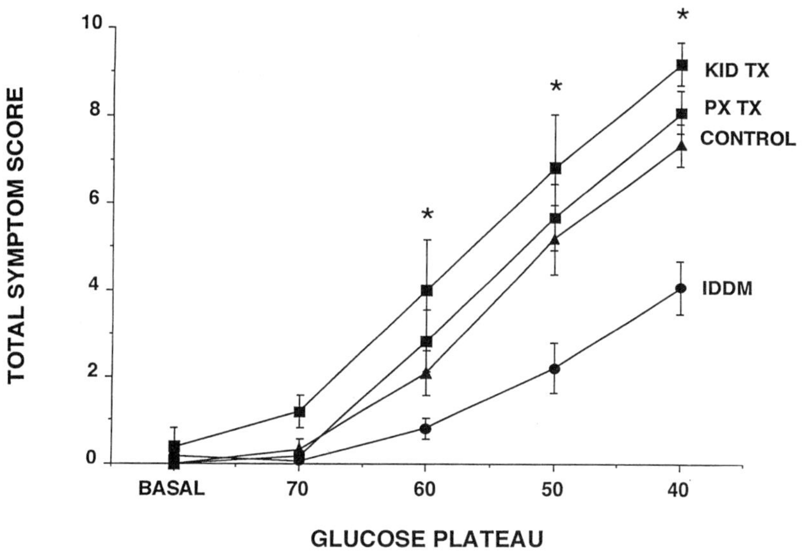

Fig. 4. Degree of symtomotology during stepped hypoglycemic clamps in nondiabetic kidney transplant recipients, type 1 diabetic pancreas transplant recipients, control subjects, and type 1 diabetic subjects. In contrast to the diminished symptom awareness of the type 1 diabetic group, diabetic patients undergoing successful pancreas transplantation have normal symptom awareness. IDDM, insulin-dependent diabetes mellitus. (Data from ref. *24*.)

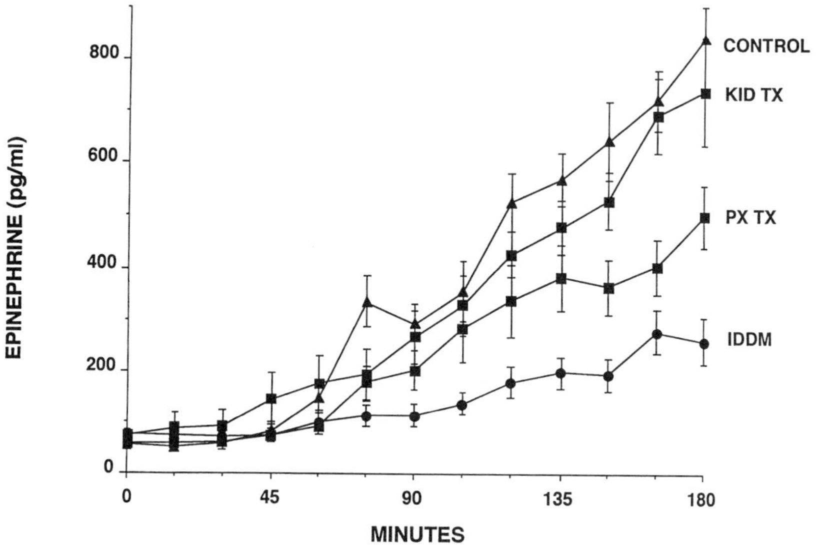

Fig. 5. Epinephrine responses during a hypoglycemic clamp in nondiabetic kidney transplant recipients, type 1 diabetic pancreas transplant recipients, and patients with type 1 diabetes mellitus. Secretion of epinephrine during the hypoglycemic clamp improves in successful recipients of pancreas transplantation, but does not return to normal levels. IDDM, insulin-dependent diabetes mellitus. (Data from ref. *24*.)

insulin-induced hypoglycemia. In recent studies, patients were subjected to progressive levels of mild hypoglycemia provided by exogenous insulin infusion. Compared to patients who did not receive a pancreas transplant, transplanted patients had normal glucagon secretion *(23)* (*see* Fig. 3) and symptom awareness *(24)* (*see* Fig. 4) and partially intact epinephrine response *(24)* (*see* Fig. 5) during hypoglycemia. Studies such as these have established that successful transplantation provides better control of glycemia than exogenous insulin treatment without running the risk of recurrent, serious hypoglycemia, and consequent diminished counterregulatory hormone secretion and symptom awareness.

BENEFICIAL EFFECTS ON CHRONIC COMPLICATIONS OF DIABETES

Although many studies have addressed the effects of pancreas transplantation on the secondary complications of chronic diabetes mellitus, no randomized studies and only few prospective studies assessing the effects of pancreas transplantation secondary to complications of diabetes have been reported. Instead, historic controls or case-controlled experimental designs have been used. Much attention has been paid to the effects of pancreas transplantation on diabetic nephropathy, diabetic neuropathy, and diabetic retinopathy. Studies on renal structure and function have shown that morphologic changes in donated kidneys of patients undergoing simultaneous kidney and pancreas transplantation have reduced rates of mesangial expansion and reduced thickening of glomerular basement membranes compared to patients undergoing kidney transplantation alone *(25)*. In both transplant groups, however, glomerular filtration is compromised because of the use of cyclosporine as an immunosuppressive agent. Most impressively, a recent report of eight patients followed for 10 yr after pancreas transplantation demonstrated reversal of established lesions of diabetic nephropathy. Significant reductions were observed in the thickness of the glomerular basement membrane and the mesangial fractional volume *(26)*.

The effects of pancreas transplantation on diabetic neuropathy have also been evaluated in detail *(27–33)*. These studies have revealed improved measures of motor and sensory nerve function in recipients of successful pancreas transplants. Stabilization or improvement in autonomic nerve function has also been reported. The caveat is, once again, that these results do not come from randomized trials and only infrequently from case-controlled trials. Most recently, motor and sensory nerve conduction velocities were found to be less abnormal in pancreas transplant recipients than nontransplanted patients in studies conducted 10 yr post-pancreas-transplantation *(33)*. Most impressively, the 5-yr life expectancy in diabetic patients with autonomic insufficiency who successfully maintained a pancreas transplant was significantly increased (from 50% to 90%) compared to matched patients with autonomic insufficiency who did not have a successful pancreas transplant *(32)*.

Studies of diabetic retinopathy have yet to conclusively demonstrate a significant benefit of pancreas transplantation. An early study *(34)* compared retinal examination data obtained from patients undergoing successful pancreas transplantation to data from a group of patients undergoing failed pancreas transplantation. Measures of retinopathy continued to progress in both groups during the first 3 yr posttransplantation. By the fifth year, there was no further progression in the patients with functioning pancreas grafts, but this difference was not statistically significant. Similar results of no improvement in the first 5 yr after pancreas transplantation have been reported by other investigators *(35,36)*. It is unfortunate that these studies have not been conducted beyond 5 yr, as have the studies of kidney and nerve function. In this regard, it is important to recall that many patients who have undergone pancreas transplantation have severe retinopathy and, as with the DCCT, as many as 10 yr may be required to show significant differences between treatment groups.

BENEFICIAL EFFECTS ON QUALITY OF LIFE

Successful pancreas transplantation clearly improves the quality of life of diabetic patients *(37–39)*. This procedure eliminates the need for exogenous insulin treatment, frequent daily blood glucose measurements, and extensive dietary restriction. In these studies, recipients of successful pancreas transplants have been compared with type 1 diabetic subjects undergoing kidney transplantation or subjects who have failed pancreas transplantation. Regardless of the comparison group, subjects undergoing successful pancreas transplantation have consistently reported higher measures of quality of life. Over 90% of patients stated that management of immunosuppression after transplantation was preferable to the management of exogenous insulin treatment. These studies have added significant momentum to the recommendation that patients scheduled for kidney transplantation for renal failure should be considered for simultaneous pancreas transplantation *(9)*. The usual benefits reported from these studies include return to employment and successful pregnancies *(34)*. However, an important factor to bear in mind when interpreting these reports is that most diabetic patients who receive pancreas transplants have had serious difficulty in avoiding extremely high and low blood glucose levels. Clearly, the worse the quality of life before transplantation, the more likely it will improve after successful surgery. Consequently, a critical criterion that must be used in deciding whether or not to transplant a pancreas in diabetic patients is the degree to which they can or cannot maintain metabolic stability with exogenous insulin-based management.

RISKS OF PANCREAS TRANSPLANTATION

There are significant risks associated with pancreas transplantation *(40)*. These include the clinical complications caused by the surgery and the immunosuppressive drugs, as well as death. Problems such as intra-abdominal infections and abscesses, vascular graft thrombosis, and anastomotic and duodenal stump leakage requiring relaparotomy have been reported to occur in approx 30% of patients. Complications caused by the immunosuppressive drugs include viral and bacterial infections and malignancy (particularly lymphoma and skin tumors). The risk of malignancy is less than 1% and appears to be no worse for pancreas transplant recipients than for recipients of other organs. Other specific drug-related complications include osteoporosis and insulin resistance secondary to the use of corticosteroids as well as decreased renal and pancreatic β-cell function associated with cyclosporine and tacrolimus.

Very little has been published about the relative cost and benefits of pancreas transplantation compared to insulin-based management. One study concluded that simultaneous pancreas–kidney transplantation, when adjusted for quality of life, is more cost-effective for diabetic patients with end-stage renal disease than kidney-alone transplantation or hemodialysis *(41)*.

SUMMARY

Over the past quarter century, pancreas transplantation has achieved placement on the list of successful organ transplants. This procedure should be reserved for diabetic patients who are experiencing unacceptable complications despite intensive medical treatment, especially recurrent hypoglycemia and symptom unawareness. An exception is made for patients with renal failure destined to receive a kidney transplant. These individuals should be considered for simultaneous pancreas and kidney transplantation. The benefits of successful pancreas transplantation include normalization of glycemia, avoidance of exogenous insulin treatment, restoration of counterregulartory responses to hypoglycemia, stabilization of diabetic neuropathy, and stabilization of diabetic nephropathy with the possibility of reversal of nephropathy. The risks inherent in pancreas transplantation and chronic immunosuppression include the immediate postoperative surgical complications as well as osteoporosis and tumors. Yet, despite these risks of pancreas transplantation, all reported studies have documented an improved quality of life for recipients. Consequently, this form of treatment should be considered for selected patients who are unable to achieve acceptable glycemic control despite intensive medical management.

REFERENCES

1. The Diabetes Control and Complications Trial Research Group. The effect of intensive treatment of diabetes on the development and progression of long-term complications in insulin-dependent diabetes mellitus. N Engl J Med 1993;329:977–986.
2. Rizza RA, Cryer PE, Gerich JE. Role of glucagon, catecholamines, and growth hormone in human glucose counterregulation. Effects of somatostatin and combined alpha- and beta-adrenergic blockade on plasma glucose recovery and glucose flux rates after insulin-induced hypoglycemia. J Clin Invest 1979;64:62–71.
3. Bolli G, de Feo P, Compagnucci P, Cartechini MG, Angeletti G, Santeusanio F, et al. Abnormal glucose counterregulation in insulin-dependent diabetes mellitus: interaction of anti-insulin antibodies and impaired glucagon and epinephrine secretion. Diabetes 1983;32:134–141.
4. Kleinbaum J, Shamoon H. Impaired counterregulation of hypoglycemia in insulin-dependent diabetes mellitus. Diabetes 1983;32:493–498.
5. Dagogo-Jack S, Rattarasarn C, Cryer PE. Reversal of hypoglycemia unawareness, but not defective glucose counterregulation, in IDDM. Diabetes 1994;43:1426–1434.
6. Fanelli CG, Epifano L, Rambotti AM, Pampanelli S, Di Vincenzo A, Modarelli F, et al. Meticulous prevention of hypoglycemia normalizes the glycemic thresholds and magnitude of most of neuroendocrine responses to, symptoms of, and cognitive function during hypoglycemia in intensively treated patients with short-term IDDM. Diabetes 1993;42:1683–1689.
7. Davis M, Mellman M, Friedman S, Chang CJ, Shamoon H. Recovery of epinephrine response but not hypoglycemic symptom threshold after intensive therapy in type 1 diabetes. Am J Med 1994;97:535–542.
8. Kelly WD, Lillehei RC, Merkel FK, Idezuki Y, Goetz FC. Allotransplantation of the pancreas and duodenum along with the kidney in diabetic nephropathy. Surgery 1967;61:827–837.
9. Robertson RP. American Diabetes Association Position Statement: Pancreas transplantation for patients with type 1 diabetes. Diabetes Care 2000;23:S85.
10. Diem P, Abid M, Redmon JB, Sutherland DE, Robertson RP. Systemic venous drainage of pancreas allografts as independent cause of hyperinsulinemia in type I diabetic recipients. Diabetes 1990;39:534–540.
11. Gruessner AC, Sutherland DE. Pancreas transplants for United States (US) and non-US cases as reported to the International Pancreas Transplant Registry (IPTR) and to the United Network for Organ Sharing (UNOS). Clin Transplant 1997;45–59.
12. International Islet Transplant Registry, Vol 6, No. 1, December 1996.
13. Robertson RP, Sutherland DE, Kendall DM, Teuscher AU, Gruessner RW, Gruessner A. Metabolic characterization of long-term successful pancreas transplants in type I diabetes. J Investig Med 1996;44:1–7.
14. Robertson RP, Sutherland DER, Lanz KJ. Normoglycemia and preserved insulin secretory reserve in diabetic patients 10 to 18 years after pancreas transplantation. Diabetes 1999;48:1737–1740.
15. Delaunay F, Kahn A, Cintra A, Davani B, Ling Z-C, Andersson A, et al. Pancreatic beta cells are important targets for the diabetogenic effects of glucocorticoids. J Clin Invest 1997;100:2094–2098.
16. Yale JF, Roy RD, Grose M, Seemayer TA, Murphy GF, Marliss EB. Effects of cyclosporine on glucose tolerance in the rat. Diabetes 1985;34:1309–1313.
17. Robertson RP. Cyclosporin-induced inhibition of insulin secretion in isolated rat islets and HIT cells. Diabetes 1986;35:1016–1019.

18. Odocha O, McCauley J, Scantlebury V, Shapiro R, Carroll P, Jordan M, et al. Posttransplant diabetes mellitus in African Americans after renal transplantation under FK 506 immunosuppression. Transplant Proc 1993;25:2433–2434.
19. Herold KC, Nagamatsu S, Buse JB, Kulsakdinun P, Steiner DF. Inhibition of glucose-stimulated insulin release from beta TC3 cells and rodent islets by an analog of FK506. Transplantation 1993;55:186–192.
20. Tamura K, Fujimura T, Tsutsumi T, Nakamura K, Ogawa T, Atumaru C, et al. Transcriptional inhibition of insulin by FK506 and possible involvement of FK506 binding protein-12 in pancreatic beta-cell. Transplantation 1995;59:1606–1613.
21. Redmon JB, Olson LK, Armstrong MB, Greene MJ, Robertson RP. Effects of tacrolimus (FK506) on human insulin gene expression, insulin mRNA levels, and insulin secretion in HIT-T15 cells. J Clin Invest 1996;98:2786–2793.
22. Drachenberg CB, Klassen DK, Weir MR, Wiland A, Fink JC, Bartlett ST, et al. Islet cell damage associated with tacrolimus and cyclosporine: morphological features in pancreas allograft biopsies and clinical correlation. Transplantation 1999;68:396–402.
23. Barrou Z, Seaquist ER, Robertson RP. Pancreas transplantation in diabetic humans normalizes hepatic glucose production during hypoglycemia. Diabetes 1994;43:661–666.
24. Kendall DM, Rooney DP, Smets YF, Salazar Bolding L, Robertson RP. Pancreas transplantation restores epinephrine response and symptom recognition during hypoglycemia in patients with long-standing type I diabetes and autonomic neuropathy. Diabetes 1997;46:249–257.
25. Bilous RW, Mauer SM, Sutherland DE, Najarian JS, Goetz FC, Steffes MW. The effects of pancreas transplantation on the glomerular structure of renal allografts in patients with insulin-dependent diabetes. N Engl J Med 1989;321:80–85.
26. Fioretto P, Steffes MW, Sutherland DE, Goetz FC, Mauer M. Reversal of lesions of diabetic nephropathy after pancreas transplantation. N Engl J Med 1998;339:69–75.
27. Navarro X, Kennedy WR, Loewenson RB, Sutherland DE. Influence of pancreas transplantation on cardiorespiratory reflexes, nerve conduction, and mortality in diabetes mellitus. Diabetes 1990;39:802–806.
28. Secchi A, Martinenghi S, Galardi G, Comi G, Canal N, and Pozza G. Effects of pancreatic transplantation on diabetic polyneuropathy. Transplant Proc 1991;23:1658–1659.
29. Aridge D, Reese J, Niehoff M, Carney K, Lindsey L, Chun HS, et al. Effect of successful renal and segmental pancreatic transplantation on peripheral and autonomic neuropathy. Transplant Proc 1991;23:1670–1671.
30. Caldara R, Sanseverino R, Lefrancois N, Martin X, Martinenghi S, Dubernard JM. Pancreas transplantation long-term results. Clin Transplant 1991;5:260–264.
31. Gaber AO, Cardoso S, Pearson S, Abell T, Gaber L, Hathaway D, et al. Improvement in autonomic function following combined pancreas-kidney transplantation. Transplant Proc 1991;23:1660–1662.
32. Allen RD, Al-Harbi IS, Morris JG, Clouston PD, O'Connell PJ, Chapman JR, et al. Diabetic neuropathy after pancreas transplantation: determinants of recovery. Transplantation 1997;63:830–838.
33. Navarro X, Sutherland DE, Kennedy WR. Long-term effects of pancreatic transplantation on diabetic neuropathy. Ann Neurol 1997;42:727–736.
34. Ramsay RC, Goetz FC, Sutherland DE, Mauer SM, Robison LL, Cantrill HL, et al. Progression of diabetic retinopathy after pancreas transplantation for insulin-dependent diabetes mellitus. N Engl J Med 1988;318:208–214.
35. Petersen MR, Vine AK. University of Michigan Pancreas Transplant Evaluation Committee. Progression of diabetic retinopathy after pancreas transplantation. Ophthalmology 1990;97:496–502.
36. Scheider A, Meyer-Schwickerath E, Nusser J, Land W, Landgraf R. Diabetic retinopathy and pancreas transplantation: a 3-year follow-up. Diabetologia 1991;34(Suppl 1):S95–S99.
37. Zehrer CL, Gross CR. Comparison of quality of life between pancreas/kidney and kidney transplant recipients: 1-year follow-up. Transplant Proc 1994;26:508–509.
38. Piehlmeier W, Bullinger M, Nusser J, Konig A, Illner WD, Abendroth D, et al. Quality of life in type 1 (insulin-dependent) diabetic patients prior to and after pancreas and kidney transplantation in relation to organ function. Diabetologia 1991;34(Suppl 1):S150–157.
39. Barrou B, Baldi A, Bitker MO, et al. Pregnancy after pancreas transplantation: report of four new cases and review of the literature. Transplant Proc 1995;27:3043–3044.
40. Gruessner RW, Sutherland DE, Troppmann C, Benedetti E, Hakim N, Dunn DL, et al. The surgical risk of pancreas transplantation in the cyclosporine era: an overview. J Am Coll Surg 1997;185:128–144.
41. Douzdjian V, Ferrara D, Silvestri G. Treatment strategies for insulin-dependent diabetics with ESRD: a cost-effectiveness decision analysis model. Am J Kidney Dis 1998;31:794–802.

30 Islet Transplantation

Thierry Berney, MD, MSc,
Norma Sue Kenyon, PhD, *Rodolfo Alejandro*, MD,
Luca Inverardi, MD, *Daniel H. Mintz*, MD,
and Camillo Ricordi, MD

CONTENTS

INTRODUCTION

Historical Perspective

A renewal of interest for the transplantation of islets of Langerhans as a means to cure diabetes is currently being observed, as clinical studies are undertaken at an expanding number of transplant centers throughout the world. This accelerated activity is the result of several significant advances achieved at the turn of the millenium. The improved clinical results in terms of graft survival were highlighted by the recent report by the Edmonton group of a series of seven consecutive recipients of allogeneic islet grafts who achieved insulin independence *(1)*. Another remarkable observation was the demonstration of long-term islet graft survival in nonhuman primates receiving T-cell signaling monoclonal antibody monotherapy alone *(2,3)*. These sentinel observations led to the notion that diabetes might be reversible by islet cell transplantation earlier in the clinical course, before complications ensue, but without the hazards associated with long-term conventional immunosuppression. The enthusiasm thus generated is best illustrated by the high priority accorded to the field of islet transplantation by the recently established Immune Tolerance Network, a collaborative effort supported by major funding organizations such as the Juvenile Diabetes Research Foundation International (JDRF) and the National Institute of Diabetes and Digestive and Kidney Diseases (NIDDK) of the United States with the mandate to advance the clinical application of effective tolerogenic therapies *(4)*.

From: *Contemporary Endocrinology: Type 1 Diabetes: Etiology and Treatment*
Edited by: M. A. Sperling © Humana Press Inc., Totowa, NJ

The recent successes in both preclinical and clinical islet transplantation are the product of long, painstaking, and often frustrating attempts to overcome numerous, seemingly immutable biologic barriers. The first "islet transplantation" procedure in a human diabetic patient was performed in 1893, in a 15-yr-old boy, who survived only 3 d after receiving chopped fragments of a sheep pancreas in the abdominal subcutaneous tissue *(5)*. Although Langerhans had discovered these unique clusters of cells in the pancreas 24 yr previously, it was not known that they played such a critical role in glucose homeostasis. It remained controversial whether the pancreas produced a "sugar-destroying substance" or not, and 30 yr of work by numerous investigators in the field would pass before the discovery that the islets of Langerhans were associated with the newly discovered hormone, insulin *(6)*.

With the availability of insulin to diabetic patients in 1922, a cure for diabetes seemed to be at hand and interest for islet transplantation was lost for awhile. It is ironic that insulin therapy saved the lives of patients destined to die because of ketoacidosis, only to permit the natural history of insulin-dependent diabetes with development of the devastating macrovascular and microvascular complications of the disease to be uncovered *(7)*. The rebirth of islet transplantation was heralded in 1967 by the description of a new method of islet isolation in rodents using collagenase digestion of the pancreas after ductal distension *(8)*. This was soon followed by the first reports of successful transplantation of isolated islets in diabetic rodents, with improved results when islets were implanted into the liver by infusion into the portal vein, which is still the preferred site of implantation in clinical islet transplantation today *(9,10)*. Isolation of human islets was the next step *(11)* and led to the first transplantation of isolated and purified human islets in a diabetic patient in 1974 at the University of Minnesota *(12)*. Results of the first allogeneic islet transplant procedures in humans were dismal, with no patient achieving insulin independence and only few instances of transient graft function as evidenced by measurable serum C-peptide being recorded. The automated method for islet isolation became available in 1988 *(13)* and proved a major advance in the primitive science of cell separation. This technical advance provided the opportunity for large numbers of human islets to be isolated and transplanted. Soon thereafter, first reports of insulin independence in recipients of islets isolated from a single donor appeared *(14,15)*.

Rationale for Islet Transplantation

The Diabetes Control and Complications Trial (DCCT) was a landmark for the demonstration that tight control of blood glucose levels could significantly delay the occurrence of the long-term complications of type 1 diabetes *(16)* and represented a fruitful long-term financial investment in terms of health care costs *(17)*. The results of the DCCT were obtained by intensive insulin therapy, a therapeutic modality that does not sustain normal blood glucose levels throughout the day, is cumbersome, and is accompanied by an increased frequency of severe hypoglycemic episodes *(18)*. The DCCT results and the observation that pancreas transplantation could reverse lesions of diabetic nephropathy *(19)* did, however, document the absolute requirement of strict metabolic control while reinforcing the notion that successful endocrine tissue replacement might be the only procedure to consistently achieve a physiological control of glycemia. Indeed, islets function for a lifetime, producing and releasing insulin in response to an intrinsic "glucose sensor" that defines an exquisite threshold sensitivity to increases or decreases in glucose levels *(20)*. Currently, whole-organ pancreas transplantation is an islet-replacing procedure that can lead to sustained euglycemia and insulin independence in a vast majority of recipients, with graft survival rates as high as 78% at 5 yr *(21)*. In addition, pancreas transplantation was calculated to be a highly cost-effective therapeutic strategy for type 1 diabetic patients *(22)*. However, despite significant progress, pancreas transplantation is still associated with perioperative mortality and significant morbidity, which still leads to early relaparotomy in almost 20% of patients *(23,24)*.

In striking contrast, islet cell transplantation can be performed as a percutaneous minimally invasive procedure, in which islets are infused into the liver via the portal vein *(25,26)*. In addition, the islet transplantation modality could circumvent the organ shortage that prevents most diabetic patients eligible for pancreas transplantation from actually receiving a graft. Islet cell availability could become unlimited, when strategies such as the use of xenogeneic islets, engineered β-cell lines, and in vitro or in vivo islet expansion reach the stage of clinical applicability *(27–31)*. Further, islet transplantation offers the possibility of maintaining the graft without chronic immunosuppression when the induction of donor-specific tolerance *(27,32)* or immunoisolation emerge as clinical strategies *(33,34)*.

ISLET ISOLATION AND PURIFICATION

Islet Isolation

The pancreas contains approximately one million islets of Langerhans *(35)*, which comprise 1% of the total mass of the gland. Thus, obtaining an islet preparation of 50 to 90% purity implies the achievement of a 50- to 90-fold enrichment during the isolation procedure. Liberation of endocrine from surrounding exocrine tissue to produce intact islets with a sufficient number, purity, and viability for transplantation was first made possible in rodent models in the late 1960s. Moskalewski was the first to use collagenase digestion to disrupt guinea pig pancreata *(36)*. Lacy and Kostianowsky improved this technique by intraductal distention of the pancreas in order to disrupt the exocrine tissue and facilitate the collagenase digestion process *(8)*. Although applicable to rodent islets, the procedure could not be scaled up for islet isolation from larger mammals, until Horaguchi and Merell combined the two methods in a dog model *(37)*. This new method involved distension of the pancreas directly with the collagenase solution to initiate the digestion process and became the basis of islet isolation protocols in all large mammals, including the human *(13,38–42)*. However, a considerable mechanical component, involving forced passage of the tissue through needles of decreasing gauge or use of a tissue macerator, was necessary to complement the enzymatic digestion. The physical insult sustained by the islets during such procedures made it generally impossible to obtain sufficient yields of endocrine tissue for transplantation. The automated method of islet isolation, in which the pancreas, fully immersed in a chamber in order to reduce the mechanical stress on the islet tissue, undergoes a continuous enzymatic digestion *(13)*, has resulted in a marked increase in the yields and reproducibility of islet isolation. This method, applicable to all mammal species studied *(2,3,13,42–46)*, led to the multiplication of clinical islet transplant procedures *(47)* and to the first reported cases of insulin independence after allotransplantation of islets isolated from a single donor *(14,15,48)*.

The necessity of applying the same standards of quality to the pancreas procurement procedure for islet isolation as for whole-organ transplantation can never be overemphasized. Indeed, the procurement team was shown to be a significant factor for the success of an islet isolation procedure in terms of yield, purity, and viability *(49,50)*. A number of donor factors have been shown to negatively affect the outcome of the isolation procedure and include young donor age (<18 yr), low body mass index, medical history, high doses of vasopressors, and duration of cardiac arrest *(49,50)*. A key parameter for a successful islet isolation is certainly the duration of cold storage prior to the procedure. In addition to better yields and in vitro function, a pancreatic cold ischemia time < 8 h was the only donor parameter identified by the International Islet Transplant Registry (ITR) as a significant determinant of insulin independence in the recipient *(47,49,50)*.

Commercially available collagenases are enzyme mixtures including metalloenzymes able to hydrolyze the collagen triple helix. Crude collagenase (clostridiopeptidase) preparations, produced in *Clostridium histolyticum* cultures, were characterized by extreme batch-to-batch variability in terms of collagenolytic activity and high endotoxin contamination *(51,52)*. Considerable progress was made to identify the critical components of the collagenase blends for optimal digestion and liberation of islets and to improve the enzyme mixtures in terms of endotoxin contents, variability, and selectivity for the exocrine tissue. These efforts led to the development of Liberase (Roche-Boehringer-Mannheim, Indianapolis, IN), a new standardized blend of highly purified enzymes, namely collagenase isoforms I and II from *C. histolyticum* and thermolysin from *Bacillus thermoproteolyticus*. The formulation of these components was selected to specifically optimize human islet isolation and was shown to significantly improve isolation yields as compared to traditional collagenase blends *(52–57)*. Endotoxin contamination of the reagents necessary for isolation was a major concern, as a large body of evidence suggested that it played a significant role in primary nonfunction of islet grafts *(57–60)*. Thus, the near-total absence of endotoxin demonstrated in Liberase *(51,57)* was an important advance. On the other hand, although initial results suggested that the need for the prescreening of enzyme lots had been eliminated, there remains uncertainty about the absence of batch-to-batch variability in the enzyme contents of the mixture.

Islet Purification

Purification addresses the need to physically separate the islets from the surrounding nonendocrine—acinar, vascular, ductal, and lymphoid—tissue. Because there is a marked difference in density between endocrine and exocrine tissues, separation by density gradient centrifugation has evolved as the preferred method of purification. Purification is usually conducted on Eurocollins–Ficoll density gradients, in which the islets are centrifuged for a time sufficient to allow them to reach their gradient of equal density *(61)*. Problems pertaining to the large volumes of pancreatic digest when dealing with human or large mammal tissue were solved by the development of a semiautomated method of islet purification, utilizing a COBE 2991 computerized cell separator *(62,63)*. The method was introduced in 1989 and was a notable addition to the automated isolation method for the recovery of greater numbers of purer islets. It undoubtedly played an additional role in the rapid increase in the number of clinical islet transplantation reported in the early 1980s *(14,15,47,48)*. The use of the COBE 2991 cell separator allowed low-temperature centrifugation of large volumes of tissue under controlled conditions in a minimal time frame, thus leading to reduced processing times, and minimal handling and risks of contamination *(62–65)*.

The optimal degree of purity for islet transplantation remains a controversial issue. Islets contaminated with exocrine tissue carry a higher immunogenic burden that can impair their engraftment *(66,67)* and ductal tissue is a significant contributor to the cytokine-induced generation of nitric oxide and free radicals to which β-cells are exquisitely sensitive *(68–70)*. In addition, lower purity implies a higher total volume of tissue to be transplanted, which raises concerns about the risks of portal hypertension, portal vein thrombosis, or even intravascular coagulation, as reported after intraportal infusion of large volumes of islet preparations in early cases of autotransplantation after pancreatectomy *(71,72)*. On the other hand, impure preparations have been infused into the portal vein with the rationale that enrichment of the islet preparation results in a substantial loss of functional endocrine tissue during the purification process *(73)*. Additionally, the presence of acinar or ductal contamination may be advantageous, considering the potential for β-cell neogenesis from pluripotent pancreatic stem cells located in the pancreatic ducts *(31,74–76)*. There is a growing body of evidence to suggest that islet–extracellular matrix interactions are critical for the survival and the functional and structural maintenance of the islets and that their absence may trigger islet cell apoptosis *(30,77,78)*. A solution combining the advantages of both the highly purified and nonpurified approaches resides in the preparation, by incomplete dissociation and purification, of islets surrounded by a layer of acinar tissue forming a mantle around the islet. In addition to the maintenance of islet–matrix interactions and to the hypothesized regeneration potential, this mantle may also confer physical protection to the islets from the graft microenvironment and enhance their survival ability *(79)*. Islets are usually cultured short term (12–48 h) at low temperature (21–24°C) prior to transplantation, in order to eliminate cells damaged during the isolation process and, thus, minimize nonspecific inflammatory phenomena at the site of implant. Longer periods of culture seemed to confer an immunological advantage because resident passenger leukocytes were deleted *(80–83)*, but concerns about loss of tissue and decrease of function during long-term islet culture obviate the use of this approach *(84,85)*. The presence of heterologous proteins, notably fetal bovine serum, in culture media is another reason for limiting the duration of culture. Heterologous proteins have been shown to reduce function and survival in vitro as compared to culture in autologous serum *(86,87)*, and attempts at culturing the islets in serum-free media have resulted in improved outcomes *(85,88,89)*. Additionally, the carryover of xenogeneic proteins, originating the from bovine serum, might significantly increase the immunogenicity of the islets. These considerations have been the rationale for the elimination of bovine serum from the isolation reagents and the immediate islet transplantation without culture in the Edmonton protocol *(1)*.

ISLET TRANSPLANTATION

Transplantation Technique

Islet graft implantation in the liver, in which the islets are infused through the portal vein, was one of the few factors demonstrated to be associated with the achievement of insulin independence by the ITR *(47)*. Other sites of implantation that have been used include the peritoneal cavity, epiploic flaps, and the spleen. Numerous advantages are associated with the choice of the liver: It is easily and safely accessible via percutaneous transhepatic catheterization of the portal vein *(90,91)*; it is considered to be an immunologically privileged site *(92)*; islets within the portal spaces are located upstream from the hepatic veins and thus limit systemic hyperinsulinization; and functioning islets have been demonstrated to survive in the liver for several years after transplantation *(15,79,93,94)*. We have, in fact, observed intact islets containing well-granulated β-cells in the liver of an insulin-independent patient who died of recurrent malignancy 5 yr after abdominal exenteration (including total pancreatectomy) and combined liver/islet transplantation *(79)*.

Implantation of the islet preparation is done via a minimally invasive procedure, requiring interventional radiology technology. The portal vein is reached by a transhepatic percutaneous approach under angiographic guidance *(91)*. Alternatively, for simultaneous islet–kidney transplantation, the portal system is usually accessed by catheterization of a colonic vein after completion of the kidney transplantation. The morbidity and mortality associated with intraportal islet infusion are minimal. Among 215 recipients of an islet allograft reported to the ITR *(47)* from 1990 through 1996, only one patient has died as a direct consequence of the procedure. This patient suffered an injury to the hepatic artery during percutaneous transhepatic catheterization of the portal vein, which provoked a fatal intra-abdominal hemorrhage *(26)*. Four nonlethal complications have been reported: perforation of the gallbladder requiring laparoscopic cholecystectomy; tear of the splenic capsule requiring splenectomy; bacteremia resulting from infusion of a contaminated islet preparation; and portal vein thrombosis in a simultaneous liver–islet transplant procedure *(26)*.

Results of Clinical Islet Transplantation: the International Islet Transplantation Registry

Through December 1998, a total of 405 islet allografts have been performed worldwide, including 306 since 1990, a relative increase in numbers related to the introduction of the automated method of islet isolation *(47)*. Cumulative 1-yr patient and graft survival of 96% and 35%, respectively, were obtained in the 200 C-peptide negative, type 1 diabetic patients transplanted from 1990 through 1997. The persistence of graft function can be assessed by measurable levels of basal serum C-peptide, at a threshold of 0.5 ng/mL. The observation that 32% of recipients lose graft function within 1 mo of transplantation (and 46% within 3 mo) indicates that primary nonfunction is a major cause of islet graft loss *(47)*. In fact, we have shown that if early graft loss was excluded from the analysis of islet allograft survival (e.g., considering only grafts that maintain function for at least 1 mo posttransplant) after a state-of-the art islet transplant procedure, the results demonstrate an approx 80% 1-yr graft survival rate *(95)*. Although the evidence of measurable C-peptide in the serum indicates unequivocal survival of the islet graft, insulin independence has, unfortunately, represented an uncommon fate following human islet allotransplantation. However, it must be emphasized that islet graft function in the absence of insulin independence is still associated with markedly improved glucose counter regulation and hypoglycemia awareness *(96,97)*. Analysis of parameters reported to the ITR has identified four features associated with persisting graft function at 1 yr and insulin independence for more than 7 d. The four criteria that now form the basis for state-of-the-art islet allotransplantation are (1) transplantation of an islet mass ≥ 6000 IEq/kg body weight; (2) cold ischemia time of the pancreas ≤ 8 h; (3) immunosuppression induction with antilymphocyte or antithymocyte globulins, or anti-interleukin (IL)-2R monoclonal antibodies, as opposed to OKT3 or none; (4) liver as the site of islet graft implantation. A significantly beneficial effect is especially obtained when all four criteria are fulfilled.

Obstacles to Success of Islet Allotransplantation

Islet grafts are exposed to a number of adverse conditions, some of which are shared with all types of transplant, and some of which are unique to the islets alone. The combined effects of these factors determines an imbalance between engrafted islet mass and metabolic demand, which explains why islet allografts do so poorly in comparison to islet autografts, on the one hand, and to whole-organ pancreatic allografts, on the other hand *(26)*.

Poor engraftment is the first of these obstacles. The number of islets infused in a transplant procedure is far from matching the number of islets composing a normal endocrine pancreas (the recommended threshold of 6000 IEq/kg represents 420,000 IEq in a 70-kg patient, i.e., less than half the one million islets of a human pancreas). Islets are an essentially avascular graft, which renders them particularly prone to hypoxia, at least during the time elapsing before neovessels revascularize the transplant *(98,99)*. As already pointed out, a vast majority of islets are lost early after transplantation. The nonspecific events leading to early graft loss are collectively termed "primary nonfunction" and are not related to classic rejection immune phenomena. Rather, they result from poor intrinsic quality of the islet preparation or from interaction of the islets with inflammatory elements of the hepatic microenvironment in which they are implanted, a situation that does not occur in whole-organ pancreatic transplantation. The isolation process itself is chronologically the first cause of islet loss. As already noted, the endotoxin contents of the various reagents necessary for the procedure is thought to be a major determinant of islet cell injury *(51,57–60)*. Apoptotic cell death was demonstrated to be responsible for significant β-cell loss as an immediate result of isolation *(100)*. Direct islet damage provoked by cytokines released by activated Kuppfer cells and sinusoidal endothelial cells, and mediated by nitric oxide and oxygen free radicals, as a result of islet implantation has been clearly demonstrated, and treatment with macrophage-depleting drugs has been shown to improve early graft survival *(101–104)*. In addition to immediate damage, new evidence suggests that the nonspecific inflammatory insult to the islets might also amplify the immune response. Briefly, macrophagic activation induces upregulation of major histocompatibility company (MHC) molecules expression, which can markedly enhance antigen presentation to host T-lymphocytes, resulting in an increased incidence of immune graft loss to acute and chronic rejection *(105,106)*.

A second set of problems arises from the high metabolic demand imposed on the islet graft, as a consequence of several factors. Because a significant number of transplanted islets are lost to the noxious inflammatory stimuli described earlier, the engrafted islet mass is, most of the time, only marginal for its insulin-release workload. Implanted islets must overcome a state of insulin resistance, as indicated by higher absolute value of hepatic glucose production during euglycemic hyperinsulinemia in nonfunctioning grafts *(107)*. Finally, islet transplantation currently necessitates conventional immunosuppression, based on the association of several drugs comprising calcineurin inhibitors (cyclosporin A [CsA] or tacrolimus) and steroids. All three drugs have long been known to have a diabetogenic effect, partially resulting from direct islet toxicity, which further increases the metabolic load on the islets *(108–112)*.

Finally, islet grafts are prone to destruction by recurrence of autoimmunity in addition to allorejection. There has not been a clear indication so far that islets are more susceptible to allorejection than whole-pancreas transplants. However, as discussed earlier, there is growing evidence that ischemia–reperfusion injury, similar to the early inflammatory events peculiar to the islet transplant situation, may upregulate specific immune mechanisms. Recurrence of islet-directed autoimmunity has been clearly demonstrated by recurrence of insulitis in recipients of segmental pancreatic grafts from an identical twin. However, the process was not observed when such recipients received full-dose immunosuppression and is rarely observed in recipients of pancreatic allografts *(113)*. Although, immune rejection and recurrence of autoimmunity are exceedingly difficult to distinguish, there is strong evidence that the latter is a significant mechanism of islet graft loss despite adequate conventional immunosuppression. Recurrence of autoimmunity was described in spontaneously diabetic Bio-Breeding (BB) rats transplanted with syngeneic intraportal islets, but not whole pancreas, despite CsA immunosuppression *(114)*. Evidence of insulitis and selective β-cell destruction was also reported after islet transplantation in a forearm muscular site in an immunosuppressed type 1 diabetic patient *(115)*. Also, a significantly lower 1-yr graft survival was demonstrated in recipients positive for anti-GAD65 or anti-islet-cell autoantibodies *(116)*.

Clinical Trials of Human Islet Allotransplantation

The demonstration that prolonged insulin independence could be achieved after transplantation of allogeneic islets was made in 1990, with the Pittsburgh trial reporting nine patients who underwent upper abdominal exenteration, including pancreatoduodenectomy, for malignancy and received a combined liver–islet transplant. Six patients who survived the extensive surgery became insulin independent *(48)*, a consistency of results that was previously only achieved with islet autotransplantation *(26,47)*. This unusual success rate could be attributed to the absence of autoimmunity, but the common identity of islets and liver from a same donor led to the intriguing notion that the islet survival was facilitated by a modification of antigen-driven immunity in a syngeneic environment. In addition, the islets were transplanted immediately after isolation and the recipients were treated with a FK506-based, steroid-free immunosuppression.

Our experience in Miami with islet allotransplantation in type 1 diabetic patients has demonstrated that long-term islet function could also be achieved in the presence of autoimmunity. Six of eight patients demonstrated graft function for more than 60 d, including two patients in whom C-peptide secretion was demonstrated for over 9 yr, and two patients were euglycemic and insulin independent for over 1 mo *(97,117)*. Although all recipients had elevated levels of HbA1c despite intensive insulin therapy and recurrent episodes of moderate to severe hypoglycemia prior to transplantation, insulin requirements and HbA1c levels were significantly reduced in all six patients with evidence of graft function. In addition, neither patient with long-term graft function has experienced hypoglycemic episodes.

Remarkable results have been reported by the Giessen group, who implemented new strategies aimed at promoting islet engraftment and transplant survival. The Giessen protocol included, in addition to fulfillment of the four criteria defined by the ITR, strategies based on observations made in experimental animal models, namely the use of endotoxin-free reagents, the use of antioxidant agents (nicotinamide), and the administration of intravenous insulin starting 2–3 d prior to transplant in order to diminish metabolic demand on the graft. With this protocol, insulin independence has been achieved in approx 30% of transplanted patients *(118,119)*. In a recent report from the Geneva group, who implemented peritransplant management along the same lines, graft function for 3 mo to 5 yr was demonstrated in all of 13 consecutive type 1 diabetic recipients of islet allografts *(120)*.

The report in early 2000 by the Edmonton group of a consecutive series of seven out of seven type 1 diabetic recipients of islet allografts with persistent insulin independence was received as a new level of achievement by the islet transplantation community *(1)*. These remarkable results were achieved in recipients of solitary islet grafts, in the absence of severe nephropathy or a need for simultaneous kidney transplantation. The Edmonton protocol uniquely combined several strategies designed to address, specifically, the various obstacles encountered in the isolation, transplantation, immunosuppression sequence. First, as in the Pittsburgh trial, cold ischemia time was kept at a minimum prior to isolation, and islet transplantation was conducted shortly after isolation without prolonged in vitro culture. Emphasis was put on utilizing state-of-the-art equipment (automated methods of isolation and purification, endotoxin-free reagents) and on obtaining high-quality, pure islet preparations. Second, the lack of pretransplant in vitro culture allowed replacement of heterologous proteins (i.e., fetal bovine serum) with human serum albumin during the isolation procedure. Third, in order to overcome the marginal mass of the first graft, all patients received a second islet transplant, within a few weeks of the initial procedure, in an effort to achieve a total transplanted islet mass of at least 10,000 IEq/kg. Finally, an improved immunosuppressive protocol was used, consisting of low-dose tacrolimus, sirolimus (rapamycin), and anti-IL-2-receptor monoclonal antibody (daclizumab) induction. The synergism of sirolimus and calcineurin inhibitors allows one to substantially reduce their dosage and, thus, islet toxicity, without increasing the occurrence of acute rejection episodes *(121,122)*. In spite of in vitro evidence that sirolimus and tacrolimus bind to the same cytosolic receptor (FKBP-12), suggesting that competition for this protein would prevent synergism *(123)*, in vivo observations in animal models have shown strong potentiation of the efficacy of both drugs *(124,125)*. The tacrolimus–sirolimus association has, in fact, shown to be extremely potent in terms of the prevention of acute rejection in a series of recipients of liver, pancreas, and kidney transplants *(126)*.

The results of the Edmonton protocol are remarkable: Seven of seven patients were able to discontinue insulin and remain so with a median follow-up of 11.9 mo; a compelling improvement of blood glucose control has been achieved, as demonstrated by marked reduction of mean amplitude of glycemic excursions and HbA1c levels; none of the patients have experienced hypoglycemic episodes; and oral glucose tolerance tests (GTT) are either normal or impaired, no patient fulfilling the criteria for a diagnosis of diabetes by the standards of the American Diabetes Association (ADA) *(127)*.

In spite of the need for two donors per recipient in human transplant clinical studies, the Edmonton immunosuppression protocol was a considerable achievement that catalyzed the funding of 10 islet transplant centers worldwide, to expand these clinical trials and investigate and develop new strategies for islet graft survival and immunological tolerance induction.

NEW STRATEGIES TOWARD TOLERANCE INDUCTION

Costimulatory Blockade

The development of therapeutic strategies that would result in donor-specific tolerance, thus obviating the need for lifelong generalized immunosuppression, is the key subject for research as we move forward. The availability of such tolerizing protocols would be particularly interesting in islet transplantation, as it would allow large-scale transplantation of diabetic patients before the occurrence of complications.

One strategy extensively explored is the blockade of costimulatory signals of T-cell activation. In order to obtain T-cell activation, proliferation and effector function upon cognate interaction with a specific antigen presented in an MHC context, three sets of signals must be delivered *(128):* The first signal results from the binding of the antigen/MHC complex to the T-cell receptor; the second signal is delivered through the engagement of costimulatory molecules on the T-cell surface by their ligand expressed on the antigen-presenting cell (APC); the third signal occurs by the binding of IL-2 and other T-cell growth factors (IL-4, IL-7, IL-9, and IL-15) to their receptor, to drive T-cell clonal expansion and functional maturation (Figs. 1 and 2).

Many efforts have focused on costimulatory blockade, because it was demonstrated that delivery of signal 1 in the absence of signal 2 could lead to T-cell clonal anergy and thus could be a way of inducing donor-specific tolerance *(129–131).* Interestingly, costimulatory blockade was shown to prevent or delay the occurrence of autoimmunity in various animal models *(132–135),* enhancing the appeal of this strategy for its application to islet transplantation.

The first costimulatory pathway ongoing intensive study was the engagement of the CD28 molecule on the T-cell surface by either member of the B7 family, B7.1 and B7.2, also termed CD80 and CD86, expressed on APCs. (Fig. 2A, B). Ligation of CD28 leads to T-cell activation, but also to the upregulation of CTLA4 (CD152), another ligand of the B7 pair that delivers inhibitory signals, counteracting the effects of B28 stimulation *(136–138).* Targeting CD28 can be achieved utilizing anti-B7 antibodies or the agent CTLA4-Ig, a soluble molecule obtained from the fusion of CTLA4 with a human immunoglobulin tail. CTLA4-Ig binds avidly to the B7 molecules, preventing their binding to CD28, but also to CTLA4, and thus results in blockade of this signaling pathway *(138).* Rodent studies involving CD28-blocking agents demonstrated an ability to prevent allograft or xenograft rejection, including in a xenogeneic islet model *(139,140),* but similar efforts in nonhuman primate models led to less encouraging results. CTLA4Ig treatment resulted in only limited kidney or islet allograft survival in monkeys *(141,142).* This could be related to the notion that CTLA4 inhibitory signals are required to optimally induce allograft tolerance *(143).*

CD40–CD154 is another major costimulatory pathway, and blockade, by targeting the CD154 molecule expressed on the surface of T-cells with monoclonal antibodies (MAb), has been effective in various models of heart, kidney, aorta, bone marrow, and skin transplantation *(144).* The interest for anti-CD154 therapy in islet transplantation has been enhanced by its ability to delay the initiation of insulitis and diabetes in nonobese diabetic (NOD) mice *(134)* and to prevent release of nonspecific inflammatory mediators *(145,146),* a phenomenon involved in early islet graft loss. Long-term graft survival (>100 d) was obtained in both allogeneic and xenogeneic islet transplantation models of chemically induced diabetes in rodents. These results were obtained when the mAb was

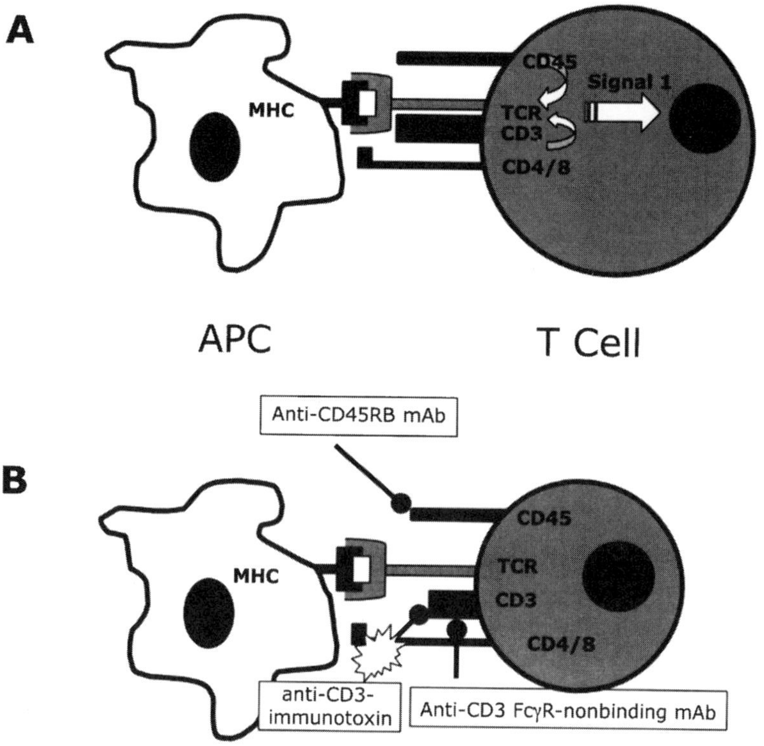

Fig. 1. **(A)** Generation of a T-cell response is initiated by the engagement of the T-cell receptor (TCR) by MHC + peptide. The delivery of "signal 1" involves a phosphorylation cascade in which the CD45 molecule and the various chains of the CD3 complex play activating and regulatory roles. **(B)** Blockade or alteration of signal 1 can be achieved using anti-CD45RB MAb or FcγR-nonbinding anti-CD3 MAb. Binding of the CD3 ε-chain by the anti-CD3 immunotoxin leads to transient but profound T-cell depletion after internalization. APC, antigen-presenting cell.

administered together with donor-specific splenocytes, but anti-CD154 treatment alone also had some effect in prolongation of graft survival *(147–149)*. In contrast, indefinite islet graft survival could not be achieved when allogeneic islets were transplanted into spontaneously diabetic autoimmune NOD mice *(150)*.

In parallel, a humanized murine anti-human CD154 was developed and tested in nonhuman primate models (*see* Fig. 2B). Indefinite kidney graft survival was achieved in rhesus monkeys with a combination of CTLA4Ig and anti-CD154 MAb *(142)* and with anti-CD154 MAb monotherapy as well, with absence of rejection >10 mo after treatment was discontinued *(151)*. This body of data suggested that anti-CD154 treatment could be especially effective in supporting islet allograft survival and led us to test the reagent in rigorous models of pancreatectomy-induced diabetic nonhuman primates. Seven of seven pancreatectomized baboons receiving islet allografts under the cover of humanized anti-CD154 MAb monotherapy achieved durable insulin independence. When rejection was encountered, a rise of postprandial blood glucose was the first sign and this could be readily reversed with anti-CD154 rescue therapy. Anti-CD154 therapy needed to be administered on a monthly basis in order to sustain islet graft survival, but a progressive reduction in the islet secretory capacity was observed.

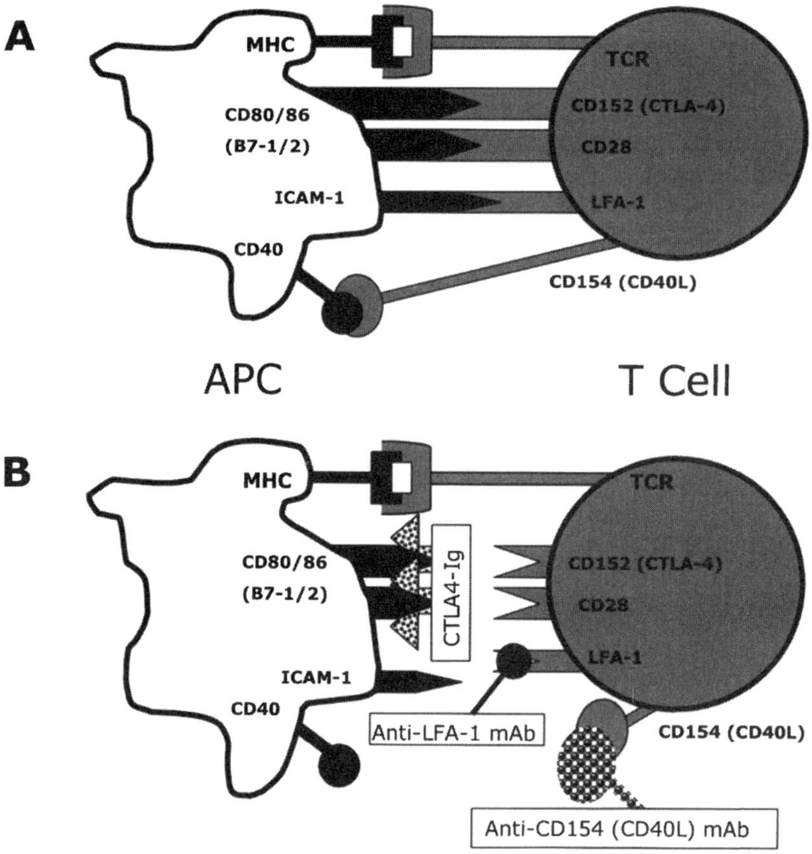

Fig. 2. **(A)** Generation of a T-cell response requires the delivery of costimulatory signals in addition to signal 1. Such signals are provided through the interaction of CD40 with CD154 (CD40L), CD80/86 (B7.1/2) with CD28, and ICAM-1 with LFA-1. CD80/86 can also bind CD152 (CTLA-4) to provide downregulatory signals. **(B)** Costimulatory blockade can be achieved using CTLA-4-Ig, a soluble form of CTLA-4 that binds to the CD80/86 molecules, or with anti-CD154 or anti-LFA-1 MAbs.

The only significant side effect was an unexpected decrease in the CD4+ population in the peripheral blood *(2)*. However, in the rhesus monkey, the same schedule of humanized anti-CD154 MAb monotherapy (induction therapy plus monthly maintenance) led to indefinite insulin independence (>125 to >476 d) in six of six pancreatectomized rhesus monkeys. In contrast to the studies in baboons, continued improvement in graft function, as determined by intravenous GTTs, was observed, no significant side effects were encountered, and donor-specific hyporesponsiveness was demonstrated in mixed lymphocyte cultures *(3)*.

Although it was acknowledged that the pancreatectomized monkey was not a perfect model of human autoimmune type 1 diabetes, these results demonstrated that blockade of the CD40/CD154 pathway could result in successful engraftment, long-term maintenance of function, and preservation of islet secretory mass. This was, in fact, so encouraging that a clinical trial of immunosuppressive monotherapy with the humanized anti-CD154 MAb was launched in 1999 for type 1 diabetic recipients of solitary islet grafts. Unfortunately, reports of unusual rates of thromboembolic complications in other clinical trials of the MAb temporarily halted all clinical studies with this promising preparation *(152,153)*. Another target for costimulatory blockade could be the LFA-1 adhesion molecule. In addition to its APC–to–T-cell adhesion function, engagement of LFA-1 by its ligand ICAM-1 enhances T-cell activation by delivering costimulatory signals *(154)*. Blockade of this pathway by anti-LFA-1 MAbs has been used in rodent models and was shown to induce long-term allograft acceptance, with a state of in vivo donor-specific unresponsiveness that could be adoptively transferred *(155,156)*. Anti-LFA-1 treatment of the recipient was also able to prolong islet xenograft survival, but addition of anti-ICAM-1 MAb directed against the donor species molecule was necessary to obtain significant prolongation *(157,158)*.

Blockade of Signal 1

Blockade of the first signal of T-cell activation can be obtained by treatment with anti-CD45RB MAbs. CD45 (also known as leukocyte common antigen) is a transmembrane protein tyrosine phosphatase critically involved in the coupling of signals from the T-cell receptor (TCR) to the proximal signaling apparatus (*see* Fig. 1A, B). Engagement of the TCR by the MHC/peptide complex triggers activation of protein tyrosine kinases, which leads to phosphorylation of chains of the CD3/TCR complex, and, in turn, of critical downstream signaling intermediates. CD45 plays a critical role in T-cell activation by regulating reversible dephosphorylation of regulatory tyrosine residues. The CD45 molecule exists in multiple isoforms obtained by alternative splicing of three exons termed A, B, and C. In mice, T-cells can be roughly divided in two populations with regard to their level of expression of exon B. $CD45RB^{Hi}$ CD4 T-cells preferentially secrete IL-2, whereas $CD45RB^{Lo}$ CD4 T-cells preferentially secrete IL-4. Treatment with anti-CD45RB MAb induces a shift from the $CD45RB^{Hi}$ to the IL-4-secreting $CD45RB^{Lo}$ phenotype, which, in turn, is responsible for the upregulation of CTLA4 (CD152), which delivers inhibitory signals for T-cell activation on ligation *(159,160)*. Treatment with anti-CD45RB MAb was shown to prevent the development of autoimmunity in experimental allergic encephalomyelitis *(161)*, and a role in the protection from diabetes of NOD mice was recognized for T-cells bearing the $CD45RB^{Lo}$ phenotype *(162)*. In addition, indefinite survival of kidney allografts and, remarkably, reversal of kidney rejection when treatment was delayed until rejection occurred were reported in anti-CD45RB-treated mice *(163)*. These protective characteristics on allorejection and autoimmunity made this antibody a good candidate for studies of islet transplantation. Indeed, indefinite islet allograft survival was achieved in 60% of chemically diabetic mice after a short induction course of the antibody *(164,165)*. Clearly, these data need to be confirmed in preclinical models or in rodent models of autoimmune diabetes, but they might represent another promising strategy for tolerance induction in islet transplantation.

Another target for the blockade of signal 1 is the CD3 molecular complex (*see* Fig. 1 A, B). OKT3 (muromonab), a murine anti-human CD3 MAb, has been used in clinical organ transplantation since the early 1980s, both as induction and as antirejection therapy. This drug is a highly effective immunosuppressant, but its broad use has been limited by two major drawbacks: the severe and potentially lethal "cytokine release syndrome" caused by the crosslinking of antibody-bound TCRs by FcγR-expressing cells of the monocyte–macrophage lineage, and the human–anti-mouse humoral response elicited by the immunogenicity of the antibody *(166)*. These considerations led to the development of a chimeric FcγR-nonbinding anti-CD3 MAb, obtained by combining the $F(ab')_2$ region of a hamster–anti-mouse CD3 with a mouse Fcγ3 portion with very low affinity for the FcγR. This MAb was first shown to have similar immunosuppressive properties as the native antibody, but prolongation of skin graft survival was observed without eliciting a cytokine storm or a humoral response against the MAb *(167)*. Further studies demonstrated that the chimeric MAb delivered incomplete TCR signals, characterized by altered phosphorylation patterns of the CD3/TCR complex and resulting in unresponsiveness of Th1 clones and a T-cell response skewed toward a Th2 phenotype *(168,169)*. This observation has important implications for islet transplantation because it is thought that enhanced Th2 activity at the expense of the Th1 subset may play a significant role in the maintenance of tolerance both to alloantigens and autoantigens *(170,171)*. In this regard, long-term remission has been achieved in overtly diabetic NOD mice by short-term treatment with anti CD3 MAb, both with the whole molecule or with noncrosslinking $F(ab')_2$ fragments *(172,173)*. Humanized, FcγR-nonbinding OKT3 antibodies were recently developed and characterized *(174)*. One of these MAbs has a γ1-chain and two point mutations in the C_H2 region, which markedly reduces the affinity for the FcγR. It has been successfully tested in a phase I trial of treatment of acute renal allograft rejection without significant side effects *(175)*. Immunosuppressive protocols including this antibody are currently being tested in clinical trials of islet transplantation. The CD3 complex can also be targeted with an anti-CD3-immunotoxin (*see* Fig. 1B) obtained by coupling an anti-CD3 MAb to a mutant diphteria toxin. Upon binding and internalization, this compound induces a transient but profound T-cell depletion, designed to "reset" the immune system so that T-cell clones re-emerging after a transplant would see the graft as self *(176)*. Tolerance to kidney allografts *(177)* and significant delay in the progress of experimental autoimmune encephalitis *(178)* were achieved by the immunotoxin in nonhuman primate models. A short-term (4 d) immunosuppressive regimen of anti-CD3 immunotoxin, cyclosporin, and steroids induced long-term survival of xenogeneic islet grafts and sustained euglycemia in monkeys with naturally occurring diabetes *(179)*.

Blockade of Signal 3

There has been much attention directed recently to apoptosis of alloresponsive T-cells as a prerequisite for the induction of peripheral tolerance *(180,181)*. Addition of a rapamycin treatment for 14 d to a costimulatory blocking induction regimen of anti-CD154 MAb and CTLA4-Ig resulted in indefinite survival of heart and skin grafts in mice, whereas the addition of CSA antagonized the effects of costimulatory blockade. The explanation for these seemingly contradictory effects of immunosuppressive agents lies in the fact that both cyclosporin A and rapamycin inhibit the proliferative component of IL-2 signaling, but only rapamycin allows the antigen-driven, IL-2-dependent, activation-induced cell death (AICD) phenomenon to occur. Enhanced skin graft tolerance in rapamycin-treated animals correlated with massive apoptosis of alloreactive T-cells *(182)*. Administration of the same regimen to mice transgenic for $Bcl\text{-}x_L$, an antiapoptotic gene, sharply reduced tolerance induction *(180)*.

T-Cell growth factor deprivation is another form of T-cell apoptosis, distinct from AICD. Targeting T-cell growth factors during clonal expansion of activated T-cells is seen as an efficient way of inducing alloreactive T-cell apoptosis and, thus, peripheral tolerance. Anti-IL-2 receptor α-chain (CD25) MAbs, such as daclizumab and basiliximab, have been efficient in preventing acute rejection episodes in clinical trials, but are unable to block other growth factors *(183)*. The fact that all receptors for T-cell growth factor (IL-2, IL-4, IL-7, IL-9, and IL-15) share a common γc-chain was exploited in a murine model, in which anti-γc-chain MAbs were administered to islet transplant recipients. This led to induction of T-cell apoptosis and indefinite allogeneic islet graft survival *(184)*. T-cell apoptosis and stable tolerance are linked by the activation of immunoregulatory mechanisms. Apoptotic lymphocytes release anti-inflammatory and inhibitory cytokines (IL-10 and transforming growth factor-β [TGF-β]) as they die. Further, phagocytosis by macrophages of apoptotic T-cells carrying their specific antigen leads to presentation of the antigen in a tolerogenic form. Thus, tolerance induced by T-cell apoptosis is stable, because deletion is followed by active regulatory pathways induced by the inhibitory properties of the apoptotic cell *(181)*. These observations present some seemingly extraordinary opportunities to exploit in tolerance-inducing protocols for clinical trials.

Donor Hematopoietic Cells

Bone marrow infusions into cytoablated recipients to induce a state of mixed chimerism is another well-established approach for the induction of donor-specific tolerance in many animal species, but it is not practical for application in the human *(185)*. However, the observation that long-term human transplant recipients who had discontinued their immunosuppressive treatment and had not rejected their graft also displayed multilineage hematopoietic microchimerism provided a rationale for continuing to explore the mixed chimerism approach *(186)*. Because bone marrow cell engraftment was demonstrated to be feasible without myeloablative conditioning, provided large numbers of marrow cells were infused *(187)*, this approach has been extensively explored. Recently, Sykes and her colleagues published a series of articles reporting the achievement of mixed chimerism without myeloablation utilizing costimulatory blockade with anti-CD154 and CTLA4Ig *(188,189)*. Remarkably, the administration of a single dose of each agent after fully MHC-mismatched bone marrow infusion in mice resulted in long-term multilineage macrochimerism and donor-specific tolerance, with skin graft acceptance for > 145 d *(190)*. The quantities of bone marrow cells necessary to achieve this state of tolerance-inducing chimerism are too high for the technique to be simply transferred to preclinical testing, but the approach of combining bone marrow infusion and costimulatory blockade appears, nonetheless, to be extremely promising. Other studies, in which anti-CD154 and CTLA4Ig were administered in combination with donor-specific transfusion (DST), have achieved permanent engraftment of allogeneic islets and skin but have also identified that the timing of administration of costimulatory blocking agents could be critical for tolerance induction *(143)*. In effect, CTLA4Ig may counteract the tolerogenic potential of anti-CD154 and DST, because of simultaneous blockade of the stimulatory CD28 and the inhibitory CTLA4 signaling pathways *(143)*.

Hematopoietic stem cell transplantation is also able to augment donor cell microchimerism *(191)* that may have a causal role in decreasing the occurrence of rejection episodes and promoting allograft survival. The dogma stating that cytoablation or cytoreduction was mandatory for the engraftment of donor bone marrow cells was challenged by the observation that chimerism and indefinite islet allograft survival could be obtained in rats by multiple bone marrow infusions, in the absence of irradiation *(192)*. Trials of donor bone marrow infusion to recipients of liver, kidney, pancreas, and multivisceral transplants in the absence of cytoablative conditioning have been initiated at the University of Miami. Preliminary analysis showed improved patient and graft survival in liver transplant recipients *(193)* and the establishment of sustained microchimerism, correlating with lower incidence of acute rejection episodes and progression toward chronic rejection *(194)*. Occurrence of graft host disease (GVHD) was reported with an incidence of 2–8%, depending on timing and schedule of bone marrow administration *(195)*.

In addition to the tolerance to alloantigens, hematopoietic stem cell transplantation (HSCT) is emerging as a feasible and efficient therapeutic modality for severe autoimmune diseases. The concept that the natural course of autoimmune disease might be altered by cytoablation and reconstitution with autologous stem cells has been tested in numerous animal models and is gaining increasing support *(196)*. A multicenter, prospective phase I/II trial of 74 patients with severe autoimmune disease treated by autologous HSCT after various conditioning protocols reported a favorable response in at least 65% of patients, but the 1-yr procedure-related mortality of 9% still needs to be reduced before this approach can be applied in indolent autoimmune disease processes *(197)*. In lethally irradiated NOD mice, autoimmune insulitis can be prevented by reconstitution with allogeneic bone marrow *(198)*, and even reversed when combined with pancreatic tissue *(199)*. More interestingly, mixed chimerism obtained by allogeneic bone marrow transplantation into sublethally irradiated NOD mice is also able to prevent diabetes and reverse insulitis *(200)*. A minimum of 5–15% chimerism may be required to prevent the onset of diabetes in autoimmune-prone NOD mice *(201)*. Protection from recurrence of autoimmunity in allogeneic islet transplant recipients was obtained in spontaneously diabetic BB rats by cotransplanting donor peripheral lymph node cells that contained an immunoregulatory T-cell subset with a direct protective action *(202)*. Otherwise, protection from islet graft loss to allorejection and recurrence of autoimmunity in diabetic NOD mice reconstituted with hematopoietic cells has necessitated lethal or sublethal irradiation and full hematopoietic chimerism *(203,204)*. Addition of anti-CD154 MAb in these models has, however, resulted in complete protection from GVHD *(204)*.

These accumulating experiences represent the rationale for upcoming trials of islet and stem cell cotransplantation to patients who do not yet have diabetic complications. The premise, in these efforts, is that $CD34^+$ enrichment of the donor bone marrow would result in elimination of T-cells responsible for GVHD. The concurrent administration of costimulatory blocking agents could play a role in facilitating bone marrow cell (BMC) engraftment and preventing GVHD. It is hoped that the establishment of a higher persisting state of chimerism would contribute to a state of functional tolerance to alloantigens and autoantigens and thus allow early weaning of the immunosuppressive regimen of islet cell transplant recipients. This is a particularly important objective for patients who receive islet transplants earlier in the clinical course of their disease before complications ensue.

CONCLUSION

Exciting opportunities for the reversal of type 1 diabetes have again resurfaced, as a product of the basic understanding of initiation signal(s) and signal transmission in immune recognition pathways. The existence of multiple steps in the immune effector pathways offer enormous possibilities for therapeutic interventions directed at the achievement of immunological tolerance.

These data indicate that an increasing list of costimulatory molecules could be targeted in the design of such tolerogenic protocols. It is likely from the experiences to date that such protocols will involve combined blockade of different costimulatory pathways, sequential blockade of signals 1, 2, and 3, or a combination of costimulatory blockade with other strategies.

The excitement generated by the achievements that have unfolded over the past few years has resulted in a renewed but cautious optimism in islet transplantation for the treatment of patients with type 1 diabetes.

REFERENCES

1. Shapiro AMJ, Lakey JRT, Ryan E, et al. Islet transplantation in seven patients with type 1 diabetes mellitus using steroid-free immunosuppression regimen. N Engl J Med 2000;343:230–238.
2. Kenyon NS, Fernandez LA, Lehmann R, et al. Long-term survival and function of intrahepatic islet in baboons treated with humanized anti-CD154. Diabetes 1999;48:1473–1481.
3. Kenyon NS, Chatzipetrou M, Masetti M, et al. Long-term survival and function of intrahepatic islet allografts in rhesus monkeys treated with humanized anti-CD154. Proc Natl Acad Sci USA 1999;96:8132–8137.
4. http://www.immunetolerance.org. Overview and Mission. Accessed Dec. 23, 2002.
5. Williams PW. Notes on diabetes treated with extract and by grafts of sheep's pancreas. Br Med J 1894;2:1303–1304.
6. Benedum J. The early history of endocrine cell transplantation. J Mol Med 1999;77:30–35.
7. Mintz DH, Alejandro R. Islet cell transplantation—A historical perspective. In: Ricordi C, ed. Pancreatic Islet Cell Transplantation. R.G. Landes, Austin, TX, 1992, pp.1–6.
8. Lacy PE, Kostianowsky M. Method for the isolation of intact islets of Langerhans from the rat pancreas. Diabetes 1967;16:35–39.
9. Ballinger WF, Lacy PE. Transplantation of intact pancreatic islets in rats. Surgery 1972;72:175–186.
10. Kemp CB, Knight MJ, Scharp D, et al. Effect of transplantation site on the results of pancreatic islet isografts in diabetic rats. Diabetologia 1973;9:486–491.
11. Sutherland DER, Steffes MW, Bauer GE, et al. Isolation of human and porcine islets of Langerhans and islet transplantation in pigs. J Surg Res 1974;16:102–111.
12. Najarian JS, Sutherland DER, Matas AJ, et al. Human islet transplantation: a preliminary report. Transplant Proc 1977;9:233–236.
13. Ricordi C, Lacy PE, Finke EH, Olack BJ, Scharp DW. Automated method for isolation of human pancreatic islets. Diabetes 1988;37:413–420.
14. Scharp DW, Lacy PE, Santiago JV, et al. Insulin independence after islet transplantation into type I diabetic patients. Diabetes 1990;39:515–518.
15. Ricordi C, Tzakis AG, Carroll PB, et al. Human islet isolation and allotransplantation in 22 consecutive cases. Transplantation 1992;53:407–414.
16. The Diabetes Control and Complications Trial Research Group. The effect of intensive treatment of diabetes on the development and progression of long-term complications in insulin-dependent diabetes mellitus. N Engl J Med 1993;329:977–986.
17. Herman WH, Eastman RC. The effects of treatment on the direct costs of diabetes. Diabetes Care 1998;21(Suppl 3):C19–C24.
18. The Diabetes Control and Complications Trial Research Group. Effects of intensive therapy on residual beta-cell function in patients with type 1 diabetes in the diabetes control and complications trial. Ann Intern Med 1998;128:517–523.
19. Fioretto P, Steffes MW, Sutherland DER, Goetz FC, Mauer M. Reversal of lesions of diabetic nephropathy after pancreas transplantation. N Engl J Med 1998;339:69–75.
20. Carroll PB. Anatomy and physiology of islets of Langerhans. In: Ricordi C, ed. Pancreatic Islet Cell Transplantation. R.G. Landes, Austin, TX, 1992, pp.7–18.
21. Sollinger HW, Odorico JS, Knechtle SJ, D'Alessandro AM, Kalayoglu M, Pirsch JD. Experience with 500 simultaneous pancreas-kidney transplants. Ann Surg 1998;228:284–296.
22. Stratta RJ. The economics of pancreas transplantation. Graft 2000;3:19–24.

23. Manske CL. Risks and benefits of kidney and pancreas transplantation for diabetic patients. Diabetes Care 1999;22 (Suppl 2):B114–B120.
24. Humar A, Kandaswamy R, Granger D, Gruessner RW, Gruessner AC, Sutherland DE. Decreased surgical risks of pancreas transplantation in the modern era. Ann Surg 2000;231:269–275.
25. Oberholzer J, Triponez F, Lou J, Morel P. Clinical islet transplantation: a review. Ann NY Acad Sci 1999;875:189–199.
26. Hering BJ, Ricordi C. Results, research priorities, and reasons for optimism: islet transplantation for patients with type 1 diabetes. Graft 1999;2:12–27.
27. Kenyon NS, Ranuncoli A, Masetti M, Chatzipetrou M, Ricordi C. Islet transplantation: present and future perspectives. Diabetes Metab Rev 1998;14:303–313.
28. Groth CG, Korsgren O, Tibell A, et al. Transplantation of porcine fetal pancreas to diabetic patients. Lancet 1994;344:1402–1404.
29. Newgard CB, Clark S, Beltrandelrio H, Hohmeier HE, Quaade C, Normington K. Engineered cell lines for insulin replacement in diabetes—current status and future prospects. Diabetologia 1997;40(Suppl 2):S42–S47.
30. Hayek A, Beattie GM, Cirulli V, Lopez AD, Ricordi C, Rubin JS. Growth factor/matrix-induced proliferation of human adult beta-cells. Diabetes 1995;44:1458–1460.
31. Ramiya VK, Maraist M, Arfors KE, Schatz DA, Peck AB, Cornelius JG. Reversal of insulin-dependent diabetes using islets generated in vitro from pancreatic stem cells. Nat Med 2000;6:278–282.
32. Waldmann H. Transplantation tolerance: where do we stand? Nat Med 1999;11:1245–1248.
33. Berney T, Ricordi C. Immunoisolation of cells and tissues for transplantation. Cell Transplant 1999;8:577–579.
34. Soon-Shiong P, Heintz RE, Merideth N, et al. Insulin independence in a type 1 diabetic patient after encapsulated islet transplantation. Lancet 1994;343:950–951.
35. Saito K, Iwama N, Takahashi T. Morphometrical analysis of topographical differences in size distribution, number and volume of islets in the human pancreas. Tohoku J Exp Med 1978;124:177–186.
36. Moskalewski S. Isolation and culture of the islets of Langerhans of the guinea pig. Gen Comp Endocrinol 1965;5:342.
37. Horaguchi A, Merrell RC. Preparation of viable islet cells from dogs by a new method. Diabetes 1981;30:455–458.
38. Noel J, Rabinovitch A, Olson L, et al. A method for large scale high yield isolation of canine pancreatic islets of Langerhans. Metabolism 1982;31:184–187.
39. Gray DWR, McShane P, Grant A, Morris PJ. A method for isolation of islets of Langerhans from the human pancreas. Diabetes 1984;33:1055–1061.
40. Ricordi C, Finke EH, Lacy PE. A method for the mass isolation of islets from the adult pig pancreas. Diabetes 1986;35:649–653.
41. Ricordi C, Lacy PE, Scharp DW. Automated islet isolation from human pancreas. Diabetes 1989;38 (Suppl 1):140–142.
42. Ricordi C, Rastellini C. Automated method for pancreatic islet separation. In: Ricordi C, ed. Methods in Cell Transplantation. R.G. Landes, Austin, TX, 1995, pp.433–438.
43. Ricordi C, Finke EH, Dye ES, Socci C, Lacy PE. Automated isolation of mouse pancreatic islets. Transplantation 1988;46:455–457.
44. Ricordi C, Socci C, Davalli AM, et al. Isolation of the elusive pig islet. Surgery 1989;107:688–694.
45. Ricordi C, Socci C, Davalli AM, et al. Application of the automated method to islet isolation in swine. Transplant Proc 1990;22:784–785.
46. Olack B, Hill A, Scharp D, Lacy P. Automated purification of canine islets. Transplant Proc 1992;24:1003–1004.
47. Brendel MD, Hering BJ, Schultz AO, Bretzel RG. International Islet Transplant Registry Newsletter No. 8, 1999.
48. Tzakis A, Ricordi C, Alejandro R, et al. Pancreatic islet transplantation after upper abdominal exenteration and liver replacement. Lancet 1990;336:402–405.
49. Benhamou PY, Watt PC, Mullen Y, et al. Human islet isolation in 104 consecutive cases. Factors affecting isolation success. Transplantation 1994;57:1804–1810.
50. Lakey JRT, Warnock GL, Rajotte RV, et al. Variables in organ donors that affect the recovery of human islets of Langerhans. Transplantation 1996;61:1047–1053.
51. Linetsky E, Inverardi L, Kenyon NS, Alejandro R, Ricordi C. Endotoxin contamination of reagents used during isolation and purification of human pancreatic islets. Transplant Proc 1998;30:345.

52. Linetsky E, Bottino R, Lehmann R, Alejandro R, Inverardi L, Ricordi C. Improved human islet isolation using a new enzyme blend, liberase. Diabetes 1997;46:1120–1123.
53. Olack BJ, Swanson CJ, Howard TK, Mohanakumar T. Improved method for the isolation of human islets of Langerhans using liberase enzyme blend. Hum Immunol 1999;60:1303–1309.
54. Brandhorst H, Brandhorst D, Hering BJ, Bretzel RG. Significant progress in porcine islet mass isolation utilizing liberase HI for enzymatic low-temperature pancreas digestion. Transplantation 1999;68:355–361.
55. Cavanagh TJ, Lakey JRT, Dwulet F, et al. Improved pig islet yield and post-culture recovery using liberase PI purified enzyme blend. Transplant Proc 1998;30:367.
56. Lakey JRT, Cavanagh TJ, Zieger MAJ, Wright M. Evaluation of a purified enzyme blend for the recovery and function of canine pancreatic islets. Cell Transplant 1998;7:365–372.
57. Berney T, Molano RD, Cattan P, et al. Endotoxin-mediated delayed islet graft function is associated with increased intra-islet cytokine production and islet-cell apoptosis. Transplantation 2001;71:125–123.
58. Vargas F, Vives-Pi M, Somoza N, et al. Endotoxin contamination may be responsible for the unexplained failure of human pancreatic islet transplantation. Transplantation 1998;65:722–727.
59. Jahr H, Pfeiffer G, Hering BJ, Federlin K, Bretzel RG. Endotoxin-mediated activation of cytokine production in human PBMCs by collagenase and Ficoll. J Mol Med 1999;77:118–120.
60. Eckhardt T, Jahr H, Federlin K, Bretzel RG. Endotoxin impairs the engraftment of rat islets transplanted beneath the kidney capsule of C57BL/6 mice. J Mol Med 1999;77:123–125.
61. Olack B, Swanson C, McLear M, Longwith J, Scharp D, Lacy PE. Islet purification using Euro–Ficoll gradients. Transplant Proc 1991;23:774–776.
62. Lake SP, Bassett D, Larkins A, et al. Large-scale purification of human islets utilizing discontinuous albumin gradient on IBM 2991 cell separator. Diabetes 1989;38(Suppl 1):143–145.
63. Alejandro R, Strasser S, Zucker P, Mintz DH. Isolation of pancreatic islets from dogs: semi automated purification on albumin gradients. Transplantation 1990;50:207–210.
64. London NJM, Robertson GSM, Chadwick DR. Purification of human pancreatic islets by large scale continuous density gradient centrifugation. Horm Metab Res 1993;25:61.
65. Robertson GSM, Chadwick DR, Contractor H, et al. The optimization of large scale density gradient human islet isolation. Acta Diabetol 1993;30:93–98.
66. Gotoh M, Maki T, Satomi S, Porter J, Monaco AP. Immunological characteristics of purified pancreatic islet grafts. Transplantation 1986;42:387–390.
67. Gray DW, Sutton R, McShane P, Peters M, Morris PJ. Exocrine contamination impairs implantation of pancreatic islets transplanted beneath the kidney capsule. J Surg Res 1988;45:432–442.
68. Pavlovic D, Chen MC, Bouwens L, Eizirik DL, Pipeleers D. Contribution of ductal cells to cytokine responses by human pancreatic islets. Diabetes 1999;48:29–33.
69. Corbett JA, Wang JL, McDaniel ML. Nitric oxide mediates cytokine-induced inhibition of insulin secretion by human islets of Langerhans. Proc Natl Acad Sci USA 1993;90:1731–1735.
70. Malaisse WJ, Malaisse-Lagae F, Sener A, Pipeleers DG. Determinants of the selective toxicity of alloxan to the pancreatic β-cell. Proc Natl Acad Sci USA 1982;79:927–930.
71. Mehigan DG, Bell WR, Zuidema GD, Eggleston JC, Cameron JL. Disseminated intravascular coagulation and portal hypertension following pancreatic islet autotransplantation. Ann Surg 1980;191:287–293.
72. Mittal VK, Toledo-Pereyra LH, Sharma M, et al. Acute portal hypertension and disseminated intravascular coagulation following pancreatic islet autotransplantation after subtotal pancreatectomy. Transplantation 1981;31:302–304.
73. Gores PF, Sutherland DER. Pancreatic islet transplantation: is purification necessary? Am J Surg 1993;166:538–542.
74. Orci L, Stefan Y, Malaisse-Lagae F, Perrelet A. Instability of pancreatic endocrine cell populations through life. Lancet 1979;i:615–616.
75. Rosenberg L, Brown RA, Duguid WP. A new model for the development of duct epithelial hyperplasia and the initiation of nesidioblastosis. J Surg Res 1983;35:63–72.
76. Rosenberg L, Duguid WP, Brown RA. Induction of islet cell proliferation will reverse diabetes in the Syrian golden hamster. Diabetes 1988;37:337–341.
77. Rosenberg L, Wang R, Paraskevas S, Maysinger D. Structural and functional changes resulting from islet isolation lead to islet cell death. Surgery 1999;126:393–398.
78. Wang RN, Rosenberg L. Maintenance of beta-cell function and survival following islet isolation requires re-establishment of the islet-matrix relationship. J Endocrinol 1999;163:181–190.

79. Ricordi C, Alejandro R, Rilo HH, et al. Long-term in vivo function of human mantled islets obtained by incomplete pancreas dissociation and purification. Transplant Proc 1995;27:3379.
80. Lacy PE, Davie JM, Finke EH. Prolongation of islet allograft survival following in vitro culture (24 degrees C) and a single injection of ALS. Science 1979;204:312–313.
81. Ricordi C, Lacy PE, Sterbenz K, Davie JM. Low-temperature culture of human islets or in vivo treatment with L3T4 antibody produces a marked prolongation of islet human-to-mouse xenograft survival. Proc Natl Acad Sci USA 1987;84:8080–8084.
82. Lacy PE, Finke EH. Activation of intraislet lymphoid cells causes destruction of islet cells. Am J Pathol 1991;138:1183–1190.
83. Warnock GL, Dabbs KD, Cattral MS, Rajotte RV. Improved survival of in vitro cultured canine islet allografts. Transplantation 1994;57:17–22.
84. Ono J, Lacy PE, Michael HE, Greider MH. Studies of the functional and morphologic status of islets maintained at 24 C for four weeks in vitro. Am J Pathol 1979;97:489–503.
85. Ling Z, Pipeleers DG. Preservation of glucose-responsive islet β-cells during serum-free culture. Endocrinology 1994;134:2614–2621.
86. Goldman H, Colle E. Human pancreatic islets in culture: effects of supplementing the medium with homologous and heterologous serum. Science 1976;192:1014–1016.
87. Sakamoto K, Hatakeyama E, Kenmochi T, et al. Improvement of porcine islet culture with porcine serum. Transplant Proc 1998;30:391–392.
88. Behboo R, Carroll PB, Memarzadeh S, et al. Improved long-term culture of functional human islets in serum-free medium. Transplant Proc 1994;26:3301.
89. Bottino R, Inverardi L, Valente U, Ricordi C. Serum-free medium and pyruvate improve survival and glucose responsiveness of islet β cells in culture. Transplant Proc 1997;29:1978–1979.
90. Alejandro R, Mintz DH, Noel J, et al. Islet cell transplantation in type I diabetes mellitus. Transplant Proc 1987;19:2359–2361.
91. Froud T, Alejandro R, Echenique AM, et al. Evaluation of the percutaneous transhepatic intraportal method of islet cell transplantation. Transplantation 2000;69 (Suppl):S208.
92. Qian JH, Kokudo S, Sato S, Hamaoka T, Fujiwara H. Tolerance induction of alloreactivity by portal venous inoculation with allogeneic cells followed by the injection of cyclophosphamide. I. Specific suppression of alloreactive cytotoxic and delayed-type hypersensitivity responses as well as allograft rejection. Transplantation 1987;43:538–543.
93. Ricordi C, Tzakis A, Alejandro R, et al. Detection of pancreatic islet tissue following islet allotransplantation in man. Transplantation 1991;52:1079–1080.
94. Carroll PB, Rilo HR, Alejandro R, et al. Long term (>3 years) insulin independence in a patient with pancreatic islet cell transplantation following upper abdominal exenteration and liver replacement for fibrolamellar hepatocellular carcinoma. Transplantation 1995;59:875–879.
95. Ricordi C. Human islet cell transplantation: new perspectives for an old challenge. Diabetes Rev 1996;4:356–369.
96. Meyer C, Hering BJ, Grossmann R, et al. Improved glucose counterregulation and autonomic symptoms after intraportal islet transplants alone in patients with long-standing type I diabetes mellitus. Transplantation 1998;66:233–240.
97. Alejandro R, Lehmann R, Ricordi C, et al. Long-term function (6 years) of islet allografts in type 1 diabetes. Diabetes 1997;46:1983–1989.
98. Menger MD, Vajkoczy P, Leiderer R, et al. Influence of experimental hyperglycemia on microvascular blood perfusion of pancreatic islet isografts. J Clin Invest 1992;90:1361–1369.
99. Mendola JF, Conget I, Manzanares JM, et al. Follow-up study of the revascularization process of purified rat islet beta-cell grafts. Cell Transplant 1997;6:603–612.
100. Paraskevas S, Maysinger D, Wang R, Duguid TP, Rosenberg L. Cell loss in isolated human islets occurs by apoptosis. Pancreas 2000;20:270–276.
101. Kaufman DB, Platt JL, Rabe FL, et al. Differential roles of Mac-1+ cells, and CD4+ and CD8+ T lymphocytes in primary nonfunction and classical rejection of islet allografts. J Exp Med 1990;172:291–302.
102. Kaufman DB, Gores PF, Field MJ, et al. Effect of 15-deoxyspergualin on immediate function and long-term survival of transplanted islets in murine recipients of a marginal islet mass. Diabetes 1994;43:778–783.
103. Rabinovitch A, Suarez-Pinzon WL, Strynadka K, Lakey JR, Rajotte RV. Human pancreatic islet beta-cell destruction by cytokines involves oxygen free radicals and aldehyde production. J Clin Endocrinol Metab 1996;81:3197–3202.

104. Bottino R, Fernandez LA, Ricordi C, et al. Transplantation of allogeneic islets of Langerhans in the rat liver: effects of macrophage depletion on graft survival and microenvironment activation. Diabetes 1998;47:316–323.
105. Halloran PF, Homik J, Goes N, et al. The "injury response": a concept linking nonspecific injury, acute rejection, and long-term transplant outcomes. Transplant Proc 1997;27:79–81.
106. Land W. Postischemic reperfusion injury to allografts: its impact on T-cell alloactivation via upregulation of dendritic cell-mediated stimulation, co-stimulation, and adhesion. Curr Opin Organ Transplant 1999;4:118–124.
107. Luzi L, Hering BJ, Socci C, et al. Metabolic effects of successful intraportal islet transplantation in insulin-dependent diabetes mellitus. J Clin Invest 1996;97:2611–2618.
108. Ricordi C, Zeng Y, Alejandro R, et al. In vivo effect of FK506 on human pancreatic islets. Transplantation 1991;52:519–522.
109. Zeng Y, Ricordi C, Lendoire J, et al. The effect of prednisone on pancreatic islet autografts in dogs. Surgery 1993;113:98–102.
110. Alejandro R, Feldman EC, Bloom AD, Kenyon NS. Effects of cyclosporin on insulin and C-peptide secretion in healthy beagles. Diabetes 1989;38:698–703.
111. Shapiro AM, Hao E, Lakey JR, Finegood D, Rajotte RV, Kneteman NM. Diabetogenic synergism in canine islet autografts from cyclosporin and steroids in combination. Transplant Proc 1998;30:527.
112. Drachenberg CB, Klassen DK, Weir MR, et al. Islet cell damage associated with tacrolimus and cyclosporine: morphological features in pancreas allograft biopsies and clinical correlation. Transplantation 1999;68:396–402.
113. Sutherland DER, Goetz FC, Sibley RK. Recurrence of disease in pancreas transplants. Diabetes 1989;38:85–87.
114. Bartlett ST, Chin T, Dirden B, et al. Inclusion of peripancreatic lymph node cells prevents recurrent autoimmune destruction of islet transplants: evidence of donor chimerism. Surgery 1995;118:392–397.
115. Stegall MD, Lafferty KJ, Kam I, et al. Evidence of recurrent autoimmunity in human allogeneic islet transplantation. Transplantation 1996;61:1272–1274.
116. Jaeger C, Brendel M, Hering BJ, et al. Progressive islet graft failure occurs significantly earlier in autoantibody-positive than in autoantibody-negative IDDM recipients of intrahepatic islet allografts. Diabetes 1997;46:1907–1910.
117. Ferreira J, Alejandro R, Kenyon NS, et al. Nine year islet allograft function in patients with type 1 DM. Transplantation 2000;69(Suppl):S208.
118. Hering BJ, Bretzel RG, Hopt UT, et al. New protocol toward prevention of human early islet allograft failure. Transplant Proc 1994;26:570–571.
119. Bretzel RG, Brandhorst D, Brandhorst H, et al. Improved survival of intraportal pancreatic islet cell allografts in patients with type-1 diabetes mellitus by refined peritransplant management. J Mol Med 1999;77:140–143.
120. Oberholzer J, Triponez F, Mage R, et al. Human islet transplantation: lessons from 13 autologous and 13 allogeneic transplantations. Transplantation 2000;69:1115–1123.
121. Kahan BD. The synergistic effects of cyclosporine and sirolimus. Transplantation 1997;63:170.
122. Kahan BD, Julian BA, Pescovitz MD, Vanrenterghem Y, Neylan J. Sirolimus reduces the incidence of acute rejection episodes despite lower cyclosporin doses in caucasian recipients of mismatched primary renal allografts: a phase II trial. Rapamune study group. Transplantation 1999;68:1526–1532.
123. Kahan BD. Cyclosporin A, FK506, rapamycin: the use of a quantitative analytic tool to discriminate immunosuppressive drug interactions. J Am Soc Nephrol 1992;2(Suppl):S222–S227.
124. Chen H, Qi S, Xu D, et al. Combined effect of rapamycin and FK 506 in prolongation of small bowel graft survival in the mouse. Transplant Proc 1998;30:2579–2581.
125. Vu MD, Qi S, Xu D, et al. Tacrolimus (FK506) and sirolimus (rapamycin) in combination are not antagonistic but produce extended graft survival in cardiac transplantation in the rat. Transplantation 1997;64:1853–1856.
126. McAlister VC, Gao Z, Peltekian K, Domingues J, Mahalati K, MacDonald AS. Sirolimus–tacrolimus combination immunosuppression. Lancet 2000;355:376–377.
127. Report of the expert committee on the diagnosis and classification of diabetes mellitus. Diabetes Care 1997;20:1183–1197.
128. Hollander GA, Zuklys S, Forster E, Krenger W. On costimulatory signals and T-cell tolerance: relevance for transplantation immunity. Transplant Proc 1999;31:25S–31S.
129. Schwartz RH. A cell culture model for T lymphocyte clonal anergy. Science 1990;248:1349–1356.
130. Schwartz RH. Costimulation of T lymphocytes: the role of CD28, CTLA-4, and B7/BB1 in interleukin-2 production and immunotherapy. Cell 1992;71:1065–1068.

131. Chen C, Nabavi N. In vitro induction of T cell anergy by blocking B7 and early T cell costimulatory molecule ETC-1/B7–2. Immunity 1994;1:147–154.
132. Griggs ND, Agersborg SS, Noelle RJ, Ledbetter JA, Linsley PS, Tung KS. The relative contribution of the CD28 and gp39 costimulatory pathways in the clonal expansion and pathogenic acquisition of self-reactive T cells. J Exp Med 1996;183:801–810.
133. Grewal IS, Foellmer HG, Grewal KD, et al. Requirement for CD40ligand in costimulation induction, T cell activation, and experimental allergic encephalomyelitis. Science 1996;273:1864–1867.
134. Balasa B, Krahl T, Patstone G, et al. CD40 ligand–CD40 interactions are necessary for the initiation of insulitis and diabetes in nonobese diabetic mice. J Immunol 1997;159:4620–4627.
135. Khoury S, Sayegh MH, Turka LA. Blocking costimulatory signals to induce transplantation tolerance and prevent autoimmune disease. Int Rev Immunol 1999;18:185–199.
136. Lenschow DJ, Walunas TL, Bluestone JA. CD28/B7 system of T cell costimulation. Annu Rev Immunol 1996;14:233–258.
137. Karandikar NJ, Vanderlugt CL, Walunas TL, Miller SD, Bluestone JA. CTLA-4: a negative regulator of autoimmune disease. J Exp Med 1996;184:783–788.
138. Slavik JM, Hutchcroft JE, Bierer BE. CD28/CTLA-4 and CD80/CD86 families: signaling and function. Immunol Res 1999;19:1–24.
139. Lenschow DJ, Zeng Y, Hathcock KS, et al. Inhibition of transplant rejection following treatment with anti-B7-2 and B7-1 antibodies. Transplantation 1995;60:1171–1178.
140. Lenschow DJ, Zeng Y, Thistlethwaite JR, et al. Long-term survival of xenogeneic pancreatic islet grafts induced by CTLA4Ig. Science 1992;257:789–792.
141. Levisetti MG, Padrid PA, Szot GL, et al. Immunosuppressive effects of human CTLA4Ig in a non-human primate model of allogeneic pancreatic islet transplantation. J Immunol 1997;159:5187–5191.
142. Kirk AD, Harlan DM, Armstrong NN, et al. CTLA4-Ig and anti-CD40 ligand prevent renal allograft rejection in monkeys. Proc Natl Acad Sci USA 1997;94:8789–8794.
143. Zheng XX, Markees TG, Hancock WW, et al. CTLA4 signals are required to optimally induce allograft tolerance with combined donor-specific transfusion and anti-CD154 monoclonal antibody treatment. J Immunol 1999;162:4983–4990.
144. Harlan MH, Kirk AD. Anti-CD154 therapy to prevent graft rejection. Graft 1998;1:63–70.
145. Kiener PA, Moran-Davis P, Rankin BM, Wahl AF, Aruffo A, Hollenbaugh D. Stimulation of CD40 with purified soluble gp39 induces preinflammatory responses in human monocytes. J Immunol 1995;155:4917–4925.
146. Dechanet J, Grosset C, Taupin JL, et al. CD40 ligand stimulates proinflammatory cytokine production by human endothelial cells. J Immunol 1997;159:5640–5647.
147. Parker DC, Greiner DL, Phillips NE, et al. Survival of mouse pancreatic islet allografts in recipients treated with allogeneic small lymphocytes and antibody to CD40 ligand. Proc Natl Acad Sci USA 1995;92:9560–9564.
148. Rossini AA, Parker DC, Phillips NE, et al. Induction of immunological tolerance to islet allografts. Cell Transplant 1996;5:49–52.
149. Gordon EJ, Markees TG, Phillips NE, et al. Prolonged survival of rat islet and skin xenografts in mice treated with donor splenocytes and anti-CD154 monoclonal antibody. Diabetes 1998;47:1199–1206.
150. Markees TG, Serreze DV, Phillips NE, et al. NOD mice have a generalized defect in their response to transplantation tolerance induction. Diabetes 1999;48:967–974.
151. Kirk AD, Burkly LC, Batty DS, et al. Treatment with humanized monoclonal antibody against CD154 prevents acute renal allograft rejection in nonhuman primates. Nat Med 1999;5:686–693.
152. Kawai T, Andrews D, Colvin RB, Sachs DH, Cosimi AB. Thromboembolic complications after treatment with monoclonal antibody against CD40 ligand. Nat Med 2000;6:114.
153. Kirk AD, Harlan DM. Thromboembolic complications after treatment with monoclonal antibody against CD40 ligand (reply). Nat Med 2000;6:114.
154. Ni HT, Deeths MJ, Li W, Mueller DL, Mescher ML. Signaling pathways activated by leukocyte function-associated Ag-1-dependent costimulation. J Immunol 1999;162:5183–5189.
155. Nishihara M, Gotoh M, Ohzato H, et al. Awareness of donor alloantigens in antiadhesion therapy induces antigen-specific unresponsiveness to islet allografts. Transplantation 1997;64:965–970.
156. Nicolls MR, Coulombe M, Yang H, Bolwerk A, Gill RG. Anti-LFA-1 therapy induces long-term islet allograft acceptance in the absence of IFN-gamma or IL-4. J Immunol 2000;164:3627–3634.
157. Buhler L, Deng S, Grau G, Mentha G, Rohner A, Morel P. Treatment with antibodies to leucocyte function-associated antigen-1 prolongs the survival of xenotransplanted islets of Langerhans. Transplant Proc 1994;26:1360–1361.

158. Ohta Y, Gotoh M, Ohzato H, et al. Direct antigen presentation through binding of donor intercellular adhesion molecule-1 to recipient lymphocyte function-associated antigen-1 molecules in xenograft rejection. Transplantation 1998;65:1094–1100.
159. Trowbridge I, Thomas ML. CD45: an emerging role as a protein tyrosine phosphatase required for lymphocyte activation and development. Annu Rev Immunol 1994;12:85–116.
160. Rothstein DM, Basadonna GP. Anti-CD45. A new approach towards tolerance induction. Graft 1999;2:239–245.
161. Schiffenbauer J, Butfiloski E, Hanley G, Sobel ES, Streit WJ, Lazarovits A. Prevention of experimental allergic encephalomyelitis by an antibody to CD45RB. Cell Immunol 1998;190:173–182.
162. Martins TC, Aguas AP. A role for CD45RBlow CD38+ T cells and costimulatory pathways of T-cell activation in protection of non-obese diabetic (NOD) mice from diabetes. Immunology 1999;96:600–605.
163. Lazarovits A, Poppema S, Zhang Z, et al. Prevention and reversal of renal allograft rejection by antibody against CD45RB. Nature 1996;380:717–720.
164. Auersvald LA, Rothstein DM, Oliveira SC, et al. Indefinite islet allograft survival in mice after a short course of treatment with anti-CD45 monoclonal antibodies. Transplantation 1997;63:1355–1358.
165. Basadonna GP, Auersvald L, Khuong CQ, et al. Antibody-mediated targeting of CD45 isoforms: a novel immunotherapeutic strategy. Proc Natl Acad Sci USA 1998;95:3821–3826.
166. Eason JD, Cosimi AB. Biologic immunosuppressive agents. In: Ginns LC, Cosimi AB, Morris PJ, eds. Immunosuppression in Transplantation. Blackwell Science, Oxford, 1999, pp.96–124.
167. Alegre ML, Tso JY, Sattar HA, et al. An anti-murine CD3 monoclonal antibody with a low affinity for Fcg receptors suppresses transplantation responses while minimizing acute toxicity and immunogenicity. J Immunol 1995;155:1544–1555.
168. Smith JA, Tso JY, Clark MR, Cole MS, Bluestone JA. Nonmitogenic anti-CD3 monoclonal antibodies deliver a partial T cell receptor signal and induce clonal anergy. J Exp Med 1997;185:1413–1422.
169. Smith JA, Tang Q, Bluestone JA. Partial TCR signals delivered by FcR-nonbinding anti-CD3 monoclonal antibodies differentially regulate individual Th subsets. J Immunol 1998;160:4841–4849.
170. Zhai Y, Ghobrial RM, Busuttil RW, Kupiec-Weglinski JW. Th1 and Th2 cytokines in organ transplantation: paradigm lost? Crit Rev Immunol 1999;19:155–172.
171. Singh VK, Mehrotra S, Agarwal SS. The paradigm of Th1 and Th2 cytokines: its relevance to autoimmunity and allergy. Immunol Res 1999;20:147–161.
172. Chatenoud L, Thervet E, Primo J, Bach JF. Anti-CD3 antibody induces long-term remission of overt autoimmunity in nonobese diabetic mice. Proc Natl Acad Sci USA 1994;91:123–127.
173. Chatenoud L, Primo J, Bach JF. CD3 antibody-induced dominant self tolerance in overtly diabetic NOD mice. J Immunol 1997;158:2947–2954.
174. Xu D, Alegre ML, Varga SS, et al. In vitro characterization of five humanized OKT3 effector function variant antibodies. Cell Immunol 2000;200:16–26.
175. Woodle ES, Xu D, Zivin RA, et al. Phase I trial of a humanized, Fc receptor nonbinding OKT3 antibody, hu OKT$3_{\gamma 1}$(Ala-Ala) in the treatment of acute renal allograft rejection. Transplantation 1999;68:608–616.
176. Neville DM Jr, Scharff J, Hu HZ, et al. A new reagent for the induction of T-cell depletion, anti-CD3-CRM9. J Immunother Emphasis Tumor Immunol 1996;19:85–92.
177. Knechtle SJ, Vargo D, Fechner J, et al. FN18-CRM9 immunotoxin promotes tolerance in primate renal allografts. Transplantation 1997;63:1–6.
178. Hu H, Stavrou S, Cairns Baker B, et al. Depletion of T lymphocytes with immunotoxin retards the progress of experimental allergic encephalomyelitis in rhesus monkeys. Cell Immunol 1997;177:26–34.
179. Thomas FT, Ricordi C, Contreras JL, et al. Reversal of naturally occurring diabetes in primates by unmodified islet xenografts without chronic immunosuppression. Transplantation 1999;67:846–854.
180. Wells AD, Li XC, Li Y, et al. Requirement for T-cell apoptosis in the induction of peripheral transplantation tolerance. Nat Med 1999;5:1303–1307.
181. Ferguson TA, Green DR. T Cells are just dying to accept grafts. Nat Med 1999;5:1231–1232.
182. Li Y, Li XC, Zheng XX, Wells AD, Turka LA, Strom TB. Blocking both signal 1 and signal 2 of T-cell activation prevents apoptosis of alloreactive T cells and induction of peripheral allograft tolerance. Nat Med 1999;5:1298–1302.
183. Blancho G, Cantarovich D, Soulillou JP. Induction therapy with new monoclonal antibodies. Curr Opin Organ Transplantation 1999;4:326–332.
184. Li XC, Ima A, Li Y, Zheng XX, Malek TR, Strom TB. Blocking the common γ-chain of cytokine receptors induces T cell apoptosis and long-term islet allograft survival. J Immunol 2000;164:1193–1199.
185. Wekerle T, Sykes M. Mixed chimerism as an approach for the induction of transplantation tolerance. Transplantation 1999;68:459–467.

186. Starzl TE, Demetris AJ, Murase N, Ildstad S, Ricordi C, Trucco M. Cell migration, chimerism and graft acceptance. Lancet 1992;339:1579–1582.
187. Stewart FM, Crittenden RB, Lowry PA, Pearson-White S, Quesenberry PJ. Long-term engraftment of normal and post-5-fluorouracil murine marrow into normal nonmyeloablated mice. Blood 1993;81:2566–2571.
188. Wekerle T, Sayegh MH, Hill J, et al. Extrathymic T cell deletion and allogeneic stem cell engraftment induced with costimulatory blockade is followed by central T cell tolerance. J Exp Med 1998;187:2037–2044.
189. Wekerle T, Sayegh MH, Ito H, et al. Anti-CD154 or CTLA4Ig obviates the need for thymic irradiation in a non-myeloablative conditioning regimen for the induction of mixed hematopoietic chimerism. Transplantation 1999;68:1348–1355.
190. Wekerle T, Kurtz J, Ito H, et al. Allogeneic bone marrow transplantation with co-stimulatory blockade induces macrochimerism and tolerance without cytoreductive host treatment. Nat Med 2000;6:464–469.
191. Fontes P, Rao AS, Demetris AJ, et al. Bone marrow augmentation of donor-cell chimerism in kidney, liver, heart, and pancreas islet transplantation. Lancet 1994;344:151–155.
192. Ricordi C, Murase N, Rastellini C, Behboo R, Demetris AJ, Starzl TE. Indefinite survival of rat islet allografts following infusion of donor bone marrow without cytoablation. Cell Transplantation 1996;5:53–55.
193. Ricordi C, Karatzas T, Nery J, et al. High dose donor bone marrow infusions in liver transplantation: the effect of timing. Transplantation 1997;63:7–11.
194. Garcia-Morales R, Carreno M, Matthew J, et al. Continuing observations on the regulatory effects of donor-specific bone marrow cell infusions and chimerism in kidney transplant recipients. Transplantation 1998;65:956–965.
195. Kenyon NS, Ranuncoli A, Masetti M, Chatzipetrou M, Ricordi C. Islet transplantation: present and future perspectives. Diabetes Metab Rev 1998;14:303–313.
196. Snowden JA, Brooks PM, Biggs JC. Haematopoietic stem cell transplantation for autoimmune diseases. Br J Haematol 1997;99:9–22.
197. Tyndall A, Fassas A, Passweg J, et al. Autologous haematopoietic stem cell transplants for autoimmune disease—feasibility and transplant-related mortality. Bone Marrow Transplant 1999;24:729–734.
198. Ikehara S, Ohtsuki H, Good RA, et al. Prevention of type I diabetes in nonobese diabetic mice by allogeneic bone marrow transplantation. Proc Natl Acad Sci USA 1985;82:7743–7747.
199. Yasumizu R, Sugiura K, Iwai H, et al. Treatment of type 1 diabetes mellitus in non-obese diabetic mice by transplantation of allogeneic bone marrow and pancreatic tissue. Proc Natl Acad Sci USA 1987;84:6555–6557.
200. Li H, Kaufman CL, Boggs SS, Johnson PC, Patrene KD, Ildstad ST. Mixed allogeneic chimerism induced by a sublethal approach prevents autoimmune diabetes and reverses insulitis in nonobese diabetic (NOD) mice. J Immunol 1996;156:380–388.
201. Mathieu C, Casteels K, Bouillon R, Waer M. Protection against autoimmune diabetes in mixed bone marrow chimeras. J Immunol 1997;158:1453–1457.
202. Bartlett ST, Schweitzer EJ, Kuo PC, et al. Prevention of autoimmune islet allograft destruction by engraftment of donor T cells. Transplantation 1997;63:299–303.
203. Li H, Kaufman CL, Ildstad ST. Allogeneic chimerism induces donor-specific tolerance to simultaneous islet allografts in nonobese diabetic mice. Surgery 1995;118:192–197.
204. Seung E, Iwakoshi N, Woda BA, et al. Allogeneic hematopoietic chimerism in mice treated with sublethal myeloablation and anti-CD154 antibody: absence of graft-versus-host disease, induction of skin allograft tolerance, and prevention of recurrent autoimmunity in islet-allografted NOD/Lt mice. Blood 2000;95:2175–2182.

31 β-Cell Replacement Therapy for Type 1 Diabetes

Shimon Efrat, PhD

CONTENTS

INTRODUCTION

β-Cell replacement is considered the optimal treatment for type 1 diabetes. Such a therapy may allow restoration of the tight regulation of blood glucose levels, avoid the daily burden to the patient of monitoring and regulating blood glucose, and prevent diabetes complications. β-Cells are uniquely equipped not only with the capacity to synthesize insulin but also with a complex sensing apparatus that integrates a large variety of signals in the continuous adjustment of insulin secretion to changing physiological needs. Ectopic insulin gene expression in non-β-cells may evade the autoimmunity directed against β-cells; however, reconstruction of regulated insulin secretion in non-β-cells is a much more difficult task. The optimal substitute for β-cells destroyed by autoimmunity in type 1 diabetes is therefore a sufficient number of functional β-cells. In principle, such cells could be obtained through β-cell regeneration in the patient or through transplantation from a foreign source of β-cells. Either way, cell therapy for type 1 diabetes faces two major obstacles: obtaining sufficient numbers of differentiated β-cells and protecting them from recurring autoimmunity without continuous immunosuppression. Genetic manipulations may help overcome both of these hurdles.

β-CELL REGENERATION

The understanding of islet development and maintenance may allow stimulation of islet renewal in patients with type 1 diabetes. The bulk of evidence suggests that the embryonic pancreas emerges by budding from the endodermal epithelium *(1)*. This process depends on expression of the homeodomain transcription factor Pdx1 and repression of sonic hedgehog signaling, induced by adjacent regions of the notochord

From: *Contemporary Endocrinology: Type 1 Diabetes: Etiology and Treatment*
Edited by: M. A. Sperling © Humana Press Inc., Totowa, NJ

(2). Subsequent branching of the initial buds depends on unknown factors secreted by mesenchymal cells. The endocrine and exocrine cells likely develop from a common progenitor cell in this branched endoderm, which later becomes the ductal epithelium of the mature pancreas *(2)*. Studies of experimental models of pancreas injury (3–5) revealed that the ductal epithelium serves as a source of cells capable of islet neogenesis in the adult and may constitute the pancreatic stem cells, from which normal renewal of islets occurs throughout life. Indeed, recent reports have demonstrated the capacity of duct cells to differentiate into β-cells in tissue culture (6,7). It is unclear to what extent β-cell regeneration occurs in type 1 diabetes. The "honeymoon period" observed in the course of the disease may result from a wave of islet regeneration. A better understanding of the extracellular and intracellular factors involved in islet neogenesis from duct cells may allow stimulation of this process in vivo.

Another potential source of cells which could be induced to develop into β-cells in vivo is represented by stem cells committed to the development of tissues other than the pancreas. Recent reports have demonstrated a remarkable plasticity in a number of stem cell types, which could be induced to transdifferentiate into a variety of other tissues *(8,9)*. The ability to induce expression of β-cell genes, including insulin, in mouse liver cells in vivo using Pdx1 adenovirus vectors *(10)*, may represent transdifferentiation of a liver progenitor cell.

If β-cell regeneration can be induced in vivo, newly-formed β-cells are likely to be targeted by the autoimmune mechanisms that destroy the original islet β-cells. Therefore, developing ways to prevent recurring autoimmunity (*see* last section) should be an integral part of any β-cell regeneration strategy. In addition, targeting of genes or proteins to specific cell types in vivo remains a difficult task. Thus, it appears more feasible at present to pursue β-cell expansion from progenitor cells in vitro for the purpose of transplantation.

β-CELL EXPANSION IN VITRO

Given the present inability to induce significant β-cell regeneration, allogeneic islet transplantation would represent the next best solution. Although clinical results in the past years have been disappointing, a recent report of islet allograft survival in type 1 diabetic patients, achieved with a novel immunosuppression protocol *(11)*, has raised new hopes for the feasibility of this treatment. However, the prospects for allogeneic islet transplantation are limited by the availability of cadaveric donors and the need to use islets from more than one pancreas for each transplant. Xenogeneic islet transplantation has been considered; however, it raises far greater immunological and physiological difficulties and remains controversial because of the risk of introducing new animal pathogens into the human population *(12)*.

The cell supply barrier to β-cell transplantation could be alleviated by β-cell expansion in tissue culture. Data from rodents suggest that pure β-cells can replace the function of intact islets *(13)*. The pancreas of type 1 diabetes patients is likely to contain sufficient numbers of α, δ, and PP cells, which could interact with β-cells transplanted outside the pancreas through endocrine feedback loops, rather than through cell-to-cell contacts.

Generation of β-Cells from Precursor Cells

Two main approaches have been taken to generate an abundant source of β-cells: expansion of mature β-cells and maturation of precursor cells. In both approaches, the main trade-off is between growth potential and functional performance. Differentiated β-cells from mature islets function well but are postmitotic and do not replicate much on their own. To expand them, one needs to stimulate their replication using elements that regulate the cell cycle, such as oncogenes. The experimental evidence suggests that induction of proliferation leads to varying degrees of dedifferentiation (*see* below). In contrast, a variety of precursor cells are relatively easy to expand in tissue culture. Their spontaneous proliferative potential varies: Embryonic stem (ES) cells can grow virtually indefinitely, as a result of expression of telomerase; tissue stem cells have a more restricted growth potential, and it may help to extend it by immortalizing them, for example by expression of telomerase. However, such cells have multiple fates to choose from, and the challenge is to find ways to direct all of them into the desired pathway. Recent reports have shown that precursor cells, such as mouse ES cells *(14)* and both murine and human pancreatic duct cells *(6,7),* can spontaneously differentiate at low rates in tissue culture into mature β-cells. The availability of human ES cell lines *(15)* raises the possibility that human β-cells could be generated in tissue culture from ES cells. With the maturation of techniques for nuclear transfer from somatic cells into oocytes *(16),* it is possible, in principle, to generate autologous ES cell lines. However, in the case of type 1 diabetes, this would not necessarily represent an advantage over allogeneic ES cells, as the autoimmune response is directed against the autologous cells.

Most probably, the closer in the lineage a precursor cell is to mature β-cells, the fewer steps will be needed to turn it into a β-cell. On the other hand, it is possible that shortcuts could be found, using master switch genes or exogenous inductive factors, that will not require passage through all the intermediate stages of natural development. It is likely that the proliferative capacity of precursor cells will decrease in inverse proportion to their degree of differentiation. The strategy for generating β-cells from precursor cells in culture would likely involve a massive expansion of undifferentiated precursor cells, followed by induction of differentiation into β-cells. An important aspect of this strategy is ensuring that differentiation into β-cells is accompanied by restriction of proliferation, to prevent unregulated cell growth following transplantation.

Expansion of Mature β-Cells

Propagation of mature islet β-cells in culture is difficult. Most of adult islet cells are postmitotic. They do not divide either in vivo or in culture, and when explanted from their tissue context, they are stressed and tend to senesce and die. Although some growth factors can induce limited replication of fetal or neonatal rodent islets *(17),* the natural growth and survival factors of β-cells, which could enable significant β-cell mass expansion in culture, remain largely unknown. Fetal islets have a larger proliferative capacity; however, they remain poorly differentiated with respect to insulin production and secretion *(18,19).*

To generate continuous rodent β-cell lines, several groups have employed oncogenes, in particular, the SV40 large T-antigen (Tag), to bypass senescence and inactivate the gatekeepers to the entrance into the cell cycle and DNA replication, such as the retinoblastoma protein, which acts at the checkpoint between the G1 and S phases (*see* ref. *20* for a recent review). Rodent β-cell lines transformed by Tag maintain low levels of insulin production and secretion. However, their secretory response to glucose is often abnormal, and they tend to lose their limited differentiation during propagation in culture *(20).* Apparently, cell transformation interferes with certain differentiated functions of β-cells. In addition, the transformed cells replicate without control and are thus not suitable for transplantation.

To overcome these drawbacks, we introduced the concept of reversible cell immortalization as a way to regulate β-cell mass and function in tissue culture and following transplantation in vivo. This was achieved by using elements of the bacterial tetracycline (tet) operon to control oncogene expression in transgenic mice *(13)*. The transformed β-cells were found to completely depend on the continuous expression of Tag for their proliferation, and the shut off of Tag expression induced growth arrest. One cell line, denoted βTC-tet, was studied in detail *(21)*. These cells produced high amounts of insulin and secreted it in response to physiological glucose concentrations. The phenotype of the proliferating cells was stable for over 60 passages in tissue culture. The βTC-tet cells were able to restore euglycemia in syngeneic streptozotocin (STZ)-diabetic mice *(13)*. Treatment of the mice with tet prevented abnormal cell expansion, and the cells remained fully functional in vivo for months in the growth-arrested state. They were capable of resuming replication if the tet block was removed. Insulin secretion in vivo was shown to be regulated by hyperglycemia in hyperglycemic clamp studies *(21)*. Thus, these cells satisfy the requirements from β-cell lines in terms of insulin biosynthesis and regulated secretion, stability, and regulation of proliferation. In addition, our data indicate that growth arrest improves βTC-tet cell function, compared with that of proliferating cells. Insulin biosynthesis is stimulated at the transcriptional and posttranslational levels, resulting in a several-fold increase in insulin mRNA and protein contents *(21,22)*. Artifacts of cell transformation, such as induction of hexokinase activity at passages >60, are reversed by growth arrest *(21)*. By employing the tet-on regulatory system *(23)*, β-cell lines may be generated that can maintain euglycemia in recipients without the need for continuous tet treatment for maintaining growth arrest following transplantation.

In contrast to the success in deriving rodent β-cell lines, induction of β-cell proliferation has been less successful with human islets. Human β-cells tend to dedifferentiate when forced to replicate and essentially lose insulin expression *(18,19)*. Application of the conditional transformation approach to human islets may help address this difficulty. In addition, human cell replication is limited by telomere length, which is much shorter compared with those of mice, and by the fact that most human cell types, unlike most somatic mouse cells, do not express telomerase *(24)*. Expression of telomerase in human β-cells may help extend their life span in culture, as has been shown for other human cell types *(25)*. Efficient gene transfer into human islet cells in culture will be facilitated by the recent development of lentivirus vectors, which allow infection of nonreplicating cells with high efficiency, and stable integration of the introduced genes into the genome of infected cells *(26)*.

The concerns regarding the use of transformed cells in humans may be addressed by enclosing them in a physical barrier through cell encapsulation (*see* the following section), by eliminating the oncogenes from the cells when the desired cell mass is achieved using approaches such as the Cre-loxP-mediated DNA recombination *(27)* and by introducing suicide mechanisms into the engineered cells, such as the herpes simplex thymidine kinase gene, which will allow cell elimination in case of escape from the encapsulation device.

β-CELL PROTECTION FROM RECURRING AUTOIMMUNITY

Once sufficient numbers of differentiated β-cells for transplantation become available, they will need to be protected from recurring autoimmunity, as well as from graft rejection. Although improved immunosuppression protocols are being developed *(11)*, the risks of lifelong immunosuppression are probably not justified by the potential improvements in insulin delivery, when compared to insulin administration. Cell encapsulation in semipermeable membrane devices may provide partial protection. The pore size of these membranes can be designed to exclude immune effector cells and large molecules, such as immunoglobulins and components of the complement system, while allowing free passage of small molecules, such as nutrients and insulin. However, in spite of successful protection of xenograft islets in experimental animals *(28–30)*, as well as survival of allogeneic insulinoma cells in a mouse model of autoimmune diabetes (the nonobese diabetic [NOD] mouse) *(31)*, β-cell encapsulation still needs to overcome a number of fundamental problems. β-Cells are highly active metabolically and require an excellent supply of oxygen for survival and function. In addition, the cells need to have a good access to insulin secretagogues to allow a continuous adjustment of the amount of secreted insulin. These requirements limit the thickness of the cell layer that can be encapsulated, which may lead to a prohibitively large device. At present, most of the devices described rely on diffusion, which requires only minor surgery for implantation and allows easy retrievability *(32)*. Vascularized devices may improve nutrient access to the cells; however, they are likely to involve invasive surgery. Another limitation of encapsulation membranes is their permeability to small cytotoxic molecules, such as cytokines and free radicals, which are released by immune effector cells and are thought to constitute the central mechanism by which autoimmunity causes apoptotic β-cell death *(33)*. β-Cells are particularly sensitive to these agents because they express relatively low levels of antioxidant enzymes *(34)*. Genetic engineering of β-cells with genes that can increase their resistance to immune effector mechanisms may improve their protection within encapsulation devices.

In principle, two types of genes can be used: those encoding proteins that act inside the β-cell to increase its resistance and those encoding secreted proteins that are small enough to pass through the membrane and affect the function of immune effector cells outside the device. A number of antioxidant proteins have been shown to protect β-cell lines exposed to cytokines in culture, as well as reduce the incidence of diabetes in NOD mice. These include the antioxidant enzymes copper/zinc superoxide dismutase (SOD) *(35)*, manganese SOD *(36)*, and catalase *(37)*, and the protein thioredoxin *(38)*. The antiapoptotic proteins Bcl-2 *(39–42)* and A20 *(43)* have also shown promising effects in protecting cultured β-cells from cytokines and oxidative stress, although Bcl-2 failed to prevent diabetes in NOD mice *(44)*.

Viruses constitute a rich source of immunomodulatory genes *(45)*. The immune system targets virus-infected cells with cellular and humoral immune responses, leading to cell death by necrosis or apoptosis, in order to stop the spread of a viral infection. Viruses must escape immune surveillance to successfully replicate in their host. Most viruses encode immunomodulatory proteins, which are among the first viral proteins to be expressed in infected cells. Among them are genes that inhibit antigen presentation, regulate cytokine activity, and prevent apoptosis. They provide the virus with a window of time in which it can replicate undisturbed. We have been studying the early region 3 (E3) genes of adenovirus as a tool for increasing β-cell resistance to immune effector molecules. These genes encode several proteins that downregulate class I major histocompatibility complex (MHC)-mediated antigen presentation on the cell surface and provide protection from apoptosis induced by tumor necrosis factor-α and by Fas *(46)*.

Expression of the E3 genes under control of the insulin promoter in β-cells in transgenic mice allowed islet transplantation into allogeneic mouse strains *(47)*. When these mice were bred with rat insulin promoter–lymphocytic choriomeningitis virus (RIP-LCMV) transgenic mice, a model of virus-induced autoimmune diabetes, the double-transgenic animals were protected from the disease *(48)*. These results suggest that E3 genes may be used to protect transplanted β-cells.

The balance between effector and suppressor T-cells is modulated by a complex array of cytokines that is not fully characterized. Expression of certain cytokines in β-cells may shift the local balance between these subsets of T-lymphocytes toward a suppressive phenotype. NOD mice expressing the suppressive cytokine interleukin-4 (IL-4) were protected from diabetes *(49,50)*. When islets from NOD/severe-combined immunodeficient mice were transduced with lentivirus vector encoding IL-4 and transplanted into syngeneic hosts together with NOD splenocytes, both the transplant and endogenous islets were protected from immune destruction *(51)*. Paracrine protection of β-cells was obtained by expression of transforming growth factor (TGF)-β_1 in islet α-cells in NOD mice, which prevented the development of both spontaneous and cyclophosphamide-induced diabetes *(52)*. In contrast, expression of TGF-β_1 in β-cells failed to inhibit autoimmunity in the RIP-LCMV model *(53)*. Expression of another cytokine, IL-10, also led to conflicting results (54), causing both a delay in the onset and a reduction in the incidence of diabetes when administered into adult NOD mice and an accelerated disease when transgenically expressed in β-cells, perhaps reflecting differences between local and systemic effects of the cytokine. Mammalian IL-10 may possess both immunosuppressive and immunostimulatory properties. A viral homolog of IL-10 (vIL-10) encoded by the Epstein–Barr virus *(55)* lacks the immunostimulatory capacity and thus may be more promising in induction of T-cell suppression *(56)*. Nonetheless, these results suggest that additional studies are needed to obtain a complete picture of the complex cytokine network, before these proteins can be safely and effectively applied to achieve local immunosuppression.

Some of the immunomodulatory and antiapoptotic agents considered for engineering β-cells for transplantation may also be effective in prevention of type 1 diabetes, if targeted by viral vectors to islets in people at risk of developing the disease. However, this prospect depends on accurate diagnosis of prediabetes by improving existing genetic and serological markers as well as the development of safe and efficient ways for gene targeting to islets in vivo.

ACKNOWLEDGMENTS

The work in my laboratory is supported by the Juvenile Diabetes Research Foundation International, the National Institute for Diabetes and Digestive and Kidney Diseases, and the Israel Science Foundation.

REFERENCES

1. Slack JMW. Developmental biology of the pancreas. Development 1995;121:1569–1580.
2. Edlund H. Pancreas: how to get there from the gut? Curr Opin Cell Biol 1999;11:663–668.
3. Bonner-Weir S, Baxter LA, Schuppin GT, Smith FE. A second pathway for regeneration of adult exocrine and endocrine pancreas: a possible recapitulation of embryonic development. Diabetes 1993;42:1717–1720.
4. Wang RN, Kloppel G, Bouwens L. Duct to islet-cell differentiation and islet growth in the pancreas of duct-ligated adult rats. Diabetologia 1995;38:1405–1411.

5. Gu D, Sarvetnick N. Epithelial cell proliferation and islet neogenesis in IFN-g transgenic mice. Development 1993;118:33–46.
6. Ramiya VK, Maraist M, Arfors KE, Schatz DA, Peck AB, Cornelius JG. Reversal of insulin-dependent diabetes using islets generated in vitro from pancreatic stem cells. Nat Med 2000;6:278–282.
7. Bonner-Weir S, Taneja M, Weir GC, et al. In vitro cultivation of human islets from expanded ductal tissue. Proc Natl Acad Sci USA 2000;97:7999–8004.
8. Watt FM, Hogan BLM. Out of Eden: stem cells and their niches. Science 2000;287:1427–1430.
9. Clarke DL, Johansson CB, Wilbertz J, et al. Generalized potential of adult neural stem cells. Science 2000;288:1660–1663.
10. Ferber S, Halkin A, Cohen H, et al. Pancreatic and duodenal homeobox gene 1 induces expression of insulin genes in liver and ameliorates streptozotocin-induced hyperglycemia. Nat Med 2000;6:568–572.
11. Shapiro AM, Lakey JR, Ryan EA, et al. Islet transplantation in seven patients with type 1 diabetes mellitus using a glucocorticoid-free immunosuppressive regimen. N Engl J Med 2000;343:230–238.
12. Bach FH, Fishman JA, Daniels N, et al. Uncertainty in xenotransplantation: individual benefit versus collective risk. Nat Med 1998;4:141–144.
13. Efrat S, Fusco-DeMane D, Lemberg H, Emran OA, Wang S. Conditional transformation of a pancreatic β-cell line derived from transgenic mice expressing a tetracycline-regulated oncogene. Proc Natl Acad Sci USA 1995;92:3576–3580.
14. Soria B, Roche E, Berna G, Leon-Quinto T, Reig JA, Martin F. Insulin-secreting cells derived from embryonic stem cells normalize glycemia in streptozotocin-induced diabetic mice. Diabetes 2000;49:157–162.
15. Thomson JA, Itskovitz-Eldor J, Shapiro SS, et al. Embryonic stem cell lines derived from human blastocysts. Science 1998;282:1145–1147.
16. Kubota C, Yamakuchi H, Todoroki J, et al. Six cloned calves produced from adult fibroblast cells after long-term culture. Proc Natl Acad Sci USA 2000;97:990–995.
17. Nielsen JH, Svensson C, Galsgaard ED, Moldrup A, Billestrup N. Beta cell proliferation and growth factors. J Mol Med 1999;77:62–66.
18. Levine F, Wang S, Beattie G, et al. Development of a cell line from the human fetal pancreas. Transplant Proc 1995;27:3410.
19. Wang S, Beattie G, Mally M, et al. Isolation and characterization of a cell line from the epithelial cells of the human fetal pancreas. Cell Transplant 1997;6:59–67.
20. Efrat S. Prospects for gene therapy of insulin-dependent diabetes mellitus. Diabetologia 1998;41:1401–1409.
21. Fleischer N, Chen C, Surana M, et al. Functional analysis of a conditionally- transformed pancreatic β-cell line. Diabetes 1998;47:1419–1425.
22. Zimmer Y, Milo-Landesman D, Svetlanov A, Efrat S. Genes induced by growth arrest in a pancreatic β-cell line: Identification by analysis of cDNA arrays. FEBS Lett 1999;457:65–70.
23. Gossen M, Freundlieb S, Bender G, Muller G, Hillen W, Bujard H. Transcriptional activation by tetracyclines in mammalian cells. Science 1995;268:1766–1769.
24. Sherr CJ, DePinho RA. Cellular senescence: mitotic clock or culture shock? Cell 2000;102:407–410.
25. Bodnar AG, Ouellette M, Frolkis M, et al. Extension of life-span by introduction of telomerase into normal human cells. Science 1998;279:349–352.
26. Naldini L, Blomer U, Gage FH, Trono D, Verma IM. Efficient transfer, integration, and sustained long-term expression of the transgene in adult rat brains injected with a lentivirus vector. Proc Natl Acad Sci USA 1996;93:11,382–11,388.
27. Sauer B, Henderson N. Cre-stimulated recombination at loxP-containing DNA sequences placed into the mammalian genome. Nucleic Acids Res 1989;17:147–161.
28. Sullivan SJ, Maki T, Borland KM, et al. Biohybrid artificial pancreas: long-term implantation studies in diabetic, pancreatectomized dogs. Science 1991;252:718–721.
29. Lacy PE, Hegre OD, Gerasimidi-Vazeou A, Gentile FT, Dionne KE. Maintenance of normoglycemia in diabetic mice by subcutaneous xenografts of encapsulated islets. Science 1991;254:1782–1784.
30. Sun Y, Ma MX, Zhou D, Vacek I, Sun AM. Normalization of diabetes in spontaneously diabetic cynomolgus monkeys by xenografts of microencapsulated porcine islets without immunosuppression. J Clin Invest 1996;98:1417–1422.
31. Loudovaris T, Jacobs S, Young S, Maryanov D, Brauker J, Johnson RC. Correction of diabetic nod mice with insulinomas implanted within Baxter immunoisolation devices. J Mol Med 1999;77:219–222.
32. Aebischer P, Schluep M, Deglon N, et al. Intrathecal delivery of CNTF using encapsulated genetically modified xenogeneic cells in amyotrophic lateral sclerosis patients. Nat Med 1996;2:696–699.

33. Mauricio D, Mandrup-Poulsen T. Apoptosis and the pathogenesis of IDDM. A question of life and death. Diabetes 1998;47:1537–1543.
34. Lenzen S, Drinkgern J, Tiedge M. Low antioxidant enzyme gene expression in pancreatic islets compared with various other mouse tissues. Free Radical Biol Med 1995;20:463–466.
35. Kubisch HM, Wang J, Luche R, et al. Transgenic copper/zinc superoxide dismutase modulates susceptibility to type I diabetes. Proc Natl Acad Sci USA 1994;91:9956–9959.
36. Hohmeier HE, Thigpen A, Tran VV, Davis R, Newgard CB. Stable expression of manganese superoxide dismutase (MnSOD) in insulinoma cells prevents IL-1 beta-induced cytotoxicity and reduces nitric oxide production. J Clin Invest 1998;101:1811–820.
37. Benhamou PY, Moriscot C, Richard MJ, et al. Adenovirus-mediated catalase gene transfer reduces oxidant stress in human, porcine, and rat pancreatic islets. Diabetologia 1998;41:1093–1100.
38. Hotta M, Tashiro F, Ikegami H, et al. Pancreatic β cell-specific expression of thioredoxin, an antioxidative and antiapoptotic protein, prevents autoimmune and streptozotocin-induced diabetes. J Exp Med 1998;188:1445–1451.
39. Iwahashi H, Hanafusa T, Eguchi Y, et al. Cytokine-induced apoptotic cell death in a mouse pancreatic β-cell line: inhibition by bcl-2. Diabetologia 1996;39:530–536.
40. Liu Y, Rabinovitch A, Suarez-Pinzon W, et al. Expression of the bcl-2 gene from a defective HSV-1 amplicon vector protects pancreatic β cells from apoptosis. Hum Gene Ther 1996;7:1719–1726.
41. Rabinovitch A, Suarez-Pinzon W, Strynadka K, et al. Transfection of human pancreatic islets with an anti-apoptotic gene (bcl-2) protects beta-cells from cytokine-induced destruction. Diabetes 1999;48:1223–1229.
42. Dupraz P, Rinsch C, Pralong WF, et al. Lentivirus-mediated Bcl-2 expression in beta TC-tet cells improves resistance to hypoxia and cytokine-induced apoptosis while preserving in vitro and in vivo control of insulin secretion. Gene Ther 1999;6:1160–1169.
43. Grey ST, Arvelo MB, Hasenkamp W, Bach FH, Ferran C. A20 inhibits cytokine-induced apoptosis and nuclear factor kB-dependent gene activation in islets. J Exp Med 1999;190:1135–1145.
44. Allison J, Thomas H, Beck D, et al. Transgenic overexpression of human Bcl-2 in islet beta cells inhibits apoptosis but does not prevent autoimmune destruction. Int Immunol 2000;12:9–17.
45. Spriggs MK. One step ahead of the game: viral immunomodulatory molecules. Ann Rev Immunol 1966;14:101–130.
46. Wold WSM, Gooding LR. Region E3 of adenovirus: a cassette of genes involved in host immunosurveillance and virus-cell interactions. Virology 1991;184:1–8.
47. Efrat S, Fejer G, Brownlee M, Horwitz MS. Prolonged survival of murine pancreatic islet allografts mediated by adenovirus early region 3 immunoregulatory transgenes. Proc Natl Acad Sci USA 1995;92:6947–6951.
48. von Herrath MG, Efrat S, Oldstone MBA, Horwitz MS. Expression of adenoviral E3 transgenes in β cells prevents autoimmune diabetes. Proc Natl Acad Sci USA 1997;94:9808–9813.
49. Mueller R, Krahl R, Sarvetnick N. Pancreatic expression of interleukin-4 abrogates insulitis and autoimmune diabetes in nonobese diabetic (NOD) mice. J Exp Med 1996;184:1093–1099.
50. Gallichman WS, Balasa B, Davies JD, Sarvetnick N. Pancreatic IL-4 expression results in islet-reactive Th2 cells that inhibit diabetogenic lymphocytes in the nonobese diabetic mouse. J Immunol 1999;163:1696–1703.
51. Gallichman WS, Kafri T, Krahl T, Verma IM, Sarvetnick N. Lentivirus-mediated transduction of islet grafts with interleukin 4 results in sustained gene expression and protection from insulitis. Hum Gene Ther 1998;9:2717–2726.
52. Moritani M, Yoshimoto K, Wong SF, et al. Abrogation of autoimmune diabetes in nonobese diabetic mice and protection against effector lymphocytes by transgenic TGF-β1. J Clin Invest 1998;102:499–506.
53. Lee M-S, Stephen S, Arnush M, et al. Transforming growth factor-β fails to inhibit allograft rejection or virus-induced autoimmune diabetes in transgenic mice. Transplantation 1996;61:1112–1113.
54. Balasa B, Sarvetnick N. The paradoxical effects of interleukin 10 in the immunoregulation of autoimmune diabetes. J Autoimmun 1996;9:283–286.
55. Moore KW, Vieira P, Fiorentino DF, Trounstine ML, Khan TQ, Mosmann TR. Homology of cytokine synthesis inhibitory factor (IL-10) to the Epstein–Barr virus gene BCRFI. Science 1990;248:1230–1234.
56. Suzuki T, Tahara H, Narula S, Moore KW, Robbins PD, Lotze MT. Viral interleukin 10 (IL-10), the human herpes virus 4 cellular IL-10 homologue, induces local anergy to allogeneic and syngeneic tumors. J Exp Med 1995;182:477–486.

32 Islet Growth Factors

Rupangi C. Vasavada, PhD,
Adolfo Garcia-Ocaña, PhD,
Karen K. Takane, PhD, Ana Cebrian, PhD,
Juan Carlos Lopez-Talavera, MD, PhD,
and Andrew F. Stewart, MD

CONTENTS

INTRODUCTION

Pancreatic islet allotransplantation has been attempted for several decades (*see* Chapter 30), but only recently has met with success. Work from the Rajotte group in Edmonton has now shown that pancreatic β-cell transplantation is possible and that adequate pharmacologic immunosuppression can be attained to permit long-term islet transplant survival *(1,2)*. Unfortunately, the balance between the numbers of diabetics and numbers of islets available for transplantation is such that available quantities of islets can service only minuscule numbers of patients with diabetes. For example, in the United States, there are approx 16 million diabetics, including approx 1.5 million type 1 diabetics. In contrast, the total numbers of pancreata available for transplant annually in the United States number in the hundreds to thousands. Moreover, the numbers of pancreata required to transplant a single diabetic ranges between two and four *(1,2)*. These considerations, together with recent advances in human and rodent embryonic stem cell research and pancreatic ductal stem cell research, have highlighted the need to identify factors that can induce β-cells or their precursors to replicate. In this review chapter, we will describe the growth factors that have been documented to date to have potential as agents that could be used to augment islet mass. Because long-term in vivo efficacy is important when considering therapy with islet growth factors, we will give particular emphasis to growth factors that have been demonstrated to be effective in vivo over the very long term in transgenic animals.

From: *Contemporary Endocrinology: Type 1 Diabetes: Etiology and Treatment*
Edited by: M. A. Sperling © Humana Press Inc., Totowa, NJ

β-Cell mass can be regulated in several fashions. One mechanism is the development of new islets, so called "islet neogenesis". This occurs via the differentiation of islet cell precursors from pancreatic stem cells. In the adult, these are believed to reside in the large, medium, and very small branches of the pancreatic duct. At present, there is no definite histochemical or molecular marker for these cells, although it has been suggested that the neuropeptide marker "nestin" may be an excellent marker *(3,4)*. In this process, β-cells differentiate in the ductular wall to express insulin, divide, and bud out into the pancreatic exocrine parenchyma to form new islets.

A second mechanism is the *induction of proliferation of existing β-cells.* There has been some resisitance to the idea that β-cells can proliferate over the years *(5),* but it is now very clear that they can. For example, β-cells can be demonstrated to proliferate in vitro and in vivo in response to glucose, pregnancy, high-fat feeding, obesity and induction of insulin resistance *(6–8).* The rate of basal β-cell replication is very slow, in the range of 2–3% of β-cells per day *(6–8),* and when "accelerated" in the above-described conditions, only 4–6% per day replicate *(9,10).* In comparison to rapidly replicating tissues such as bone marrow cells, intestinal epithelial cells, keratinocytes, and malignant tumor cells, these proliferative rates are very slow. This slow rate of replication, together with the small numbers of β-cells in the pancreas and the difficulty of obtaining pure β-cell populations has made the study of β-cell replication difficult.

A third and final mechanism of enhancing β-cell mass is through the regulation of β-cell life span or survival. It is now clear that accelerating β-cell death plays an important part in the reduction of β-cell mass in conditions such as sustained fasting, hypoglycemia in rodent models of insulinoma, and in the immediate postpartum period in maternal rodents (and presumably humans) to reverse the upregulation of β-cell mass associated with pregnancy and insulin resistance *(11,12).* Similarly, cell death plays an important role in the modeling and remodeling of the islet in the neonatal period in some rodent models *(6,7,11,12).* Of course, accelerated, cell- and cytokine-mediated cell death is a central feature of β-cell death in type 1 diabetes (*13; see* Chapter 4). Finally, reducing the rate of cell death has been demonstrated to be effective in upregulating islet mass and function in some animal models such as the rat insulin promoter (RIP)–parathyroid hormone-related protein (PTHrP) mouse described in more detail on p. 566.

MOLECULAR CONTROL OF REPLICATION IN THE β-CELL

Thus, total islet mass reflects components of the three above-described processes. With regard to β-cell proliferation or replication, surprisingly little is known. This reflects (1) the long-standing dogma that β-cells could not replicate; (2) the difficulty described earlier in obtaining large quantities of pure β-cells for careful biochemical and molecular study; and (3) the extremely slow rate of normal β-cell replication. On the other hand, a surprising amount of information, when culled from the literature and examined in the aggregate, point to the G1–S checkpoint of the cell cycle and the corresponding gatekeeper molecule, Rb (for retinoblastoma), as critical sites of regulation of β-cell replication.

The retinoblastoma protein Rb, plays a critical role in inducing and maintaining growth arrest at the G1–S checkpoint in the cell cycle of all cells *(14,15).* Under basal conditions of growth arrest, Rb serves as a transcriptional repressor of the E2F family of generalized transcription factors that are believed to be central in the G1–S transition *(14,15)*. Understandably, therefore, loss of Rb results in activation of the cell cycle in many cell types, and homozygous loss at this locus in humans is associated with familial retinoblastoma. Homozygous loss of Rb in knockout mice is lethal early in embryonic life. Hemizygous Rb loss in mice is associated with an increase in the frequency of pituitary and thyroid tumors *(14,15)*. Phosphorylation of Rb by the cyclin D1–cdk4 complex causes dissociation of Rb from the E2F family of generalized transcriptional activators, thereby allowing progression of the cell cycle in essentially all cell types. Upregulation of the activity of the cyclin D1–cdk4 complex may result from upregulation of either of these proteins or an increase of their enzymatic activity.

Cyclin D1 and cdk4 activity are, in turn, regulated in a negative fashion through transcriptional repression by a family of proteins that include p16 (also known as Ink4a) and p27 (also known as Kip1) as well as by p21 (also known as Cip1) *(14)*. p21 is, in turn, transcriptionally activated by p53, which is maintained at steady-state levels by an association with a protein named mdm2, a chaperone protein that targets excessive accumulation of p53 for ubiquitinization and proteasomal degradation *(14)*. As with the other proteins described, imbalance of any of these proteins is associated with inappropriate proliferation or inappropriate growth arrest in virtually every cell type. With this background, what is the evidence that this pathway is relevant to islet proliferation? A recent series of publications, together with an older literature on T-antigen, make it inescapably clear that this pathway is likely to be central to the control of β-cell proliferation.

First, the very first β-cell-targeted transgenic mouse, prepared by Hanahan, employed the rat insulin II promoter to target the SV40 T-antigen to β-cells *(16)*. T-antigen interacts with both p53 as well as well Rb, inactivating both. Not surprisingly, these RIP–TAg mice developed islet hyperplasia followed by frank β-cell malignancies *(16, 17)*. Over the years, Hanahan and Efrat have prepared a variety of rodent cell lines, such as the βTC3 cell line, based on the constitutive or regulatable delivery of TAg to β-cells *(16–18)*. On the positive side, RIP–TAg mice display accelerated β-cell proliferation, increases in islet mass, and insulin-mediated hypoglycemia. On the negative side, these mice develop lethal malignant insulinomas. In the current context, they illustrate that freeing β-cells from Rb- and p53-mediated growth arrest leads to β-cell tumors and, therefore, indicates that this is a key cell cycle checkpoint in β-cells, as in so many other cell types. Of course, these results are predictable and convey no sense of β-cell specificity for the p53–Rb pathway: TAg overexpression causes tumors in many different tissues.

The apparent specificity of this pathway in β-cells begins to be highlighted by the observation that mice that are homozygously null for p53 and also heterozygously null for Rb (Rb-null homozygotes are nonviable) develop a very restricted profile of oncogenesis: They develop soft tissue sarcomas and lymphomas and pituitary, thyroid, pineal, and islet tumors *(19,20)*. Although most of the tumors are also present in either singly mutant p53 or Rb mutant mice, islet tumors are present only in mice doubly mutant for Rb and p53 *(19,20)*. These findings make it very clear that p53 and Rb are critical regulators of β-cell replication and that their combined absence has a surprisingly tissue-specific effect on β-cells.

Further evidence for a critical, cell-type specific role of this pathway in β-cell replication is provided by the work of Barbacid and Tsutsui and their collaborators *(21,22)*. These two groups of investigators created mice that lacked cdk4. The investigators expected to find a generalized reduction in cell proliferation rates. To their surprise, they found that null homozygosity for cdk4 yielded a very restricted phenotype. These mice displayed abnormalities in only three tissues: the ovary, the testis, and the β-cell. The animals displayed β-cell dropout and developed diabetes and ketoacidosis. These findings indicate marked specificity for, and lack of redundancy in, the actions of the cdk4–cyclin D pathway in the control of the cell cycle in β-cells.

The Barbacid group took these observations further, creating a knock-in mouse in which the normal cdk4 was replaced by a constitutively active form of cdk4 *(21)*. This constitutively active cdk4 employed its own promoter and was presumably expressed in all tissues. The surprise again was that these mice, with generalized expression of a constitutively active cdk4, demonstrated significant abnormalities in only one tissue: the β-cell. The β-cell abnormality was marked islet hyperplasia (unaccompanied by hypoglycemia). These observations make the very clear point that the cdk4–cyclin D1–p53–Rb pathway is, indeed, very specifically involved in the regulation of the cell cycle in β-cells.

One final observation provides additional evidence of the key role of this pathway in the control of β-cell replication. Arnold and his group have reported recently on a series of 64 human pancreatic endocrine tumors in which they sought abnormalities in the p53–Rb–cdk4–cyclin D1 pathway *(23)*. Interestingly, 43% of the 64 tumors demonstrated upregulation of cyclin D1 at the protein, mRNA, and histochemical level, and this applied to the insulinoma subset as well: Eight of 22 insulinomas also displayed upregulation of cyclin D1. The cellular mechanisms responsible for the upregulation did not appear to include structural alterations in the cyclin D1 gene, but rather likely resulted from abnormal transcriptional or posttranscriptional regulation of cyclin D1 in islet tumors. This degree of association of a single oncogene with a single tumor type is unusual outside the setting of heritable tumors and again points a very specific finger at the central importance of this pathway in the control of the cell cycle in β-cells.

It is important to point out that these observations in no way exclude other cell cycle checkpoints or cell cycle regulatory molecules in β-cell proliferation. Of course, other cyclins and cyclin-dependent kinases and their upstream regulatory molecules are obviously essential to the completion of the cell cycle in β-cells. However, they make the point that this is likely a particularly important control mechanism in the β-cell and strongly suggest that it is an important avenue to explore in any study of the regulation of the cell cycle in the β-cell.

β-CELL GROWTH FACTORS

Hepatocyte Growth Factor

Hepatocyte growth factor (HGF) was identified in the regenerating liver and plays a role in recovery from hepatic injury or resection *(24–26)*. A mesenchyme-derived factor, HGF is synthesized and secreted as an inactive single-chain precursor and requires activation by proteolytic enzymes. The resulting disulfide- linked heterodimeric glycoprotein is composed of a 69-kDa α-subunit containing four kringle domains and a 34-kDa β-subunit with an inactive serine protease-like motif *(27–30)*. Recently, it has been demonstrated that HGF is a pleiotropic factor capable of promoting cell growth (mitogenesis), cell motility (motogenesis), and organ development (morphogenesis) in a wide variety of cells and tissue types *(31,32)*. Northern blot studies have also revealed the presence of several HGF transcripts in total RNA from different tissues *(33,34)*. Some of the variants encoded by these transcripts display different activities compared to the full-length form of the molecule.

HGF binds with high affinity to its specific membrane-spanning tyrosine kinase receptor encoded by the proto-oncogene, c-met *(32,35,36)*. Like HGF, the receptor is widely distributed, and the pancreatic β-cell is one of the sites of expression. In mouse embryos lacking either HGF or the c-met receptor, placenta, liver, and skeletal muscle in the limb and diaphragm are developmentally impaired, resulting in early intrauterine death *(37,38)*. HGF signals via mitogen-activated protein (MAP) kinase and PI3 kinase pathways in many tissues, including the liver and kidney. Its signaling mechanisms in the islet have been less well studied, but there is evidence for signaling via the PI3 kinase pathway in the β-cell *(39)*.

HGF and c-met mRNA are coexpressed during the early development of the pancreas, then decline to a lower level during puberty and adult life *(40–42)*. HGF immunoreactivity has been localized in rabbit exocrine pancreas and in rat, mouse, and human islets *(43–45)*. HGF-activating proteases have also been detected in the exocrine and endocrine rat and human pancreas *(46,47)*. Additionally, c-met receptor protein has been colocalized to insulin-containing cells in the islet *(42)* as well as the apical membrane of ductal cells *(48)* by confocal immunofluorecent studies. The fetal lethality that occurs in mice lacking HGF or c-met has been an impediment in defining the exact role of these molecules in pancreatic development, but in vitro studies suggest that HGF may be essential in fetal mesenchyme-induced pancreatic β-cell growth *(42)*. In addition, HGF is able to increase the expression of Reg (regenerating gene) (*see* p. 570), a protein implicated in pancreatic regeneration *(49)*. In combination with activin A, HGF is able to convert pancreatic acinar AR42J cells into insulin-producing cells *(50)*. HGF and c-met expression seems to be upregulated in the regenerating pancreas after acute pancreatitis *(51,52)*. All of this indirect evidence suggests that HGF could have an important role in pancreatic development, and conditional pancreatic knockouts of HGF or its receptor would be useful in helping to better define this role.

Many studies have shown that HGF is a mitogenic and an insulinotropic agent for fetal and adult islet cells in vitro *(53,54)*. On the other hand, Lefebvre and collaborators have suggested that HGF is able to stimulate the proliferation of human adult pancreatic ductal cells, but not of the underlying β-cells *(5)*. To determine if localized overexpression of HGF in the islet would result in an increase in islet mass and function in vivo, we developed transgenic mice overexpressing HGF in the islet under the control of the rat insulin II promoter (RIP) *(9)*. Interestingly, RIP–HGF mice show a dramatic increase in islet mass, because of an increase in both islet size and number. The principal mechanism responsible for the increase in islet size is a dramatic twofold to threefold augmentation of β-cell proliferation in these transgenic mice. Proliferation definitely occurs within β-cells, as evidenced by labeling of β-cells with the cell division marker, bromodeoxyuridine (BrdU) *(9)*. Associated with this increase in islet mass, RIP–HGF mice have lower blood glucose levels than their normal littermates under fasting and nonfasting conditions, as well as inappropriate hyperinsulinemia *(9)*. Overexpression of HGF in the islet was accompanied by an increase in the levels of insulin mRNA and insulin peptide content in the islet. Studies of the molecular mechanisms responsible for these effects are underway. RIP–HGF mice have also been shown to be more resistant to the development of STZ-induced diabetes than their normal littermates *(9)*.

A recent study has demonstrated that a daily intraperitoneal injection of HGF ameliorates hyperglycemia in STZ-induced diabetic mice receiving a marginal mass of intrahepatic islet grafts *(55)*. The authors suggest that the beneficial effects of HGF may be caused by the prevention of apoptotic cell death of β-cells in the islet grafts.

All these results suggest that HGF is an excellent candidate for future strategies aimed at treating diabetes mellitus. One of these strategies could be the delivery of HGF to isolated islets to enhance their mass and function. These islets would then be transplanted into patients with diabetes. We have recently demonstrated using adenovirus-encoding HGF cDNA that this growth factor can be delivered into isolated human islets and causes a dramatic increase in islet cell proliferation *(56)*. These results give strong support to the hypothesis that this factor, delivered by gene transfer to transplanted islets at the time of transplant, may very well enhance the quantity, function, and survival of transplanted human islets.

Parathyroid Hormone-Related Protein

As will become clear, parathyroid hormone related protein (PTHrP) is not, in formal terms, a growth factor for the β-cell in the sense that it stimulates β-cell proliferation. However, it is clearly a growth factor in many other cell types and is included here for completeness. PTHrP was initially identified as the factor responsible for the majority of cases of the common paraneoplastic syndrome humoral hypercalcemia of malignancy *(57,58)*. PTHrP undergoes extensive posttranslational processing to generate a family of daughter peptides. Extensive reviews of this process are available *(59,60)*. PTHrP gene expression has subsequently been detected in almost every normal tissue and organ of the body, and the pancreatic islet is no exception *(60)*. Within the islet, PTHrP is produced in all four cell types (α-, β-, δ- and pancreatic polypeptide cells) and in the cells of the pancreatic duct *(61,62)*. It does not appear to be produced by the exocrine cells of the pancreas. A receptor for PTHrP is present on β-cells as well, suggesting that in the islet, as in other tissues, PTHrP may play a paracrine or autocrine role *(61,63)*.

Disruption of the PTHrP or the PTH receptor genes in mice results in embryonic or perinatal lethality, which appears to have a skeletal basis *(64,65)*. The islets are still forming at this time of development, but appear grossly normal in PTHrP- or PTH receptor-null mice. These observations preclude a clear understanding, to date, of the normal physiological role of PTHrP within the β-cell. In order to gain some insight into a possible physiologic role for PTHrP in the pancreatic islet, we prepared transgenic mice in which PTHrP was overexpressed in the pancreatic islet using the RIP II promoter *(66,67)*. These RIP–PTHrP mice display islet cell hyperplasia, significant hypoglycemia, both under fasting and nonfasting conditions, as well as inappropriate hyperinsulinemia.

The primary effect of PTHrP overexpression appears not to be developmental, but postnatal, because transgenic mice at 1 wk of age are normoglycemic and display normal islet mass despite expression of the PTHrP transgene *(67)*. In contrast, by 8–12 wk of age, islet mass increases approximately twofold *(66,67)*. This continues through the life of the animals, such that by 1 yr of age, islet mass has increased approximately threefold to fourfold. Both an increase in the number of β-cells per islet as well as an increase in total islet number contribute to the enhancement of islet mass in RIP–PTHrP mice. This increase in islet mass clearly does not result from an increase in the proliferation rates of pre-existing β-cells within the islet, as BrdU incorporation rates are normal in RIP–PTHrP mice in vivo and PTHrP fails to stimulate β-cell proliferation in vitro *(67)*. Instead, the increased islet mass in RIP–PTHrP mice appears to result from a decline in the rate of β-cell death in RIP–PTHrP mice *(67)*. In other cell types such as chondrocytes, neuronal cells, and prostate carcinoma cells, PTHrP has been shown to have an antiapoptotic or protective effect against cell death. In line with this, β-cells of the RIP–PTHrP mice have also shown to be more resistant to the cytotoxic effects of high doses of the diabetogenic agent streptozotocin (STZ): RIP–PTHrP transgenic mice remain relatively euglycemic, unlike their normal littermates, which become severely diabetic following STZ injection *(67)*. The molecular mechanisms responsible for this enhanced β-cell survival are under study.

These findings suggest that PTHrP, like HGF, may have potential in gene therapeutic strategies designed to increase β-cell mass and function. Specifically, this peptide could prove to be valuable in islet transplant survival in type 1 diabetes.

Prolactin, Growth Hormone, and Placental Lactogen

Several studies have demonstrated that prolactin (PRL) and growth hormone (GH) secreted by the pituitary and the closely related placental lactogen (PL) secreted by the placenta during pregnancy may play an important role in the regulation of pancreatic islet growth and function. In homologous systems, islet β-cells respond to PRL and PL via an increase in cell proliferation as well as an enhancement of β-cell function, through a lowering of the threshold for glucose-stimulated insulin secretion (GSIS) *(68,69)*. This has been demonstrated in vivo by PRL infusion into rats *(69)*, and in vitro by exposing islets from several different species to these peptides *(70)*. Among the several islet growth factors studied to date, PL and PRL seem to be among the most potent in their ability to stimulate β-cell proliferation.

Although synthesis of PRL and PL occurs in two very different organs, these proteins are closely related and interact with a common receptor, the PRL receptor, the long form of which is expressed in β-cells. Binding of PRL or PL to this receptor in islets stimulates the Jak-2/Stat-5 intracellular signaling pathway *(71,72)*. PRL receptor activation in the islet results in an upregulation of a number of genes in the glucose metabolism pathway, including glucokinase, GLUT-2, insulin, as well as a number of other transcription factors and cell-cycle-related genes *(73)*.

Several studies performed in rats using heterologous human GH that binds PRL and GH receptors have reached the erroneous conclusion that GH is as potent as PRL or PL as an islet growth factor. However, studies with homologous GH have demonstrated that the actions of this hormone in the islet β-cells are very modest when compared to those induced by PRL-receptor activation *(70)*. This limited effect of GH in the islet may be the result of a rapid downregulation of its receptor activity *(70)*.

The actions of PRL and GH on the islet are likely primarily surrogate responses to what is the normal ligand, PL, for the PRL/GH receptor. In vivo, PL has been implicated as the primary factor responsible for the enhanced islet mass and function that occurs during pregnancy *(68)*. The temporal correlation between the appearance of circulating PL and the onset of changes in islet cell proliferation and insulin secretion during pregnancy *(68,74)*, as well as the proliferative and insulin secretory effects of PL on islets in vitro *(70)*, give credence to this argument. However, during late pregnancy, islet proliferation and function return to normal levels despite continued elevated serum PL levels. This reduction in islet mass and function is postulated to be the result of an increase in the level of progesterone and other steroids during late pregnancy, as progesterone has been shown to have an inhibitory effect on PRL-stimulated islet proliferation and insulin secretion in vitro *(75)*.

To evaluate whether overexpression of PL in the islet could stimulate islet growth and function in vivo, we generated transgenic mice expressing mouse PL-I cDNA in β-cells *(10)*. Three different lines of RIP–mPL-1 transgenic mice, expressing PL in the range of 16 to 200 pg/μg of protein in islets, were generated and all exhibited a similar phenotype. These mice, like the RIP–HGF and RIP–PTHrP mice, display islet hyperplasia, mild hypoglycemia, and inappropriate hyperinsulinemia. The increase in islet mass seen in the RIP–mPL-1 transgenic mice appears to be largely the result of enhanced β-cell proliferation, as measured by BrdU labeling in vivo, and also, to a minor degree, to an increase in individual islet cell size *(10)*. Surprisingly, in contrast to islets treated with PL in vitro, which secrete higher amounts of insulin at any given glucose concentration, RIP–mPL-1 transgenic islets respond normally to glucose, both in vivo as assessed by the intraperitoneal glucose tolerance test (IPGTT) *(76)* and in vitro in glucose-stimulated insulin secretion perifusion experiments *(10)*.

Thus, PL has a sustained effect on islet function and proliferation in vivo, which fits nicely with the long-term adaptive changes demanded in pregnancy. Importantly, given its efficacy in vivo in rodent islets, it may, like HGF and PTHrP, prove to be useful in gene-transfer strategies for the treatment of diabetes.

GLP-1/Exendin-4

As with the PTHrP gene and those of many other neuroendocrine peptides, the glucagon gene encodes a number of active peptide hormones, including glucagon, glicentin, and the glucagonlike peptides (GLPs). GLP-1(7–36), acting through the seven transmembrane-spanning G-coupled protein GLP-1 receptor on the β-cell, has been shown to be a potent stimulator of β-cell replication in vitro *(77–85)*. It also stimulates the expression of the critical islet-specific transcription factor, PDX-1 *(80)*. Similarly, a homologous peptide, exendin-4, derived from the salivary glands of the gila monster lizard, also binds to the GLP-1 receptor and stimulates β-cell replication *(77)*. GLP-1(7–36) is susceptible to cleavage and inactivation by the serum protease dipeptidyl peptidase IV, and this has limited its use in in vivo settings *(82)*. In any case, both GLP-1(7–34) and exendin-4 have been shown in studies to stimulate adenylyl cyclase within β-cells and in some studies to accelerate the growth and/or recovery of β-cells in subtotal pancreatectomy models *(83–85)*.

Recently, Baggio et al. have described a transgenic mouse model in which exendin-4 was overexpressed using the generic metallothionein promoter *(81)*. Surprisingly, despite clear evidence of widespread expression in multiple tissues and systemic increases in circulating concentrations of exendin-4, these mice have no striking phenotype relating to the β-cell and glucose homeostasis is essentially normal. This does not appear to be the result of failure of exendin-4 expression or to secretion of an inactive form of exendin-4. These observations raise the possibility that sustained responses to GLP-1(7–34) and/or exendin-4 may become desensitized or downregulated with time. Nonetheless, these molecules are interesting and should remain in the potential armamentarium of islet mass-enhancing factors. Pharmacological small-molecule analogs of GLP-1 and exendin-4 may also hold promise therapeutically.

Insulin and Insulin-Like Growth Factors 1 and 2

Insulin may not intuitively seem a growth factor for the pancreatic islet, but it has recently become clear through the conditional knockout of the insulin receptor in the β-cell (the β-cell insulin receptor knockout or "βIRKO" mouse), that insulin action is required for the maintenance of normal islet mass and function *(86)*. βIRKO mice display reductions in first-phase insulin secretion and associated glucose intolerance. In addition, they demonstrate a 20–40% reduction in β-cell mass by 4 mo of age. In a sense, this is rational because insulin is required for the normal growth and maintenance of many different cell types, and the β-cell should be no exception.

Insulin-like growth factor-1 (IGF-1) has been shown to have minor effects, if any, on isolated pancreatic islets or pancreatic β-cell lines as studied in vitro using tritiated thymidine incorporation *(87,88)*. On the other hand, IGF-2 is expressed at higher levels in the islet and has been shown in several in vitro and in vivo systems with some regularity to enhance β-cell proliferation *(89)*. Devedjiain et al have prepared transgenic mice that overexpress IGF-2 in the β-cell under the control of the RIP-I promoter *(90)*. To their surprise, although the mice developed islet hyperplasia and some degree of accentuated glucose-stimulated insulin secretion from islets in vitro, the mice were not hypoglycemic, but, in fact, were either glucose intolerant or frankly diabetic. The authors hypothesize that this is the result of systemic insulin oversecretion inducing insulin resistance. This seems unlikely, however, as other transgenic models of insulin overproduction, such as the RIP–HGF mouse, the RIP–PL mouse and the RIP–PTHrP mouse, all of which have lifelong insulin overproduction, are hypoglycemic, not diabetic *(9,10,66)*. Thus, this phenomenon requires further explanation. Circulating IGF-2 concentrations were elevated in the RIP–IGF-2 mouse *(90)*, and perhaps this led to insulin resistance in some fashion.

Fibroblast Growth Factors

The fibroblast growth factor (FGF) family of proteins is composed of at least 19 related peptides with actions that include mitogenesis, angiogenesis, and morphogenesis in a variety of fetal, neonatal, and adult tissues. FGF-1 (also called acid FGF) and FGF-2 (also called basic FGF) are present in normal adult human pancreas and are highly expressed in pancreatic tumors *(91)*. FGF-1 has been detected in α-cells and in acinar and ductal epithelial cells, and FGF-2 mRNA has been localized in α- and β-cells and also in ductal cells *(92)*. Both FGFs strongly increase proliferation in isolated rat islets *(92)*. In addition, FGF-1 is able to increase the insulin content of rat fetal islet-like structures *(93)*. On the other hand, FGF-2 induces pancreatic epithelial cell proliferation during embryonic life *(94)* and also increases the formation of islet-like cell clusters in culture *(93)*. Interestingly, exogenous FGF-7 (also called keratinocyte growth factor or KGF) is also a potent inducer of islet cell proliferation in vitro *(92)*, although overexpression of this factor in transgenic mice using the human insulin promoter induces the formation of hepatocytes within islets and intraislet duct cell proliferation *(95)*. This suggests that this factor could induce the differentiation of uncommitted stem cells present in the pancreas. Recently, Hart and collaborators have expanded the repertoire of FGFs observed in the islet, demonstrating that the islet also produces FGF-4, FGF-5, and FGF-10 *(96)*.

Fibroblast growth factors effects are mediated by FGF receptors (FGFRs), four high-affinity receptors designated FGFR1 through FGFR4. These receptors are abundant and widespread in the developing pancreas *(93,94,96)*. Hart et al. demonstrated, using dominant negative FGFR1 under the control of the PDX1 promoter (a duct, islet, and exocrine pancreas promoter), that FGFR1, but not FGFR2, is required for normal islet development and function *(96)*. Mice deficient in FGFR1 have a 25% reduction in β-cell mass and also display other β-cell defects, including reduced prohormone convertase function and GLUT-2 expression *(96)*. These data provide clear evidence that the FGF family is required for normal attainment of normal β-cell mass in rodents.

Islet Neogenesis-Associated Protein and the Reg Family

From a regenerating islet-derived cDNA library, Okamoto et al. isolated a novel gene called *reg* that may be involved in β-cell regeneration following 90% pancreatectomy in the rat *(97,98)*. The *reg* sequence is identical to that of pancreatic stone protein (PSP) *(99,100)*, and *reg* and PSP proteins are derived from the same gene *(101)*. PSP was originally discovered as an exocrine gene product and shown to comprise up to 10% of the protein in pancreatic exocrine secretion. The *reg* gene is expressed in regenerating islets but not in normal pancreatic islets or insulinomas. More recently, it has been discovered that *reg* and *reg*-related genes constitute a multigene family. Based on the primary structures of the encoded proteins, the members of this family have been grouped in three different subclasses: type I, II, and III *(102–104)*. Recently, a *reg* protein receptor cDNA has been isolated from a rat islet cDNA library *(105)*. This receptor appears to be highly homologous with a human multiple exostosislike gene, the function of which has not yet been clarified.

Administration of recombinant rat *reg* protein stimulates β-cell replication in vitro, increases β-cell mass in 90% pancreatectomized rats and also in nonobese diabetic (NOD) mice, resulting in the amelioration of diabetes in both cases *(106,107)*. However, the absence of *reg* I protein in the *reg* I protein knockout mouse does not seem to induce any phenotypic abnormality under normal physiological conditions *(108)*. In addition, transgenic mice overexpressing the *reg* I gene in islet β-cells using the RIP II, did not show any enhancement of islet size *(109)*.

Islet neogenesis-associated protein (INGAP), a protein homologous with the type III *reg* proteins, was recently cloned by differential display using mRNA from a regenerating hamster pancreas *(110)*. INGAP is produced in acinar cells but not in the islets, and it is absent in normal mouse pancreas. The expression of this gene is confined to the first 2 d after the treatment and is not detectable after that time. It has been also observed that INGAP is mitogenic for primary-cultured epithelial cells of pancreatic ducts, but not for a hamster insulinoma tumor cell line. Because ductal cell proliferation seems to be prerequisite for islet neogenesis, it has been postulated that this protein could be involved in the islet neogenesis process after partial duct obstruction. Although these results were exciting when first presented, little recent progress has been made in this area.

Betacellulin

Betacellulin (BTC) is a member of the epidermal growth factor (EGF) family of proteins *(111)*. Like other members of the EGF family, BTC is synthesized as a 177-amino-acid transmembrane precursor containing 6 conserved cysteine residues. The 80-amino-acid mature peptide was initially identified in conditioned media from a mouse pancreatic β-cell carcinoma cell line that was mitogenic for Balb/C 3T3 cells *(112)*. BTC is expressed in the βTC-3 mouse insulinoma cell line, implying a possible regulatory role of BTC in the proliferation of pancreatic β-cells *(113)*.

Members of the EGF/BTC family bind to and activate four tyrosine kinase receptors encoded by the erbB gene family *(114)*. BTC stimulates complex patterns of erbB family receptor tyrosine phosphorylation and coupling to cellular signaling pathways that are distinct from the patterns stimulated by EGF and neuregulin-β (NRG-β) *(115)*. Thus, BTC exhibits activities that are distinct from those displayed by EGF, which activates EGF receptor alone, as well as NRG-β, which activates erbB-3 and erbB-4. On this basis, BTC stimulates a pattern of receptor transmodulation that is qualitatively distinct from the patterns stimulated by EGF and NRG-β *(115)*.

The mitogenic effect of BTC on the mouse insulinoma cell line INS-1 confirms that this growth factor is capable of stimulating the proliferation of at least some β-cell types *(116)*. BTC has also been shown to convert clonal pancreatic exocrine/ductal cells of the AR42J line into insulin-expressing cells *(117)*. BTC is also required for the induction of insulin gene expression in clonal α-cells transfected with the *pdx-1* gene *(118)*. Recently, Yamamoto et al. have demonstrated that BTC administered subcutaneously to alloxan-treated diabetic mice stimulated β-cell neogenesis from ductular cells and accelerated islet recovery from alloxan-induced diabetes *(119)*.

Transforming Growth Factor-α and Gastrin

Transforming growth factor-α (TGF-α) is a member of the EGF family and is a ligand for the EGF receptor, a tyrosine kinase receptor. TGF-α is synthesized as a 160-amino-acid transmembrane precursor. The 50-amino-acid mature form is generated by proteolytic cleavage of a soluble form from a membrane-bound domain. Pro-TGF-α is able to bind to EGFR on adjacent cells and is biologically active, albeit at a reduced level. TGF-α overexpression in pancreatic acinar cells of transgenic mice, under the control of the metallothionein 1 promoter (MT), resulted in proliferation of acinar cells and fibroblasts, eventually leading to interstitial fibrosis *(120,121)*. There was also a development of multifocal pseudoductular acinar metaplasia. However, expression of TGF-α in pancreatic islets was not detected.

Gastrin is synthesized as a preprohormone of 101 amino acids and is rapidly processed into its mature forms. Gastrin is transiently expressed in the developing pancreas. In the neonatal rat, maximal gastrin mRNA expression occurs in the islet prior to the rise in somatostatin, insulin, and glucagon mRNA levels *(122)*. In transgenic mice overexpressing preprogastrin in islets under the control of the RIP I, there appeared to be no change in pancreatic histology, nor was islet mass increased *(123)*.

However, crossing MT–TGF-α mice with RIP I–gastrin mice, thereby overexpressing both transgenes, led to a decrease in ductular proliferation and interstitial fibrosis *(124)*. Gastrin and TGF-α also acted synergistically to significantly increase the islet mass in the double transgenics compared to the control animals. Despite the greater islet mass, these animals displayed no difference in blood glucose levels nor in insulin mRNA levels. The importance of these events physiologically and therapeutically is uncertain.

Platelet-Derived Growth Factor

Platelet-derived growth factor (PDGF) is a disulfide-bonded heterodimer composed of A and B polypeptide chains. The effects of PDGF are mediated by two different transmembrane receptors with intrinsic tyrosine kinase activity: A-type and B-type. In the normal pancreas, PDGF immunoreactivity has been detected in islet cells and the B-type receptor is present in acinar cells and, at very low levels, in islet cells *(125,126)*. PDGF seems to induce very modest proliferative effects in fetal rat islet cells, with no changes in insulin release *(127)*. Furthermore, the growth response of isolated mouse pancreatic islet cells transfected with PDGF and/or its receptors seems to be very small *(126)*.

Nerve Growth Factor

Nerve growth factor (NGF) has been demonstrated to be produced, along with its receptor, TrkA, in the β-cell, and there is some evidence that it may drive neuritelike outgrowths from β-cells *(128,129)*. However, targeted overexpression of NGF in the β-cell causes no abnormality in β-cell morphology or function, and immunoneutralization of NGF in mice resulted in no β-cell abnormalities *(129,130)*. Thus, there seems little reason for enthusiasm for NGF as a potential islet growth factor.

SUMMARY

Enormous progress has been made in identifying effective islet growth factors, as summarized in the chapter. On the other hand, there is equally enormous room for additional investigation in this arena. For example, what other currently unknown growth factors are required for normal islet development and which new growth factors may prove effective therapeutically in enhancing β-cell mass? What is the optimal target for these growth factors: the mature β-cell/islet? The intraislet β-cell precursor? The ductal β-cell precursor? Circulating marrow-derived stem cells? Embryonic stem cells? And how do they work across species: Simply because one finds a certain phenotype in a murine knockout or transgenic model, does that imply that the human homolog of the growth factor in question functions identically in human islets? And how about their use in porcine and primate islets? And should these growth factors be used in combination, and if so, what combinations and what ratios? And how should they be delivered? Systemically, following transplant of islets? Or using gene therapy strategies at the time of islet isolation? And how will islets engineered or stimulated using these growth factors hold up in response to immunosuppressant cocktails employed in islet transplantation schemes? And what about their malignant potential: Will they lead to the development of insulinomas (as does T-antigen) or other types of tumors? And, finally, what are the signaling mechanisms and cell-cycle-regulatory events that transduce the growth factor signals into replication? These questions will keep islet biologists busy for some time to come. There is reason to be optimistic that mass- and function-enhanced human islets will be derived from these types of study.

REFERENCES

1. Shapiro AMJ, Lakey JRT, Ryan EA, et al. Islet transplantation in seven patients with type 1 diabetes mellitus using a glucocorticoid-free immunosuppressive regimen. N Engl J Med 2000;343:230–238.
2. Ryan EA, Lakey JRT, Rajotte RV, et al. Clinical outcomes and insulin secretion after islet transplantation with the Edmonton protocol. Diabetes 2001;50:710–719.
3. Lumelsky N, Blondel O, Laeng P, Velasco I, Ravin R, McKay R. Differentiation of embryonic stem cells to insulin-secreting structures similar to pancreatic islets. Science 2001;292:1389–1394.
4. Zulewski H, Abraham EJ, Gerlach MJ, et al. Multipotential nestin-positive stem cells isolated from adult pancreatic islets differentiate ex vivo into pancreatic endocrine, exocrine and hepatic phenotypes. Diabetes 2001;50:521–533.
5. Lefebvre VH, Otonkoski T, Ustinov J, Huotari M-A, Pipeleers DG, Bouwens L. Culture of adult human islet preparations with hepatocyte growth factor and 804G matrix is mitogenic for duct cells but not for β-cells. Diabetes 1998;47:134–137.

6. Finegood DT, Scaglia L, Bonner-Weir S. Dynamics of β-cell mass in the growing rat pancreas. Estimation with a simple mathematical model. Diabetes 1995;44:249–256.
7. Bonner-Weir S. Postnatal pancreatic beta cell growth. Endocrinology 2000;141:1926–1929.
8. Kassem SA, Ariel I, Thornton PS, Scheimberg I, Glaser B. Beta cell proliferation and apoptosis in the developing normal human pancreas and in hyperinsulinism of infancy. Diabetes 2000;49:1325–1333.
9. García-Ocaña A, Takane K, Syed MA, Vasavada RC, Stewart AF. Hepatocyte growth factor overexpression in the islet of transgenic mice increases beta cell proliferation and induces hypoglycemia. J Biol Chem 2000;275:1226–1232.
10. Vasavada RC, Garcia-Ocana A, Zawalich WS, et al. Targeted expression of placental lactogen in the beta cells of transgenic mice results in beta cell proliferation, islet mass augmentation, and hypoglycemia. J Biol Chem 2000;275:15,399–15,406.
11. Scaglia L, Smith FE, Bonner-Weir S. Apoptosis contributes to the involution of beta cell mass in post partum rat pancreas. Endocrinology 1995;136:5461–5468.
12. Blume N, Skouv J, Larsson L-I, Holst JJ, Madsen OD. Potent inhibitory effects of transplantable rat glucagonomas and insulinomas on the respective endogenous islet cells are associated with pancreatic apoptosis. J Clin Invest 1995;96:2227–2235.
13. Benoist C, Mathis D. Cell death mediators in autoimmune diabetes. Cell 1997;89:1–3.
14. Pestell RG, Albanese C, Reutens AT, Segall JE, Lee RJ, Arnold A. The cyclins and cyclin-dependent kinase inhibitors in hormonal regulation of proliferation and differentiation. Endocr Rev 1999;20:501–534.
15. Lee W-H, Bookstein R, Hong F, Young L-J. Human retinoblastoma susceptibility gene: cloning, identification and sequence. Science 1987;235:1394–1399.
16. Hanahan D. Heritable formation of pancreatic β-cell tumors in transgenic mice expressing recombinant insulin/simian virus 40 oncogenes. Nature 1985;315:115–122.
17. Efrat S. Genetic engineering of beta cells for cell therapy of diabetes: cell growth, function and immunogenicity. Diabetes Rev 1996;4:224–234.
18. Efrat S, Linde S, Kofod H, et al. Beta-cell lines derived from transgenic mice expressing a hybrid insulin gene-oncogene. Proc Natl Acad Sci USA 1988;85:9037–9041.
19. Harvey M, Vogel H, Lee EY-P, Bradley A, Donehower LA. Mice deficient in both p53 and Rb develop tumors primarily of endocrine origin. Cancer Res 1995;55:1146–1151.
20. Williams BO, Remington L, Albert DM, Mukai S, Bronson RT, Jacks T. Cooperative tumorigenic effects of germline mutations in Rb and p53. Nat Genet 1994;7:480–484.
21. Rane S, Dubus P, Mettus RV, et al. Loss of expression of cdk4 causes insulin-deficient diabetes and cdk4 activation results in beta cell hyperplasia. Nat Genet 1999;22:44–52.
22. Tsutsui T, Hesabi B, Moons D, et al. Targeted disruption of cdk4 delays cell cycle entry with enhanced p27–kip activity. Mol Cell Biol 1999;19:7011–7019.
23. Chung DC, Brown SB, Grahme-Cooke F, et al. Overexpression of cyclin D1 occurs frequently in human pancreatic endocrine tumors. J Clin Endocrinol Metab 2000;85:4373–4378.
24. Nakamura T, Nishizawa T, Hagiya M, et al. Molecular cloning and expression of human hepatocyte growth factor. Nature 1989;342:440–443.
25. Nakamura T, Nawa K, Ichihara A. Partial purification and characterization of hepatocyte growth factor from serum of hepatectomized rats. Biochem Biophys Res Commun 1984;122:1450–1459.
26. Gohda E, Tsubouchi H, Nakayama H, et al. Purification and partial characterization of hepatocyte growth factor from plasma of a patient with fulminant hepatic failure. J Clin Invest 1988;88:414–419.
27. Shimomura T, Miyazawa K, Komiyaza Y, et al. Activation of hepatocyte growth factor by two homologous proteases, blood-coagulation factor XIIa and hepatocyte growth factor activator. Eur J Biochem 1995;229:257–261.
28. Naldini L, Tamagnone L, Vigna E, et al. Extracellular proteolytic cleavage by urokinase is required for activation of hepatocyte growth factor/scatter factor. EMBO J 1992;11:4825–4833.
29. Mars WM, Zarnegar R, Michalopoulos GK. Activation of hepatocyte growth factor by the plasminogen activators uPA and tPA. Am J Pathol 1993;143:949–958.
30. Miyazawa K, Shimomura T, Kitamura A, Kondo J, Morimoto Y, Kitamura N. Molecular cloning and sequence analysis of the cDNA for a human serine protease responsible for activation of hepatocyte growth factor. J Biol Chem 1993;268:10,024–10,028.
31. Zarnegar R, Michalopoulos GK. The many faces of hepatocyte growth factor: from hepatopoiesis to hematopoiesis. J Cell Biol 1995;129:1177–1180.
32. Matsumoto K, Nakamura T. Emerging multipotent aspects of hepatocyte growth factor. J Biochem (Tokyo) 1996;119:591–600.

33. Miyazawa T, Kiatmura T, Naka D, Kitamura N. An alternatively processed mRNA generated from human HGF gene. Eur J Biochem 1991;197:15–22.
34. Rubin JS, Chan AM, Bottaro DP, et al. A broad-spectrum human lung fibroblast-derived mitogen is a variant of HGF. Proc Natl Acad Sci USA 1991;88:415–419.
35. Bottaro DP, Rubin JS, Faletto DL, et al. Identification of the hepatocyte growth factor receptor as the c-met proto-oncogene product. Science 1991;251:802–804.
36. Prat M, Narsimhan RP, Crepaldi T, Nicotra MR, Natali PG, Comoglio PM. The receptor encoded by the human c-MET oncogene is expressed in hepatocytes, epithelial cells and solid tumors. Int J Cancer 1991;49:323–328.
37. Uehara Y, Minowa O, Mori C, et al. Placental defect and embryonic lethality in mice lacking hepatocyte growth factor/scatter factor. Nature 1995;373:702–705.
38. Bladt F, Riethmacher D, Isenmann S, Aguzzi A, Birchmeler C. Essential role for the c-met receptor in the migration of myogenic precursor cells into the limb bud. Nature 1995;376:768–771.
39. Ptasznik A, Beattie GM, Mally MI, Cirulli V, Lopez A, Hayek A. Phosphatidyl 3-kinase is a negative regulator of cellular differentiation. J Cell Biol 1997;137:1127–1136.
40. Sonnenberg E, Meyer D, Weidner M, Birchmeier C. Scatter factor/hepatocyte growth factor and its receptor, the c-met tyrosine kinase, can mediate a signal exchange between mesenchyme and epithelia during mouse development. J Cell Biol 1993;123:223–235.
41. Calvo EL, Boucher C, Pelletier G, Morisset J. Ontogeny of hepatocyte growth factor and c-met/hgf receptor in rat pancreas. Biochem Biophys Res Commun 1996;229:257–263.
42. Otonkoski T, Cirulli V, Beattie GM, et al. A role for hepatocyte growth factor/scatter factor in fetal mesenchyme-induced pancreatic β-cell growth. Endocrinology 1996;137:3131–3139.
43. Zarnegar R, Muga S, Rahija R, Michalopoulos G. Tissue distribution of hepatopoietin-A: a heparin-binding polypeptide growth factor for hepatocytes. Proc Natl Acad Sci USA 1990;87:1252–1256.
44. Tsuda H, Iwase T, Matsumoto K, et al. Immunohistochemical localization of hepatocyte growth factor protein in pancreas islet A-cells of man and rats. Jpn J Cancer Res 1992;83:1262–1266.
45. Furukawa T, Duguid WP, Kobari M, Matsuno S, Tsao M-S. Hepatocyte growth factor and Met receptor expression in human pancreatic carcinogenesis. Am J Pathol 1995;147:889–895.
46. Kristensen P, Nielsen JH, Larsson LI, Dano K. Tissue-type plasminogen activator in somatostatin cells of rat pancreas and hypothalamus. Endocrinology 1987;121:2238–2244.
47. Friess H, Cantero D, Graber H, et al. Enhanced urokinase plasminogen activation in chronic pancreatitis suggests a role in its pathogenesis. Gastroenterology 1997;113:904–913.
48. Vila MR, Nakamura T, Real FX. Hepatocyte growth factor is a potent mitogen for normal human pancreas cells in vitro. Lab Invest 1995;73:409–418.
49. Otonkoski T, Mally MI, Hayek A. Opposite effects of β-cell differentiation and growth on reg expression in human fetal pancreatic cells. Diabetes 1994;43:1164–1166.
50. Mashima H, Shibata H, Mine T, Kojima I. Formation of insulin-producing cells from pancreatic acinar AR42J cells by hepatocyte growth factor. Endocrinology 1996;137:3969–3976.
51. Menke A, Yamaguchi H, Giehl K, Adler G. Hepatocyte growth factor and fibroblast growth factor 2 are overexpressed after cereulin-induced acute pancreatitis. Pancreas 1999;18:28–33.
52. Otte J-M, Kiehne K, Schmitz F, Fölsch UR, Herzig K-H. C-Met protooncogene expression and its regulation by cytokines in the regenerating pancreas and in pancreatic cancer cells. Scan J Gastroenterol 2000;35:90–95.
53. Otonkoski T, Beattie GM, Rubin JS, Lopez AD, Baird A, Hayek A. Hepatocyte growth factor/scatter factor has insulinotropic activity in human fetal pancreatic cells. Diabetes 1994;43:947–953.
54. Hayek A, Beattie GM, Cirulli V, Lopez AD, Ricordi C, Rubin JS. Growth factor/matrix-induced proliferation of human adult β-cells. Diabetes 1995;44:1458–1460.
55. Nakano M, Yasunami Y, Maki T, et al. Hepatocyte growth factor is essential for amelioration of hyperglycemia in streptozotocin-induced diabetic mice receiving a marginal mass of intrahepatic islet grafts. Transplantation 2000;69:214–221.
56. Garcia-Ocaña A, Takane KK, Reddy VT, et al. Growth factor expression in mouse islets. J Biol Chem, 2003;278:343–351.
57. Stewart AF, Broadus AE. Malignancy-associated hypercalcemia. In: DeGroot L, Jameson LJ, eds. Endocrinology, 4th ed. WB Saunders, Philadelphia, 2001, pp. 1093–1100.
58. Strewler GJ. The physiology of parathyroid hormone-related protein. N Engl J Med 2000;342:177–185.
59. Wu T, Vasavada R, Yang K, et al. Structural and physiologic characterization of the mid-region secretory form of PTHrP. J Biol Chem 1996;271:24,371–24,381.

60. Philbrick WM, Wysolmerski JJ, Galbraith S, et al. Defining the physiologic roles of parathyroid hormone-related protein in normal physiology. Physiol Rev 1996;76:127–173.
61. Gaich G, Orloff JJ, Atillasoy EJ, Burtis WJ, Ganz MB, Stewart AF. Amino-terminal parathyroid hormone-related protein: specific binding and cytosolic calcium responses in rat insulinoma cells. Endocrinology 1993;132:1402–1409.
62. Drucker DJ, Asa SL, Henderson J, Goltzman D. The parathyroid hormone-like peptide gene is expressed in the normal and neoplastic human endocrine pancreas. Mol Endocrinol 1989;3:1589–1595.
63. Villanueva-Penacarrillo ML, Cancelas J, de Miguel F, et al. Parathyroid hormone-related protein stimulates DNA sytnhesis and insulin secretion in pancreatic islets. J Endocrinol 1999;163:403–408.
64. Karaplis AC, Luz A, Glowacki J, et al. Lethal skeletal dysplasia from targeted disruption of the parathyroid hormone-related peptide gene. Genes Dev 1994;8:277–289.
65. Lanske B, Karaplis AC, Lee K, et al. PTH/PTHrP receptor in early development and indian hedgehog-regulated bone growth. Science 1996;273:663–666.
66. Vasavada RC, Cavaliere C, D'Ercole AJ, et al. Overexpression of parathyroid hormone-related protein in the pancreatic islets of transgenic mice causes islet hyperplasia, hyperinsulinemia, and hypoglycemia. J Biol Chem 1996;271:1200–1208.
67. Porter SE, Sorenson RL, Dann P, Garcia-Ocana A, Stewart AF, Vasavada RC. Progressive pancreatic islet hyperplasia in the islet-targeted, parathyroid hormone-related protein-overexpressing mouse. Endocrinology 1998;139:3743–3751.
68. Sorenson RL, Brelje TC. Adaptation of islets of Langerhans to pregnancy: beta-cell growth, enhanced insulin secretion and the role of lactogenic hormones. Horm Metab Res 1997;29:301–307.
69. Sorenson RL, Johnson MG, Parsons JA, Sheridan JD. Decreased glucose stimulation threshold, enhanced insulin secretion, and increased beta cell coupling in islets of prolactin-treated rats. Pancreas 1987;2:283–288.
70. Brelje TC, Scharp DW, Lacy PE, et al. Effect of homologous placental lactogens, prolactins, and growth hormones on islet B-cell division and insulin secretion in rat, mouse, and human islets: implication for placental lactogen regulation of islet function during pregnancy. Endocrinology 1993;132:879–887.
71. Stout LE, Svensson AM, Sorenson RL. Prolactin regulation of islet-derived INS-1 cells: characteristics and immunocytochemical analysis of STAT5 translocation. Endocrinology 1997;138:1592–1603.
72. Sorenson RL, Stout LE. Prolactin receptors and JAK2 in islets of Langerhans: an immunohistochemical analysis. Endocrinology 1995;136:4092–4098.
73. Weinhaus AJ, Stout LE, Sorenson RL. Glucokinase, hexokinase, glucose transporter 2, and glucose metabolism in islets during pregnancy and prolactin-treated islets in vitro: mechanisms for long term up-regulation of islets. Endocrinology 1996;137:1640–1649.
74. Parsons JA, Brelje TC, Sorenson RL. Adaptation of islets of Langerhans to pregnancy: increased islet cell proliferation and insulin secretion correlates with the onset of placental lactogen secretion. Endocrinology 1992;130:1459–1466.
75. Sorenson RL, Brelje TC, Roth C. Effects of steroid and lactogenic hormones on islets of Langerhans: a new hypothesis for the role of pregnancy steroids in the adaptation of islets to pregnancy. Endocrinology 1993;133:2227–2234.
76. Garcia-Ocana A, Vasavada RC, Takane K, Reddy VT, Batt A, Stewart AF. Transgenic islets overexpressing hepatocyte growth factor (HGF) demonstrate superior glucose and insulin responses in vitro and in vivo as compared to transgenic PTH-related protein (PTHrP), placental lactogen (PL) and normal islets. Diabetes 2000;49(Suppl 1):A43.
77. Xu G, Stofffers DA, Habener JF, Bonner-Weir S. Exendin-4 stimulates both beta cell replication and neogenesis, resulting in increased beta cell mass and improved glucose tolerance in diabetic rats. Diabetes 1999;48:2270–2276.
78. Perfetti R, Zhou J, Doyle ME, Egan JM. Glucagon-like peptide-1 induces cell proliferation and pancreatic-duodenum homeobox-1 expression and increases endocrine cell mass in the pancreas of old, glucose intolerant rats. Endocrinology 2000;141:4600–4605.
79. Keiffer TJ, Habener JF, The glucagon-like peptides. Endocr Rev 1999;20:876–913.
80. Stoffers DA, Kieffer TJ, Hussain MA, et al. Insulinotropic glucagon-like peptide 1 agonists stimulate expression of homeodomain protein IDX-1 and increase islet size in mouse pancreas. Diabetes 2000;49:741–748.
81. Baggio L, Adatia F, Troels B, Brubaker PL, Drucker DJ. Sustained expression of exendin-4 does not perturb glucose homeostasis, beta cell mass, or food intake on metallothionine–preproxendin transgenic mice. J Biol Chem 2000;275:34,471–477.

82. Deacon CF, Danielsen P, Klarskov L, Olesen M, Holst JJ. Dipeptidyl peptidase IV inhibition reduces the degradation and clearance of GIP and potentiates its insulinotropic and antihyperglycemic effects in anesthetized pigs. Diabetes 2001;50:1588–1597.
83. Flamez D, Gilon P, Moens K, et al. Altered cAMP and Ca2+ signaling in pancreatic islets with glucagon-like peptide-1 receptor null phenotype. Diabetes 1999;48:1979–1986.
84. Young AA, Gedulin BR, Bhavsar S, et al. Glucose-lowering and insulin-sensitizing actions of exendin-4. Diabetes 1999;48:1026–1034.
85. Tourrel C, Bailbe D, Meile M-J, Kergoat M, Portha B. Glucagon-like peptide and exendin-4 stimulate beta cell neogenesis in streptozotocin-treated newborn rats resulting in persistently improved glucose homeostasis at adult age. Diabetes 2001;50:1562–1570.
86. Kulkarni RN, Burnning JC, Winnay JN, Postic C, Magnuson MA, Kahn CR. Tissue-specific knockout of the insulin receptor on beta cells creates and insulin secretory defects similar to that in type 2 diabetes. Cell 1999;96:329–339.
87. Rhodes CJ. IGF-I and GH post-receptor signaling mechanisms for pancreatic beta-cell replication. J Mol Endocrinol 2000;24:303–311.
88. Otonkoski T, Beattie GM, Rubin JS, Lopez AD, Baird A, Hayek A. Hepatocyte growth factor/scatter factor has insulinotropic activity in human fetal pancreatic cells. Diabetes 1994;43:947–953.
89. Petrik J, Pell JM, Arany E, et al. Overexpression of insulin-like growth factor-II in transgenic mice is associated with pancreatic islet cell hyperplasia. Endocrinology 1999;140:2353–2363.
90. Devedjian JC, George M, Casellas A, et al. Transgenic mice overexpressing insulin-like growth factor-II in beta cells develop type 2 diabetes. J Clin Invest 2000;105:731–740.
91. Kornmann M, Beger HG, Korc M. Role of fibroblast growth factors and their receptors in pancreatic cancer and chronic pancreatitis. Pancreas 1998;17:169–175.
92. Arany E, Hill DJ. Ontogeny of fibroblast growth factors in the early development of the rat endocrine pancreas. Pediatr Res 2000;48:389–403.
93. Oberg-Welsh C, Welsh M. Effects of certain growth factors on in vitro maturation of rat fetal islet-like structures. Pancreas 1996;12:334–339.
94. Le Bras S, Miralles F, Basmaciogullari A, Czernichow P, Scharfmann R. Fibroblast growth factor 2 promotes pancreatic epithelial cell proliferation via functional fibroblast growth factor receptors during embryonic life. Diabetes 1998;47:1236–1242.
95. Krakowski ML, Kritzik MR, Jones EM, et al. Pancreatic expression of keratinocyte growth factor leads to differentiation of islet hepatocytes and proliferation of duct cells. Am J Pathol 1999;154:683–691.
96. Hart AW, Baeza N, Apelqvist A, Edlund H. Attenuation of FGF signaling in mouse beta cells leads to diabetes. Nature 2000;408:864–888.
97. Terazono K, Yamamoto H, Takasawa S, et al. A novel gene activated in regenerating islets. J Biol Chem 1988;263:2111–2114.
98. Terazono K, Uchiyama Y, Ide M, Watanabe T, Yonekura H, Okamoto H. Expression of reg protein in rat generating islets and its co-localization with insulin in the beta-cell secretory granules. Diabetologia 1990;33:250–252.
99. Stewart TA. The human *reg* gene encodes pancreatic stone protein. Biochem J 1989;260:622–623.
100. Rouquier S, Giorgi D, Iovanna J, Dagorn J-C. Sequence similarity between the *reg* transcript and pancreatic stone protein mRNA. Biochem J 1989;264:621–624.
101. Watanabe T, Yonekura H, Tarazono K, Yamamoto H, Okamoto H. Complete nucleotide sequence of human *reg* gene and its expression in normal and tumoral tissues: the *reg* protein, pancreatic stone protein, and pancreatic thread protein are one and the same product of the gene. J Biol Chem 1990;265:7432–7439.
102. Unno M, Yonekura H, Nakagawara K, et al. Structure, chromosomal localization, and expression of mouse reg genes, reg I and reg II. A novel type of Reg gene, Reg II, exists in the mouse genome. J Biol Chem 1993;268:15,974–15,982.
103. Narushima Y, Unno M, Nakagawara K, et al. Structure, chromosomal localization and expression of mouse genes encoding type III Reg, Reg IIIα, Reg IIIβ, Reg IIIγ. Gene 1997;185:159–168.
104. Miyashita H, Nakagawara K, Mori M, et al. Human REG family genes are tandemly ordered in a 95-kilobase region of chromosome 2p12. FEBS Lett 1995;377:429–433.
105. Kobayashi S, Akiyama T, Nata K, et al. Identification of a receptor for Reg (regenerating gene) protein, a pancreatic β-cell regenerating factor. J Biol Chem 2000;275:10,723–10,726.
106. Watanabe T, Yonemura Y, Yonekura H, et al. Pancreatic beta-cell replication and amelioration of surgical diabetes by Reg protein. Proc Natl Acad Sci USA 1994;91:3589–3592.

107. Gross DJ, Weiss L, Reibstein I, et al. Amelioration of diabetes in NOD mice with advanced disease by Linomide-induced immunoregulation combined with Reg protein treatment. Endocrinology 1998;139:2369–2374.
108. Okamoto H. The role of Reg genes: genetic introduction of human REG I and/or administration of REG I product may be effective in the prevention and cure of diabetes in man. Exp Clin Endocrinol Diabetes 1997;105:A12–A13.
109. Okamoto H. The reg gene family and reg proteins: with special attention to the regeneration of pancreatic beta cells. J Hepatobiliary Pancreat Surg 1999;6:254–262.
110. Rafaeloff R, Pittenger GL, Barlow SW, et al. Cloning and expression of the pancreatic islet neogenesis-associated protein (INGAP) gene and its expression in islet neogenesis in hamsters. J Clin Invest 1997;99:2100–2109.
111. Watanabe T, Shintani A, Nakata M, et al. Recombinant human betacellulin. Molecular structure, biological activities and receptor interaction. J Biol Chem 1994;269:9966–9973.
112. Shing Y, Christofori G, Hanahan D, et al. Betacellulin: a mitogen from pancreatic β-cell tumors. Science 1993;259:1604–1607.
113. Sasada R, Ono Y, Taniyama Y, Shing Y, Folkman J, Igarashi K. Cloning and expression of cDNA encoding human betacellulin, a new member of the EGF family. Biochem Biophys Res Commun 1993;190:1173–1179.
114. Groenen LC, Nice EC, Burgess AW. Structure–function relationships for the EGF/TGF-alpha family of mitogens. Growth Factors 1994;11:235–257.
115. Riese DJ, Bermingham Y, van Raaij TM, Buckley S, Plowman GD, Stern DF. Betacellulin activates the epidermal growth factor receptor and erbB-4, and induces cellular response patterns distinct from those stimulated by epidermal growth factor or neuregulin-β. Oncogene 1996;12:345–353.
116. Huotari M, Palgi J, Otonkoski T. Growth factor-mediated proliferation and differentiation of insulin-producing INS-1 and RINm5F cells: identification of betacellulin as a novel β-cell mitogen. Endocrinology 1998;139:1494–1499.
117. Mashima H, Ohnishi H, Wakabayashi K, et al. Betacellulin and activin A coordinately convert amylase-secreting pancreatic AR42J cells into insulin-secreting cells. J Clin Invest 1996;97:1647–1654.
118. Watada H, Kajimoto Y, Miyagawa J, et al. PDX-1 induces insulin and glucokinase gene expressions in αTC1 clone 6 cells in the presence of betacellulin. Diabetes 1996;45:1826–1831.
119. Yamamoto K, Miyagawa J-I, Waguri M, et al. Recombinant human betacellulin promotes neogenesis of beta cells and ameliorates glucose intolerance in mice with diabetes induced by selective alloxan perfusion. Diabetes 2000;49:2021–2027.
120. Eric P. Sandgren, Noreen C, et al. Overexpression of TGFα in transgenic mice: induction of epithelial hyperplasia, pancreatic metaplasia, and carcinoma of the breast. Cell 1990;61:1121–1135.
121. Jhappan C, Stahle C, Harkins RN, et al. TGFα overexpression in transgenic mice induces liver neoplasia and abnormal development of the mammary gland and pancreas. Cell 1990;61:1137–1146.
122. Brand SJ, Fuller PJ. Differential gastrin Gene expression in rat gastrointestinal tract and pancreas during neonatal development. J Biol Chem 1988;263:5341–5347.
123. Wang TC, Koh TJ, Varro A, et al. Processing and proliferative effects of human progastrin in transgenic mice. J Clin Invest 1996;98:1918–1929.
124. Wang TC, Bonner-Weir S, Oates PS, et al. Pancreatic gastrin stimulates islet differentiation of transforming growth factor alpha-induced ductular precursor cells. J Clin Invest 1993;92:1349–1356.
125. Ebert M, Kasper HU, Hernberg S, et al. Overexpression of platelet-derived growth factor (PDGF) B chain and type beta PDGF receptor in human chronic pancreatitis. Dig Dis Sci 1998;43:567–574.
126. Welsh M, Claesson-Welsh L, Hallberg A, et al. Coexpression of the platelet-derived growth factor (PDGF) B chain and the PDGF β receptor in isolated pancreatic islet cells stimulates DNA synthesis. Proc Natl Acad Sci USA 1990;87:5807–5811.
127. Swenne I, Heldin CH, Hill DJ, Hellerstrom C. Effects of platelet-derived growth factor and somatomedin-C/insulin-like growth factor I on the deoxyribonucleic acid replication of fetal rat islets of Langerhans in tissue culture. Endocrinology 1988;122:214–218.
128. Kanaka-Gantenbein C, Dicou E, Czernichow P, Scharfmann R. Presence of nerve growth factor and its receptors in an in vitro model of islet cell development: implications for normal islet morphogenesis. Endocrinology 1995;136:3154–3162.
129. Rosenbaum T, Sanchez-Soto MC, Hiriart M. Nerve growth factor increases insulin secretion and barium current in pancreatic beta cells. Diabetes 2001;50:1755–1756.
130. Boyd AE. The nerve of them beta cells and nerve growth factor. Endocrinology 1994;134:2319–2320.

INDEX

From: *Contemporary Endocrinology: Type 1 Diabetes: Etiology and Treatment*
Edited by: M. A. Sperling © Humana Press, Totowa, NJ

K

L

M

X

About the Editor

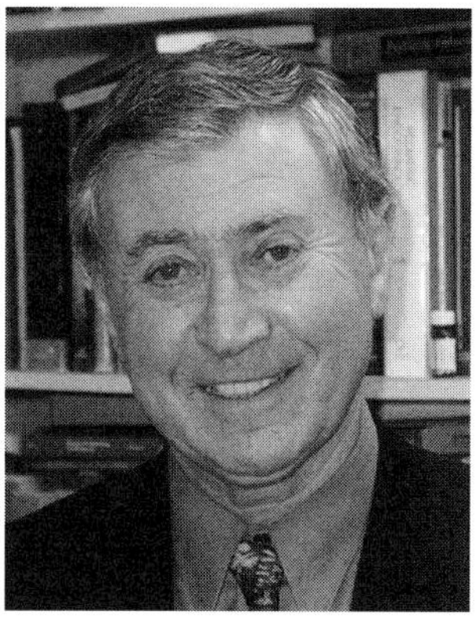

Dr. Sperling is a Professor of Pediatrics in the Division of Endocrinology at the University of Pittsburgh School of Medicine and Children's Hospital of Pittsburgh, where he served as Vira I. Heinz Professor, chair of the department, and pediatrician-in-chief from 1988 through 1999. He received his medical degree and training in Pediatrics at the University of Melbourne, Australia. After a fellowship in Pediatric Endocrinology and Diabetes in the United States, he was on the faculty at UCLA, assuming the position of Chief of Pediatric Endocrinology and Diabetes at Children's Hospital Medical Center and was Professor of Pediatrics at the Medical College in Cincinnati in 1978.

Dr. Sperling has a distinguished record in research, patient care, and teaching related to pediatric endocrinology and childhood diabetes. He has served as a member of the editorial boards of *Diabetes* and the *Journal of Clinical Endocrinology and Metabolism,* as well as several other leading pediatric journals. Currently he is editor-in-chief of the journal, *Pediatric Diabetes,* and is editor of the textbook, *Pediatric Endocrinology* (second edition, Saunders, an imprint of Elsevier Science, June 2002). His research and training of future academic pediatricians has been continuously funded from the National Institutes of Health (NIH) and other funding agencies since 1972. He has served on NIH study sections and was a member of the National Diabetes Advisory Board, as well as serving on the Research Advisory Board of the Juvenile Diabetes Research Foundation International (JDRF) and the research committee and program committees of the American Diabetes Association (ADA). He is a member of several scientific organizations, including the Association of American Physicians, American Society for Clinical Investigation, American Pediatric Society, Society for Pediatric Research, Endocrine Society, and the American Diabetes Association (ADA). He served as president of the Lawson Wilkins Pediatric Endocrine Society from 2002 to 2003. He has lectured extensively and published numerous peer-reviewed articles as well as chapters and reviews by invitation.

This extensive experience has been brought to bear in the production of this book, intended for all those interested in the field of type 1 diabetes mellitus, incorporating research and practice.